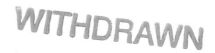

When to Screen in Obstetrics and Gynecology

Second edition

Edited by

Hajo I.J. Wildschut, MD, PhD

Consultant in Obstetrics and Gynaecology
Department of Obstetrics and Gynaecology
Erasmus University Medical Center
Rotterdam, The Netherlands

Carl P. Weiner, MD, MBA, FACOG

Professor, Obstetrics, Gynecology and Reproductive Sciences
Professor, Physiology
University of Maryland School of Medicine
Baltimore, Maryland, USA

Tim J. Peters, PhD, CStat, FFPH

Professor of Primary Care Health Services Research
Department of Community Based Medicine
University of Bristol
Bristol, UK

SAUNDERS

ELSEVIER

SAUNDERS
ELSEVIER

1600 John F. Kennedy Boulevard
Suite 1800
Philadelphia, PA 19103-2899

WHEN TO SCREEN IN OBSTETRICS AND GYNECOLOGY

ISBN 13: 978-1-4160-0300-7
ISBN 10: 1-4160-0300-2

NOTICE

Knowledge and best practice in this field are constantly changing. As new research and experience broaden our knowledge, changes in practice, treatment and drug therapy may become necessary or appropriate. Readers are advised to check the most current information provided (i) on procedures featured or (ii) by the manufacturer of each product to be administered, to verify the recommended dose or formula, the method and duration of administration, and contraindications. It is the responsibility of the practitioner, relying on his or her own experience and knowledge of the patient, to make diagnoses, to determine dosages and the best treatment for each individual patient, and to take all appropriate safety precautions. To the fullest extent of the law, neither the Publisher nor the Editors assume any liability for any injury and/or damage to persons or property arising out or related to any use of the material contained in this book.

Second Edition
Library of Congress Cataloging-in-Publication Data
Wildschut, H. I. J. (Hajo I. J.)
   When to screen in obstetrics and gynecology/Hajo Wildschut, Carl Weiner, Tim J. Peters.–2nd ed.
      p.; cm.
   Includes bibliographical references and index.
   ISBN 1-4160-0300-2
      1. Gynecology–Diagnosis. 2. Obstetrics–Diagnosis. 3. Pregnancy–Complications–Diagnosis. 4. Generative organs, Female–Diseases–Diagnosis. 5. Generative organs, Female–Cancer–Diagnosis. I. Weiner, Carl P. II. Peters, Tim J. (Timothy James), 1958-III. Title.
      [DNLM: 1. Genital Diseases, Female–diagnosis. 2. Gynecology–methods. 3. Obstetrics–methods. 4. Pregnancy Complications–diagnosis. WP 141 W674w 2006]
   RG107.W47 2006
   618.1'075–dc22

2005044230

Acquisitions Editor: Todd Hummel
Project Manager: Mary Stermel
Marketing Manager: Dana Butler

Working together to grow
libraries in developing countries

www.elsevier.com | www.bookaid.org | www.sabre.org

ELSEVIER BOOK AID International Sabre Foundation

Printed in the United States of America.

Last digit is the print number: 9 8 7 6 5 4 3 2 1

There is good reason why the second edition is twice the size of the first—much has changed since the first edition of *When to Screen in Obstetrics and Gynecology* was published. The complexity posed to both the caregiver and patient has increased dramatically. This edition is dedicated to them in hopes of simplifying important health care decisions with life/death potential.

The editors would also like to acknowledge Stephanie Donley for her support to bringing this effort forward.

Contents

Contributors   xiii

Introduction   xix

Chapters

1 **Epidemiologic Considerations in Screening**   1
Tim J. Peters • Hajo I. J. Wildschut • Carl P. Weiner

2 **Maternal Red Blood Cell Group and Antibody Screen**   15
Charlene M. Elbert • Ronald G. Strauss

3 **Antepartum Assessment of Hemoglobin, Hematocrit, and Serum Ferritin**   22
Christine Kirkpatrick • Sophie Alexander •
Hajo I. J. Wildschut

4 **Postpartum Assessment of Hemoglobin, Hematocrit, and Serum Ferritin**   34
Christine Kirkpatrick • Sophie Alexander

5 **Asymptomatic Bacteriuria in Pregnancy**   40
Francis S. Nuthalapaty • Dwight J. Rouse

6 **Neonatal Group B Streptococcal Disease**   48
Walter Foulon • Anne Naessens

7 **Rubella During Pregnancy**   55
Walter Foulon • Anne Naessens

8 **Congenital Toxoplasmosis**   61
Walter Foulon • Anne Naessens

9 **Congenital Cytomegalovirus Infection**   68
Walter Foulon • Anne Naessens

10 **Hepatitis A, B, and C During Pregnancy**   75
Lise Jensen

11 **Syphilis**   90
R. Phillip Heine • Michael J. Paglia

12   **Gonorrhea** 97
R. Phillip Heine • Michael J. Paglia

13   **Chlamydial Infection** 103
R. Phillip Heine • Michael J. Paglia

14   **HIV Infection** 112
R. Phillip Heine • Michael J. Paglia

15   **Screening for Cystic Fibrosis Carrier Status** 121
Darren A. Shickle • Adrienne R. Hunt

16   **Screening for Hemoglobinopathies** 138
Joan S. Henthorn • Sally C. Davies

17   **Early-onset Genetic Diseases** 147
Grazia M.S. Mancini

18   **Screening for Fragile X Syndrome** 163
Anneke Maat-Kievit • Ben A. Oostra

19   **Screening for Huntington Disease** 175
Anneke Maat-Kievit

20   **Routine Ultrasound for Dating** 191
Heiner C. Bucher • Johannes G. Schmidt • William L. Martin •
Khalid S. Khan

21   **First Trimester Screening for Aneuploidy** 201
Kevin Spencer

22   **Second Trimester Screening for Aneuploidy (Ultrasound
and Biochemistry)** 217
Lami Yeo • Anthony M. Vintzileos

23   **Biochemical Screening for Fetal Abnormalities** 232
George J. Knight • Glenn E. Palomaki • James E. Haddow

24   **Routine Ultrasonography for the Detection of Fetal
Structural Anomalies** 244
Juriy W. Wladimiroff

25   **Molecular Tests for Antenatal Detection of Aneuploidy** 253
Gill M. Grimshaw

26 **Thrombophilia and Pregnancy Complications: Preeclampsia, (Late) Intrauterine Fetal Death, and Thrombosis** 268
Christianne J.M. de Groot • Eric A. P. Steegers

27 **Screening for Autoimmune Diseases in Pregnancy** 279
Lorin Lakasing • Catherine Williamson

28 **Gestational Diabetes Mellitus** 303
Seth C. Brody

29 **Screening for Low Birth Weight Using Maternal Height and Weight** 320
Lambert H. Lumey

30 **Fundal Height Measurement** 326
Jeanne C. McDermott

31 **Fetal Growth Restriction** 344
Jason Gardosi • Kate Morse • Jill Wright

32 **Doppler Velocimetry for the Detection of Intrauterine Growth Restriction** 360
Sicco A. Scherjon

33 **Preterm Delivery** 378
Jay D. Iams • David N. Hackney

34 **Preeclampsia: Blood Pressure, Weight Gain, and Edema** 394
Peter von Dadelszen • Thomas R. Easterling

35 **Uterine Artery Doppler as Screening Tool for Preeclampsia** 408
Antoinette C. Bolte • Gustaaf A. Dekker

36 **Preeclampsia and Uric Acid** 420
Antoinette C. Bolte • Gustaaf A. Dekker

37 **Fetal Hypoxia** 429
Caterina M. Bilardo • Ahmet Alexander Baschat • Gerard H. A. Visser

38 **Peripartum Coagulopathy** 466
Jamie Star • Jeffrey F. Peipert

39 **Postpartum Umbilical Cord Blood Testing** 476
Charlene M. Elbert • Ronald G. Strauss

40 When to Screen for Neonatal Hypoglycemia 483
Diva D. DeLeón • Charles A. Stanley

41 Neonatal Hyperbilirubinemia 491
Vinod K. Bhutani • Lois H. Johnson

42 Screening for Neonatal Genetic Disorders 503
Monique Williams

43 The Annual Bimanual Examination 529
Susan R. Johnson • Ann Laros

44 Dyslipidemia 536
Eric J. G. Sijbrands • Janneke G. Langendonk

45 Diabetes Mellitus 549
Hajo I. J. Wildschut

46 Screening Tests for Contraceptive Users 558
Donna M. LaFontaine • Jeffrey F. Peipert

47 Genetic Predisposition to Gynecologic Cancers 574
Hanne Meijers-Heijboer

48 Screening for Breast Cancer 591
Jacques Fracheboud • Harry J. de Koning

49 Pap Smear 603
Clare Wilkinson • Roy Farquharson

50 High-Risk Human Papillomavirus Testing in Cervical Cancer Screening 612
Mariëlle A. E. Nobbenhuis • Theo J. M. Helmerhorst

51 Transvaginal Ultrasound as a Screening Method for Ovarian Cancer 622
Paul D. DePriest • Frederick R. Ueland • John R. van Nagell, Jr.

52 Serum CA-125 Screening for Ovarian Cancer 629
Kees A. Yedema • Peter Kenemans

53 Screening for Colorectal Cancer 649
Mehul Lalani • Robert E. Schoen

54 **The Electrocardiogram** 658
Rudolph W. Koster • Patrick M. M. Bossuyt

55 **Intravenous Pyleography** 666
Michelle L. Kush • Joanne T. Piscitelli • David L. Simel

56 **Osteoporosis** 673
Susan R. Johnson

Index 683

Contributors

Sophie Alexander, MD, PhD
Senior Lecturer in Public Health, Reproductive Health Unit, School of Public Health, Université Libre de Bruxelles, Brussels, Belgium

Ahmet Alexander Baschat, MD
Department of Obstetrics, Gynecology and Reproductive Sciences, Center for Advanced Fetal Care, University of Maryland, Baltimore, Maryland, USA.

Vinod K. Bhutani, MD
Clinical Professor of Pediatrics, Newborn Pediatrics, Pennsylvania Hospital, University of Pennsylvania, Philadelphia, Pennsylvania, USA

Caterina M. Bilardo, MD, PhD
Head of the Division, Prenatal Diagnosis of the Department of Obstetrics and Gynecology, Academic Medical Center, Amsterdam, The Netherlands

Antoinette C. Bolte, MD, PhD
Associate Professor, Department of Obstetrics and Gynaecology, Vrije Universiteit Medical Center, Amsterdam, The Netherlands

Patrick M.M. Bossuyt, MD, PhD
Professor, Department of Clinical Epidemiology and Biostatistics, Academic Medical Center, Amsterdam, The Netherlands

Seth C. Brody, MD, MPH
Associate Professor, Department of Obstetrics and Gynecology, University of North Carolina School of Medicine, Chapel Hill, North Carolina, USA

Heiner C. Bucher, MD, MPH
Professor, Basel Institute for Clinical Epidemiology, University Hospital Basel, Basel, Switzerland

Sally C. Davies, MB, FRCP, FRCPath
Professor, Deputy Director of Research and Development, Department of Health, London, UK

Christianne J.M. de Groot, MD, PhD
Consultant in Obstetrics and Gynaecology, Department of Obstetrics and Gynaecology, Erasmus University Medical Center Rotterdam, Rotterdam, The Netherlands

Gustaaf A. Dekker, MD, PhD
Professor, Department of Obstetrics and Gynaecology, University of Adelaide, Lyell McEwin Health Service, South Australia, Australia

Harry J. de Koning, MD, PhD
Senior Lecturer in Public Health, Department of Public Health, Erasmus University Rotterdam, Rotterdam, The Netherlands

Diva D. De León, MD
Assistant Professor of Pediatrics, Department of Pediatrics, University of Pennsylvania, Philadelphia, Pennsylvania, USA, Attending Physician, Department of Pediatric Endocrinology, The Children's Hospital of Philadelphia, Philadelphia, Pennsylvania, USA

Paul D. DePriest, MD
American Cancer Society Clinical Oncology Fellow, Department of Obstetrics and Gynecology, University of Kentucky Medical Center, Lexington, Kentucky, USA

Thomas R. Easterling, MD
Professor, Department of Obstetrics and Gynecology, University of Washington, Seattle, Washington, USA

Charlene M. Elbert, MT (ASCP) SBB
Professor of Pathology and Pediatrics, University of Iowa College of Medicine, Iowa City, Iowa, USA

Roy Farquharson, MD, FRCOG
Clinical Director, Department of Gynaecology, Liverpool Women's Hospital, Liverpool, UK

Walter Foulon, MD
Professor, Division of Maternal Fetal Medicine, Department of Obstetrics and Gynecology, Akademisch Ziekenhuis Vrije Universiteit Brussels, Brussels, Belgium

Jacques Fracheboud, MD
Department of Public Health, Erasmus University Rotterdam, Rotterdam, The Netherlands

Jason Gardosi, MD, FRCOG, FRCSED
Professor, Director, West Midlands Perinatal Institute, Birmingham, UK

Gill M. Grimshaw, BSc, MSc, PhD, CPhys, MinstP
Principal Research Fellow, Warwick Medical School, Medical Teaching Center, University of Warwick, Coventry, UK

David N. Hackney, MD
Division of Maternal Fetal Medicine, Department of Obstetrics and Gynecology, and Division of Transfusion Medicine, Department of Pathology, The Ohio State University College of Medicine and Public Health, Columbus, Ohio

James E. Haddow, MD, PhD
Associate, Foundation for Blood Research, Scarborough, Maine, USA

R. Phillip Heine, MD
Assistant Professor, Obstetrics, Gynecology and Reproductive Science, University of Pittsburgh, Magee-Women's Research Institute, Pittsburgh, Pennsylvania, USA

Theo J.M. Helmerhorst, MD, PhD
Professor and Chairman, Department of Obstetrics and Gynecology, Erasmus University Medical Center, Rotterdam, The Netherlands

Joan S. Henthorn, FIMBS, CSci
Department of Haematology, Central Middlesex Hospital, London, UK

Adrienne R. Hunt
Research Associate, Section of Public Health, University of Sheffield, Sheffield, UK

Jay D. Iams, MD
Professor and Frederick P. Zuspan Endowed Chair, Department of Obstetrics and Gynecology, The Ohio State University, Columbus, Ohio, USA

Lise Jensen, MD
Pediatric Clinic II, Rigshospitalet, Copenhagen, Denmark

Lois H. Johnson, MD
Clinical Professor of Pediatrics, University of Pennsylvania School of Medicine, Philadelphia, Pennsylvania, USA

Susan R. Johnson, MD, MPH
Professor/Associate Dean, Department of Obstetrics and Gynecology, University of Iowa Hospitals and Clinics, Iowa City, Iowa, USA

Peter Kenemans, MD, PhD
Professor, Department of Obstetrics and Gynaecology, Akademisch Ziekenhuis Vrije Universiteit, Amsterdam, The Netherlands

Khalid S. Khan, MRCOG MSc
Professor in Obstetrics and Gynaecology and Clinical Epidemiology, Education Resource Centre, Birmingham Women's Hospital, Birmingham, UK; Birmingham Women's Healthcare NHS Trust, Birmingham, UK

Christine Kirkpatrick, MD, PhD
Senior Lecturer in Obstetrics and Gynecology, Department of Obstetrics and Gynecology, Hospital Erasme, Université Libre de Bruxelles, Brussels, Belgium

George J. Knight, PhD
Director, Prenatal Screening Laboratory, Foundation for Blood Research, Scarborough, Maine, USA

Rudolph W. Koster, MD, PhD
Senior Lecturer in Cardiology, Department of Cardiology, Academic Medical Center, Amsterdam, The Netherlands

Michelle L. Kush, MD
Assistant Professor, Department of Maternal and Fetal Medicine, University of Maryland, Baltimore, Maryland, USA

Donna M. LaFontaine, MD
Clinical Assistant Professor, Department of Obstetrics and Gynecology, Women and Infants' Hospital, Brown University School of Medicine, Providence, Rhode Island, USA

Lorin Lakasing, MD, MRCOG
Consultant in Obstetrics, Harris Birthright Center for Fetal Medicine, King's College Hospital, London, UK

Mehul Lalani, MD
Gastroenterology Fellow, Division of Gastroenterology, Hepatology, and Nutrition, University of Pittsburgh Medical Center, Pittsburgh, Pennsylvania, USA

Janneke G. Langendonk, MD, PhD
Assistant Professor, Departments of Internal Medicine and Metabolic and Vascular Diseases, Erasmus Medical Center, Rotterdam, The Netherlands

Ann Laros, MD
Clinical Assistant Professor, Department of Obstetrics and Gynecology, University of Iowa Hospitals and Clinics, Iowa City, Iowa, USA

Lambert H. Lumey, MD, MPH, PhD
Department of Epidemiology, Columbia University Mailman School of Public Health, New York, New York, USA

Anneke Maat-Kievit, MD, PhD
Clinical Geneticist, Department of Clinical Genetics, Erasmus Medical Center Rotterdam, Rotterdam, The Netherlands

Grazia M.S. Mancini, MD, PhD
Clinical Geneticist, Department of Clinical Genetics, Erasmus Medical Center Rotterdam, Rotterdam, The Netherlands

William L. Martin, MRCOG, MD
Department of Fetal Medicine, Birmingham Women's Hospital, Birmingham, UK

Jeanne C. McDermott, CNM, PhD
Medical Epidemiologist, Centers for Disease Control and Prevention, WHO Collaborating Center in Perinatal Care and Health Services Research in Maternal and Child Health, Atlanta, Georgia, USA

Hanne Meijers-Heijboer
Senior Lecturer in Clinical Genetics, Department of Clinical Genetics, Erasmus University Medical Center, Rotterdam, The Netherlands

Kate Morse, Bsc (Hons), DPSM, RM, RGN
Specialist Midwife, West Midlands Perinatal Institute, Birmingham, UK

Anne Naessens, MD
Department of Microbiology, Akademisch Ziekenhuis, Vrije Universiteit Brussel, Brussels, Belgium

Mariëlle A.E. Nobbenhuis, MD, PhD
Senior Registrar, Department of Obstetrics and Gynecology, Erasmus University Medical Center, Rotterdam, The Netherlands

Francis S. Nuthalapathy, MD
Fellow, Maternal-Fetal Medicine, Center for Research in Women's Health, University of Alabama at Birmingham, Birmingham, Alabama, USA

Ben A. Oostra, PhD
Professor, Department of Clinical Genetics, Erasmus University Medical Center, Rotterdam, The Netherlands

Michael J. Paglia, MD, PhD
Clinical Instructor, Obstetrics, Gynecology & Reproductive Science, University of Pittsburgh, Magee-Women's Research Institute, Pittsburgh, Pennsylvania, USA

Glenn E. Palomaki, BS
Director, Biometry, Foundation for Blood Research, Scarborough, Maine, USA

Jeffery F. Peipert, MD, MPH
Assistant Professor of Obstetrics and Gynecology, Department of Obstetrics and Gynecology, Brown University School of Medicine, Women and Infants' Hospital, Providence, Rhode Island, USA

Tim J. Peters BSc, MSc, PhD
Professor of Primary Care Health Services Research, Department of Community Based Medicine, University of Bristol, Bristol, UK

Joanne T. Piscitelli, MD, FACOG
Associate Clinical Professor, Chief, Division of General Obstetrics-Gynecology, Duke University Medical Center, Durham, North Carolina, USA

Dwight J. Rouse, MD
Assistant Professor, Department of Obstetrics and Gynecology, Division of Maternal-Fetal Medicine, University of Alabama at Birmingham, Birmingham, Alabama, USA

Sicco A. Scherjon, MD, PhD
Senior Lecturer in Obstetrics and Gynecology, Department of Obstetrics and Gynecology, Leiden University Medical Center, Leiden, The Netherlands

Johannes G. Schmidt, MD
Professor, Institute für klinische Epidemiologie, Einsiedeln, Switzerland

Robert E. Schoen, MD, MPH
Associate Professor, School of Medicine; Associate Professor, School of Public Health, University of Pittsburgh, Pittsburgh, Pennsylvania, USA

Darren A. Shickle, MPH, MFPHM
Senior Lecturer in Public Health Medicine, University of Sheffield, Sheffield, UK

Eric J.G. Sijbrands, MD, PhD
Associate Professor, Departments of Internal Medicine and Metabolic and Vascular Diseases, Erasmus Medical Center, Rotterdam, The Netherlands

David L. Simel, MD, MHS
Associate Professor, Co-Director, Women's Veterans Healthcare Center, Durham, Veterans Affairs Medical Center, Duke University, Durham, North Carolina, USA

Kevin Spencer, BSc, MSc, DSc, FRSC, FRCPath
Consultant Biochemist, Prenatal Screening Unit, Department of Clinical Biochemistry, Harold Wood Hospital, Romford, Essex, UK; Honorary Senior Lecturer, Harris Birthright Research Center for Fetal Medicine, Kings College Hospital, London, UK

Charles A. Stanley, MD
Professor of Pediatrics, Department of Endocrinology, University of Pennsylvania School of Medicine, Philadelphia, Pennsylvania, USA; Division Chief, Department of Endocrinology, The Children's Hospital of Philadelphia, Philadelphia, Pennsylvania, USA

Jamie Star, MD
Associate Professor, Maternal-Fetal Medicine Specialist, Department of Obstetrics and Gynecology, University of Massachusetts, Worcester, Massachusetts, USA; Maternal-Fetal Medicine Specialist, Department of Obstetrics and Gynecology, University of Massachusetts Memorial Medical Center, Worcester, Massachusetts, USA

Eric A.P. Steegers, MD, PhD
Professor, Department of Obstetrics and Gynecology, Erasmus University Medical Center Rotterdam, Rotterdam, The Netherlands

Ronald G. Strauss, MD
Professor of Pathology and Pediatrics, University of Iowa College of Medicine, Iowa City, Iowa, USA

Frederick R. Ueland, MD
Department of Obstetrics and Gynecology, Division of Gynecologic Oncology, University of Kentucky Medical Center, Lexington, Kentucky, USA

John R. van Nagell, Jr., MD
American Cancer Society Professor of Clinical Oncology, Department of Obstetrics and Gynecology, Division of Gynecologic Oncology, University of Kentucky Medical Center, Lexington, Kentucky, USA

Anthony M. Vintzileos, MD
Professor and Chair, Department of Obstetrics, Gynecology and Reproductive Sciences, UMDNJ-Robert Wood Johnson Medical School/Saint Peter's University Hospital, New Brunswick, New Jersey, USA

Gerard H.A. Visser, MD, PhD
Professor, Department of Obstetrics and Gynaecology, University Medical Center, Utrecht, The Netherlands

Peter von Dadelszen, MBChB, Dphil
Associate Professor, Department of Obstetrics and Gynaecology, University of British Columbia, Vancouver, British Columbia, Canada; Consultant in Maternal-Fetal Medicine, Department of Obstetrics and Gynaecology, BC Women's Hospital and Health Center, Vancouver, British Columbia, Canada

Carl P. Weiner, MD
Professor, Obstetrics, Gynecology and Reproductive Sciences; Professor, Physiology, University of Maryland School of Medicine, Baltimore, Maryland, USA

Hajo I.J. Wildschut, MD, PhD
Consultant in Obstetrics and Gynaecology, Department of Obstetrics and Gynaecology, Erasmus University Medical Center, Rotterdam, The Netherlands

Clare Wilkinson, MD, BCh, DRCOG, MRCGP
Senior Lecturer in General Practice, Department of General Practice, University of Wales College of Medicine, Department of General Practice, Llanedeyrn Health Center, Cardiff, UK

Monique Williams, MD, PhD
Consultant in Pediatrics, Sophia Children's Hospital, Erasmus University Medical Center, Rotterdam, The Netherlands

Catherine Williamson, BSc, MD, MRCP
Senior Lecturer in Obstetric Medicine, Institute of Reproductive and Developmental Biology, Imperial College London, London, UK

Juriy W. Wladimiroff, MD, PhD
Emeritus Professor, Department of Obstetrics and Gynaecology, Erasmus University Medical Center, Rotterdam, The Netherlands

Jill Wright, RM, BSc (Hons), MSc
Specialist Midwife, West Midlands Perinatal Institute, Birmingham, UK

Kees A. Yedema, MD, PhD
Consultant in Obstetrics and Gynecology, Department of Obstetrics and Gynecology, Westeinde Ziekenhuis, The Hague, The Netherlands

Lami Yeo, MD
Associate Professor of Obstetrics and Gynecology, Director of Perinatal Ultrasound, Director of Fetal Cardiovascular Unit, Department of Obstetrics, Gynecology, and Reproductive Sciences, Division of Maternal-Fetal Medicine, UMDNJ-Robert Wood Johnson Medical School, Robert Wood Johnson University Hospital, New Brunswick, New Jersey, USA

Introduction

Introduction to the First Edition

Both the complexity and the cost of modern medicine continue to rise while societal resources to pay for it fall further behind. A growing number of tests are routinely performed in the name of advanced medical care before their advantages and disadvantages have been clearly demonstrated. This is especially true in obstetrics and gynecology, where the risk of litigation is high and physicians fear being held responsible for either an unpreventable or an unpredictable event. However, many screening tests lead to unnecessary interventions that pose a health risk to the patient. Since a screening test is performed on asymptomatic individuals, it must be accurate and safe. Too often, though, the medical practitioner is ill-prepared to evaluate its value. Limited resources require the practitioner to seek the greatest return on investment.

The purpose of this book is to examine objectively many of the screening tests used in obstetrics and gynecology. It was neither pragmatic nor feasible to cover all screening tests. We have focused on more common ones in everyday practice plus a few 'future' screening tests such as that for cystic fibrosis.

Objective evaluation requires that the sensitivity, specificity, and positive and negative predictive values be quantified before even considering the cost of testing and its potential impact. Such an appraisal requires a heavy dose of epidemiology, a subject capable of sedating the most lively individual. As a result, the information often fails to reach those in greatest need of it. Those seeking the typical, in-depth epidemiological approach to screening issues should look elsewhere. We asked our expert contributors to digest the available information and present it in the following standardized format, addressing the fundamental questions the practitioner should consider to make an informed decision:

1 ■ What Is the Problem that Requires Screening?

   a. What is the incidence/prevalence of the target condition?

   b. What are the sequelae of the condition that are of interest in clinical medicine?

2 ■ The Tests

   a. What is the purpose of the tests?

   b. The nature of the tests

c. Implications of testing

    1.What does an abnormal test result mean?
    2.What does a normal test result mean?

d. What is the cost of testing?

3 ■ Conclusions and Recommendations

Our goal was to produce an easily read text which would help the practitioner to make everyday decisions. The three editors bring a diverse scientific and international background to this effort. Two are obstetricians and gynecologists (one with an interest in public health), while the third is a medical statistician. The authors represent many countries and were asked to take an international approach considering both how the costs of testing and the frequency of the target disorder might vary among locations. Perhaps to the disgruntlement of some contributors, all chapters were heavily edited to give the feel of a 'single author' text. Preparation of the book was truly an educational experience for the editors. Several of the screening tests commonly used in obstetrics and gynecology are unjustified. The usefulness of many remains unclear despite widespread application. In other cases, the tests were adopted before an appropriate evaluation was even attempted. We believe established practitioners, trainees, midwives and nurse practitioners will find the text valuable as they reexamine their current (and plan for their future) practices. In many instances, they will find their practice differs from the recommendations. Considering the need for evidence-based practice, the divergence provides a challenge—confirm the value of a screening test, or cease to use it.

Hajo I.J. Wildschut
Carl P. Weiner
Tim J. Peters

Introduction to the Second Edition

Screening tests have become increasingly incorporated into women's health care since the publication of our first edition in 1996. This growth was particularly marked in obstetrics, with the introduction of large-scale screening tests for Down syndrome and cystic fibrosis (as predicted in the 1st edition) during the last decade. Screening has also gained momentum in other areas of women's health care. Health care providers are therefore increasingly being called upon to make complex decisions regarding screening, and the need for a reference text is clear.

Though the number and scope of applications have grown, the concept of screening has not changed. While diagnostic tests are usually intended for patients seeking health care, screening tests are aimed at asymptomatic individuals who are typically not familiar with the condition of interest. As a consequence, an inherent feature—indeed, one of the many challenges—of screening programs is that the majority of individuals involved may derive reassurance through negative test results but they will ultimately experience no obvious personal health gain. In addition to the important issue of economic costs, this characteristic of screening gives rise to some disquieting problems pertaining to the generation of false positive and false negative screening test results. These concepts and measures have continued to be the focus of the contributions to this book.

In compiling this book we too have had to respond to the growth of screening in women's health care. The first edition contained 28 chapters pertaining principally to obstetrics and gynecology. The second edition has doubled to 56 chapters covering a much broader field of both women's and children's health. Moreover, these chapters have been laid out in a manner to match the way caregivers actually practice and encounter patients.

New topics include screening for hemoglobinopathies, early and late onset genetic diseases, thrombophilia, neonatal hypoglycemia and hyperbilirubinemia, diabetes, hyperlipidemia, osteoporosis and colon cancer. Each chapter from the 1st edition has been extensively redesigned and updated. As before, each chapter was heavily edited to give the feel of a 'single author' text. We have focused on the applicability of testing in both developed and developing settings.

We have thoroughly enjoyed the development and production of this 2nd edition. We are extremely grateful to the authors for their fine contributions, and sincerely hope that this text serves the needs of those providing preventive health care to women in both developed and developing regions of the world. We solicit their feedback and pledge to incorporate their growing needs in future editions.

Hajo I.J. Wildschut
Carl P. Weiner
Tim J. Peters

1

Epidemiologic Considerations in Screening

Tim J. Peters

Hajo I. J. Wildschut

Carl P. Weiner

■ Definitions and Objectives

Screening is defined as a procedure to help identify, in an organized way, a specified disease or condition among asymptomatic individuals. Because most screened individuals will be unaffected, the test must be safe to be acceptable. A **diagnostic test** is defined as the application of a variety of examinations or tests to patients who have actively sought health care services to identify the exact cause for their complaints.[1] The two are not mutually exclusive (e.g., genetic screening). The distinction between the two is whether or not that individual would have sought service for that particular problem. Diagnostic tests are also applied to individuals who seek medical care because of positive or suspicious findings resulting from a screening test. Diagnostic tests should be highly accurate, and there are important initiatives designed to improve the quality and consistency of the reporting of the relevant statistics.[2] In addition, there is guidance available about obtaining information from the literature about diagnostic studies.[3]

Compared with diagnostic procedures, screening tests should be relatively simple and quick to perform. For this reason, screening tests are allowed to possess higher error rates and thus may be less accurate than diagnostic tests.[1,4] **Population (or mass) screening programs** are applied to a general population to detect disease early to facilitate effective treatment. Such programs may also be applied for the purpose of separating seemingly healthy individuals into groups with high and low probabilities for a given disorder so that further health care resources can be targeted more efficiently.[1] The initiative for screening comes from either an investigator or an agency and involves participants with no known and/or reported symptoms or complaints related to the condition sought.[5] Individuals with positive or suspicious findings are referred for further investigation, diagnosis, and appropriate management.

The objectives of population screening programs are to reduce morbidity and mortality and to improve quality of life.[5,6,7] Prerequisites for a successful screening program include a safe and acceptable test, an adequate infrastructure in terms of administrative setting, quality control measures, systematic data handling, adequate health care services at the referral level that are accessible to those who need it, and clear targets in terms of delineating the problem to be screened. The condition should be amenable to treatment or prevention, with the timing of screening reflecting the opportunities for effective intervention. Finally, the severity and/or frequency of the target condition should be sufficient to justify the cost of screening.

Targeted screening programs involve the systematic testing of a selected group considered to be at increased risk. Targeted screening programs can be situation dependent (for example, screening in pregnancy), age dependent (mammography), inheritance dependent (for example, screening of family members because the individual has a specified genetic disorder), or ethnic/race dependent (for example, screening for sickle cell disease in black populations).

■ What Is the Problem that Requires Screening?

A clear, well-defined statement of the target condition being screened for is critical in assessing the value of any screening program. In practice, the true status is often not known for certain and hence effectively the test is evaluated in comparison with some other, more accurate classification—the "gold standard."[8,9]

What is the nature of the screening test result?

Because the test result is to be used as an indication of the presence or absence of the target condition, the simplest and most common situation is that the test itself classifies individuals into just two groups—those with a positive test result and those with a negative test result. For example, a woman may either be positive or negative for hepatitis B surface antigen. Alternatively, test results may be presented as continuous variables, where the value of a measurement can take any number in a range—for example, the blood glucose level. Given the objective of identifying a subgroup of individuals for further investigation, these measures are usually simplified to a dichotomy according to whether the measurement is above or below a cutoff. In this situation, the selection of the cutoff is critical and often controversial.

The proper evaluation of a screening program should address the following questions (Table 1–1; derived from[1,4,7]):

Is the condition being screened for an important health problem?

Perception of the importance of a health problem needs to be considered from the point of view of the individual, health care personnel, and community. Con-

Table 1–1	**Desirable characteristics for a successful screening program**

1. Is the condition being screened for an important health problem?
2. Is the screening test (and its consequences in terms of further diagnostic testing and subsequent treatment) acceptable to the population?
3. Does the target condition have a recognizable latent or early symptomatic phase? Is the natural history of the target condition well understood?
4. How valid and reliable is the screening test?
5. Are there adequate facilities for confirming the diagnosis and for adequate treatment?
6. Is the screening program a continuing process and not just a one-off activity?
7. Is "early" treatment of the target condition effective?
8. Do the objectives of the screening program justify the costs?

From Sackett DL, Holland WW. Controversy in the detection of disease. *Lancet* 1975;ii:357–359; Wilson JMG, Jungner G. Principles and practice of screening for disease. Public Health Papers, No. 34. Geneva: World Health Organization, 1968; and Hannigan VL. The periodic health examination. In: Diehl AK, ed., *Prevention and Screening in Office Practice: Contemporary Management in Internal Medicine.* New York: Churchill Livingstone, 1991:3–26.

ceptually, the benefits of screening may signify "reassurance" to the individual, "prolonging life" to the physician and "reduced cost" to policy makers. The following five principles have been suggested: (a) considerable weight should be accorded to community priorities, preferences, and concerns; (b) common problems should have higher priority than ones that occur rarely; (c) serious problems should be given higher priority than minor ones; (d) easily preventable health problems should be given higher priority than ones difficult to prevent; and (e) health problems whose frequencies show upward trends should generally be given higher priority than those that are static or decreasing.[10] These principles, however, are to some extent open to interpretation.

As indicated earlier, the importance of a health problem is closely associated with its frequency in the general population. In this context, the terms *incidence* and *prevalence* are often used. Incidence and prevalence are related but different terms and should not be used interchangeably.

Incidence (Table 1–2)[8] measures the occurrence of newly diagnosed events, occurring among previously unaffected persons. Typically, incidence rates are calculated from follow-up studies (cohort studies), where a fixed number of apparently healthy people are observed over a given period of time (usually a year) to determine the number of new events that occur during that period.[5]

Prevalence (Table 1–2) measures the extent to which the condition of interest exists among a specified group of people at a given point (or period) in time. Prevalence is usually given as a proportion—that is, the total number of affected persons per total number of subjects. For example, the annual incidence of pancreatic cancer is likely to be similar to its prevalence because most patients die within a year of diagnosis. In contrast, the prevalence of diabetes in a particular group of individuals will continue to grow even if its incidence remains stable because most patients will live more than a year with disease.

Table 1-2 **Characteristics of incidence and prevalence**		
	Incidence	**Prevalence**
Numerator	New cases occurring during a period of time among a group initially free of disease	All cases counted on a single survey or examination of a group
Denominator	All susceptible persons present at the beginning of the period	All persons examined, including affected and nonaffected
Time	Duration of period	Gven point or period
How measured	Cohort study	Cross-sectional study

From Fletcher RH, Fletcher SW, Wagner EH. *Clinical Epidemiology: The Essentials*, 2nd edition. Baltimore: Williams & Wilkins, 1988.

Thus, the prevalence depends on the incidence and duration of the disease. Incidence has been described as the water flowing into a lake and prevalence as the water in the lake.[11] Incidence and prevalence are frequently confused in obstetrics. For example, the proportion of newborns with trisomy 21 is generally referred to as a birth incidence, whereas to be correct, it should be termed the birth prevalence.

Is the screening test and its consequences acceptable to the population?

The individual (or community) has a free choice to participate in a screening program. The screening test itself must be safe and acceptable. The individual should be adequately informed before testing about the potential benefits and hazards of the program. For instance, therapeutic options may not be acceptable because of ethical concerns, regarding for example termination of pregnancy in the case of Down syndrome or unwanted side effects such as unnecessary surgery in ovarian cancer screening programs. Furthermore, with respect to screening programs for certain medical conditions, such as sexually transmitted diseases, it is well known that noncompliance is high, especially among those who would benefit most from the program. If a large proportion of the population does not comply with the medical advice following positive test results, any potentially beneficial effects of the screening program will be undermined. For screening tests, attention needs to be paid both to the technical issues of risk assessment and the risk perceptions of those for whom the screening program is being designed.[12]

Does the target condition have a recognizable latent or early symptomatic phase? Is the natural history of the target condition well understood?

Survival rates may appear to improve if earlier diagnosis is achieved as a result of screening—that is, before signs or symptoms of the condition of interest become manifest. This so-called *lead time* is dependent on both the biologic rate of disease progression and on the ability of the screening test to detect disease at an early stage. If the lead time is short, screening is unlikely to be of value because treatment of the target condition following detection by screening will be essentially the same as treatment following overt disease.[8]

Overestimation of survival time due to detection of disease in the early—asymptomatic—stage is known as lead time bias.[8] It is important not to be misled by lead time bias. For example, if screening could successfully identify women with stage 1 ovarian cancer but no therapy was instituted, and success was measured by survival time from diagnosis, it might appear that survival was improved by screening, although in reality it was unaltered. In practical circumstances where there is no effective treatment, screening only provides an early death sentence. Knowledge of the natural history of the target condition is clearly important for the assessment of the results of early treatment.

How valid and reliable is the screening test?

Validity is a summary measure of test performance, which is determined by both the underlying quality of the test and by the way the test is carried out. Validity refers to the degree to which a test measures what it purports to measure. It therefore requires an independent standard of reference.[8,9] Both internal and external validity must be considered.

Internal validity is synonymous with accuracy (i.e., the degree to which the test result corresponds to the true state of the phenomenon being measured).[8] The two components of internal validity are sensitivity and specificity.[11]

Sensitivity is defined as the proportion of individuals with the target condition who screened positive (Table 1–3).[8,13] Sensitivity is a measure of how good the test is at identifying patients with the disease. High sensitivity implies that a large proportion of individuals with the target condition have a positive result on the screening test. Highly sensitive tests are needed when there is an important penalty for missing the disorder.[8] This is particularly true when "false-negative" test results (category "c" in Table 1–3) create harm. Any test that is not 100% sensitive will inevitably result in false reassurance and possibly delay the seeking of medical care once symptoms of the target disorder do appear.[7] Moreover, the physician or midwife may fear litigation when the target disorder is not detected by the test.

Specificity is defined as the proportion of individuals without the disease who have a negative result on the screening test. Specificity is a measure of how good the test is at identifying unaffected individuals (Table 1–3).[8,13] It assesses how good it is at excluding the condition of interest. Hence, specificity is related to reassurance about health. High specificity thus reflects a low proportion of individuals falsely labeled as having the disease when they are in fact free of disease (the "false positives," category "b" in Table 1–3). In contrast, low specificity implies a high proportion of healthy individuals who are labeled as test positive (high false-positive rate). In screening programs, false-positive test results produce most of the problems because healthy indi-

Table 1-3	**Formulas for sensitivity, specificity, prevalence, positive predictive value (PPV), and negative predictive value (NPV)**	
	Target Condition[1]	
Test Result	**Present**	**Absent**
positive	a	b
negative	c	d

[1]True state of the individual, as determined by a relevant "gold standard"

sensitivity = a/(a+c)   PPV = a/(a+b)

Specificity = d/(b+d)   NPV = d/(c+d)

Prevalence = (a+c)/(a+b+c+d)   (For detailed definitions see text.)

viduals are subjected to often expensive, time-consuming, and potentially dangerous diagnostic procedures that would not be experienced without the screening test.[7] Moreover, false-positive test results may create unnecessary anxiety for patient.

The receiver operating characteristic (ROC) curve is useful for a test involving a continuous measurement with many possible cutoff values, such as serum bilirubin.[13] As shown for example in Chapter 40, the ROC curve is a graphical representation, where sensitivity is plotted against the false-positive rate (1-specificity). As is illustrated by such curves, the sensitivity and specificity are inversely related to each other. In a given situation, false-positive results are decreased at the cost of increasing false-negative results and vice versa. Sensitivity and specificity, and therefore the ROC curve, do not take into account the prevalence of the condition sought.

The general performance of a test is often expressed using the area under the ROC curve, with 0.5 reflecting a test no better than chance, 1.0 a perfect test, and 0 a "perfectly" imperfect test. In practice, though, it is more useful to consider particular cutoff values that reflect acceptable levels of sensitivity and specificity. One possible guideline for this approach is that where the condition is uncommon, then 1-specificity (the "false-positive rate" b/(b+d) in Table 1-3) is very close to the proportion that would be test positive in the target population. Between them, feasibility, costs, and the potential for psychological problems among those testing positive may indicate what test positive rate would be acceptable. Thus the ROC curve will immediately yield the anticipated sensitivity corresponding to this level. This is best accompanied by a sensitivity analysis in its general sense. That is, it is helpful to conduct an investigation of the impact on the sensitivity of the test by altering the proportion of test positives in the population—either directly using the ROC if the condition is rare, or in general, in relation to various potentially acceptable false-positive rates.

Table 1–4 Predictive values of a test with a sensitivity of 90% and a specificity of 99% when the prevalence of the disease is 10%

Test Result	Disease/Condition Present	Absent	Total
Positive	90	9	99
Negative	10	891	901
Total	100	900	1000

PPV: 90/99=90.9%
NPV: 891/901=98.9%

In clinical practice, **predictive values** are important because they are the probabilities in a particular setting that someone testing positive has the condition and someone testing negative does not. In this context, the **positive predictive value** (PPV) is the probability of disease in subjects with a positive test result, whereas **negative predictive value** (NPV) is the probability of absence of the disease in subjects with a negative test result (Table 1–3). Predictive values are affected by test performance, in terms of sensitivity and specificity, *and* by the prevalence of the condition in the target population. As illustrated in Table 1–4, in settings with a relatively high prevalence of disease (e.g., 10%), the probability of disease among the test-positive subjects is high (the PPV is 91%). On the other hand, in settings with a lower prevalence (e.g., 1%) the probability of disease among test-positive subjects is reduced (in Table 1–5, the PPV is 47%). This occurs despite the fact that sensitivity (90%) and specificity (99%) are identical in each setting. A further general point to be emphasized when considering these performance statistics is that we are considering the ability of the test to detect *prevalent* cases, whether at a given point in time or over a period

Table 1–5 Predictive values of a test with a sensitivity of 90% and a specificity of 99% when the prevalence of the disease is 1%

Test Result	Disease/Condition Present	Absent	Total
positive	9	10	19
negative	1	980	981
Total	10	990	1000

PPV = 9/19 = 47.4%
NPV = 980/981 = 99.9%

of time; hence, the relevant measure of frequency in situations such as those in Tables 1–3, 1–4, and 1–5 is prevalence not incidence.

Likelihood ratios (LRs) are an alternative way of looking at test performance. LRs are a reflection of sensitivity and specificity and are given by the formulas presented in Table 1–6.[8,13] LRs can be used to calculate "posttest probabilities," which are the probabilities of disease after either a positive or negative test result. For example, LRs allow us to update the pretest probability of intrauterine growth restriction (IUGR) from about 10% of all deliveries to 20% of those with an abnormal uterine artery Doppler ratio and 7% of those with a normal Doppler ratio (see Chapter 25).

First, the value of the pretest odds is computed from the pretest probability (prevalence), using the following formula:

$$\text{Pretest odds} = \frac{\text{Pretest probability}}{1 - \text{Pretest probability}}$$

Note that odds and probability are not the same and should not be used interchangeably. For example, a probability of $\frac{1}{3}$ would correspond to odds of $\frac{1}{2}$. These pretest odds are then converted to posttest odds by applying the likelihood ratios in the following way:

$$\text{Posttest odds}^{(pos)} = \text{Pretest odds} \times \text{LR}^{(pos)}$$
$$\text{Posttest odds}^{(neg)} = \text{Pretest odds} \times \text{LR}^{(neg)}$$

and the posttest odds values converted to probabilities by:

$$\text{Prob.(disease/pos.test)} = \frac{\text{Posttest odds}^{(pos)}}{1 + \text{Postest odds}^{(pos)}}$$
$$\text{Prob.(disease/neg.test)} = \frac{\text{Posttest odds}^{(neg)}}{1 + \text{Postest odds}^{(neg)}}$$

In summary, the prevalence is first expressed as a single odds. In turn, this is converted via the $\text{LR}^{(pos)}$ and $\text{LR}^{(neg)}$ to two posttest odds, which are then re-expressed as posttest probabilities of disease given, respectively, a positive or a negative test result. This procedure is equivalent to obtaining the positive and

Table 1–6	**Formulas for the likelihood ratio (LR) associated with a positive (Abnormal) test result (LR^{pos}) and the LR associated with a negative (Normal) test result (LR^{neg})**		
LR(pos) =	$\dfrac{\text{Prob.(pos.test/disease)}}{\text{Prob.(pos.test/no disease)}}$	=	$\dfrac{\text{Sensitivity}}{1\text{-Specificity}}$
LR(neg) =	$\dfrac{\text{Prob.(neg.test/disease)}}{\text{Prob.(neg.test/no disease)}}$	=	$\dfrac{1\text{-Sensitivity}}{\text{Specificity}}$

Prob.(pos.test/disease), probability of a positive test result among those with the disease (e.g., sensitivity); prob.(neg.test/no disease) = probability of a negative test result among those without the disease (e.g., specificity).

negative predictive values from the sensitivity, specificity, and prevalence using Bayes theorem.[13] The purpose is to allow the calculation of predictive values in various clinical settings with different prevalences given the underlying sensitivity and specificity of the test. As illustrated in Table 1–4, even if the sensitivity and the specificity do not change, the predictive values are dependent on the prevalence. Of course, sensitivity and specificity may vary in different clinical settings (e.g., due to varying skills in carrying out the test and varying durations of follow-up—see Chapter 52).

In conclusion, a likelihood ratio different from one demonstrates that a test is potentially useful, but does not necessarily imply that the test is a good indicator of disease, especially when the target condition is rare. In this situation, someone testing positive is still more likely to be unaffected than affected.[13] Nevertheless, where test positives are uncommon, the LR$^{(pos)}$ will approximately equal the odds ratio (OR=[a/c]/[b/d] or, equivalently, ad/bc from Table 1–3), and likewise the LR$^{(neg)}$ will approximately equal 1. The OR approximates to the risk ratio (or relative risk, RR=[a/(a+c)]/[b/(b+d)] from Table 1–3) if the disease is rare.[13] In any case, whatever the prevalence, the OR is the same as the ratio of the two likelihood ratios—that is, OR=LR$^{(pos)}$/LR$^{(neg)}$. The implication of this is that a high OR does not necessarily imply that a test will be useful in practice; it is a prerequisite, but the practical value of the test will also depend on the prevalence of the condition and the frequency of positive test results.

External validity (generalizability) is the degree to which test results hold true in other settings.[8] Sensitivity estimates are usually derived from carefully controlled research settings and may not apply to everyday situations. Published sensitivity values for a given test or examination tend to be overestimates because the findings are often based on special expertise and novel technologies applied to an atypical clinical population.

Reliability is also a measure of a test's performance. It is synonymous with reproducibility, repeatability, transferability, precision, and consistency. Reliability refers to the degree of stability when a measurement is repeated under the same conditions.[5] The extent to which a test is reproducible is affected by variation arising from three main sources: the examination (laboratory facilities or equipment), the examiner (skill), and the examined (characteristics).[1] Lack of reliability may be the result of measurement errors and/or instability of the attribute being studied.

Are there adequate facilities for confirming the diagnosis and for treatment?

Several aspects of screening procedures are demanding. These include the recording of the screening result, the proper interpretation of the result, communication between the screening program and the patient/caregiver, and quality control. Results, in particular when abnormal, should be communicated to the individual being screened and to the physician responsible for further evaluation and management. For this purpose, adequate facilities should be accessible to those who need it. Adequate facilities include hospitals and laboratories, which need to be properly staffed and technically equipped to meet the demands of confirmatory testing, diagnosis, and subsequent treatment where indicated. For the optimal use of resources, a carefully designed and agreed upon referral system is imperative for a successful screening program. The total burden on medical, diagnostic, and therapeutic resources, therefore, could well be increased by the introduction of a screening program.

Is testing a continuing process and not a one-off activity?

In some situations, screening is best served by the performance of examinations at regular intervals. An ongoing reminder system should be part of the screening program.

Is "early" treatment of the target condition effective?

Will "early" treatment—in the asymptomatic phase—be more effective than "delayed" treatment —that is, when symptoms appear? The question of whether treatment can work is one of both efficacy and effectiveness.[5,8] Efficacy is the performance of an intervention under ideal circumstances, whereas effectiveness is performance under everyday circumstances.[5,8] The randomized controlled trial (RCT) is generally accepted as the ideal method to ascertain efficacy.[14] By the use of pragmatic RCTs,[15] it is possible to bring efficacy as close as possible to effectiveness. Random allocation to intervention groups eliminates the possibility that differences in outcome between the groups are due to differences in underlying risks between the groups.

Of course, the justification for screening requires more than evidence of effective early treatment. In general, the proper evaluation of screening programs should involve an RCT of the screening program compared with an appropriate unscreened group where disease is detected in the usual way. Such RCTs would normally involve randomization of groups rather than individuals. Because such a trial should incorporate all the complexities that would occur in practice—such as variations in attendance, compliance, acceptability, and quality of procedures among others—a pragmatic approach would invariably be needed. Furthermore, comprehensive evidence about screening is not possible without full attention to cost-effectiveness.

Do the objectives of the screening program justify the costs?

What are the important and relevant costs?

The costs of screening can be both psychological and economic. Psychological costs include the anxiety engendered by participation in the screening program, the wait for test results and subsequent treatment, and knowledge of one's risk status or the future likelihood of overt disease (in particular the unnecessary anxiety produced by a false-positive screen). In addition, there may be other psychological stresses caused by indicated follow-up tests and therapy.

Economic costs include direct costs to the health care system (such as organizational and operating costs), direct costs borne by individuals being screened and their families (for example, travel expenses), and any indirect costs such as lost work time. In economic evaluations of health care programs, marginal (extra) costs should be used. Marginal cost refers to the extra costs of producing one extra unit of the desired health outcome. For example, the desired outcome might be years of life gained or the number of abnormalities avoided. Hence, when making a comparison of two or more programs, the question is what the extra costs and consequences are of the alternative program over and above the costs of the existing program. In screening, as in many other contexts, marginal costs depend on the size of the program. For example, the introduction of a small-scale screening program targeted at high-risk groups may show a low cost per case detected. If the screening program were to be expanded to groups at lower risk, the number of screening tests required to detect a positive case would rise, resulting in a net increase in the cost per case detected.[16]

Why is an economic evaluation important?

Choices have to be made concerning the deployment of health care programs, services, and procedures because resources in terms of manpower, time, facilities, and equipment are limited. Decisions on where to allocate resources should be based on explicit criteria. A systematic economic evaluation is important to identify clearly the costs and consequences of alternative programs.[17] Only with systematic evaluation is it possible to estimate and compare the various costs and benefits. In this context, the term efficiency is defined as maximizing the benefit derived from available resources.[16] Hence, costs incurred finding a case, which includes both identification and treatment, should be weighed against the costs of an alternative program.[18]

What strategies are used for a full economic evaluation?

There are two prerequisites for a full economic evaluation. First, two or more alternative programs, services, or procedures need to be compared. Second, both costs and health outputs need to be compared. The five basic types of full economic evaluation considered are cost-minimization analysis, cost-effectiveness analysis, cost-utility analysis, cost-benefit analysis, and cost-consequences analysis.[17,19]

Comparative evaluation of health programs solely in terms of costs is called **cost-minimization analysis**. For this approach to be appropriate, some preceding evidence is required to rule out differences in effectiveness of the programs being compared. An example of cost-minimization analysis is the comparison of progesterone versus danazol antagonists for the treatment of endometriosis. They are similar in effectiveness, but one is considerably more expensive than the other. Although attractive as a simple approach to economic evaluations, it is rare that there is sufficient evidence to rule out a difference between interventions or programs; certainly the failure to detect a statistically significant difference between them is not sufficient to justify a cost-minimization analysis given the wide confidence intervals for measures of effectiveness that are commonly obtained.[20]

Cost-effectiveness analysis is concerned with determining the least cost to achieve a specified level of effectiveness or the greatest effectiveness for a given level of expenditure.[5] Cost-effectiveness analysis is relevant to programs that produce health effects directly and to those that achieve clinical objectives that can be linked to improvements in patient outcome.[17] It implicitly assumes that the output in terms of health effects (e.g., preventing death, increasing life years gained, or disability days saved) is worth having.[17] For instance, the different diagnostic strategies for breast cancer can be compared in terms of the cost per case detected.

In **cost-utility analysis**, utilities are used as measures of the effects of a program. Utility refers to the perceived value, or worth, of a particular health status. It can be quantified by elucidating individual or societal preferences in relation to specific health outcomes.[17] The results of a cost-utility analysis are expressed in terms of the costs per unit of health-related utility, or cost per quality adjusted life year (QALY) gained under one program compared with another.[17]

Cost-benefit analysis is the evaluation of health care programs by valuing benefits as well as costs in terms of money. This means that costs and benefits can be compared directly, which in principle allows the assessment of a program's worth in absolute terms rather than just relative to an alternative program.[17] In practice, however, cost-benefit analyses almost always involve the comparison of at least two programs, even if one is a "do-nothing" alternative with more or less minimal intervention.[17] In evaluations of screening programs, the do-nothing option includes all the clinical management of patients that will take place even in the absence of screening. For example, in a cost-benefit analysis of screening for neural tube defects, it would be assumed that therapy is given to children with spina bifida under the "no screening" alternative.

A **cost-consequence analysis** is a variation of cost-effectiveness analysis where a comprehensive list of the expected costs and health outcomes is presented in a tabular form without totaling the various costs or placing value on the outcomes. This disaggregated approach provides greater flexibility to users in applying the relevant findings to other settings, including the imputation of different costs and of different values (and/or value judgments) for the various consequences.[19]

Is an economic evaluation always needed?

Evaluation is in itself a costly activity; indeed it has been said that even a cost-benefit analysis should itself be subjected to a cost-benefit analysis.[17] In addition, economic evaluations are difficult to accomplish, requiring a variety of subjective and qualitative decisions that may greatly impact the final result. When the analysis is mainly descriptive, the term *partial evaluation* is used. Partial evaluation indicates that the analysis will not allow us to determine definitively whether the health program is worth doing.[17] A full economic evaluation, however, only seems reasonable in situations where program objectives require clarification, where the competing alternatives are markedly different in nature, or where large resource commitments are under consideration.[17] In any case, all economic evaluations should be subjected to a sensitivity analysis, where the assumptions and valuations used are varied within appropriate bounds of uncertainty in order to ascertain the robustness of the conclusions. One of the objectives of the sensitivity analysis will be to assess the generalizability of the results of the economic evaluation—in particular, how the implications of the evaluation may vary across different local settings.

■ Conclusions and Recommendations

The ultimate objective of screening is to reduce mortality and/or morbidity.[7] Conditions screened for should therefore include important causes of mortality or morbidity, in terms of prevalence, severity, or both. Moreover, such conditions should be amenable to either treatment or prevention when detected early. The screening procedure itself should be safe and easy to perform to maximize compliance. The ideal screening test should be capable of identifying a large group of individuals with—or susceptible to—disease and should also be capable of excluding the majority of those without disease. Harm should be avoided and adverse psychological effects kept to a minimum. A full description of the screening program should be given: Who does what, to whom, where, how often, and what are the results.[17] Precise definitions of the condition and the target population are essential.

Appropriate action should be taken on the basis of explicit criteria when an abnormal test result is obtained. For this reason, adequate health care services should be available for the diagnosis and treatment of confirmed disease. These services should be accessible and affordable. Screening programs are demanding in various respects, including data handling, continuity, and communication. Adequate infrastructure and health care facilities at the referral level are essential if a screening program is to be successful.

Finally, individuals should be motivated to comply with medical advice. There is widespread ethical, legal, and medical agreement that screening should be preceded—and followed—by counseling, even if a screening test becomes routine. The individual should be adequately informed about the potential benefits and limitations of screening in terms of primary objectives, results, and implications. Screening should always be offered as an option that may be accepted or rejected.

References

1. Sackett DL, Holland WW. Controversy in the detection of disease. *Lancet* 1975;ii:357–359.
2. STAndards for Reporting of Diagnostic Accuracy: The STARD Initiative. http://www.consort statement.org.
3. Haynes RB, Wilczynski NL. Optimal search strategies for retrieving scientifically strong studies of diagnosis from Medline: analytical survey. *BMJ* 2004;328:1040.
4. Wilson JMG, Jungner G. Principles and practice of screening for disease. Public Health Papers, No. 34. Geneva: World Health Organization, 1968.
5. Last JM. *A Dictionary of Epidemiology*, 4th edition. Oxford: Oxford University Press, 2001.
6. Morrison AS. *Screening in Chronic Disease*, 2nd edition. New York: Oxford University Press, 1985.
7. Hannigan VL. The periodic health examination. In: Diehl AK, ed., *Prevention and Screening in Office Practice: Contemporary Management in Internal Medicine*. New York: Churchill Livingstone, 1991:3–26.
8. Fletcher RH, Fletcher SW, Wagner EH. *Clinical Epidemiology: The Essentials*, 2nd edition. Baltimore: Williams & Wilkins, 1988.
9. Editorial. Instructions for authors. *JAMA* 1992;268:43–44.
10. Backett EM, Davies AM, Petros-Barvazian A. The risk approach in health care. With special reference to maternal and child health care planning. *World Health Organization Public Health Reports* 1984;76.
11. Barker DJP, Rose G. *Epidemiology in Medical Practice*, 4th edition. Churchill Livingstone, Edinburgh, 1990.
12. World Health Organization. The world health report: chapter 2—defining and assessing risks to health. Available at http://www.who.int/whr/2002/chapter2/en/.
13. Altman DG. *Practical Statistics for Medical Research*. London: Chapman & Hall, 1991:409–419.
14. Thacker SB. Quality of controlled clinical trials: the case of imaging ultrasound in obstetrics—a review. *Br J Obstet Gynaecol* 1985;92:437–444.
15. Schwartz D, Lellouch J. Explanatory and pragmatic attitudes in therapeutical trials. *J Chron Dis* 1967;20:637–648.
16. Cohen D. Marginal analysis in practice: an alternative to needs assessment for contracting health care. *BMJ* 1994;309:781–784.
17. Drummond MF, Stoddard GL, Torrance GW. *Methods for the Economic Evaluation of Health Care Programmes*. Oxford: Oxford University Press, 1987.
18. Hakama M. Screening. In: Holland WW, Detels R, Knox G (eds.). *Oxford Textbook of Public Health*. 2nd edition. Applications in Public Health (vol. 3). Oxford: Oxford University Press 1991; pp. 91–106.
19. Coast J. Is economic evaluation in touch with society's health values? *BMJ* 2004;329:1233–1236.
20. Briggs A, O'Brien B. The death of cost-minimisation analysis. *Health Economics Letters* 2000; 4.

Maternal Red Blood Cell Group and Antibody Screen

Charlene M. Elbert

Ronald G. Strauss

■ What Is the Problem that Requires Screening?

Hemolytic disease of the fetus and newborn (HDN) secondary to red blood cell (RBC) antigens other than to the ABO systems; possible maternal transfusion at delivery.

What is the incidence/prevalence of the target condition?

Two to five percent of pregnant women exhibit RBC alloimmunization (isoimmunization)[1]; 1% to 3% of vaginal and 3% to 5% of cesarean deliveries undergo RBC transfusions.[2]

What are the sequelae of the condition that are of interest in clinical medicine?

RBC alloimmunization is the production of antibodies against antigens not present on the maternal RBCs but expressed on the fetal RBCs due to paternal inheritance. It can cause fetal hemolytic anemia leading to stillbirth, hydrops, preterm delivery, and kernicterus if the neonate develops severe hyperbilirubinemia. Although the most severe HDN occurs with anti-Rh (D), many other anti-RBC immunoglobulin G (IgG) antibodies can cause life-threatening disease. The incidence of alloimmunization to Rh (D) is greatly reduced by the timely administration of anti-D immunoglobulin during pregnancy and postpartum. RBC alloimmunization can delay or even prevent the availability of compatible blood for maternal transfusion.

Because the severity of HDN cannot be precisely predicted, all women should be tested during early pregnancy for the presence and identity of potentially significant RBC antibodies.[3] Only IgG isotype antibodies, which cross the placenta from mother to fetus and are directed against antigens on fetal/neonatal RBCs, can cause HDN. Management of women and their fetuses varies with local practices. The decision for an intervention such as amniocentesis, cordocentesis, or intrauterine RBC transfusion is based on antibody specificity, baseline levels and changes in antibody titer, and the severity of hemolytic disease in the neonates of preceding pregnancies.[4,5] Although often available only in specialized laboratories, genetic testing of maternal serum free RNA, fetal blood, or amniotic fluid cells provides knowledge of whether or not the fetus possesses the RBC antigen in question.[6]

Less than 3% of women receive an RBC transfusion postpartum. Thus, it is unnecessary to routinely cross-match women in labor, providing that the ABO and Rh (D) typing and RBC antibody screening were normal antenatally, unless a risk factor such as placenta previa or cesarean delivery occurs.[3] Instead, a blood sample for compatibility testing is obtained at the time a transfusion is deemed necessary.

■ The Tests

What is the purpose of the tests?

Antenatal maternal blood grouping identifies Rh (D)–negative women who are candidates for RhIG prophylaxis (e.g., completion of pregnancy and those undergoing invasive prenatal diagnosis). RBC antibody screening detects IgG alloantibodies to RBC antigens other than ABO, which, if present, could cause HDN. In addition, prior knowledge of unexpected antibodies (i.e., other than to ABO antigens) can facilitate the issuance of compatible RBC units to transfuse either mothers or their infants during the perinatal period. Testing women for ABO antibody isotype or titers is not predictive of HDN and should not be done.

What is the nature of the tests?

Blood grouping consists of determining both ABO group and Rh (D) type. These tests should be performed as early as possible in pregnancy. These need not be repeated for subsequent pregnancies, providing the testing facility has records of concordant results on two samples obtained on different occasions.[3]

ABO grouping tests distinguish RBCs of four distinct phenotypes: A, B, O, and AB. The ABO group of most adult individuals can be determined by direct agglutination tests (forward grouping) using RBC typing antibodies prepared from serum of hyperimmunized human subjects (polyclonal antisera) or immunoglobulin-secreting mouse hybridoma cells (monoclonal antisera). All reagents used for both ABO and Rh grouping are required to meet potency and specificity requirements of regulatory agencies, such as the US Food and Drug Administration.

The ABO system is the only blood group system in which individuals older than 6 months of age predictably produce "natural" antibodies to antigens they lack. Serum grouping (reverse grouping) tests are routinely used to confirm the results of RBC antigen grouping procedures. A test accuracy approaching 100%

can be assumed if the RBC antigen and serum antibody results are complementary. However, discrepancies can occur between the results of antigen and serum grouping when the RBCs either possess unexpected antigens or lack expected ones and when serum antibodies do not complement the antigens expressed. Certain subgroups of A and B (less than 1%) may exhibit weaker reactions than normally seen, and depending on the subgroup, may appear nonreactive (i.e., fail to exhibit the presence of the antigen) in normal testing procedures. In addition, antigen expression may be altered by infection and malignancy, and plasma antibodies may be absent in immunodeficiency states. These discrepancies must be resolved before a final ABO group can be assigned with confidence.

The terms "Rh-positive" and "Rh-negative" refer in Rh typing to the presence or absence of the Rh (D) RBC antigen. RBCs from approximately 85% of whites and 92% of blacks express the Rh (D) antigen. Some Rh-positive RBCs fail to directly agglutinate with anti-D typing reagent. Additional testing for the weak D (formerly called Du) and partial D can be performed to distinguish between RBCs possessing an apparent Rh (D) antigen from those that are truly Rh-negative. The decision to perform a test for weak D is at the discretion of the transfusion service medical director. If the decision is made to include a test for weak D and the test is clearly positive, the woman should be regarded as D-positive and treated as such. Testing for weak expression of D should be done using anti-IgG rather than anti-IgG+C3 antiglobulin reagents to prevent false-positive tests due to complement coating of the RBCs. The test for weak D should not be read microscopically. There must be mechanisms and interpretation criteria to prevent mistyping of the D-woman as D-positive if Rh typing is performed during the third trimester or at delivery due to a large fetomaternal hemorrhage (FMH). Only when the prenatal tests for Rh are clearly reactive (>2+) is the woman considered D-positive. If testing for weak D is not performed, women whose RBCs do not react in direct tests with anti-D (i.e., those labeled as being Rh-negative) are considered candidates for RhIG therapy during pregnancy and at delivery.[3]

RBC antibody screening tests are used to detect unexpected clinically relevant antibodies (i.e., other than "expected" anti-A or anti-B). The woman's serum is reacted with RBC screening cells that must bear the following antigens: D, C, E, c, e, M, N, S, s, P_1, Le^a, Le^b, K, k, Fy^a, Fy^b, Jk^a, and JK^b. Detected antibodies in the antiglobulin test are more likely IgG and clinically significant, compared with those reactive only at room temperature or below. However, antibody screening tests do not detect all antibodies of clinical significance. Antibodies to antigens not present on the screening cells (e.g., low-prevalence antigens) and those that manifest dosage (i.e., react only with RBCs from homozygotes) are likely to be missed.

What are the implications of testing?

What does an abnormal test result mean? When screening tests for unexpected RBC antibodies are positive, the antibody must be identified to determine its clinical significance. The woman should be asked about previous blood transfusions. All IgG antibodies pose a potential risk of causing fetal hemolytic anemia. The biologic father, if available, should be typed and, where appropriate, genotyped. The purpose of titrating potentially significant antibodies detected in pregnancy is not to predict the severity of HDN, but to determine when to monitor for HDN by nonserologic means. This requires referral for additional management according to local practice (antibody titration, ultrasound, amniocentesis, or cordocentesis). Such an evaluation is initiated if there is a twofold or greater increase in titer during pregnancy or if the titer exceeds a critical level. A value of 8 to 32 is used as a critical titer in most centers.

Anti-D is the major antibody for which titration is appropriate, because it is the antibody for which intrauterine intervention or early delivery is most likely to be considered.[3] Occasionally, other Rh antibodies act similarly.[7] In contrast, non-Rh antibodies cause HDN, but early delivery is almost never undertaken. Thus, routine serial titration of non-Rh antibodies is of questionable value.[3] Moreover, the predictive value of titration results for antibodies other than anti-D is quite poor or variable among institutions.

What does a normal test result mean? A clearly defined ABO and Rh (D) type and a negative RBC antibody screening test are the normal results. Although this does not guarantee absence of alloimmunization and/or eliminate the possibility of HDN, clinically significant disease is unlikely. Women who are Rh negative should receive anti-D immunoglobulin (125–300 µg, the practice varies among countries) at 28 weeks' gestation and again at delivery if the newborn is D-positive. No additional testing is required.

What is the cost of testing?

Charges do not reflect a true picture because of incomplete reimbursement due to capitation and other negotiated pay structures. Though institutional *charges* to the woman vary markedly, actual laboratory costs to perform testing should be comparable. As an example, current reagent and supply costs at our center are approximately $3.50 for each blood type and antibody screen. If the antibody screen is negative, labor is about $5, based on ¼ hour per test at $20 per hour. When the antibody screen is positive, the antibody identification can take 30 minutes to several hours. Thus, laboratory costs can range from $8.50 up to $50 or higher. The total charges to the woman include the sum of the reagent and supply costs, labor costs, and an overhead cost (space, utilities, insurance, etc.), and often exceed laboratory costs by several-fold.

It is not necessary to repeat ABO and Rh (D) typing after the initial prenatal visit providing the testing facility has records of concordant results on two samples obtained on different occasions.[3] Rh-positive women should be screened for RBC antibodies once during pregnancy, at the initial visit. Rh-negative women should be screened for RBC antibodies at the initial visit and again at 28 to 30 weeks' gestation before administering anti-D immunoglobulin.

Repeated antibody screening and identification are recommended during the third trimester whenever unexpected antibodies are detected.[3] Titrations need not be repeated after other means of fetal monitoring are initiated in alloimmunized patients. If one assumes 95% of pregnant women initially tested have a negative antibody screen, repeated testing of 85% of them who are Rh-positive is unnecessary.

■ Conclusions and Recommendations

A maternal blood sample should be obtained early in pregnancy from all pregnant women to determine their ABO and Rh (D) types and to detect unexpected anti-RBC antibodies. Women who are Rh (D) antigen–negative and who exhibit no anti-RBC antibodies should be tested for anti-RBC antibodies a second time at 28 to 30 weeks' gestation, following which anti-D immunoglobulin is administered to those women not immunized to Rh (D). No further testing is needed during a normal pregnancy for these "low-risk" women. Women who are Rh (D)–negative and who are immunized to Rh (D) antigen (exhibit anti-D) at the time of initial testing should be referred for additional management according to local practice (antibody titration, ultrasound, amniocentesis, or cordocentesis).

Rh (D)–positive women who on initial testing exhibit no anti-RBC antibodies require no further testing during normal pregnancy. Women who are Rh (D)–positive on initial testing and who exhibit clinically significant anti-RBC antibodies should be retested at least once. Paternal testing may be an appropriate next step. Depending on the specificity and titer of the anti-RBC antibody detected on initial testing, the women should be referred to an appropriate center for management.

■ Summary

1 ■ What Is the Problem that Requires Screening?

Hemolytic disease of the fetus and newborn (HDN); possible maternal transfusion at delivery.

a. *What is the incidence/prevalence of the target condition?*

Three to five percent of pregnant women exhibit RBC alloimmunization; 1%–3% of vaginal and 3%–5% of cesarean deliveries undergo RBC transfusions.

Continued

■ **Summary—cont'd**

b. *What are the sequelae of the condition that are of interest in clinical medicine?*
RBC alloimmunization can cause fetal hemolytic anemia leading to hydrops, stillbirth, preterm delivery, and kernicterus. RBC alloimmunization can delay or even prevent the availability of compatible blood for maternal transfusion.

2 ■ The Tests

a. *What is the purpose of the tests?*
Antenatal maternal blood grouping identifies women who are Rh (D)–negative and thus candidates for RhIG prophylaxis. Prior knowledge of unexpected antibodies can facilitate obtaining compatible units of RBCs to transfuse mothers or their infants during the perinatal period.

b. *What is the nature of the tests?*
RBC grouping and antibody screening

c. *What are the implications of testing?*
1. What does an abnormal test result mean?
When screening tests for unexpected RBC antibodies are positive, the antibody must be identified to determine its clinical significance.
2. What does a normal test result mean?
A clearly defined RBC group and a negative RBC antibody screening test are the normal results. An Rh (D)–negative woman with a negative screen should be retested at 28 weeks' gestation.

3 ■ Conclusions and Recommendations

A maternal blood sample should be obtained early in pregnancy from all pregnant women to determine their RBC ABO and Rh (D) groups and to detect unexpected anti-RBC antibodies.

References

1. Geifman-Holtzman O, Wojtowycz M, Kosmas E, Artal R. Female alloimmunization with antibodies known to cause hemolytic disease. *Obstet Gynecol* 1997;89:272–275.
2. Combs CA, Murphy EL, Laros RK Jr. Cost-benefit analysis of autologous blood donation in obstetrics. *Obstet Gynecol* 1992;80:621–625.
3. Judd WJ, for the Scientific Section Coordinating Committee of the AABB. Practice guidelines for prenatal and perinatal immunohematology, revisited. *Transfusion* 2001;41:1445–1452.
4. Bowman JM. Treatment options for the fetus with alloimmune hemolytic disease. *Transfusion Med Rev* 1990;4:191–207.
5. Weiner CP, Williamson RA, Wenstrom KD, et al. Management of fetal hemolytic disease by cordocentesis, I: prediction of fetal anemia. *Am J Obstet Gynecol* 1991;165:546–553.
6. Bennett PR, LeVan KC, Colin Y, et al. Prenatal determination of fetal RhD type by DNA amplification. *N Engl J Med* 1993;329:607–610.
7. Bowell PJ, Allen DL, Entwistle CC. Blood group antibody screening tests during pregnancy. *Br J Obstet Gynecol* 1968;93:1038–1043.

Antepartum Assessment of Hemoglobin, Hematocrit, and Serum Ferritin

Christine Kirkpatrick

Sophie Alexander

Hajo I. J. Wildschut

■ What Is the Problem that Requires Screening?

Antepartum abnormalities of the maternal red blood cell mass

What is the incidence/prevalence of the target condition?

About 8% to 40% of pregnant women in developed countries are classified as having anemia,[1] while the reported prevalence of iron deficiency anemia among women of reproductive age in developing countries approximates 60%.[2] Apart from geographic variations, the wide range in reported prevalences likely reflects differences in the definition of anemia. From 8% to 10% of women have an elevated red blood cell count.

In recent years, both the World Health Organization (WHO) criteria—hemoglobin less than 11 g/dL (6.8 mmol/L) and a hematocrit less than 33%[3]—have become widely accepted definitions of anemia during pregnancy. However, the arbitrary dividing line between dilutional and true anemia ranges from 10 g/dL (6.2 mmol/L) to 11 g/dL (6.8 mmol/L).[4] It is suggested that a more physiologic threshold would be the fifth percentile for gestational age.[3] It is also possible that the distribution of hemoglobin values varies among populations.[5] To what extent this reflects nutritional habits or other extrinsic factors has not been explored.

What are the sequelae of the condition that are of interest in clinical medicine?

The levels of hemoglobin and hematocrit decrease in most healthy pregnant women during the second trimester due to a rapid increase in plasma volume. As red cell production catches up with intravascular volume, hemoglobin and hematocrit rise in the third trimester (Figure 3–1).[1,6] The initial decline in hemoglobin and hematocrit is often described as a physiologic or dilutional anemia. Iron deficiency is the most common cause of pathologic anemia during pregnancy. Iron deficiency usually evolves slowly, progressing through several stages before presenting as frank anemia.[7] In the earliest stage (iron storage depletion), iron reserves are low, but there is adequate iron supply for the developing red cell. The second stage begins when the supply of iron available for erythropoiesis is diminished. The circulating hemoglobin content is not markedly decreased, but the red blood cell size is smaller (decreased mean corpuscular volume [MCV]). The final stage of iron deficiency is overt iron deficiency anemia.

The evidence that marked iron deficiency is associated with severe maternal and perinatal problems is compelling in developing countries.[1,2,8,9] In these countries, anemia during pregnancy often results from poor nutritional status, micronutrient deficiencies, infection with hookworm and other intestinal helminths, HIV infection, hemoglobinopathies, and malaria.[10,11] These underlying conditions have important adverse effects on maternal and child health.[2] Further, chronic anemia will have an adverse effect on physical health, leading to productivity losses arising from poor endurance in physically demanding jobs, and on mental health, in particular cognitive development.[2] Not surprisingly, these factors may be enough in the setting of suboptimal health care to contribute to the more than 20-times greater mater-

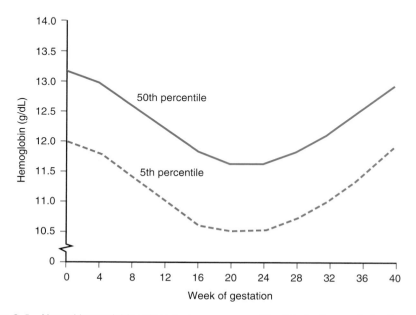

Figure 3–1 Normal hemoglobin values during pregnancy. Reprinted with permission from *Nutrition During Pregnancy*. Copyright 1990 by the National Academy of Sciences. Courtesy of the National Academy Press, Washington, DC.

nal mortality in developing compared with that of developed countries. However, the evidence of adverse effects of iron deficiency on maternal and child health is less convincing in developed countries. The underlying assumption pervading the literature is that a low hemoglobin content is associated with adverse perinatal outcome,[12] and that the maintenance of an optimal hemoglobin and iron store is bound to be advantageous for mother and child.[13] However, few studies actually address this issue in developed countries. There are no maternal physical symptoms secondary to mild anemia[14] and the evidence for adverse neonatal effects is conflicting. Rios and colleagues[15] and Sweet et al.[16] found no difference in the umbilical cord ferritin measurements of infants born to iron-deficient and iron-replete women. Thus, the fetus is efficient at extracting iron from its mother. In contrast, two other investigators observed either a limit to the iron-extracting capacity of the placenta or a correlation between the maternal and neonatal ferritin levels.[17,18] Another study of children between the ages of 10 and 12 years old concluded that the child's mean systolic blood pressure adjusted for current weight rose by 2.6 mm Hg for each 1 g/dL (0.6 mmol/L) fall in the mother's lowest hemoglobin level during pregnancy.[19] These results parallel findings in animal experiments and suggest that impaired maternal nutrition may influence the origin of adult hypertension during fetal life.

In contrast to low hemoglobin/hematocrit, a high hemoglobin/hematocrit (polycythemia) is a marker for an increased risk of preeclampsia, intrauterine growth restriction, and preterm delivery.[12,13,20–25] Duvekot et al.[26] observed that the likelihood of poor intravascular volume expansion in early pregnancy is increased in those pregnancies subsequently complicated by fetal growth restriction. Thus, the increase in hematocrit is not the result of excess red blood cell synthesis compared with that of normal pregnancy, but to decreased dilutional expansion.

■ The Tests

What is the purpose of the tests?

Antepartum identification of women with pathologic anemia or polycythemia for the purpose of initiating therapy to reduce their risk of an adverse pregnancy outcome.

What is the nature of the tests?

The antepartum measurement of maternal red blood cell mass and/or iron stores. The assessment of hemoglobin, hematocrit, and MCV in developed countries is usually performed with automated equipment. The principle limitation of hemoglobin as an index of iron deficiency is the marked overlap in frequency distribution curves of anemic and nonanemic individuals. As a result, the use of the WHO criteria for pathologic anemia (i.e., a hemoglobin level of less than 11 g/dL (6.8 mmol/L) and a hematocrit of less than 33%) results in large numbers of false-negative and false-positive findings. There is a debate about the timing of testing. An approach often recommended is to test at the first antenatal visit and again some time in the mid-second and third trimesters because anemia may manifest over time.

The three erythrocyte indices (i.e., the MCV, the mean corpuscular hemoglobin concentration [MCHC], and the mean corpuscular hemoglobin [MCH]) are commonly used to screen for the various types of anemia, including microcytic anemia due to iron deficiency and macrocytic anemia due to folate or B_{12} deficiency. These indices remain within the normal range in women with dilutional anemia. The MCV is regarded as the *most sensitive red cell index* for the identification of iron deficiency. Values below 70 fL occur only with iron deficiency anemia or thalassemia minor. A normal MCV in an anemic woman argues against both iron deficiency anemia and thalassemia.

A high hemoglobin level (> 13 g/dL or 8.1 mmol/L) is associated with adverse pregnancy outcomes.[13,27] The red blood cell indices are not usually affected by polycythemia.

Serum ferritin is most accurate indicator of available iron stores.[28] However, the sensitivity of serum ferritin for true depletion of iron reserves is low. A concentration below 12 µg/L is diagnostic of depleted iron stores in white males.[7] A low serum ferritin level in combination with low hemoglobin is strongly suggestive of iron-deficiency anemia. However, ferritin behaves as an acute phase reactin. Several pathologic conditions, such as infection, chronic disease, and liver disease, increase serum ferritin levels independent of the iron stores. Thus, a normal ferritin level does not exclude iron deficiency anemia. Methods for the measurement of serum ferritin include immunoradiometric assays (IRMAs) using labeled antibody, radioimmunoassays (RIAs) using labeled antigen, and enzyme-linked immune assays (EIAs), which eliminate the need for radioisotopes. Interlaboratory comparisons reveal that the differences between laboratories are not substantially greater than the intra-assay differences within the same laboratory.[7] An important advantage of serum ferritin measurements is its reliability on serial study. In one study, day-to-day variability in serum ferritin in the same subject was 15%. This compares favorably with the 28% day-to-day variability in serum iron and transferrin levels.[29]

What are the implications of testing?

What does an abnormal test result mean? *Screening for anemia:* Hemoglobi below 11 g/dL (6.8mmol/L) and a hematocrit below 33% suggest the presence of a pathologic anemia. Low hemoglobin levels and low hematocrit should prompt MCV testing to seek iron deficiency anemia. Hemoglobin and hematocrit testing is typically performed during the first antenatal visit and repeated at some point in the mid-second or third trimesters because anemia may develop over time. Some researchers suggest that serum ferritin also be measured routinely at the start of antenatal care, or by 20 to 24 weeks' gestation and at 6- to 8-week intervals thereafter.[30] There is no evidence to support this recommendation. There are at least two therapeutic routes to take once a pathologic anemia associated with a low MCV is identified: Confirm the presence of iron deficiency anemia by measuring the serum ferritin or proceed directly with iron replacement therapy. A reticulocytic response to iron replacement confirms the diagnosis of iron deficiency anemia. When there is no response to iron supplementation, other causes of anemia should be ruled out.

Iron supplementation has a beneficial effect on the maternal hematologic indices in women with iron deficiency anemia.[31,32] However, any evidence for a beneficial effect of iron supplementation on relevant birth outcomes is lacking.[31–34] The treatment of iron deficiency anemia in developing countries should be targeted at the underlying disorder.[11] Because the impact, if any, of anemia on pregnancy outcome in developed countries is unclear, it is impossible to evaluate the possible benefits of iron replacement therapy in terms of improvement of maternal and perinatal outcome.

It has been suggested that women begin iron supplementation if their hemoglobin level continues to fall in the third trimester or if they have low serum ferritin at the first antenatal visit.[35] For the treatment of anemia during pregnancy the WHO currently recommends a daily dose of 60 mg elemental iron (300 mg ferrous sulfate). Most randomized controlled trials have concluded that supplemented women are less likely to develop anemia, in particular when folate is added to the iron tablets.[36] Parenteral treatment with iron sucrose is justified in women with malabsorption or intolerance to oral therapy or when the iron loss exceeds the maximum oral replacement. However, in terms of clinical efficacy, there is no evidence that parenteral treatment with iron is superior to oral iron supplementation.[37] Blood transfusion is not warranted for the treatment of iron deficiency anemia per se.

Screening for preterm birth and low birth weight: A relationship between an elevated hemoglobin or hematocrit and poor pregnancy outcome is well documented, but it is difficult to determine whether the relationship is direct or indirect. Overall, the sensitivity of an elevated hemoglobin or hematocrit for the prediction of an adverse pregnancy outcome ranges from 5% to 36%, and specificity varies from 79% to 97%. Although there is no known therapy for polycythemia to reduce the risk of an adverse outcome, increased maternal and fetal surveillance seems warranted. Both high and low hematocrit levels are risk factors for intrauterine growth restriction and preterm birth.[13] Many studies, however, have failed to consider either the timing of the hematocrit measurements or the physiologic U-shaped relationship between hematocrit and pregnancy duration (Figure 3–1).[12,24,38] Blankson and colleagues[5] suggested that a mean hematocrit above 40% is associated with an increased risk of intrauterine growth restriction and elective preterm delivery, the latter resulting mainly from hypertension with or without fetal growth restriction. Studies that did not control for gestational age at sampling have tended to find a strong association between low hematocrit and preterm birth especially among black women. However, a low hematocrit is not associated with adverse pregnancy outcome when adjusted for confounding factors.

What does a normal test result mean? Women with normal red blood cell mass and iron stores do not have anemia or polycythemia. A 3% to 5% decline is typical between the first measurement at booking and the second measurement later in pregnancy (Figure 3–1.).

Routine iron supplementation of 30 to 60 mg Fe daily is advocated in several countries including the United States. Most randomized controlled trials conclude that supplemented women are less likely to develop anemia. However, this is the only difference in terms of outcome.[31,34,39] Iron supplementation targeted at pregnant women should be considered in countries with a high prevalence of anemia.[2] A reduction of the prevalence of anemia in developing countries could also be achieved by fortifying food products consumed by the poor and children. It is argued that iron fortification of food products, such as flour or salts, could have a major impact on maternal and child health in developing countries.[2]

Routine iron supplementation has potential risks. Iron supplements can cause unpleasant gastrointestinal symptoms (e.g., nausea and constipation), which are typically dose-related and usually occur at higher than recommended doses for supplementation.[40] It is recommended that iron supplements be taken between meals and not with tea or coffee.[41] Iron supplements may also exacerbate preexisting gastrointestinal disorders such as ulcerative colitis. Complications of excessive iron storage, such as hemochromatosis and hemosiderosis, are possible but uncommon in women taking oral supplements. There is a documented risk of accidental iron over dosage in young children.[42]

Perhaps because of the lack of evidence, patient and physician compliance is a potential problem when recommending routine iron supplementation.[41] In Norway, where routine iron supplementation is officially recommended, only 11% of care givers and 25% of the pregnant women comply.[43] In fact, increased absorption of iron from food is a physiologic consequence of normal pregnancy. The increase is large enough to meet the requirements of pregnancy, provided the dietary intake is adequate.[44] Although the routine use of folate in multivitamins has virtually eliminated macrocytic anemia resulting from a folic acid deficiency, this category of anemia is still a problem in the developing world and in populations not receiving antenatal care.

What is the cost of testing?

The cost of testing either red cell mass and/or iron stores in most developed countries is similar or even higher than the cost of routine iron supplementation. The cheapest preparation of combined iron and folate supplementation for an entire pregnancy costs £3.57 ($5.70, 1995) and a serum ferritin assay cost £2.50 ($4.00, 1995).[45] However, the price of testing is considerably higher in the United States where a complete blood profile approximates $17 and a serum ferritin $36 (1995). These costs have increased only modestly over the last decade. If routine screening of red cell mass is performed at the initial prenatal visit and in the early third trimester, and 15% of the women have iron deficiency anemia on initial prenatal visit and 5% of the remaining women are anemic when tested later in pregnancy, the cost per case identified (per 1,000 women, exclusive of treatment) is $164 (1995) if ferritin is not checked. In contrast to routine testing, the cost of iron and folate supplementation to the pregnant woman for 1 year approximates $17 (1995). Thus, the cost of routine supplementation to prevent one case of iron deficiency anemia is $89 without laboratory screening (1995). Considering the lack of an identifiable improvement in maternal or child health outcomes in developed nations, neither routine testing nor routine iron supplementation is necessary in women at low risk of iron deficiency anemia.

Targeted iron supplementation at pregnant women in developing countries is more cost-effective than iron fortification in terms of saving lives at the least cost, although fortification may be more sustainable in the long run.[2]

■ Conclusions and Recommendations

In contrast to the developing countries where the prevalence of iron deficiency anemia is high, there is no scientific justification for the age-old practice in developed countries of routine supplementation of iron in pregnancy.[36] Furthermore, the practice carries theoretic risk and real costs. Routine iron supplementation/testing is advised only for pregnant women who are at increased risk of developing iron deficiency anemia (e.g., multiple-fetus pregnancy, recurrent pregnancies within a 2-year interval, low socioeconomic status, and pregnant adolescents). In the future, any endorsement for routine testing or treatment of pregnant women in developed countries must be based on a properly conducted randomized trial. In contrast, there are strong arguments for supporting a policy of targeting either iron supplements or fortification of food products at poor women and children, as these measures clearly have a beneficial effect of on maternal and child health in the developing world.[2]

What form of enhanced surveillance can be offered to women who have high hematocrits in pregnancy remains unclear. We suggest that if hemoglobin level is more than 13 g/L (8.1 mmol/L), the pregnancy should be considered at risk of an unfavorable outcome.

■ Summary

1 ■ What Is the Problem that Requires Screening?

Antepartum abnormalities of the maternal red blood cell mass.

a. *What is the incidence/prevalence of the target condition?*

Eight to forty percent of pregnant women are classified as having anemia. The reported prevalence of iron deficiency anemia among reproductive age women in developing countries approximates 60%. Apart from geographic variations, the wide range in prevalences likely reflects differences in the definition of anemia. Eight to ten percent of women have an elevated red blood cell count.

b. *What are the sequelae of the condition that are of interest in clinical medicine?*

In developing countries, moderate and severe anemias are associated with poor maternal and child health. In these countries, iron deficiency anemia is typically the result of poor nutrition, an underlying disorder, or both. However, in developed countries, there is little evidence that iron deficiency is an important health problem for women and their offspring. Polycythemia is indirectly associated with an increased risk of preeclampsia, intrauterine growth restriction, and preterm delivery.

2 ■ The Tests

a. *What is the purpose of the tests?*

To identify women antenatally with either pathologic anemia or polycythemia for the purpose of initiating therapy to reduce their risk of an adverse pregnancy outcome.

b. *What is the nature of the tests?*

The measurement of maternal red blood cell mass and/or iron stores.

Continued

c. *What are the implications of testing?*

   1. What does an abnormal test result mean?

      A hemoglobin value below 11 g/dL (6.8 mmol) suggests the presence of a pathologic iron deficiency anemia, particularly when associated with an abnormal MCV value (<70 fL). If anemia is associated with a low MCV, serum ferritin should be measured or iron replacement therapy instituted. Iron supplementation does have a beneficial effect on maternal hematologic indices in women with iron deficiency anemia. However, evidence about beneficial effects of iron supplementation on relevant birth outcomes is lacking.

      A high hemoglobin value (> 13 g/dL or 8.1 mmol/L) or a high hematocrit (> 40%) warrants increased maternal and fetal surveillance.

   2. What does a normal test result mean?

      Women with normal red blood cell mass and iron stores do not have anemia or polycythemia. A 3% to 5% decline is typical between the first measurement during the initial prenatal visit and the second measurement later in pregnancy.

      Routine iron supplementation is advocated in a number of countries. A reduction in the prevalence of anemia may also be achieved by targeting fortified food products at pregnant women and young children. It is argued that iron fortification of food products, such as flour or salts, will have a major impact on maternal and child health in developing countries. Iron supplements may cause unpleasant gastrointestinal symptoms. These are dose-related and usually occur at higher-than-recommended doses for iron supplementation. As a result, there are problems with therapy compliance.

d. *What is the cost of testing?*

   Considering the lack of an identifiable improvement in maternal or child health outcomes in developed nations, neither routine testing nor routine iron supplementation is necessary in women at low risk of iron deficiency anemia. For saving lives at least cost, targeted iron supplementation at pregnant women in developing countries is more cost-effective than iron fortification, although the latter is a more sustainable solution.

3 ■ Conclusions and Recommendations

There is no scientific justification for the age-old practice in developed countries of routine supplementation of iron in pregnancy, in contrast to the developing countries where the prevalence of iron deficiency anemia is high. The practice carries theoretic risk and real costs. Routine iron supplementation/testing is advised only for pregnant women who at increased risk of developing iron deficiency anemia (e.g., multiple pregnancies, recurrent pregnancies within a 2-year interval, low socioeconomic status, and pregnant adolescents). In developed countries, any endorsement for routine testing or treatment in the future should be based on a randomized controlled trial. There are adequate scientific data to conclude that either iron supplementation or food fortification is beneficial for pregnant women in the developing world.

References

1. Leeuw NKM de, Brunton L. Maternal hematologic changes, iron metabolism, and anaemias in pregnancy. In: Goodwin JW, Godden JO, Chance GH, eds., *Perinatal Medicine*. Baltimore: Williams & Williams, 1979: 425–447.
2. Hunt JM. Reversing productivity losses from iron deficiency: the economic case. *J Nutr* 2002;132:794S–801S.
3. Yip R. Centers for Diseases Control (CDC) Criteria for anaemia in children and childbearing-aged women. *MMWR Recomm Rep* 1989;38:400–404.
4. Mahomed K, Hytten F. Iron and folate supplementation in pregnancy. In: Chalmers I, Enkin M, Keirse M, eds. *Effective Care in Pregnancy and Childbirth*. Oxford: Oxford University Press, 1989:301–317.
5. Blankson ML, Goldenberg RL, Cutter G, et al. The relationship between maternal haematocrit and pregnancy outcome: black-white differences. *J Natl Med Assoc* 1993;85:130–134.
6. Scott DE, Pritchard JA. Anaemia in pregnancy. *Clin Perinata* 1974;1:491–506.
7. Cook JD. Clinical evaluation of iron deficiency. *Semin Hematol* 1982;19:6–18.
8. Griswold DM, Cavanagh D. Prematurity: the epidemiologic profile of the "high risk" mother. *Am J Obstet Gynecol* 1996;96:878–882.
9. Royston E, Armstrong S. *Preventing Maternal Deaths*. Geneva: World Health Organization, 1989.
10. Harrison KA. Anaemia, malaria and sickle cell disease. *Clin Obstet Gynaecol* 1982;9:445–477.
11. Crawley J. Reducing the burden of anemia in infants and young children in malaria-endemic countries of Africa: from evidence to action. *Am J Trop Hyg* 2004;71:25–34.
12. Garn SM, Keating MT, Falkner F. Hematological status and pregnancy outcomes. *Am J Clin Nutr* 1981;34:115–117.
13. Murphy JF, O'Riordan J, Newcombe RG, et al. Relation of haemoglobin levels in first and second trimesters to outcome of pregnancy. *Lancet* 1986;1:992–994.
14. Elwood PC. Evaluation of the clinical importance of anaemia. *Am J Clin Nutr* 1973;26:958–964.
15. Rios E, Lipschitz DA, Cook JD, et al. Relationship of maternal and iron stores as assessed by determination of plasma ferritin. *Pediatrics* 1975;55:694–699.
16. Sweet DG, Savage G, Tubman TRJ, et al. Study of maternal influences on fetal iron status at term using cord blood transferring receptors. *Arch Dis Child Fetal Neonatal Ed* 2001;84:F40–F43.

17. Colomer J, Colomer C, Gutierrez D, et al. Anaemia during pregnancy as a risk factor for infant iron deficiency: report from the Valencia Infant Anaemia Cohort (VIAC) study. *Paediatr Perinat Epidemiol* 1990;4:196–204.
18. Puolakka J, Jänne O, Vihko R. Evaluation by serum ferritin assay of the influence of maternal iron stores on the iron status of newborns and infants. *Acta Obstet Gynecol Scand Suppl* 1980;95:53–56.
19. Godfrey KM, Forrester T, Barker DJ. et al. Maternal nutritional status in pregnancy and blood pressure in childhood. *Br J Obstet Gynaecol* 1994;101:398–403.
20. Koller O, Sagen N, Ulstein M, et al. Fetal growth retardation associated with inadequate haemodilution in otherwise uncomplicated pregnancy. *Acta Obstet Gynecol Scand* 1979;58:9–13.
21. Koller O, Sandvei R, Sagen N. High haemoglobin levels during pregnancy and fetal risk. *Int J Gynaecol Obstet* 1980;18:53–56.
22. Koller O. The clinical significance of hemodilution during pregnancy. *Obstet Gynecol Surv* 1982;37:649–652.
23. Klebanoff MA, Shiono PH, Berendes HW, Rhoads GG. Facts and artefacts about anaemia and preterm delivery. *JAMA* 1989;262:511–515.
24. Lieberman E, Ryan KJ, Monson RR, et al. Association of maternal haematocrit with premature labor. *Am J Obst Gynaecol* 1988;159:107–114.
25. Mau A. Hemoglobin changes during pregnancy and growth disturbances in the neonate. *J Perinat Med* 1977;5:172–177.
26. Duvekot JJ, Cheriex EC, Pieters FAA, et al. Maternal volume homeostasis in early pregnancy in relation to fetal growth restriction. *Obstet Gynecol* 1995;85:361–367.
27. Mitchell MC, Lerner E. Maternal hematologic measures and pregnancy outcome. *J Am Diet Assoc* 1992;92:484–486.
28. Lipschitz DA, Cook JD, Finch CA. A clinical evaluation of serum ferritin as an index of iron stores. *N Engl J Med* 1974;290:1213–121
29. Pilon VA, Howanitz PJ, Howanitz JH, et al. Day-to-day variation in serum ferritin concentration in healthy subjects. *Clin Chem* 1981;27:78–82.
30. Romslo I, Haram K, Sagen N, et al. Iron requirement in normal pregnancy as assessed by serum ferritin, serum transferrin saturation and erythrocyte protoporphyrin determinations *Br J Obstet Gynaecol* 1983; 90:101–107.
31. Cuervo LG, Mahomed K. Treatment for iron deficiency anaemia in pregnancy: the Cochrane Database of Systematic Reviews 2001;2:CD003094.
32. Sloan NL, Jordan E, Winikoff B. Effects of iron supplementation on maternal hematologic status in pregnancy. *Am J Public Health* 2002;92:288–293.
33. Rasmussen KM. Is there a causal relationship between iron deficiency or iron-deficiency anemia and weight at birth, length of gestation and perinatal mortality? *J Nutr* 2001;131:590S–603S.
34. Cogswell ME, Parvanta I, Ickes L, et al. Iron supplementation during pregnancy, anemia, and birth weight: a randomized controlled trial. *Am J Clin Nutr* 2003;78:772–781.
35. Bentley DP. Iron metabolism and anaemia in pregnancy. *Clin Haematol* 1985;14:613–628.
36. Juarez-Vazquez J, Bonizzoni E, Scotti A. Iron plus folate is more effective than iron alone in the treatment of iron deficiency anaemia in pregnancy: a randomised, double blind clinical trial. *Br J Obstet Gynaecol* 2002;109:1009–1014.
37. Bayoumeu F, Subiran-Buisset C, Baka NE, et al. Iron therapy in iron deficiency anemia in pregnancy: intravenous route versus oral route. *Am J Obstet Gynecol* 2002;186:518–522.
38. Ogambode O. The relationship between hematocrit levels in gravidae and their newborns. *Int J Gynaecol Obstet* 1980;18:57–60.
39. US Preventive Services Task Force. Routine iron supplementation during pregnancy. *JAMA* 1993;270:2846–2854.
40. Markides M, Crowther CA, Gibson RA, et al. Efficacy and tolerability of low-dose iron supplements during pregnancy: a randomized controlled trial. *Am J Clin Nutr* 2003;78:145–153.
41. Beard JL. Effectiveness and strategies of iron supplementation during pregnancy. *Am J Clin Nutr* 2000;71:1288S–1294S.
42. Berkovitch M, Matsui D, Lamm SH, et al. Recent increases in numbers and risk of fatalities in young children ingesting iron preparations. *Vet Hum Toxicol* 1994;36:53–55.

43. Rytter E, Forde R, Andrew M, et al. Graviditet og jerntilskudd-blir de offisielle retningslinjene fulgt? *Tidsskrift for den Norske Laegeforening* 1993;113:2416–2419.
44. Barrett JF, Whittaker PG, Williams JG, et al. Absorption of non-haem iron from food during normal pregnancy. *BMJ* 1994;309:79–82.
45. Horn E. Iron and folate supplements during pregnancy: supplementing everyone treats those at risk and is cost effective. *BMJ* 1988;297:1325–1327.

4

Postpartum Assessment of Hemoglobin, Hematocrit, and Serum Ferritin

Christine Kirkpatrick

Sophie Alexander

■ What Is the Problem that Requires Screening?

Anemia secondary to either pregnancy or delivery that will delay the woman's recovery and potentially place her at increased risk of disease.

What is the incidence/prevalence of the target condition?

The frequency of iron deficiency anemia in postpartum women who were not iron supplemented is high. In one Danish study, 40% of women not supplemented with oral iron had a serum ferritin measurement below 20 µg/L and 4% had a hemoglobin level of less than 12.1 g/L (7.5 mmol/L). The corresponding frequencies in women who received iron were 16% and 0%, respectively.[1] These findings are in agreement with earlier observations.[2]

What are the sequelae of the condition that are of interest in clinical medicine?

Delayed recovery from pregnancy and health sequelae secondary to severe, untreated anemia. The estimated normal blood loss at delivery varies greatly. Mathie and Snodgrass[3] reported a blood loss between 5 mL and 1600 mL with a mean of 186 mL. Careful investigation using reliable laboratory techniques to actually measure blood loss reveals a mean blood loss at delivery of 339 mL.[4] Much of the loss represents excess red blood cell mass synthesized during pregnancy and need not be replaced. Nonetheless, the red blood cell loss constitutes a drain on iron stores, which are typically low in menstruating women. Iron loss via lactation is insignificant.[5]

Massive postpartum hemorrhage is a serious problem in both the developed and developing worlds.[6] In fact, hemorrhage, primarily postpartum, accounts for approximately 25% of maternal deaths globally.[7] Postpartum anemia secondary to iron deficiency and acute blood loss are intimately related. It is estimated that it takes the average woman approximately 1 year to recover her iron losses without supplementation. However, it remains unknown whether women who end their pregnancy with a serum ferritin below normal, or who suffer a modest blood loss anemia, are in worse health during the first year postpartum than women with normal values. Such information is crucial for the formulation of informed public health policy.

■ The Tests

To identify women with postpartum anemia for the purpose of initiating therapy to reduce their risk of an adverse health outcome.

What is the purpose of the tests?

The purpose of the tests is to estimate the severity of anemia secondary to blood loss at delivery and to evaluate the woman's iron stores.

What is the nature of the tests?

The tests are discussed in the previous chapter on antepartum screening. Internationally accepted criteria for abnormal hemoglobin, hematocrit, and mean corpuscular volume (MCV) levels in the puerperium have not been adopted, nor is there any agreement on the optimal day for postpartum testing. This is important because there is a 400 mL increase in plasma volume within 48 hours after delivery followed by a fall in plasma volume with hemoconcentration.[8] There is no practical way to assess and correct for plasma volume routinely. The measurement of serum ferritin to determine iron stores is not useful since ferritin rises during the first 2 to 4 days postpartum.[9] Moreover, serum ferritin levels may be normal in women who are mildly anemic because of iron release precipitated by the acute decline in red cell mass.[2,10]

What are the implications of testing?

What does an abnormal test result mean? An abnormal test means that the woman has a pathologic anemia. Anemia following blood loss during delivery and following postpartum hemorrhage is usually assessed by estimation of hemoglobin and hematocrit levels. This approach was challenged by Goodlin[11] who pointed out that the hematocrit is a poor index of blood loss, as women with hematocrit levels of less than 35% may actually have increased red cell masses. In addition, there are very few published data on criteria for iron supplementation of asymptomatic anemic women. As a result, there is no consensus on whom to treat. There is some evidence of favorable outcomes for treatment of postpartum anemia with erythropoietin. However, most of the available literature focuses on laboratory hematologic indices rather than clinical outcomes.[12]

There is also no consensus on when to transfuse the profoundly anemic woman postpartum. The literature is remarkable for the absence of carefully controlled trials that would permit definitive conclusions. A major factor associated with maternal death after obstetric hemorrhage is the underestimation of total blood loss and, subsequently, inadequate volume replacement. An accurate assessment of blood loss is an important guide to management of postpartum hemorrhage. Certainly, massive hemorrhage associated with hypoperfusion requires immediate blood replacement with blood components, whole blood, or blood volume expanders adequate to restore and maintain adequate perfusion of vital organs. In healthy individuals, cardiac output does not increase dramatically until the hemoglobin level decreases to approximately 7.0 g/dL (4.3 mmol/L). The same conclusion probably applies to women with a hemorrhage large enough to produce postural hypotension. It is essential to recognize that the combination of hypovolemia and anemia may lead to mortality or severe maternal morbidity due to insufficient tissue oxygenation. Sheehan's syndrome (i.e., hypopituitarism following ischemia and infarction of the pituitary gland) is a rare but well-known late complication of obstetric hemorrhage. The potential benefits of maternal transfusion should be balanced against the potential risks of adverse outcome, including red cell alloimmunization and chronic viral infection. Usually the amount of blood replaced does not completely restore the hemoglobin deficit after hemorrhage. Once dangerous hypovolemia has been treated and hemostasis achieved, however, any residual anemia can be treated by oral iron supplementation. Transfusion is not normally indicated in hemodynamically stable postpartum women with moderate anemia (e.g., hemoglobin levels from 7 to 10 g/dL [4.3 to 6.2 mmol/L]). Oral iron therapy for at least 3 months should restore the lost iron.[12,13]

What does a normal test result mean? Postpartum women with normal red cell masses need no further evaluation. Because most women who breast feed do not menstruate, dietary iron is usually sufficient to meet daily iron requirements.[15]

What is the cost of testing?

The costs of these tests are discussed in the previous chapter on antepartum screening. There is inadequate information to allow a cost-benefit analysis for the practice of routine postpartum screening. Because there are no known sequelae of asymptomatic postpartum anemia, however, such expenditure is not likely to be necessary.

■ Conclusions and Recommendations

Blood loss at delivery can be considerable. Postpartum hemorrhage may lead to maternal death or severe maternal morbidity. No single laboratory test currently available can replace sound clinical judgment as the basis for the optimal management of excessive blood loss during the postpartum period.

There is no rationale in the developed world for the widespread practice of routinely prescribing postpartum iron. This is true for lactating and nonlactating women. The estimated iron loss from lactation is about 1 mg/day.[16] On empirical grounds, iron supplementation is reasonable if the hemoglobin level is less than 10 g/dL (6.2 mmol/L) 4 days postpartum and/or the MCV is abnormal (<70 fL), the diet is deficient of iron-containing foods, pregnancy within 1 year is likely, or the woman will breast feed for more than 6 months.

■ Summary

1 ■ What Is the Problem that Requires Screening?

Anemia secondary to either pregnancy or delivery that will delay the woman's recovery and potentially place her at increased risk of disease.

a. What is the incidence/prevalence of the target condition?

The frequency of iron deficiency anemia postpartum is high in particular in women who were not given iron supplementation during pregnancy. In one study, 40% of women who did not receive supplements had a serum ferritin below 20 µg/L and 4% had a hemoglobin level of less than 12.1 g/L (7.5 mmol/L). The corresponding frequencies in women who received iron supplements were 16% and 0%, respectively.

b. What are the sequelae of the condition that are of interest in clinical medicine?

Delayed recovery from pregnancy and health sequelae secondary to severe, untreated anemia or excessive blood loss. It remains unknown whether women with moderate blood loss postpartum have longterm health sequelae.

2 ■ The Tests

a. What is the purpose of the tests?

The purpose of the tests is to estimate the severity of anemia secondary to blood loss at delivery and to evaluate the woman's depletion of iron stores.

b. What is the nature of the tests?

The measurement of maternal red blood cell mass and/or iron stores.

Continued

■ **Summary—cont'd**

c. *What are the implications of testing?*
   1. What does an abnormal test result mean?
      An abnormal test means that the woman has a pathologic anemia and therapy is indicated. There is some evidence of favorable outcomes for treatment of postpartum anemia with erythropoietin. However, the clinical usefulness of erythropoietin therapy for postpartum anemia is questionable. There is also no consensus on when to transfuse the profoundly anemic woman postpartum.
   2. What does a normal test result mean?
      Postpartum women with normal red cell mass need no further evaluation if they are hemodynamically stable.

d. *What is the cost of testing?*
   There is inadequate information to allow a cost-benefit analysis for the practice of routine postpartum screening. Because there are no known sequelae of asymptomatic postpartum anemia, however, such expenditure is not likely to be necessary.

3 ■ Conclusions and Recommendations

No single laboratory test can replace sound judgement as the basis for the optimal management of excessive postpartum blood loss.

References

1. Milman N, Agger AO, Nielsen OJ. Iron supplementation during pregnancy. *Dan Med Bull* 1991;38:471–476.
2. Taylor DJ, Mallen C, Mc Dougall N, et al. Effect of iron supplementation on serum ferritin levels during and after pregnancy. *Br J Obstet Gynaecol* 1982;89:1011–1017.
3. Mathie IK, Snodgrass CA. The effect of prophylactic oxytocic drugs on blood loss after delivery. *J Obstet Gynaecol Br Commonw* 1967;74:653–662.
4. Newton M, Mosey LM, Egli GE, et al. Blood loss during and immediately after delivery. *Obstet Gynecol* 1961;17:9–18.
5. Underwood EJ. *Trace Elements in Human and Animal Nutrition,* 4th edition. New York: Academic Press, 1977:23.
6. Duthie SJ, Ven D, Yung GLK, et al. Discrepancy between laboratory determination and visual estimation of blood loss during normal delivery. *Eur J Obstet Gynecol Reprod Biol* 1990;38: 119–124.
7. Tsu VD, Langer A, Aldrich T. Postpartum hemorrhage in developing countries: is the public health community using the right tools? *Int J Gynaecol Obstet* 2004;85:S42–51.

8. Dewhurst CJ. *Integrated Obstetrics and Gynaecology for Postgraduates,* 2nd edition. Oxford: Blackwell Scientific Publications, 1976:316–339.

9. Haram K, Sandberg S, Ulstein M. High serum ferritin postpartum: an acute phase reaction. *Acta Obstet Gynecol Scand* 1993;72:50–51.

10. Puolakka J, Jänna O, Vihko J. Evaluation by serum ferritin assay on the influence of maternal iron stores on the iron status of newborns and infants. *Acta Obstet Gynecol Scand Suppl* 1980;95:53–56.

11. Goodlin RC. Need for plasma volume estimation. *Am J Obstet Gynecol* 1990;162:601.

12. Dodd J, Dare M, Middleton P. Treatment for women with postpartum iron deficiency anemia. Cochrane Database of Systematic Reviews 2004;CD 004222.

13. Cunningham FG, Mac Donald PC, Gant NF, et al. Hematologic disorders. In: Appleton & Lange, eds., *Williams Obstetrics,* 19th edition. Upper Saddle River, NJ: Prentice Hall International, 1993; pp.1171–1199.

14. Inglie S, Stevens L, Udom-Rice I, et al. Is observation of severe acute anemia in women safe? *Am J Obstet Gynecol* 1995;172:290.

15. Leeuw NKM de, Brunton L. Maternal hematologic changes, iron metabolism, and anemias in pregnancy. In: Goodwin JW, Godden JO, Chance GH, eds., *Perinatal Medicine.* Baltimore: Williams & Williams, 1976:425–447.

16. Fairbanks VF. Is the peripheral blood film reliable for the diagnosis of iron deficiency anaemia? *Am J Clin Pathol* 1971;55:447–451.

5

Asymptomatic Bacteriuria in Pregnancy

Francis S. Nuthalapaty

Dwight J. Rouse

■ What Is the Problem that Requires Screening?

Asymptomatic bacteriuria, which may lead to symptomatic upper and/or lower urinary tract infection, preterm birth, or both.

What is the incidence/prevalence of the target condition?

Asymptomatic bacteriuria is defined as more than 100,000 bacteria per milliliter of urine in an individual without symptoms of urinary tract infection.[1] The condition is present in 2% to 10% of women at their first antenatal visit.[2,3] Pregnancy does not predispose to acquisition of asymptomatic bacteriuria, as only 1% of initially screen-negative pregnant women develop asymptomatic bacteriuria subsequently.[4,5] The likelihood of asymptomatic bacteriuria varies inversely with socioeconomic status and directly with age[6] and certain maternal conditions such as sickle cell trait and diabetes mellitus.[7,8,9]

What are the sequelae of the condition that are of interest in clinical medicine?

Asymptomatic bacteriuria in healthy nongravid women poses little or no significant health risk.[10] However, 30% of gravid women with untreated asymptomatic bacteriuria develop symptomatic urinary tract infection.[2] This increased risk may be due to the physiologic obstruction of urine flow and stasis that occurs during pregnancy.[11] Many of these acute infections are classified as pyelonephritis on the basis of fever, costovertebral tenderness, and pyuria. Conversely, only 0.2% to 2.0% of gravidas who are screened early in gestation and found not to have bacteriuria will subsequently develop symptomatic urinary tract infection during pregnancy.[3,12] Pyelonephritis can be life-threatening during pregnancy: both adult respiratory distress syndrome and septic shock can occur.[13,14] Asymptomatic bacteriuria is also associated with an increased risk of preterm delivery or low birth weight.[7,15,16]

■ The Tests

What is the purpose of the tests?

To identify women with asymptomatic bacteriuria because they are at high risk of symptomatic urinary tract infection during pregnancy.

What is the nature of the tests?

Urine culture remains the standard for detection of asymptomatic bacteriuria against which all other tests are judged. As originally defined, two consecutive clean-voided urine specimens with more than 100,000 bacteria per milliliter of the same organism, or one specimen with more than 100,000 bacteria per milliliter obtained by catheterization were required to diagnose asymptomatic bacteriuria.[17,18] Subsequent studies used one clean-voided specimen with more than 100,000 bacteria per milliliter for diagnosis.[12] To decrease the cost and shorten the time required for screening, other tests have been evaluated. These include urinalysis, urine dipstick studies for leukocyte esterase and/or nitrites, and Gram staining. Table 5–1 (adapted from Bachman et al.[12]) summarizes the results of a comprehensive evaluation of screening methods for asymptomatic bacteriuria of pregnancy.

The optimal time to screen for asymptomatic bacteriuria is unknown but because the risks of asymptomatic bacteriuria progression to symptomatic infection are continuous throughout pregnancy, it is reasonable to conclude that screening should be accomplished as early in gestation as possible.

What are the implications of testing?

The sensitivities and specificities in Table 5–1 are, for the most part, in accordance with the results from multiple previous investigations.[10] However, better results are reported for combined leukocyte esterase and nitrite testing in pregnancy. Defining a positive result as one where either test is positive, sensitivity and specificity for asymptomatic bacteriuria were 92% and 95% respectively, in one investigation[19] and 73% and 86%, respectively, in another.[20]

What does an abnormal test result mean? A positive urine culture or one combination of the tests listed in Table 5–1 suggests the woman has asymptomatic bacteriuria. The bacterial pathogens responsible for asymptomatic bacteriuria during pregnancy are similar to those that most commonly cause cystitis and pyelonephritis in the general population, the most common being *Escherichia coli*.[21] A meta-analysis of 14 randomized clinical trials comparing antibiotic treatment with placebo or no treatment in pregnant women with asymptomatic bacteriuria concluded that antenatal screening followed by antibiotic treatment effectively reduced the incidence of pyelonephritis (odds ratio [OR] 0.24; 95% confidence interval [CI], 0.19–0.32) and the incidence of preterm delivery or low birth weight (OR, 0.60; 95% CI, 0.45–0.80).[16]

Table 5–1   Test results of urine samples obtained on initial visit from 1,047 pregnant women*

Test	No. positive samples	No. positive by culture	Sensitivity (%)	Specificity (%)	PPV (%)
Urine dipstick					
Leukocyte esterase activity	33	4	16.7	97.2	12.1
Nitrites present	14	11	45.8	99.7	78.6
Leukocyte activity or nitrites present	44	12	50.0	96.9	27.3
Leukocytes and nitrites present	3	3	12.5	100	100
Gram stain					
Borderline or positive	133	22	91.7	89.2	16.5
Positive	72	20	83.3	94.9	27.8
Urinalysis					
> 10 leukocytes	16	6	25.0	99.0	37.5
> 50 leukocytes	5	2	8.3	99.7	40.0
Bacteria present	432	18	75.0	59.7	4.2
Bacteria present or leukocytes > 20	440	20	83.3	58.9	4.5
Urine culture positive	24	24			

* Of 1047 pregnant women, 24 were diagnosed with asymptomatic bacteriuria by urine culture.
PPV, positive predictive value

Numerous antimicrobial agents and varying durations of therapy can be used to treat asymptomatic bacteriuria in pregnancy. Several effective regimens are described in Table 5–2. Short-course therapy (either 3 or 7 to 10 days) appears more effective than single-dose therapy in eradicating bacteriuria in nonpregnant and pregnant women.[22] Follow-up urine culture and repeat treatment are recommended if the bacteriuria persists.[7,23] Approximately one third of women with asymptomatic bacteriuria will experience recurrent infection during pregnancy. Continuous antibiotic suppression is recommended after treatment of a recurrence.

What does a normal test result mean? Only 0.2% to 2.0% of gravidas develop a symptomatic urinary tract infection during pregnancy after a negative culture for asymptomatic bacteriuria.[3,12] No follow-up urine screening is recommended. However, gravidas screened only by nonculture methods have higher rates of symptomatic urinary tract infection as a result of lower test sensitivity. The optimal follow-up of women screened for asymptomatic bacteriuria by nonculture methods has not been established.

What is the cost of testing?

The cost-effectiveness of asymptomatic bacteriuria screening during pregnancy has been comprehensively evaluated. Bachman et al.[12] analyzed four asymptomatic bacteriuria detection techniques using the following cost estimates (US$, 1993):

- Dipstick: $1
- Gram stain: $15
- Urinalysis: $15
- Urine culture: $25

These investigators assumed a urine culture would be performed for each positive screen. Assuming only one screening test is used, these investigators

Table 5–2	**Antimicrobial agents used to treat asymptomatic bacteriuria in pregnancy**	
3- to 7 Day Course of Therapy		
Nitrofurantoin	100 mg PO qid	
Amoxicillin	250 mg PO tid	
Sulfisoxazole	500 mg PO qid	
Trimethoprim/sulfamethoxazole	320/100 mg PO	
Single-dose therapy		
Nitrofurantoin	200 mg PO	
Amoxicillin	3 g PO	
Cephalexin	3 g PO	
Sulfisoxazole	2 g PO	
Prophylaxis		
Nitrofurantoin macrocrystals	100 mg PO qhs	

concluded that testing for nitrites was the single most cost-effective approach ($127 per case of asymptomatic bacteriuria detected). However, more than half of the cases of asymptomatic bacteriuria would be missed by using only measuring nitrites.

Wadland and Plante[24] and Rouse et al.[25] conducted cost-benefit analyses of screening and immediate treatment for asymptomatic bacteriuria in pregnancy using decision analysis models. Rouse et al.[25] found that no screening resulted in 23 cases of pyelonephritis per 1,000 pregnancies versus 16 cases with a leukocyte esterase-nitrite dipstick strategy and 11 with a culture strategy. Wadland and Plante[24] considered a culture-based strategy alone and concluded that screening and treatment for asymptomatic bacteriuria resulted in a cost savings of $28.85 (1989) per patient screened as compared with no screening. Noting that leukocyte-esterase and nitrite testing was previously shown[12] to be a more cost-effective approach to asymptomatic bacteriuria detection as compared with culture, Rouse et al.[25] directly compared the cost-effectiveness of these two screening strategies with immediate treatment for the prevention of pyelonephritis. They concluded both the dipstick and culture strategies were cost-effective for the prevention of pyelonephritis compared with no screening. The culture-based strategy resulted in a cost of $3,492 (1995) to prevent each additional case of pyelonephritis not prevented by dipstick, compared with an estimated cost of treatment per case of polynephritis of $2,485 (US). Therefore, the culture strategy was not cost-beneficial compared to the dipstick strategy.

■ Conclusions and Recommendations

Two to ten percent of pregnant women have asymptomatic bacteriuria; 30% of these women will develop acute and often serious urinary tract infection in pregnancy. The diagnosis and treatment of asymptomatic bacteriuria by any of the aforementioned methods prevent the progression of asymptomatic bacteriuria to symptomatic infection and is cost saving. Therefore, all pregnant women should be screened for asymptomatic bacteriuria at their first antenatal visit. Screening can be accomplished in a cost-effective manner by culture or with dipstick testing for leukocyte esterase and nitrites (with the presence of either substance defining a positive test). Individual practice situations will influence the optimal method of screening.

Women with a positive screen result should be treated with a short course of oral antibiotic therapy with activity against E. coli. After completion of therapy, the urine should be reassessed to document cure. Finally, certain gravidas at high risk of urinary tract infection (e.g., those with insulin-dependent diabetes mellitus, sickle cell trait, nephrolithiasis, a history of frequent urinary tract infections or a known urinary tract abnormality) may benefit from periodic screening for asymptomatic bacteriuria throughout their pregnancy, although the optimal timing and frequency of assessment have not been established by controlled investigations.

■ Summary

1 ■ **What Is the Problem that Requires Screening?**

Asymptomatic bacteriuria.

a. What is the incidence/prevalence of the target condition?
Two to ten percent of women at their first antenatal visit.

b. What are the sequelae of the condition that are of interest in clinical medicine?
Thirty percent of gravid women with untreated asymptomatic bacteriuria develop symptoms. Only 0.2% to 2.0% of women who are screened early in gestation and found not to have bacteria will subsequently develop symptomatic urinary tract infection during pregnancy. Asymptomatic bacteriuria is associated with an increased risk of preterm birth, but whether it plays a causative role is controversial.

2 ■ **The Tests**

a. What is the purpose of the tests?
To identify women with asymptomatic bacteriuria during pregnancy.

b. What is the nature of the tests?
Urine culture remains the standard against which all other tests are judged. Other tests that have been evaluated include urinalysis, urine dipstick studies for leukocyte esterase and or nitrites, and Gram staining.

c. What are the implications of testing?
1. What does an abnormal test result mean?
Either a positive urine culture of a combination of tests (Table 5–1) suggests the woman has asymptomatic bacteriuria. A 7-day course of oral antibiotics will sterilize the urine 65% to 90% of patients and prevent 80% of the cases of pyelonephritis.
2. What does a normal test result mean?
Only 0.2% to 2.0% of gravidas develop a symptomatic urinary tract infection during pregnancy after a negative culture for asymptomatic bacteriuria.

Continued

■ **Summary—cont'd**

c. *What is the cost of testing?*
Most screening modalities are predicted to be cost-beneficial in terms of preventing pyelonephritis.

3 ■ Conclusions and Recommendations

From 2% to 10% of pregnant women have asymptomatic bacteriuria; 30% of these will develop acute and often serious urinary tract infection in pregnancy. The diagnosis and treatment of asymptomatic bacteriuria by any of the methods listed prevents the development of symptomatic infection and is cost saving. All pregnant women should be screened for asymptomatic bacteriuria at their first antenatal visit.

References

1. Kass EH. Bacteriuria and the diagnosis of infection of the urinary tract. *Arch Intern Med* 1957;100:709–714.
2. Whalley PJ. Bacteriuria of pregnancy. *J Obstet Gynecol* 1967;97:723–738.
3. Norden CW, Kass EH. Bacteriuria of pregnancy—a critical appraisal. *M Rev Med* 1968;19:431–470.
4. Savage WE, Hajj SN, Kass EH. Demographic and prognostic characteristics of bacteriuria in pregnancy. *Medicine* 1967;46:385–407.
5. Stenqvist K, Dhalen-Nilsson I, Lidin-Janson G, et al. Bacteriuria in pregnancy: frequency and risk of acquisition. *Am J Epidemiol* 1989;129:372–379.
6. Foxman B. Epidemiology of urinary tract infections: incidence, morbidity, and economic costs. *Am J Med* 2002;113:5S–13S.
7. Androile VT, Patterson TF. Epidemiology, natural history, and management of urinary tract infections in pregnancy. *Med Clin North Am* 1991;75:359–373.
8. Zhanel GG, Harding GKM, Nicolle LE. Asymptomatic bacteriuria in patients with diabetes mellitus. *Rev Infect Dis* 1991;3:150–154.
9. Pastore LM, Savitz DA, Thorp JM Jr: Predictors of urinary tract infections at the first prenatal visit. *Epidem* 1999;10:282–287.
10. Pels RJ, Bor DH, Wolhandler S, et al. Dipstick urinalysis screening of asymptomatic adults for urinary tract disorders. *JAMA* 1989;262:1220–1224.
11. Lindheimer MD, Katz AI. The kidney in pregnancy. *N Engl J Med* 1970;183:1095–1097.
12. Bachman JW, Heise RH, Nassems JM, et al. A study of various tests to detect asymptomatic urinary tract infections in an obstetric population. *JAMA* 1993;270:1971–1974.
13. Cunningham FG, Leveno KJ, Hankins GDV, et al. Respiratory insufficiency associated with pyelonephritis during pregnancy. *Obstet Gynecol* 1984;63:121–125.
14. Hankins GDV, Whalley PJ. Acute urinary tract infections in pregnancy. *Clin Obset Gynecol* 1985;28:266–278.
15. Romero R, Oyarzun E, Mazor M, et al. Meta-analysis of the relationship between asymptomatic bacteriuria and preterm delivery/low birth weight. *Obstet Gynecol* 1989;73:576–582.

16. Smaill F. Antibiotics for asymptomatic bacteriuria in pregnancy. Cochrane Pregnancy and Childbirth Group. Cochrane Database of Systematic Reviews, 2004:2.
17. Kass EH. Pyelonephritis and bacteriuria: a major problem in preventive medicine. *Ann Int Med* 1962;56:46–53.
18. Kass EH. Maternal urinary tract infection. *N Y State J Med* 1962;62:2822–2826.
19. Robertson AW, Duff P. Nitrite and leukocyte esterace tests for the evaluation of asymptomatic bacteriuria in obstetric patients. *Obstet Gynecol* 1988;71:878–881.
20. Etherington IJ, James DK. Reagent strip testing of antenatal urine specimens for infection. *Br J Obstet Gynaecol* 1993;100:806–808.
21. Millar LK, Cox SM. Urinary tract infections complicating pregnancy. *Infect Dis Clin North Am* 1997;11:13–26.
22. Patterson TF, Andriole VT. Detection, significance, and therapy of bacteriuria in pregnancy. *Infect Dis Clin North Am* 1997;11:593–608.
23. Gordon MC, Hankins GDV. Urinary tract infections and pregnancy. *Comp Ther* 1989;15:52–58.
24. Wadland WC, Plante DA. Screening for asymptomatic bacteriuria in pregnancy. *J Fam Pract* 1989;29:372–376.
25. Rouse DJ, Andrews WW, Goldenberg RL, et al. Screening and treatment of asymptomatic bacteriuria of pregnancy to prevent pyelonephritis: a cost-effectiveness and cost-benefit analysis. *Obstet Gynecol* 1995;86:119–123.

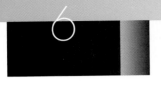
Neonatal Group B Streptococcal Disease

Walter Foulon

Anne Naessens

■ What Is the Problem that Requires Screening?

Neonatal group B streptococcal disease

What is the incidence/prevalence of the target condition?

Group B streptococcus (GBS) colonizes the gastrointestinal or genital tract in 15% to 30% of pregnant women and is transmitted to 40% to 70% of their infants[1] (Table 6–1). Colonization with GBS is often intermittent.[2] Fewer than 1% of the neonates of GBS carriers are affected with early-onset GBS sepsis absent peripartal antibiotic treatment.

GBS is transmitted vertically into the amniotic fluid during labor and is then aspirated by the fetus or acquired during passage through the birth canal. Early-onset GBS infection of the neonate is defined as a GBS sepsis within 7 days of birth, and the prevalence of early-onset GBS infection depends on the colonization rate. Without intervention, the microorganism causes early-onset septicemia in 1–2 per 1,000 live births in the United States[3] and 0.5 per 1,000 live births in the United Kingdom.[4] Several risk factors are associated with the occurrence of early-onset GBS disease: gestational age less than 37 completed weeks, prolonged rupture of the membranes (18 hours or more), heavy maternal colonization, intrapartum temperature of 38°C (100.4°F), previous infant with invasive GBS disease, and GBS bacteriuria during this pregnancy.[5]

What are the sequelae of the condition that are of interest in clinical medicine?

Early-onset GBS is recognized as the most serious newborn infection causing fulminant septicemia, pneumonia, meningitis, and shock. The most (about 90%) occurs within hours of delivery, demonstrating that the infection is acquired prior to birth.[1] The clinical picture of early-onset GBS is often characterized by rapid clinical deterioration. The fatality rate among neonates with

Table 6-1	**Public health consequences of maternal group B streptococcal (GBS) infection**		
Number		**Probability**[a]	**Range**[b]
1000	Pregnant women		
200	GBS colonized women	0.20	0.15–0.30
100	Vertical transmission	0.50	0.40–0.75
2	Neonatal GBS infection	0.02	0.01–0.02

[a]Crude estimates.
[b]See text.

early-onset GBS approximates 10% to 15% despite appropriate therapy. Those who survive may suffer long-term visual, hearing, or cognitive impairment.

Preterm infants constitute up to 30% of GBS deaths. Term babies also develop early-onset GBS, and though their individual risk is ten times lower than that of preterm infants, they are numerically important because of their large number.[5]

■ The Tests

What is the purpose of the tests?

To identify pregnant women colonized with GBS.

What is the nature of the tests?

All strategies aimed at decreasing early-onset GBS infection are based on the selection of women for intrapartum antibiotic treatment. Because women colonized with GBS have no symptoms of disease, the standard test for GBS colonization consists of culturing a combined vaginal and anal swab on a selective medium. Although such cultures are the standard, their clinical use is somewhat limited by the 24 to 48 hours required for a definite result. Gram stain of a vaginal smear is insensitive. The rapid antigen detection tests also have poor sensitivity (15% to 30%).[6,7] Therefore, more rapid, sensitive, and easy-to-use diagnostic tests for GBS have been developed and studied. Some polymerase chain reaction (PCR) assays meet these requirements.[8] If these tests perform equally well in routine practice, they might replace the classical culture. Intrapartum screening with these tests would eliminate the need for empirical antibiotic prophylaxis and reserve treatment for women and infants who actually need it.

The site for GBS culture is an important aspect of delineating the pregnancies at risk for developing early-onset GBS. Culture specimens should be collected from both the maternal vagina and the rectum. If only vaginal swabs are collected, up to 39% of the women colonized with GBS may be missed.[8]

Vaginal and rectal swabs are taken between 35 and 37 weeks' gestation for the most accurate prediction of colonization status at delivery. Yancey et al.[9] found that 87% of women with positive cultures within 6 weeks of delivery are still positive at delivery. However, Hager et al.[10] found a positive predictive value of only 67% for such cultures. As a result, some women at very low risk for developing early-onset GBS will receive unnecessary antibiotic agents during labor, whereas others with a negative culture for GBS at 35–37 weeks' gestation may become colonized at the moment of delivery.

What are the implications of testing?

Neonatal early-onset GBS disease may develop so rapidly that antibiotic therapy begun at birth is too late. Intrapartum antibiotics are effective in decreasing neonatal colonization and early-onset GBS disease.[11,12]

There are two strategies used. Each approach reduces the incidence of GBS disease, but not necessarily to the same degree. The first strategy is based on antenatal (35–37 weeks) vaginal and rectal culture for GBS and the treatment during labor of all women positive for GBS and for those for whom GBS status is unknown and the existence of at least one of the following risk factors: delivery at less than 37 weeks' gestation, amniotic membrane rupture after 18 hours or more of labor, and intrapartum temperature of 38°C (100.4°F). Pregnant women with GBS bacteriuria during the current pregnancy or those who have had a prior infant with invasive GBS disease are also considered at high risk and should receive intrapartum chemoprophylaxis.[13,14]

The second strategy is to restrict treatment to pregnancies with at least one of the following risk factors: preterm delivery, preterm rupture of membranes, intrapartum fever of 38°C (100.4°F), prolonged rupture of membranes (18 hours), a prior child with neonatal GBS disease, or GBS bacteriuria in the current pregnancy.[15]

The two strategies have not been compared directly in a clinical trial because of the large sample size required. On the basis of the analysis of different cohort studies, the Centers for Disease Control and Prevention (CDC) in the United States concluded that the screening approach was at least 50% more effective at preventing neonatal GBS disease than the risk-based approach.[13] This conclusion was supported by the results of a retrospective cohort study in which GBS sepsis was significantly lower in the screening group (0.33/1,000 births) compared with the group managed on the basis of risk factors (0.59/1,000 births; relative risk [RR], 0.48; 95% confidence interval [CI], 0.37–0.63).[16]

Conversely, antenatal screening and intrapartum chemoprophylaxis could have adverse effects based on the widespread use of antibiotic agents during labor and delivery. There is strong evidence that the increasing use of antibiotics is associated with an increase in the incidence of "other causes" of neonatal sepsis,[17] mainly gram-negative microorganisms.[18,19] Another concern is the risk of allergic reactions to antibiotic agents during labor. The risk of fatal anaphylaxis secondary to penicillin is estimated at one per 100,000.[14] Avoidance of "unnecessary" antibiotics might favor risk-based screening because it is estimated a strategy based on risk factors results in 18% of women receiving intrapartum antibiotics compared with the 27% for antenatal screening.[20] However, in the CDC review, intrapartum antibiotic use was similar for the two strategies (24%).[13] This may reflect a high incidence of risk factors in the United States, which cannot be generalized to other Western countries.

What does an abnormal test result mean? Women considered at risk of transmitting GBS to their neonate on the basis of either screening approach should receive intrapartum chemoprophylaxis. The recommended antibiotic agent is intravenous (IV) penicillin G 5 million units as a loading dose, and then 2.5 million units every 4 hours until delivery. For women who are allergic to penicillin, cefazolin 2 g IV as a loading dose, then 1 g every 8 hours can be given. Women at high risk for anaphylaxis should receive clindamycin 900 mg IV every 8 hours until delivery, or erythromycin 500 mg IV every 6 hours until delivery.

What does a normal test result mean? Pregnant women with vaginal and rectal cultures negative for GBS need not to be treated during labor because the likelihood of early-onset GBS is very low.

What is the cost of testing?

Mohle-Boetani et al.[21] examined how the cost of intervention varied with the incidence of early-onset GBS septicemia. The cost of introducing a strategy on the basis of risk factors exceeded the cost of disease until the incidence of early-onset GBS infection exceeded 0.6/1,000 live births. The cost of a strategy based on culture is greater than the cost of disease until the incidence of infection exceeds 1.2/1,000 live births. In such a classic cost-benefit analysis, costs of screening are balanced against the lifetime costs of caring for people with sequelae from early-onset GBS. The cost per case prevented for the risk-based strategy was estimated to be $3,067 compared with $11,925 for the antenatal culture screening–based strategy. The higher expense of universal screening methodology reflects the cost of the antenatal GBS cultures.

■ Conclusions and Recommendations

GBS is a commensal organism of the vagina and gastrointestinal tract. Ten to thirty percent of pregnant women are colonized with the microorganism. Vertical transmission from colonized mother to infant occurs in 40% to 75%. The incidence of early-onset GBS infection approximates 1% of colonized newborns.

The core recommendation for the prevention of early-onset GBS septicemia is the intrapartum use of IV penicillin G. Two strategies are used to identify which women should receive intrapartum chemoprophylaxis. The first is based on a rectovaginal GBS culture taken at 35 to 37 weeks' gestation with intrapartum antibiotics administered to all carriers. The second strategy recruits women on the basis of risk factors for early-onset GBS absent antenatal GBS cultures. These at risk women should receive the same antibiotic treatment as those who are known culture positive prior to labor. Considerable evidence exists that implementation of either guideline reduces but cannot eliminate the risk of early-onset GBS.

There is no consensus on the best approach to prevent early-onset GBS. The CDC and the American College of Obstetrics and Gynecology recommend the culture based screening policy, while other expert guidelines advocate peripartal antibiotic treatment based on the presence of well-defined risk factors. Whichever strategy is chosen, the most important determinant of effectiveness is compliance.

■ Summary

1 ■ What Is the Problem that Requires Screening?

Neonatal GBS disease.

a. *What is the incidence/prevalence of the target condition?*
GBS colonizes the gastrointestinal or genital tract in 15% to 30% of pregnant women and is transmitted to 40% to 70% of their infants. The prevalence of early-onset disease is less than 2/1,000.

b. *What are the sequelae of the condition that are of interest in clinical medicine?*
GBS infection can cause fulminate sepsis, pneumonia, meningitis, and shock. It is frequently accompanied by respiratory distress. The mortality is 10% to 15% despite appropriate antibiotic therapy. Surviving infants often develop long-term sequelae such as neurologic deficits.

2 ■ The Tests

a. *What is the purpose of the tests?*
To identify pregnant women colonized with GBS.

b. *What is the nature of the tests?*
The gold standard is culture of the vagina, cervix, and rectum at 35 to 37 weeks' gestation. The rapid antigen test has too low a sensitivity to be clinically useful.

c. *What are the implications of testing?*
   1. What does an abnormal test result mean?
      Maternal colonization indicates the need for either universal or targeted chemoprophylaxis.
   2. What does a normal test result mean?
      The women are at very low risk for having a child with GBS disease.

d. *What is the cost of testing?*
   Screening based on risk factors is cost beneficial when the likelihood of early-onset GBS exceeds 0.6/1,000, and a strategy based on routine culture is cost beneficial when the likelihood exceeds 1.2/1,000.

3 ■ Conclusions and Recommendations

Intrapartum chemoprophylaxis reduces the rates of both neonatal colonization and early-onset GBS. Unless the likelihood of disease is extremely low, either targeted or universal screening is recommended.

References

1. Backer CJ, Edwards MS. Group B streptococcal infections. In: Remington JS, Klein JO, eds. *Infectious Diseases of the Fetus and Newborn Infant*, 4th edition. Philadelphia: WB Saunders, 1995:880–1054.
2. Gilbert GL, Hewitt MC, Turner CM, et al. Epidemiology and predictive values of risk factors for neonatal group B streptococcal sepsis. *Aust N Z J Obstet Gynaecol* 2002;42:497–503.
3. McKenna DS, Jand JD. Group B streptococcal infections. *Sem Perinatol* 1998;22:267–276.
4. Heath PT, Balfour G, Weisner AM, and the PHLS Group B Streptococcus Working Group. Group B streptococcal disease in UK and Irish infants younger than 90 days. *Lancet* 2004;363:292–294.
5. Benitz W, Gould J, Druzin M. Risk factors for early-onset group B streptococcal sepsis: estimation of odds ratios by critical literature review. *Pediatrics* 1999;3:1–23.
6. Greenspoon JS, Fishman A, Wilcox JG, et al. Comparison of culture for group B streptococcus versus enzyme immunoassay and latex agglutination rapid tests: results in 250 patients during labor. *Obstet Gynecol* 1991;77:97–100.
7. Skoll MA, Mercer BM, Baselski V, et al. Evaluation of two rapid group B streptococcal antigen tests in labor and delivery patients. *Obstet Gynecol* 1991;77:322–326.
8. Bergeron MG, Ke D, Menard C, et al. Rapid detection of group B streptococci in pregnant women at delivery. *N Engl J Med* 2000;343:175–179.
9. Yancey MK, Schuchat A, Brown LK, et al. The accuracy of late antenatal screening cultures in predicting genital group B streptococcal colonization at delivery. *Obstet Gynecol* 1996;88:811–815.

10. Hager WD, Schuchat A, Gibbs R, et al. Prevention of perinatal group B streptococcal infection: current controversies. *Obstet Gynecol* 2000;96:141–145.

11. Yow MD, Mason EO, Leeds LJ, et al. Ampicillin prevents intrapartum transmission of group B streptococcus. *JAMA* 1979;241:1245–1247.

12. Schrag SJ, Zywicki S, Farley MM, et al. Group B streptococcal disease in the era of intrapartum antibiotic prophylaxis. *N Engl J Med* 2000;342:15–20.

13. Centers for disease-control and prevention of perinatal group B streptococcal disease. *MMWR Recomm Rep* 2002;51:1–24.

14. ACOG. Prevention of early-onset group B streptococcal disease in newborns. ACOG Committee Opinion, no. 279, 2002, 1405–1412.

15. Prevention of early-onset neonatal group B streptococcal disease. Royal College of Obstetricians and Gynaecologists. Guideline No. 2003:1–9.

16. Schrag SJ, Zell ER, Lynfield R, et al. A population-based comparison of strategies to prevent early-onset group B streptococcal disease in neonates. *N Engl J Med* 2002;347:233–239.

17. Rouse DJ, Goldenberg RL, Cliver SP, et al. Strategies for the prevention of early-onset neonatal group B streptococcal sepsis: a decision analysis. *Obstet Gynecol* 1994;83:483–494.

18. Towers CV, Carr MH, Padilla G, Asrat T. Potential consequences of widespread antepartum use of ampicillin. *Am J Obstet Gynecol* 1998;179:879–883.

19. Stoll BJ, Hanssen N, Fanaroff AA, et al. Changes in pathogens causing sepsis in very-low-birth-weight infants. *N Engl J Med* 2002;347:240–247.

20. O'Reilly GC, Hitte JE, Benedetti TJ. Group B streptococcus infection in pregnancy: an update. *Fetal Matern Med Rev* 1998;10:231–239.

21. Mohle-Boetani JC, Suchat A, Plikaytis BD, et al. Comparison of prevention strategies for neonatal group B streptococcal infection: a population-based economic analysis. *JAMA* 1993;270:1442–1448.

7

Rubella During Pregnancy

Walter Foulon

Anne Naessens

■ What Is the Problem that Requires Screening?

Congenital rubella infection

What is the incidence/prevalence of the target condition?

Only seronegative women are at risk because the fetus becomes infected during the maternal viremia associated with primary infection. There is a strong relationship between the gestation period at infection and the sequelae. Eighty-five percent of fetuses are infected when maternal infection occurs early (8 weeks); 50% to 55% of fetuses become infected in the period of 9 to 16 weeks (Table 7–1).[1]

Vaccination programs in Western countries have had a major impact on the epidemiology of rubella and the incidence of congenital rubella syndrome (CRS). The World Health Organization (WHO) recommends vaccination of children of both sexes and seronegative adult women. Restricting vaccination to the population at risk (i.e., teenage girls) reduces the prevalence of seronegative pregnant women from 20% to 5% and can decrease the likelihood of a large rubella epidemic to some extent.[2] However, it will not eliminate smaller outbreaks during which susceptible pregnant women can become infected.

There are great inequalities both between and within countries. Reports form Finland,[3] Denmark,[4] the United Kingdom,[5] France[6] and the United States[7] demonstrate that long-standing immunization programs have successfully interrupted domestic rubella transmission, and CRS is now rare. In Italy,[8] however, vaccination coverage remains suboptimal, and a high proportion of pregnant women (>5%) are susceptible. Not surprisingly, the rate of CRS in Southern Italy is 6/100,000 live births. The problem is greater in central and Eastern Europe where large epidemics still occur. A Romanian epidemic in 2002 to 2003 resulted in more than 115,000 reported cases nationwide and a rate of 531 CRS cases per 100,000 live births.[9] A 1993 epidemic of rubella in Greece[10] was followed by a CRS rate of 24.6/100,000. Moreover, a new phenomenon has occurred in some countries with the arrival of large numbers of nonimmunized people from other countries. Small outbreaks of rubella have been reported within these groups.[10]

Table 7-1	Public health consequences of maternal rubella infection		
Number		**Probability[a]**	**Range[b]**
300,000	Pregnant women	1.00	
30,000	Seronegative women	0.10	0.02–0.12
17	Maternal infection[c]	0.0006	?
10	Vertical transmission[d]	0.60	0.40–0.80
1	Congenital rubella syndrome at birth	0.10	0.00–0.10

[a]Crude estimates.
[b]See text.
[c]Maternal infection in ongoing pregnancy (no figures are currently available on the number of pregnancy terminations for maternal rubella infection).
[d]Dependent on the stage of pregnancy at which infection occurs.

In many countries, rubella vaccination is incorporated into the childhood vaccination schedule, allowing a growing number of countries to meet the WHO target for CRS prevention: less than one case of CRS per 100,000 live births. In light of the successful programs,[2] there is now an impetus to extend vaccination programs to the developing world. According to WHO, there are more than 100,000 cases of CRS every year in the developing world. It is encouraging that rubella vaccination has increased from 71 countries in 1996 to 123 in 2002.[11]

What are the sequelae of the condition that are of interest in clinical medicine?

Fetal damage reflects a combination of viral-induced cellular damage and its effect on dividing cells. As a result, the number of cells in most organs of infected offspring is lower than in healthy neonates. Severe sequelae such as cataracts, deafness, cardiac abnormalities, and neurologic damage are almost universal in fetuses infected prior to 12 weeks' gestation. Between 13 and 16 weeks, the risk of CRS declines to about 35%, and the sequelae are mostly deafness and to a lesser extent mild neurologic abnormalities.[12] Maternal infection after this period does not usually result in long-term defect.

■ The Tests

What is the purpose of the tests?

To detect pregnant women who are seronegative for rubella and thus at risk for primary infection.

What is the nature of the tests?

Enzyme immunoassays for immunoglobulin G (IgG) and IgM antibodies. The clinical diagnosis of an acute rubella infection is based on the presence of fever and malaise followed by a maculopapular rash. Arthralgia occurs in up to 60%. Rubella-like illnesses can also be induced by other viruses such as parvovirus B19 and human herpes virus 6. The clinical diagnosis of rubella is unreliable and laboratory confirmation is essential. In the past, rubella-specific IgG antibodies were detected using the hemagglutination test. This test has now been replaced by commercially available enzyme immunoassays for IgG and IgM antibodies. Typically, an IgG antibody level of 10 IU/mL is indicative of past immunity.

Recent rubella infection is diagnosed by the finding of rubella-specific IgM antibodies or by the detection of a rubella IgG seroconversion. Rubella IgM antibodies typically persist for 8 to 12 weeks, although low concentrations may be detectable for up to 6 months after a primary infection. Moreover, a positive IgM assay may be the result of a cross-reaction with other viral IgM antibodies. It is therefore important to confirm all positive IgM results with other methods and the testing of follow-up serum samples to distinguish an acute rubella infection from a residual IgM titer of a past infection.

What are the implications of testing?

What does an abnormal test result mean? If confirmed, the presence of maternal rubella-specific IgM antibodies in the mid-second trimester indicates first-trimester infection and the woman is at risk of delivering a child with CRS. She should be offered either pregnancy termination or antenatal diagnosis. Antenatal diagnosis is based on either a polymerase chain reaction (PCR) test to detect rubella-specific RNA in amniotic fluid and/or the detection of specific IgM antibodies in fetal blood.[13,14] There is a possibility of false-negative results if the invasive tests are performed less than 6 weeks after the maternal infection or before 21 weeks.[14]

IgG seronegative women should be retested between 16 and 20 weeks to detect a rubella infection in the critical period for development of a CRS.

What does a normal test result mean? The presence of rubella-specific IgG without IgM indicates immunity. No further investigation is required. Seronegative women should be vaccinated after delivery to protect subsequent pregnancies and to reduce the subject pool available for wild virus.

What is the cost of testing?

The 1994 cost for a single test for IgM and IgG antibodies in Belgium is estimated at $7. Perhaps more relevant is the patient cost, rather than the cost of the test itself. The 1994 patient cost in a large medical center in the United States for rubella-specific IgG is $32.50. If we assume all women register for care by 10 weeks' gestation (an unlikely event in many geographic areas), 90% of women are immune, and seronegative women are rescreened between 16 and 18 weeks' gestation, the cost per case of CRS identified is approximately $154,000 if the incidence is 1/4,300 pregnancies, or $10,725,000 if the incidence is 1/300,000. This excludes the cost of antenatal testing for diagnosis of fetal disease.

Most children with CRS require round-the-clock supervision and help for the rest of their lives. The annual cost per individual was estimated in 1985 to be at least $31,000.[9,15] This amount is likely tripled in 2005 adjusting for inflation. Furthermore, this cost does not include societal costs such as the loss of income and patient suffering. If we assume an average 50-year lifespan, CRS would add a minimum of $310,000 in excess medical costs.

Maternal screening for rubella is probably no longer cost-effective in many Western countries where the rate has dropped below 1/100,000 live births. However, the importance of maintaining high coverage with rubella vaccination of the seronegative susceptible population is important to control local outbreaks. Rubella screening during pregnancy should be regarded as part of a comprehensive CRS prevention strategy for the elimination of rubella in the population.

■ Conclusions and Recommendations

Congenital rubella is a preventable disease. Vaccination is effective, safe, and inexpensive. Maternal rubella has become rare in many countries that have adopted universal vaccination programs. However, CRS remains a major cause of severe handicap in some developing countries. The maternal–fetal transmission rate during the critical period for developing CRS of 1 to 16 weeks' gestation is high (>50%) and the consequences often devastating.

It is advisable to screen with IgG antibodies in early pregnancy in countries where rubella has been successfully controlled by universal vaccination policy. There is no need to include IgM antibodies in the screening test. Indeed, this avoids needless anxiety due to the presence of residual IgM antibodies in some patients because the risk of a rubella infection during pregnancy has become so rare. Seronegative women should be retested between 16 and 20 weeks' gestation to detect seroconversion. Those that remain seronegative should be vaccinated in the postpartum period.

In countries where CRS remains a problem, it is appropriate to continue screening for IgG and IgM rubella antibodies in early pregnancy. Women with positive IgM antibodies should be fully evaluated to exclude an acute rubella infection in the first 16 weeks of pregnancy.

■ Summary

1 ■ What Is the Problem that Requires Screening?

Congenital rubella syndrome (CRS).

a. What is the incidence/prevalence of the target condition?
1/5500 to 1/300,000 depending on the country's vaccination policy.

b. What are the sequelae of the condition that are of interest in clinical medicine?
Congenital rubella syndrome includes cataracts, deafness, cardiac abnormalities, and neurologic damage that occur in about 80% of infected fetuses.

2 ■ The Tests

a. What is the purpose of the tests?
To detect women at risk for rubella during early pregnancy.

b. What is the nature of the tests?
Measurement of rubella-specific IgG and IgM levels where appropriate.

c. What are the implications of testing?
1. What does an abnormal test result mean?
   Rubella-specific IgM indicates a recent infection. If infection occurs during the first 16 weeks' gestation, the woman is at risk of delivering a child with CRS and should be offered either antenatal diagnosis or pregnancy termination.
2. What does a normal test result mean?
   The presence of rubella-specific IgG without IgM indicates immunity. Persistently seronegative women should be vaccinated in the postpartum period.

Continued

■ **Summary—cont'd**

d. **What is the cost of testing?**

Assuming all women register for care by 10 weeks' gestation, 90% are immune, and seronegative women are rescreened between 16 and 18 weeks, the cost per case of CRS identified ranges from $154,000 (1/4,300 pregnancies) to $10 million (1/300,000 pregnancies), excluding the cost of antenatal testing.

3 ■ **Conclusions and Recommendations**

Congenital rubella is a preventable disease. Vaccination is effective, safe, and inexpensive. Maternal rubella-specific IgG and IgM antibodies if appropriate should be screened for during the first prenatal visit. Although congenital rubella is no longer considered a problem of high priority in developed countries, it is a major problem in less developed countries where vaccination programs are insufficient or nonexistent.

References

1. Centers for Disease Control and Prevention. Measles, mumps, and rubella vaccine use and strategies for elimination of measles, rubella, and congenital rubella syndrome and control of mumps. Recommendations of the Advisory Committee on Immunization Practices (ACIP). *MMWR Morb Mortal Wkly Rep* 1998;47:1–57.
2. Noah ND, Fowle SE. Immunity to rubella in women of childbearing age in the United Kingdom. *BMJ* 1988;297:1301–1304.
3. Davidkin I, Peltola H, Leinikki P. Epidemiology of rubella in Finland. *Euro Surveill* 2004;9:11–12.
4. Glismann S. Rubella in Denmark. *Euro Surveill* 2004;9:9–10.
5. Tookey P. Rubella in England, Scotland and Wales. *Euro Surveil* 2004;9:21–22.
6. Levy-Bruhl D, Six C, Parent I. Rubella control in France. *Euro Surveill* 2004; 9:13–4.
7. Centers for Disease Control and Prevention. Rubella and congenital rubella syndrome: United States, January 1, 1991–May 7, 1994. *MMWR Morb Mortal Wkly Rep* 1994;43:391–401.
8. Ciofi Degli Atti M, Filia A, et al. Rubella control in Italy. *Euro Surveill* 2004;9:17–18.
9. Rafila A, Marin M, Pistol A, et al. A large rubella outbreak, Romania: 2003. *Euro Surveill* 2004;9:7–8.
10. Lemos C, Ramirez R, Ordobas M, et al. New features of rubella in Spain: the evidence of an outbreak. *Euro Surveill* 2004;9:19–20.
11. Banatvala JE, Brown DWG. Rubella. *Lancet* 2004;363:1127–1137
12. Miller E, Cradock-Watson JE, Pollock TM. Consequences of confirmed maternal rubella at successive stages of pregnancy. *Lancet* 1982;2:781–784.
13. Enders G, Jonatha W. Prenatal diagnosis of intrauterine rubella. *Infection* 1987;15:162–164.
14. Revello MG, Baldanti F, Sarasini A, et al. Prenatal diagnosis of rubella virus infection by direct detection and semiquantitation of viral RNA in clinical samples by reverse transcription-PCR. *J Clin Microbiol* 1997;35:708–713.
15. Appel MW. The multihandicapped child with congenital rubella: impact on family and community. *Rev Infect Dis* 1985;7:17–21.

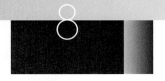

8

Congenital Toxoplasmosis

Walter Foulon

Anne Naessens

■ What Is the Problem that Requires Screening?

Congenital toxoplasma infection

What is the incidence/prevalence of the target condition?

The prevalence of toxoplasmosis acquired in pregnancy varies greatly according to geographic location. The estimated incidence in France and Belgium is 8/1,000[1,2] susceptible pregnancies; in Scotland 2 to 3 per 1,000[3] and 2/1,000 in Norway.[4] It is lower yet in the United States.

Apart from immune compromised women, seropositive women do not transmit the parasite to the fetus absent maternal immune compromise. Transplacental infection occurs after primary infection. The stage of pregnancy at which the maternal infection is acquired greatly impacts the transmission rate. It approximates 5% to 10% in the first trimester, 25% in the second trimester, and more than 50% in the third trimester.[5] The seroprevalence indicative of past infection varies considerably ranging from 3–30% in the US,[6,7] 13% in Norway,[8] 20% in Scotland,[3] 51% in Belgium,[9] and 54% in France.[1]

The parasite may be transmitted from mother to fetus when infection occurs during pregnancy. Rates of congenital infection with toxoplasmosis vary from 1/10,000 births in the Boston area,[10] 2/10,000 in Alabama,[11] Perth[12] (Australia), 70/10,000 in Brussels,[2] and between 70 and 10 per 10,000 in France.[1]

What are the sequelae of the condition that are of interest in clinical medicine?

Congenital toxoplasmosis causes marked morbidity in the children. The risk of sequelae is inversely related to gestation at the time of maternal infection. Early maternal infection can cause hydrocephalus, intracranial calcifications, and chorioretinitis. Other clinical manifestations include icterus, hepatosplenomegaly, and thrombocytopenia. These severe sequelae occur in less that 10% of cases, but nearly all of these children develop long-term neurologic and/or ophthalmologic sequelae (Table 8–1).[8]

Over 90% of congenitally infected infants are asymptomatic at birth. The risk of subclinical congenital toxoplasmosis should not be underestimated because 50% of these infants will develop chorioretinitis with vision impairment during adolescence if untreated.[8]

■ The Tests

What is the purpose of the tests?

To detect seronegative pregnant women at risk of primary infection during pregnancy.

What is the nature of the tests?

Toxoplasma infection can be detected by demonstration of specific immunoglobulin G (IgG) and IgM antibodies. If seroconversion is detected in serial blood samples, primary infection has occurred between the last negative and the first positive samples.

What are the implications of testing?

What does an abnormal test result mean? IgM antibodies appear first in the maternal plasma, as soon as 5 days after acute toxoplasma infection. Depending on the serological test used, IgM antibodies may persist for up to several years. In most instances of persistence, the levels are low, but in others they remain high.

IgG antibodies appear within a few weeks of infection, and, depending on the serological test used, may take 2 to 6 months to peak. In some women, high

Table 8–1	**Public health consequences of *Toxoplasma gondii* infection**		
Number		**Probability[a]**	**Range[b]**
10,000	Pregnant women	1.00	
5000	Seronegative women	0.50	0.30–0.97
200	Maternal infection	0.04	0.02–0.16
100	Vertical transmission[c,d]	0.50	0.15–0.80
10	Neonatal symptoms at birth	0.10	0.00–0.10
	Longterm sequelae in asymptomatic children:		
45	Chorioretinitis	0.50	?
18	Mental subnormality	0.20	?

[a]Crude estimates.
[b]See text.
[c]Dependent on the stage of pregnancy at which infection occurs.
[d]From: Klapper and Morris (1990).

levels of IgG antibodies may be detected years after acute infection. This makes the interpretation of serological data for toxoplasmosis difficult at times (e.g., when the sera at the beginning of pregnancy reveal high levels of IgG antibodies and/or the presence of IgM antibodies). The specific IgM antibody may have been present before the current pregnancy, and consequently the fetus is protected against infection. Supplementary tests are necessary to estimate whether the infection occurred during the current pregnancy or before. IgA and IgG avidity are frequently used. IgG avidity is low during the first phase of infection and increases over time. Although high avidity excludes a recent toxoplasma infection, a low avidity does not prove that the infection occurred within the last 20 weeks.[13]

Women without detectable toxoplasmosis antibodies are susceptible and should be instructed to adopt the following hygienic measures throughout gestation: Never eat raw or insufficiently cooked meat; avoid touching the mouth or eyes after handling raw meat, and always wash hands thoroughly; and avoid contact with cat feces (or possibly contaminated items by cat feces, e.g., during gardening). These measures should be fully explained in a leaflet and preferably reiterated mid gestation during antenatal classes. Applying this strategy, the incidence of toxoplasmosis seroconversion during pregnancy was reduced by 92%.[7]

The woman should be treated with antibiotics when the diagnosis of toxoplasmosis during pregnancy is confirmed (seroconversion in IgG antibodies). Desmonts and Couvreur[14] and Hohlfeld et al.[15] assert that the aim of antenatal treatment for toxoplasma infection during pregnancy is to prevent neurological or visual impairment in infected children by either preventing mother to child transmission, or after the fetal infection, by decreasing the severity of the disease. Spiramycin (3 g/d), a macrolide antibiotic, has been used extensively in Europe. Spiramycin concentrates in the placenta and is believed to reduce the incidence of congenitally infected infants from 61% to 23%.[14] However, a recent study failed to confirm the effect of antenatal spiramycin on the transmission rate, although there was a significant decrease in the sequelae in affected children (odds ratio [OR], 0.3; 95% confidence interval [CI], 0.1–0.9).[16]

All women at risk of delivering a congenitally infected child should be offered antenatal diagnosis. Amniocentesis is generally performed at around 20 weeks' gestation. The definite diagnosis of fetal infection relies on the isolation of the parasite from the amniotic fluid (mouse inoculation) (sensitivity 58%, specificity 98%) and on a polymerase chain reaction (PCR) test to detect toxoplasma DNA in amniotic fluid (sensitivity 81%, specificity 96%).[17] If fetal infection is diagnosed, pregnancy termination may be offered, especially if sonographic abnormalities such as hydrocephalus or brain necrosis are seen. When the ultrasound examination findings are normal and the parents wish to continue pregnancy, the women should receive pyrimethamine 25 mg/d combined with sulfadiazine 3 g/d and folinic acid 5 mg twice weekly. Most experts recommend alternating this treatment regime at 3-week intervals with spiramycin 3 g daily for the duration of pregnancy.

All infected children need specific therapy. The child considered uninfected on the basis of the results of the antenatal testing must be retested with serial blood samples until 11 months of age to exclude congenital toxoplasmosis.

What does a normal test result mean? Pregnant women with specific IgG antibodies and the absence of IgM antibodies in their first serum sample can be considered toxoplasma immune. There is no need to retest these women during pregnancy. Seronegative women should be retested around 20 and 30 weeks' gestation.

What is the cost of testing?

Using a hospital fee of $40 per specimen, it has been calculated that the initial screening of all pregnant women in the United States would cost $160 million.[18] If 70% of US women are seronegative, monthly titer assessment would cost $1 billion annually, exclusive of the costs for confirmatory testing, diagnostic evaluation, and treatment. This cost estimate is outdated for at least three reasons. First, the laboratory methodology has changed dramatically. The increased sensitivity and specificity of the enzyme-linked immunosorbent assays (ELISAs) coupled with the ability to automate testing reduces the cost of screening. Second, the monthly titer assessment of seronegative women as advocated originally is unnecessary. More recent approaches screen thrice (in the first trimester, between 16 and 20 weeks, and around 30 weeks). Third, the cost of antenatal diagnosis has decreased with the development of the PCR methodology.

It is difficult to quantify and compare the preventable costs of congenital toxoplasmosis with screening and costs of treatment. The preventable costs depend on the occurrence of congenital toxoplasmosis, which varies greatly from one country to another. Based on a serological screening program in Norway, retesting the seronegative population once in the second and once in the third trimester, Stray-Pedersen et al.[19] concluded that screening is of economic benefit when the incidence of maternal toxoplasmosis exceeds 10 to 15 per 10,000 pregnancies.

■ Conclusions and Recommendations

Congenital toxoplasmosis is a potentially preventable disease. Knowledge of the life cycle of the parasite allows physicians to focus on the prevention of toxoplasmosis. The mode of acquiring toxoplasmosis from meat, cat feces, and contaminated soil is so well circumscribed that very simple hygienic measures are extremely effective.

Primary prevention of toxoplasmosis should become standard obstetric care. In an area with a high prevalence of toxoplasmosis such as Brussels, a simple preventive program can decrease the infection rate during pregnancy by 92%. If this result is confirmed prospectively, the utility of any screening program for toxoplasmosis during pregnancy may become questionable. Until then, we recommend that screening programs continue in regions with a high prevalence of the disease: once in the beginning of pregnancy, a control serology in seronegative women around 20 to 30 weeks' gestation, and postpartum on the umbilical cord blood. Early treatment after seroconversion reduces the odds of sequelae in affected children by 70%.[17,20] The focus should be on health education in regions with a low prevalence of toxoplasmosis during pregnancy.

■ Summary

1 ■ What Is the Problem that Requires Screening?

Congenital toxoplasma infection

a. What is the incidence/prevalence of the target condition?
The prevalence of toxoplasma during pregnancy ranges widely by geographic location. Recent data from serological studies indicate that the congenital infection rate varies from 0.2/1,000 births to 2/1,000 births.

b. What are the sequelae of the condition that are of interest in clinical medicine?
Less than 10% of infected neonates have symptoms at birth. Early maternal infection may lead to spontaneous abortion or severe sequelae such as hydrocephalus, chorioretinitis, and mental retardation. Other clinical manifestations include icterus, hepatosplenomegaly, and thrombocytopenia. Congenital infections occurring after the 24th week of pregnancy are usually subclinical. Nearly all symptomatic newborns have long-term neurologic and/or ophthalmologic sequelae.

2 ■ The Tests

a. What is the purpose of the tests?
To detect seronegative pregnant women at risk of primary infection during pregnancy.

Continued

■ **Summary—cont'd**

b. **What is the nature of the tests?**
A variety of serologic tests, none of which is definitive alone.

c. **What are the implications of testing?**
1. What does an abnormal test result mean?
When seroconversion is confirmed or suspected (high antibody level in a first serum sample), the woman should be offered antenatal diagnosis. If fetal infection is diagnosed, pregnancy termination may be offered, especially if sonographic abnormalities are seen. If the parents wish to continue the pregnancy, the woman should be treated with antibiotics.
2. What does a normal test result mean?
Pregnant women with IgG antibodies and absence of IgM antibodies are considered immune. Women without detectable antibodies are at risk. They should be instructed on potentially preventive measures and retested at 20 and again at 30 weeks' gestation in geographic areas of high risk.

d. **What is the cost of testing?**
Dependent on the geographic prevalence and the frequency of retesting.

3 ■ Conclusions and Recommendations

Maternal screening for toxoplasmosis using an automated ELISA at first prenatal visit with retesting of seronegative women once in the second and once in the third trimesters is likely to be cost-effective when the prevalence of maternal toxoplasmosis is more than 1 to 1.5 per 1,000.

References

1. Ancelle T, Goulet V, Tirard-Fleury V, et al. La Toxoplasmose chez la femme enceinte en France en 1995: Résultats d'une enquête nationale périnatale. *Bull Epidémiol Hebdomadaire* 1996;51:227–229.
2. Foulon W, Naessens A, Volckaert M, et al. Congenital toxoplasmosis:a prospective survey in Brussels. *Br J Obstet Gynaecol* 1984;91:419–423.
3. Joss AW, Skinner LJ, Chatterton JM, et al. Simultaneous serological screening for congenital cytomegalovirus and toxoplasma infection. *Public Health* 1988;102:409–417.
4. Stray-Pedersen B. A prospective study of acquired toxoplasmosis among 8,043 pregnant women in the Oslo area. *Am J Obstet Gynecol* 1980;136:399–406.

5. Desmonts G, Couvreur J. Congenital toxoplasmosis: a prospective study of 378 pregnancies. *N Engl J Med* 1974;1:417–422.

6. Hershey DW, McGregor JA. Low prevalence of toxoplasma infection in a Rocky Mountain prenatal population. *Obstet Gynecol* 1987;70:900–902.

7. Remington JS, McLeod R, Desmonts G. Toxoplasmosis. In: Remington JS, Klein JO, eds., *Infectious Diseases of the Fetus and Newborn*. Philadelphia: WB Saunders, 1995.

8. Jenum PA, Kapperud G, Stray-Pedersen B, et al. Prevalence of *Toxoplasma gondii* specific immunoglobulin G antibodies among pregnant women in Norway. *Epidemiol Infect* 1998;1:87–92.

9. Breugelmans M, Naessens A, Foulon W. Prevention of toxoplasmosis during pregnancy—an epidemiologic survey over 22 consecutive years. *J Perinat Med* 2004;32:211–214.

10. Guerina NG, Hsu HW, Meissner HC, et al. Neonatal serologic screening and early treatment for congenital *Toxoplasma gondii* infection. *N Engl J Med* 1994;330:1858–1863.

11. Hunter K, Stagna S, Capps E, et al. Prenatal screening of pregnant women for infections caused by cytomegalovirus, Epstein-Barr virus, herpesvirus, rubella and *Toxoplasma gondii*. *Am J Obstet Gynecol* 1983;145:269–273.

12. Walpole IR, Hodgen N, Bower C. Congenital toxoplasmosis: a large survey in Western Australia. *Med J Aust* 1991;154:720–724.

13. Jenum PA, Stray-Pedersen B, Gundersen AG. Improved diagnosis of primary *Toxoplasma gondii* infection in early pregnancy by determination of antitoxoplasma immunoglobulin G avidity. *J Clin Microbiol* 1997;35:1972–1977.

14. Desmonts G, Couvreur J. Toxoplasmose congénitale. Etude prospective de l'issue de la grossesse chez 542 femmes atteintes de toxoplasmose acquise en cours de gestation. *Ann Pédiatr* 1984;31:805–809.

15. Hohlfeld P, Daffos F, Costa JM, et al. Prenatal diagnosis of congenital toxoplasmosis with a polymerase-chain-reaction test on amniotic fluid. *N Engl J Med* 1994;331:695–699.

16. Foulon W, Villena I, Stray-Pedersen B, et al. Treatment of toxoplasmosis during pregnancy: a multicenter study of impact on fetal transmission and children's sequelae at age 1 year. *Am J Obstet Gynecol* 1999;180:410–415.

17. Foulon W, Pinon JM, Stray-Pedersen B, et al. Prenatal diagnosis of congenital toxoplasmosis: a multicenter evaluation of different diagnostic parameters. *Am J Obstet Gynecol* 1999;181:843–847.

18. Thorpe JM, Seeds JW, Herbert WNP, et al. Prenatal management of congenital toxoplasmosis. *N Engl J Med* 1988;319:372–373.

19. Stray-Pedersen B and Jemin P. Economic evaluation of preventive programs against congenital toxoplasmosis. *Second J Infect Dis* 1992;84[Suppl]:86–92.

20. Foulon W, Naessens A, Ho-Yen D. Prevention of congenital toxoplasmosis. *J Perinat Med* 2000;28:337–345.

21. Klapper PE and Morris DJ. Screening for viral and protozoal infection in pregnancy. A review. *Br J Obstet Gynaecol* 1990;97:974–983.

9

Congenital Cytomegalovirus Infection

Walter Foulon

Anne Naessens

■ What Is the Problem that Requires Screening?

Congenital cytomegalovirus infection

What is the incidence/prevalence of the target condition?

Cytomegalovirus (CMV) infection is a ubiquitous human herpes virus. It is transmitted by direct contact with infected excretions such as saliva and urine. Congenital CMV infection is one of the most common fetal viral infections, occurring in 0.2 to 2.2% of live-born infants[1] (Table 9–1). The rate of congenital CMV infections varies widely among countries as indicated by serologic surveys showing that the prevalence of maternal CMV antibodies ranges from 30% of women in the upper socioeconomic group in industrialized countries to nearly 100% in the lower socioeconomic group of developing countries.[2] In the Brussels area, 43% of pregnant women have no antibodies in their first serum sample. Seroconversion occurs in 1.4% of these women during pregnancy. The transmission rate from mother to fetus approximates 50%.[3]

Cytomegalovirus may also be transmitted by seropositive women to the fetus after reactivation or reinfection with a different strain of CMV.[4] Pregnant women with preexisting immunity have a lower rate of congenital infection: 0.27%.[3]

What are the sequelae of the condition that are of interest in clinical medicine?

Ten percent of congenitally infected infants are symptomatic at birth. Neonatal symptoms include hepatosplenomegaly, thrombocytopenia, purpura, jaundice, hemolytic anemia, hepatitis, microcephaly, chorioretinitis, and intracerebral calcifications. The mortality for symptomatic forms is high; approximately 20% die in the following days or weeks. More than 90% of all symptomatic newborns who survive develop long-term sequelae, mostly hearing loss and psychomotor retardation.[5]

Table 9–1	**Public health consequences of primary cytomegalovirus infection**		
Number		**Probability**[a]	**Range**[b]
100,000	Pregnant women	1.00	
40,000	Seronegative women	0.40	0.40–0.50
400	Maternal infection[c]	0.01	
140	Vertical transmission	0.35	0.20–0.50
14	Symptomatic defects at birth	0.10	
	Mortality ($n = 3$)	0.20	
	Late sequelae ($n = 10$)	0.70	
126	Asymptomatic at birth;	0.90	
32	sequelae after mean follow-up of 5 years[c,d]		
	($n = 32$)	0.25	0.09–0.30

[a]Crude estimates.
[b]See text.
[c]Fowler et al., 1992.
[d]Logan et al., 1992.

Ninety percent of all congenital CMV children are asymptomatic at birth. Five to 17% of these asymptomatic newborns will develop symptoms usually in the form of hearing deficits and subtle neurodevelopmental problems.[6,7]

The timing of infection and the serologic status of the mother play an important role in defining the transmission rate and sequelae in affected children. If the maternal CMV infection occurs in the first half of pregnancy, there is a higher incidence of sequelae than infections occurring later in gestation.[8] Primary maternal infection carries a much higher risk to the fetus in terms of long term handicap.[9] After a mean follow-up of all congenitally infected children for nearly 5 years, one or more sequelae were seen in 25% of the primary infection group and 8% of the secondary infection group. In the latter group, sequelae were usually limited to sensorineural hearing loss that develops over several years. Other studies suggest the sequelae of congenital CMV children secondary to recurrent maternal infection are more frequent than previously thought.[10,11]

■ The Tests

What is the purpose of the tests?

To identify pregnant women at risk of primary CMV infection.

What is the nature of the tests?

CMV specific IgG and IgM antibodies can be measured using commercially available enzyme immunoassays. The IgM response to a primary CMV infection is variable: most women will have IgM antibodies, but occasionally there is no IgM response.[12] Those IgM antibodies may persist for 4–7 months. Furthermore, reactivation or reinfection with a different strain of CMV can trigger a secondary IgM response. Therefore, IgM testing cannot be used as the sole indicator of primary infection. Primary infection can be diagnosed with certainty only if there is a seroconversion in IgG antibodies during pregnancy. As a result, CMV screening programs require the retesting of seronegative women to search for seroconversion. The measurement of CMV IgG binding avidity can be useful distinguishing primary from recurrent infection since[13] the avidity of IgG antibodies increases over time. Though low avidity does not necessarily mean recent infection as it may persist longer than 1 year, high avidity does indicate the primary infection occurred at least 4–5 months earlier.

What are the implications of testing?

What does an abnormal test result mean? Seroconversion during pregnancy means the fetus is at risk of congenital CMV. Proof of seroconversion would lead to invasive fetal studies. The best way to determine whether a fetus is infected is to demonstrate CMV in the amniotic fluid, either by culture or by a PCR test. The overall sensitivity for prenatal diagnosis is 80–90% when the amniocentesis is performed more than 6 weeks after maternal seroconversion and after 20 weeks' gestation.[14] Whether the remaining 10–20% are false negatives, or fetuses that become infected subsequently is unclear. The sensitivity is substantially less (approximately 50%) if the sampling is performed prior to 20 weeks or less than 6 weeks after seroconversion.[15]

Not all infected fetuses will develop adverse sequelae. Recent studies indicate that the viral load as measured by quantitative PCR can identify those fetuses at greatest risk for developing adverse sequelae.[16] However, the amniotic fluid viral load may also be dependent on other factors such as the gestational age at sampling and the time elapsed between the maternal infection and the time of sampling.[17] Additional studies are needed before using amniotic fluid viral load clinically as a prognostic marker for symptomatic CMV infection. And while sonographic abnormalities in affected fetuses are highly predictive of an adverse outcome,[14] there are rare case reports of infants born with antenatal ultrasound or MRI evidence of abnormalities who appear to develop normally.[18] Pregnancy termination is a reasonable option should an affected fetus have an abnormal ultrasound.

What does a normal test result mean? In the absence of concurrent IgM positivity, IgG-positive women are considered to have become infected before the current pregnancy. While they are protected from primary infection, they remain at risk of delivering a child infected from a recurrence or reactivation. Seronegative women have not had a CMV infection, but a negative test does not exclude primary infection as there is a small window for incubation. Implicit in screening is the assumption that seronegative women can significantly reduce their risk of CMV acquisition by adhering to simple, hygienic measures as there is no effective antenatal treatment. It is well established that CMV is transmitted through contamination of oropharyngeal or genital secretions. The optimal approach to prevention during pregnancy pending vaccine development is primary prevention. Theoretically, careful hand washing and minimal contact with toddler urine and saliva should reduce the infection rate during pregnancy. However, the efficacy of a primary prevention campaign to reduce the rate of CMV seroconversion during pregnancy has not been established.

What is the cost of testing?

The costs of treating CMV infection complications are high, perhaps $2 billion annually (1995).[19] It is difficult to evaluate the cost-efficacy of CMV screening, because key variables differ in countries. CMV seropositivity rates, type of screening tests, and the screening interval in seronegative women all influence the costs of a screening policy. The cost of monthly serology for seronegative women and amniocentesis for women with seroconversion plus the management of infected fetuses was estimated at 20,000 euros per affected fetus identified in France.[20]

■ Conclusions and Recommendations

Congenital CMV infection is a common congenital infection and an important cause of major long-term sequelae such as hearing loss and mental retardation. In most Western countries, 1% of all live births are CMV infected. Primary infection in mothers can be confirmed by CMV IgG seroconversion, and supporters of screening agree that sequelae could be prevented by antenatal screening and subsequent pregnancy termination of an affected fetus. While the identification of intrauterine CMV infection is possible with high sensitivity and specificity, the prediction of fetal damage especially when the ultrasound is normal remains a difficult task, creating problems for appropriate antenatal counseling. No fetal treatment has proven effective and safe.

Many issues regarding the usefulness of a screening strategy remain unsettled.[20] As a result, routine antenatal screening for CMV infection is not currently recommended. In the absence of an effective vaccine, the optimal available approach to CMV infection in pregnancy is the prevention of infection by hygienic measures. The impact of such a primary prevention program has not been established.

■ Summary

1 ■ What Is the Problem that Requires Screening?

Congenital CMV infection

a. *What is the incidence/prevalence of the target condition?*

1–2/1,000 deliveries. Maternal seropositivity varies by location and socioeconomic status. Approximately 40% of reproductive age women from industrialized countries are seronegative. About 1% of these develop a primary infection during pregnancy causing fetal infection in about 20 to 50 percent of those cases.

b. *What are the sequelae of the condition that are of interest in clinical medicine?*

Most congenitally infected infants are asymptomatic at birth. 10% experience severe sequelae including thrombocytopenia, hemolytic anemia, hepatitis, microcephaly, and chorioretinitis. Late sequelae such as hearing loss, mental retardation, or both occur in 90% of these survivors. The majority of asymptomatic children remain normal, but 10% develop sensorineural hearing loss over several years.

2 ■ The Tests

a. *What is the purpose of the tests?*

To identify women at risk of primary CMV infection.

b. *What is the nature of the tests?*

The measurement of maternal CMV-specific IgG and IgM antibodies

c. *What are the implications of testing?*

1. What does an abnormal test result mean?
   Women who seroconvert have had a primary CMV infection during pregnancy and should be offered antenatal diagnosis and subsequent appropriate counseling.
2. What does a normal test result mean?
   Women with CMV antibodies at their initial screen have previously been infected. They are not at risk of primary infection, but remain at risk of reactivation or reinfection.

Women without CMV antibodies have not been infected, and are at risk of a primary episode during pregnancy. In the absence of contrary evidence, all women are encouraged to practice high caliber oral-digital hygiene since CMV is transmitted through contamination of oropharyngeal and/or genital secretions.

c. *What is the cost of testing?*
It is difficult to evaluate the cost-efficacy of CMV screening in the absence of clinical efficacy.

3 ■ Conclusions and Recommendations

Although congenital CMV infection is an important health issue, there are too many unsolved problems to recommend mass screening of pregnant women.

References

1. Gaytant MA, Steegers EA, Semmekrot BA, et al. Congenital cytomegalovirus infection: review of the epidemiology and outcome. *Obstet Gynecol Surv* 2002;57:445–456.
2. Stagno S, Pass RF, Dworsky ME, et al. Maternal cytomegalovirus infection and perinatal transmission. *Clin Obstet Gynecol* 1982;25:563–576.
3. Naessens A, Casteels A, De Catte L,. A serologic strategy for detecting neonates at risk for congenital cytomegalovirus infection. *J Pediatr* Foulon W. 2005;146:194–197.
4. Boppana SB, Rivera LB, Fowler KB, et al. Intrauterine transmission of cytomegalovirus to infants of women with preconceptional immunity. *N Engl J Med* 2001;344:1366–1371.
5. Stagno S, Whitley RJ. Herpesvirus infections of pregnancy. I: cytomegalovirus and Epstein-Barr virus infections. *N Engl J Med* 1985;313:270–274.
6. Peckham CS, Stark O, Dudgeon JA, et al. Congenital cytomegalovirus infection: a cause of sensorineural hearing loss. *Arch Dis Child* 1987;62:1233–1237.
7. Hanshaw JB. Congenital cytomegalovirus infection. *Pediatr Ann* 1994;23:124–128.
8. Stagno S, Pass RF, Cloud G, et al. Primary cytomegalovirus infection in pregnancy: incidence, transmission to fetus, and clinical outcome. *JAMA* 1986;256:1904–1908.
9. Fowler KB, Stagno S, Pass RF, et al. The outcome of congenital cytomegalovirus infection in relation to maternal antibody status. *N Engl J Med* 1992;326:663–667.
10. Griffiths PD, Baboonian C, Rutter D, et al. Congenital and maternal cytomegalovirus infections in a London population. *Br J Obstet Gynaecol* 1991;98:135–140.
11. Casteels A, Naessens A, Gordts F, et al. Neonatal screening for congenital cytomegalovirus infections. *J Perinat Med* 1999;27:116–121.
12. Stagno S, Whitley RJ. Herpesvirus infections of pregnancy, I: cytomegalovirus and Epstein-Barr virus infections. *N Engl J Med* 1985;313:1270–1274.
13. Lazzarotto T, Varani S, Spezzacatena P, et al. Maternal IgG avidity and IgM detected by blot as diagnostic tools to identify pregnant women at risk of transmitting cytomegalovirus. *Viral Immunol* 2000;13:137–141.

14. Enders G, Bader U, Lindemann L, et al. Prenatal diagnosis of congenital cytomegalovirus infection in 189 pregnancies with known outcome. *Prenat Diagn* 2001;21:362–377.
15. Liesnard C, Donner C, Brancart F, et al. Prenatal diagnosis of congenital cytomegalovirus infection: prospective study of 237 pregnancies at risk. *Obstet Gynecol* 2000;95:881–888.
16. Lazzarotto T, Varani S, Guerra B, et al. Prenatal indicators of congenital cytomegalovirus infection. *J Pediatr* 2000;137:90–95.
17. Gouarin S, Gault E, Vabret A, et al. Real-time PCR quantification of human cytomegalovirus DNA in amniotic fluid samples from mothers with primary infection. *J Clin Microbiol* 2002;40:1767–1772.
18. Grangeot-Keros L, Simon B, Audibert F, Vial M. Should we routinely screen for cytomegalovirus antibody during pregnancy? *Intervirology* 1998;41:158–162.
19. Daniel Y, Gull I, Peyser MR, et al. Congenital cytomegalovirus infection. *Eur J Obstet Gynecol Reprod Biol* 1995;63:7–16.
20. Audibert F. For or against routine CMV screening in the pregnant woman? Are there arguments for routine screening for maternal-fetal CMV infection? *Gynecol Obstet Fertil* 2002;30:994–998.
21. Logan S, Tookey P, Ades T. Congenital cytomegalovirus infection and maternal antibody status (letter). *N Engl J Med* 1992;326:663–667.

10

Hepatitis A, B, and C During Pregnancy

Lise Jensen

Hepatitis A

■ What Is the Problem that Requires Screening?

Hepatitis A virus infection.

What is the incidence/prevalence of the target condition?

Hepatitis A virus infection is a common cause of acute hepatitis and has a worldwide distribution. An estimated 1.5 million clinical cases occurs annually.[1] The incidence varies geographically and is related to socioeconomic development.[2, 3] The principle mode of transmission is via the fecal–oral route from person-to-person contact or by exposure to contaminated food or water. Almost 100% of the adult population in developing countries are immune, and the infection is mostly acquired during childhood.[1] In low-prevalence countries, around 15% have antibodies. In the United States, one third of the population has had the infection.[1] Vertical transmission is very rare.[4]

What are the sequelae of the condition that are of interest in clinical medicine?

Hepatitis A virus infection is an acute viral infection with a clinical spectrum ranging from no symptoms to severe disabling disease with a recovery period lasting for months. The incubation period is 15 to 50 days with an average of 25 to 30 days. Symptoms include fever, malaise, anorexia, nausea, and abdominal pain followed by jaundice. Acute liver failure is rare. Infection with hepatitis A virus gives life-long immunity, and chronic infection does not occur.[5] Hepatitis A virus infection is usually symptomatic in adults (>70%). In contrast, the infection is asymptomatic in most children, and the morbidity rises with age.[6] There is no specific treatment available for persons with hepatitis A virus. The case fatality rate among reported cases of all ages approximates 0.3%, but is higher among older persons.[6]

In the Western World, hepatitis A virus infection during pregnancy does not seem to cause complications and it is not teratogenic.[7,8]

Passive immunization with immunoglobulin is recommended for pregnant women traveling to developing countries during pregnancy. Hepatitis A vaccination is made of formalin-inactivated virus and has no known teratogenic effect.[6] It is not contraindicated during pregnancy.

■ The Tests

What is the purpose of the tests?

To identify hepatitis A virus–susceptible women.

It may be useful to test women who have moved from a high-prevalence country to a low-prevalence country before vaccinating them for travel to avoid unnecessary vaccination.[9]

What is the nature of the tests?

Serologic testing for antibodies (IgG and IgM) is performed using commercially available third-generation radioimmune assay (RIA) and enzyme-linked immune assay (EIA) techniques. Immunoglobulin M (IgM) antibodies are present at the time symptoms appear; IgG antibodies are present shortly thereafter.[5,6]

What are the implications of testing?

What does an abnormal test result mean? A positive IgM test indicates current or recent infection. Newborn infants of hepatitis A virus–infected mothers whose symptoms first manifest between 2 weeks before and 1 week after delivery should also receive immunoglobulin.[9,10]

It is recommended that susceptible pregnant women exposed to hepatitis A virus receive postexposure prophylaxis with immunoglobulin. Immunoglobulin given within 2 weeks of exposure to hepatitis A virus is more than 85% effective in preventing symptomatic infection.[11] Hepatitis A virus vaccination has not yet been evaluated as postexposure prophylaxis.

What does a normal test result mean? A person without antibodies to hepatitis A virus either has not had the infection or could be in the incubation period (window phase) before the onset of symptoms. A positive IgG anti–hepatitis A virus test with a negative IgM anti–hepatitis A virus test indicates past infection or earlier vaccination. No further testing is indicated.

What is the cost of testing?

There is only one scenario where screening may be cost-effective. This relates to women born in a high-prevalence area but presently living in a low-prevalence area and now planning travel to a high-prevalence area.[12]

■ Conclusions and Recommendations

Pregnancy does not alter the course of hepatitis A virus, and the risk to the mother and fetus reflects the severity of symptoms. Hepatitis A virus is only rarely transmitted to the newborn child. There are no teratogenic implications of hepatitis A virus. Standard recommendations for the prophylaxis of hepatitis A virus infection should be followed. Pregnant women, like other exposed persons, should receive immunoglobulin as postexposure prophylaxis; those traveling to high-prevalence areas should receive immunoglobulin or possibly hepatitis A virus vaccination.

■ Summary

1 ■ What Is the Problem that Requires Screening?

Hepatitis A virus infection.

a. What is the incidence/prevalence of the target condition?

Almost 100% of the adult population in developing countries are immune. In low-prevalence countries, around 15% have antibodies. In the United States, one third of the population has been infected. Vertical transmission is very rare.

b. What are the sequelae of the condition that are of interest in clinical medicine?

Hepatitis A virus infection is an acute viral infection with a clinical spectrum ranging from no symptoms to severe disabling disease with a recovery period lasting for months.

2 ■ The Tests

a. What is the purpose of the tests?

To identify hepatitis A virus–susceptible women.

Continued

■ **Summary—cont'd**

b. ***What is the nature of the tests?***
Serologic testing for antibodies (IgG and IgM) is performed using commercially available third-generation RIA and EIA.

c. ***What are the implications of testing?***
1. What does an abnormal test result mean?
   A positive IgM test indicates current or recent infection.
2. What does a normal test result mean?
   A woman without antibodies to hepatitis A virus either has not had the infection or is in the incubation period before the onset of symptoms. A positive IgG anti-hepatitis A virus test with a negative IgM indicates past infection or earlier vaccination.

d. ***What is the cost of testing?***
Generally not considered cost beneficial.

3 ■ Conclusions and Recommendations

Pregnancy does not alter the course of hepatitis A virus, and the risk to the mother and fetus reflect the severity of symptoms. Hepatitis A virus is only rarely transmitted to the newborn child.

Hepatitis B

■ What Is the Problem that Requires Screening?

Perinatal transmission of hepatitis B virus from mother to child.

What is the incidence/prevalence of the target condition?

Hepatitis B virus infection occurs worldwide. The prevalence of a chronic carrier state ranges from less than 2% in some areas (Northwestern Europe, North America, and Australia) up to 20% in other areas (Africa and Asia).[13,14] It is estimated that 350 million people are chronic carriers of hepatitis B virus infection, and two billion have been infected.[15] Symptomatic acute hepatitis B virus infection occurs most commonly in adults. More than 500,000 people die annually due to hepatitis B virus infection.[14,15] Hepatitis B virus is transmitted through the exchange of blood and body fluids. Worldwide perinatal transmission accounts for up to 40% of chronic hepatitis B carriers.[16]

What are the sequelae of the condition that are of interest in clinical medicine?

Hepatitis B surface antigen (HBsAg) appears during the incubation period in acute hepatitis B virus infection, typically 1 to 6 weeks before clinical or biochemical illness develops, and disappears during convalescence. Transmission of hepatitis B virus from mother to child at birth results in chronic infection for more than 90% of the children.[16,17] HBeAg-positive mothers have a 70% to 90% risk of transmitting disease, whereas HBsAg-positive HBeAg-negative mothers have a risk of 5 % to 20 %.[17] Although these children have no acute signs of infection, they are at increased risk of cirrhosis and hepatocellulary carcinoma later in life.[18]

Screening of the mother for HBsAg and vaccination of the newborn prevents more than 95% of perinatal transmission of hepatitis B virus.[19,20] A small proportion (2%) of children are infected in utero.[21,22] The risk of transmission by breast feeding is negligible if the child has received postexposure prophylaxis and the follow-up vaccinations.[23]

Pregnancy does not seem to influence the clinical course of chronic hepatitis B infection.[24,25]

■ The Tests

What is the purpose of the tests?

The identification of pregnant women with hepatitis B virus infection before delivery to vaccinate the newborn soon after delivery. In many countries, all pregnant women are screened for HBsAg (universal screening); in others, only selected groups with special risk factors (e.g., origin in a high-prevalence area) are screened during pregnancy (selective screening). Selective screening of pregnant women with risk factors for hepatitis B virus infection misses a significant proportion of infected persons. About one third of persons with chronic hepatitis B virus infection in low-prevalence countries do not belong to a risk group.[23]

The World Health Organization (WHO) recommended universal childhood immunizations for hepatitis B virus in the 1990s to reduce the global burden of hepatitis B virus infection. In 2001, 66% of 191 WHO member countries had universal infant or childhood hepatitis B vaccination programs.[6] However, it will take years before this initiative can reduce the risk of perinatal transmission of hepatitis B virus.

What is the nature of the tests?

Commercially available serologic tests are used for the screening of HBsAg in maternal blood.

What are the implications of testing?

What does an abnormal test result mean? The sensitivity and specificity of HBsAg tests are 99% to 100%. A positive test may be confirmed by a neutralization test. A positive HBsAg test indicates that the woman has acute or chronic hepatitis B. The definition of chronic hepatitis B virus infection requires the presence of HBsAg in serum for at least 6 months without immunoglobulin M (IgM) anti-HBc (anti–hepatitis B core). Further blood tests to evaluate the stage of hepatitis B virus infection are needed. The risk of transmission secondary to an invasive procedure such as amniocentesis or chorion villus seems very low.[26] A fetal scalp electrode is probably best avoided during labor though the neonate should be protected if appropriately vaccinated.

Hepatitis B e antigen is a viral protein secreted by hepatitis B virus–infected cells. Its presence indicates high levels of virus in the blood, and it is a reflection of the infectiousness of the carrier. The relatively small group of women with a high viral load during pregnancy may benefit from lamivudine therapy.[27–29] Several studies suggest that treatment markedly reduces the risk of vertical transmission. Chronic active hepatitis B can develop even with a negative HBeAg test. A positive anti–HBc-IgM indicates acute infection and generally becomes undetectable 6 months after the onset of the infection.

The Centers for Disease Control and Prevention (CDC) and the American Academy of Pediatrics both recommend that newborns of HBsAg-positive mothers receive hepatitis B immunoglobulins and the first dose of vaccine within 12 hours after birth.[30,31] Most countries currently recommend administration of both, although recent evidence suggests that the vaccine alone may be almost as effective. Two effective regimens of follow-up vaccinations are currently used. The vaccination is repeated either at 1 and 6 months or at 1, 2, and 12 months after birth. The follow-up vaccinations are important for long-term protection, as the HBsAg-positive mother will still have a risk of transmitting the disease to the child.

Household contacts and sexual partners to HBsAg carriers should be tested for HBsAg and vaccinated if not immune to hepatitis B virus.

What does a normal test result mean? A negative HBsAg test means that the person is not infected and no further clinical precautions need be taken unless the person has been exposed to hepatitis B virus very recently (the window period from transmission to a positive HBsAg tests). If the mother has an at-risk behavior, a negative screening test from early pregnancy should be repeated closer to the delivery. Anti-HBs (hepatitis B surface antibody) indicates past infection or vaccination.

What is the cost of testing?

The cost efficacy of hepatitis B virus screening has been intensively studied. Screening of all pregnant women for HBsAg and immunization of the neonates at risk is estimated cost-effective when the prevalence for HBsAg is at least 0.06%.[32] (Universal screening has been recommended in the United States since 1988, but implementation was relatively slow. Even now, recent unpublished data indicate the current testing rates approximate 90%.) Neonatal vaccination will decrease the number of the hepatitis B virus carriers, thus reducing the transmission rate of the virus in the population.

New prevention strategies are being implemented to further reduce the transmission of hepatitis B virus. These include the selective vaccination of at-risk adolescents and adults, and universal hepatitis B virus vaccination of all children as part of the childhood vaccination program.[33,34] Universal vaccination of infants has been implemented in most countries in the industrialized part of the world. Immunization programs to ensure that all women of child-bearing age are immune to hepatitis B virus infection are cost-effective in some studies.[35,36]

■ Conclusions and Recommendations

The prevention of perinatal transmission of hepatitis B virus at birth has an important role in the elimination of chronic HBsAg carriage. Transmission of hepatitis B virus infection can be prevented if pregnant women are screened for HBsAg before delivery and if children of HBsAg-positive mothers receive immunizations within 12 hours of delivery. Infants born to HBsAg-positive mothers should complete the vaccination schedule within 6 to 12 months of delivery to obtain long-term protection. Breast feeding does not increase the risk of hepatitis B virus acquisition in neonates who have been given immunoprophylaxis and should not be discouraged.

■ Summary

1 ■ **What Is the Problem that Requires Screening?**

Perinatal transmission of hepatitis B virus infection.

a. *What is the incidence/prevalence of the target condition?*

There is wide variation in the prevalence of the maternal carrier state by geographic location ranging from 0.5% to 20%. Transmission depends on the antigen status of the mother: In HBsAg-positive mothers, neonatal infection occurs in 5% to 20%. The risk is much higher if the woman is also HBeAg positive.

Continued

■ **Summary—cont'd**

b. *What are the sequelae of the condition that are of interest in clinical medicine?*

Neonatal HBV infection is usually asymptomatic. Transmission of hepatitis B virus from mother to child results in more than 90% of newborns with hepatitis B virus infection becoming chronic carriers, placing them at risk for serious long-term sequelae. Chronic active hepatitis develops in 40%. These individuals are at risk of either cirrhosis or hepatocellular carcinoma. As many as 25% of chronic carriers of hepatitis B virus will die of complications.

2 ■ The Tests

a. *What is the purpose of the tests?*

The identification of pregnant women with hepatitis B virus infection before delivery in order to vaccinate the newborn soon after delivery.

b. *What is the nature of the tests?*

The detection of the HBsAg is the cornerstone in the prevention of perinatal transmission of hepatitis B virus.

c. *What are the implications of testing?*

1. What does an abnormal test result mean?

   Infants whose mothers are infected with hepatitis B virus are exposed to infected secretions at the delivery. Hepatitis B vaccination and hepatitis B immunoglobulin should be given within 12 hours of birth. The efficacy of the treatment decreases with a longer time interval. Furthermore, hepatitis B virus vaccination is administered at 1 and 6 months of age or at 1, 2 and 12 months of age.

2. What does a normal test result mean?

   The mother has not been previously exposed to hepatitis B virus unless there is a history of recent exposure, and the newborn is not at risk for hepatitis B virus infection.

d. *What is the cost of testing?*

Universal screening for maternal HBsAg and immunization of the neonates at risk is cost-effective if the prevalence rate of HBsAg is at least 0.06%.

3 ■ Conclusions and Recommendations

All pregnant women should be screened for HBsAg at their first antenatal visit. All infants born to HBsAg-positive mothers should receive a hepatitis B vaccination and hepatitis B immunoglobulin (at different sites) within 12 hours of birth, followed by vaccinations at 1 and 6 months or 1, 2 and 12 months of age.

Hepatitis C

■ What Is the Problem that Requires Screening?

Hepatitis C virus infection.

What is the incidence/prevalence of the target condition?

Hepatitis C virus infection is a major global health problem. It is estimated by WHO that 170 million people have the infection, corresponding to an overall prevalence 3%.[37] Hepatitis C virus is transmitted by infected blood (before screening of blood products was introduced in the early 1990s, intravenous drug use, contaminated hospital equipment, and other percutaneous procedures). Sexual transmission is rare, but occurs.[38] In some parts of the world, the prevalence is relatively high, in great part due to the use of contaminated hospital equipment (needles, surgical equipment).[39] Most infected individuals in the Western world belong to at-risk groups. The prevalence is 70% to 90% among drug users.[40] It is estimated to be less than 1% among pregnant women in the United Kingdom,[5] around 2% in Southern Europe,[41] and 1% to 2% in the United States.[42] In the Western world, blood banks have screened their products since the early 1990s, reducing the risk of infection in the general and the pediatric population.

The risk of vertical transmission is 3% to 5% and is associated with hepatitis C virus viremia in the mother.[43,44] The risk is higher with human immunodeficiency virus (HIV) co-infection, reflecting the associated high hepatitis C viral loads.

What are the sequelae of the condition that are of interest in clinical medicine?

The incubation period is 7 weeks (range, 4–20 weeks).[45] Most cases of hepatitis C virus infection are asymptomatic for years, but 60% to 85% of infected individuals will develop chronic hepatitis. Hepatitis C infection is the leading cause for liver transplantation in adults in the Western world. Twenty percent of infected individuals develop cirrhosis, and 1% to 4% progress to hepatocellulary carcinoma. Antiviral treatment generates a sustained response in 10% to 40% of adults depending on the treatment regimen and subtype of hepatitis C virus.[46–49]

Chronic hepatitis C virus infection in pregnant women does not appear to alter the course of the pregnancy.[43]

Hepatitis C infection acquired perinatally is usually asymptomatic. Children born to hepatitis C virus–positive women should be tested for anti–hepatitis C virus at 1 year of age, when the mothers' antibodies have declined.[50] The long-term course of hepatitis C virus infection acquired perinatally is not well described, but early identification of infected children allows evaluation of the course and the possible treatment of liver disease.

■ The Tests

What is the purpose of the tests?

To identify pregnant women with hepatitis C virus infection. Universal antenatal screening is not cost beneficial at the moment in populations with low prevalence.[51] There is no intervention during pregnancy that has been shown to alter outcome. Invasive procedures such as chorion villus sampling, amniocentesis, and forceps and scalp electrode for heart rate monitoring are relatively contraindicated because of the theoretical risk of vertical transmission. Women with a high viral load may be evaluated for pharmacologic therapy after delivery when the unimmunized woman should be offered vaccination for hepatitis A and B. The utility and safety of pharmacologic therapy to reduce the viral load during pregnancy in hopes of lowering the rate of perinatal transmission has not been evaluated. The child can be examined at 1 year of age and, if infected, monitored and treated as appropriate.

In targeted screening, pregnant woman who abuse intravenous drugs or have a positive transfusion or organ transplant history before the routine screening of blood for hepatitis C virus and women undergoing long-term hemodialysis treatment are considered at high risk.[50] Testing may also be considered for women with a hepatitis C virus–positive partner or women with piercing or tattooing.[50]

What is the nature of the tests?

Serologic tests are used to screen for hepatitis C virus infection. Initially, an antibody assay such as an enzyme-linked immunosorbent assay (ELISA) or EIA is used and when positive, a confirmatory RIBA (recombinant immunoblot assay) test performed. If both are positive, a reverse transcriptase–polymerase chain reaction (RT-PCR) test for hepatitis C virus RNA and a test for liver disease (alanine aminotransferase [ALT]) are performed to distinguish between active and past infection. Positive hepatitis C virus RNA indicates active infection, but a single negative test does not exclude active infection as viremia can be intermittent.

What are the implications of testing?

What does an abnormal test result mean? The anti–hepatitis C virus test (IgG) does not distinguish between acute, chronic, or resolved infection. A relatively high proportion of false-positive or inconclusive results can occur especially in low-prevalence populations, requiring retesting and counseling of the woman. There are only a limited number of publications investigating the sensitivity and specificity of anti–hepatitis C virus assays in pregnant women. A confirmatory RIBA test should be performed; if negative the person can be considered uninfected. Detection of hepatitis C virus RNA by PCR indicates current infection.

It has been suggested that elective caesarean delivery reduces the risk of perinatal transmission, but there is no clear supporting evidence. A protective effect of cesarean delivery is, however, observed with hepatitis C virus and HIV co-infection.[52] Very few studies address other procedures and circumstances during delivery other than the mode of delivery, but it seems advisable to avoid invasive procedures whenever possible. There is limited experience during pregnancy with the antiviral therapy currently available for treatment of hepatitis C virus infection: peg interferon-α2b, interferon-α2a and 2b, or ribavirin. Rodent studies suggest teratogenic effects especially at high doses arguing that these drugs should be avoided in the first trimester.

Breast feeding is not considered a risk factor for transmission in asymptomatic and HIV-negative mothers[52] unless the nipples are cracked and bleeding.

What does a normal test result mean? The sensitivity of all available anti–hepatitis C virus tests is high (97%–99%). Thus, there are two possibilities. A woman with negative antibodies is unlikely to be infected. Nor is a woman with antibodies but who is asymptomatic with a normal ALT level and a repeatedly negative PCR.

What is the cost of testing?

There is little information available on the cost-effectiveness of universal screening[53] and none on screening during pregnancy. Targeted screening is likely to be effective in high-risk populations.[51]

■ Conclusions and Recommendations

The prevalence of hepatitis C virus infection in pregnant women is relatively high. There is little information on possible interventions during pregnancy to reduce mother-to-infant transmission. The risk of perinatal transmission is 5%. It is likely cost beneficial to screen women in at-risk groups (e.g., intravenous drug use), and it has been argued that universal screening may also be beneficial. Further research is needed.

■ Summary

1 ■ What Is the Problem that Requires Screening?

Hepatitis C virus infection that may be transmitted perinatally.

a. *What is the incidence/prevalence of the target condition?*

The overall prevalence is about 3%, though it is between 70% and 90% among drug users. It is estimated to be less than 1% among pregnant women in the United Kingdom, around 2% in Southern Europe, and 1% to 2% in the United States.

b. *What are the sequelae of the condition that are of interest in clinical medicine?*

From 60% to 85% of infected individuals develop chronic hepatitis. Hepatitis C infection is the leading cause for liver transplantation in adults. Twenty percent of infected individuals develop cirrhosis, and 1% to 4% progress to hepatocellulary carcinoma.

2 ■ The Tests

a. *What is the purpose of the tests?*

To identify pregnant women with hepatitis C virus infection.

b. *What is the nature of the tests?*

Serologic tests are used. An antibody assay such as an ELISA or EIA is used initially, and when positive, a confirmatory RIBA (recombinant immunoblot assay) performed.

c. *What are the implications of testing?*

1. What does an abnormal test result mean?

   When a positive ELISA is confirmed by PCR, the woman has active infection. An elevated ALT is consistent with chronic hepatitis.

It has been suggested that elective cesarean section reduces the risk of perinatal transmission, but there is no clear supporting evidence presently.

2. What does a normal test result mean?

A woman with negative antibodies is not likely to be infected if she is out of the incubation period. Nor is a woman with antibodies but who is asymptomatic with a normal ALT level and a repeatedly negative PCR.

d. *What is the cost of testing?*

Universal hepatitis C screening is not regarded cost-beneficial at the moment.

3 ■ Conclusions and Recommendations

The prevalence of hepatitis C virus infection in pregnant women is relatively high among at-risk groups. Universal screening is not recommended, but screening among women at risk is recommended. There is little information on possible interventions during pregnancy to reduce mother-to-infant transmission. The risk of perinatal transmission is 5%.

References

1. World Health Organization. Hepatitis A vaccines: WHO position paper. *Wkly Epidemiol Rec* 2000;75:38–44.
2. Gust ID. Epidemiological patterns of hepatitis A in different parts of the world. *Vaccine* 1992;10[Suppl 1]:S56–S58.
3. Feinstone SM. Hepatitis A: epidemiology and prevention. *Eur J Gastroenterol Hepatol* 1996;8:300–305.
4. Leikin E, Lysikiewicz A, Garry D, Tejani N. Intrauterine transmission of hepatitis A virus. *Obstet Gynecol* 1996;88:690–691.
5. Koff RS. Clinical manifestations and diagnosis of hepatitis A virus infection. *Vaccine* 1992;10[Suppl 1]:S15–S17.
6. Centers for Disease Control and Prevention. Prevention of hepatitis A through active or passive immunization: recommendations of the Advisory Committee on Immunization Practices (ACIP). *MMWR Morb Mortal Wkly Rep* 1999;48:1–37.
7. Michielsen PP, Van Damme P. Viral hepatitis and pregnancy. *Acta Gastroenterol Belg* 1999;62:21–29.
8. Duff P. Hepatitis in pregnancy. *Semin Perinatol* 1998;22:277–283.
9. Duff B, Duff P. Hepatitis A vaccine: ready for prime time. *Obstet Gynecol* 1998;91:468–471.
10. Prevention of hepatitis A infections: guidelines for use of hepatitis A vaccine and immune globulin: American Academy of Pediatrics Committee on Infectious Diseases. *Pediatrics* 1996;98:1207–1215.

11. Winokur PL, Stapleton JT. Immunoglobulin prophylaxis for hepatitis A. *Clin Infect Dis* 1992;14:580–586.
12. Fishbain JT, Eckart RE, Harner KC, et al. Empiric immunization versus serologic screening: developing a cost-effective strategy for the use of hepatitis A immunization in travelers. *J Travel Med* 2002;9:71–75.
13. www.who.int/vaccines-surveillance/graphics/htmls/hepbprev.htm.
14. Alter MJ. Epidemiology and prevention of hepatitis B. *Semin Liver Dis* 2003;23:39–46.
15. Kane MA. Global programme for control of hepatitis B infection. *Vaccine* 1995;13[Suppl 1]: S47–S49.
16. Edmunds WJ, Medley GF, Nokes DJ, et al. The influence of age on the development of the hepatitis B carrier state. *Proc R Soc Lond B* 1993; 253:197–201.
17. Beasley RP, Trepo C, Stevens CE, et al. The e antigen and vertical transmission of hepatitis B surface antigen. *Am J Epidemiol* 1977; 105:94–98.
18. McMahon BJ, Alward WLM, Hall DB, et al. Acute hepatitis B virus infection: relation of age to clinical expression of disease and subsequent development of the carrier state. *J Infect Dis* 1985;151:599–603.
19. Wong VC, Ip HM, Reesink HW, et al. Prevention of the HBsAg carrier state in newborn infants of mothers who are chronic carriers of HBsAg and HBeAg by administration of hepatitis B-vaccine and hepatitis B immunoglobulin. *Lancet* 1984;I:921–926.
20. Stevens CE, Toy PT, Taylor PE, et al. Prospects for control of hepatitis B virus infection: implications of childhood vaccination and long term protection. *Pediatrics* 1992;90S:170–173.
21. Lin H-H, Lee T-Y, Chen D-S, et al. Transplacental leakage of HBeAg-positive maternal blood as the most likely route in causing intrauterine infection with hepatitis B virus. *J Pediatr* 1987;111: 877–881.
22. Ghendon Y. Perinatal transmission of hepatitis B virus in high incidence countries. *J Virol Methods* 1987;17: 69–79.
23. Boxall E. Screening of pregnant women for hepatitis B. *Vaccine* 1998;16[Suppl]:S30–S33.
24. Dinsmoor MJ. Hepatitis in the obstetric patient. *Infect Dis Clin North Am* 1997;11:77–91.
25. Michielsen PP, Van Damme P. Viral hepatitis and pregnancy. *Acta Gastroenterol Belg* 1999;62:21–29.
26. Grosheide PM, Quartero HW, Schalm SW, Heijtink et al. Early invasive prenatal diagnosis in HBsAg-positive women. *Prenat Diagn* 1994;14:553–558.
27. van Zonneveld M, van Nunen AB, Niesters HG, et al. Lamivudine treatment during pregnancy to prevent perinatal transmission of hepatitis B virus infection. *J Viral Hepat* 2003;10:294–297.
28. Su GG, Pan KH, Zhao NF, et al. Efficacy and safety of lamivudine treatment for chronic hepatitis B in pregnancy. *World J Gastroenterol* 2004;10:910–912.
29. Ranger-Rogez S, Denis F. Hepatitis B mother–to–child transmission. *Expert Rev Anti Infect Ther* 2004;2:133–145.
30. Centers for Disease Control and Prevention. Update: recommendations to prevent hepatitis B virus transmission—United States. *JAMA* 1999;281:790.
31. No authors. American Academy of Pediatrics Committee on Infectious Diseases: Universal hepatitis B immunization. *Pediatrics* 1992;89:795–800.
32. Arevalo JA, Washington AE. Cost-effectiveness of prenatal screening and immunization for hepatitis B virus. *JAMA* 1988;259:365–369.
33. Anonymous. Hepatitis B virus: A comprehensive strategy for eliminating transmission in the United States through universal childhood vaccination: recommendations of the Immunization Practices Advisory Committee. *MMWR Recomm Rep* 1991; 40:1–25.
34. Kraus DM, Campbell MM, Marcinak JF. Evaluation of universal hepatitis B immunization practices of Illinois pediatricians. *Arch Ped Adolesc Med* 1994;148:936–942.
35. Bloom BS, Hillman AL, Fendrick AM, et al. A reappraisal of hepatitis B virus vaccination strategies using cost-effectiveness analysis. *Ann Int Med* 1993;118:298–306.
36. Margolis HS, Coleman PJ, Brown RE, et al. Prevention of hepatitis B virus transmission by immunization. An economic analysis of current recommendations. *JAMA* 1995t ;274:1201–1208.
37. Weekly Epidemiological Record. No. 49, 1999, WHO.

38. Ackerman Z, Ackerman E, Paltiel O. Intrafamilial transmission of hepatitis C virus: a systematic review. *J Virol Hepat* 2000;7:93–103.
39. Frank C, Mohamed MK, Strickland GT et al. The role of parenteral antischistosomal therapy in the spread of hepatitis C virus in Egypt. *Lancet* 2000;335:887–891.
40. Goldberg D, Cameron S, McMenamin J. Hepatitis C virus antibody prevalence among injecting drug users in Glasgow has fallen but remains high. *Commun Dis Public Health* 1998;1:25–27.
41. Conte D, Fraquelli M, Prati D et al. Prevalence and clinical course of chronic hepatitis C virus (HCV) infection and rate of HCV vertical transmission in a cohort of 15,250 pregnant women. *Hepatology* 2000;31:751–755.
42. Dinsmoor MJ. Hepatitis C in pregnancy. *Curr Womens Health Rep* 2001;1:17–30.
43. Roberts EA, Yeung L. Maternal-infant transmission of hepatitis C virus infection. *Hepatology* 2002;36[5 Suppl 1]:S106–113.
44. Saez A, Losa M, Lo Iacono O, et al. Diagnostic and prognostic value of virologic tests in vertical transmission of hepatitis C virus infection: results of a large prospective study in pregnant women. *Hepatogastroenterology* 2004;51:1104–1108.
45. Hoofnagle JH. Hepatitis C: the clinical spectrum of disease. *Hepatology* 1997;26[Suppl 1]:15S–20S.
46. Hoofnagle JH. Management of hepatitis C: current and future perspectives. *J Hepatol* 1999;31[Suppl 1]:264–268.
47. Sarbah SA, Younossi ZM. Hepatitis C, an update on the silent epidemic. *J Clin Gastroenterol* 2000;30:125–143.
48. NIH Consensus Statement on Management of Hepatitis C: 2002. *NIH Consens State Sci Statements* 2002;19:3–46.
49. Lindsay KL. Introduction to therapy of hepatitis C. *Hepatology* 2002;36[5 Suppl 1]:S114–120.
50. Centers for Disease Control and Prevention. Recommendations for prevention and control of hepatitis C virus (HCV) infection and HCV-related chronic disease. *MMWR Recomm Rep* 1998;47:1–39.
51. Gordon FD. Cost-effectiveness of screening patients for hepatitis C. *Am J Med* 1999;27;107:36S–40S.
52. Pembrey L, Tovo PA, Newell ML. European Paediatric HCV Network. Effects of mode of delivery and infant feeding on the risk of mother-to-child transmission of hepatitis C virus. *Br J Obstet Gynaecol* 2001;108:371–377.
53. Loubiere S, Rotily M, Moatti JP. Prevention could be less cost-effective than cure: the case of hepatitis C screening policies in France. *Int J Technol Assess Health Care* 2003;19:432–445.

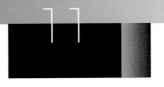

Syphilis

R. Phillip Heine

Michael J. Paglia

■ What Is the Problem that Requires Screening?

Infectious and congenital syphilis.

What is the incidence/prevalence of the target condition?

The prevalence of infectious syphilis in the United States is 2.4/100,000 population, with 6,862 new cases of primary and secondary syphilis reported in 2002.[1] The rate of infectious syphilis in the adult female population has decreased in recent years.[1] This decrease occurred mainly in heterosexual non-Hispanic blacks and American Indians/Alaska Natives.[2] The rate among black women is still much higher than in white women.[1]

Importantly, the decreased rate of infectious syphilis has led to a decrease in the rate of congenital syphilis. The prevalence has declined from 107.3/100,000 in 1991 to 10.2/100,000 in 2002. There were only 412 reported cases of congenital syphilis in 2002.[1] The rates of congenital syphilis are highest in the South, among young women (age less than 19) and black American and Hispanic women.[3] Over one fourth of these cases occur among women receiving no antenatal care.

What are the sequelae of the condition that are of interest in clinical medicine?

The clinical sequelae of infection with the spirochete *Treponema pallidum* are well described. They include primary, secondary, latent, and tertiary stages. After an incubation period of approximately 21 days from exposure, a painless chancre develops at the site of the inoculum. This is the primary stage. The chancre disappears spontaneously in 1 to 4 months and is followed by spirochetemia—the second stage. Symptoms of secondary syphilis typically begin 4 to 10 weeks after the chancre first appears. Clinical manifestations of the second stage include a generalized maculopapular rash of the palms and soles (50% to 80% of cases), mucus patches, condyloma latum, and generalized lymphadenopathy. Within 2 to 6 weeks, these findings clear spontaneously, and the latent stage begins. This period is characterized by a lack of clinically evident disease. If treatment of the primary, secondary, or latent stages is not provided, 25% to 30% of patients develop tertiary syphilis, which includes cardiovascular syphilis, neurosyphilis, and gummatous disease.[4,5]

Syphilis can infect the fetus at any gestational age, including the first trimester, and can be transmitted during any stage of maternal disease.[6] Untreated primary syphilis is associated with a 70% to 100% probability of congenital syphilis and up to a 30% risk of stillbirth.[7] The risk of intrauterine infection is highest in the early maternal infectious stages of the disease and rare in later stages.[7,8] Manifestations of fetal infection include preterm birth, stillbirth, neonatal death, and disorders including deafness, neurologic impairment, and bone deformities.[3] Fetal mortality is highest in younger women (younger than 25 years) and in women with no antenatal care.[9]

■ The Tests

What is the purpose of the tests?

To identify women with infectious syphilis. Most cases of syphilis are diagnosed by the routine screening of asymptomatic persons, including pregnant women at their first antenatal care visit. Universal screening is especially important for women where most cases of primary syphilis are asymptomatic. Women identified with syphilis should be screened for other sexually transmitted diseases including gonorrhea, chlamydia, and human immunodeficiency virus (HIV).

What is the nature of the tests?

Visualization of spirochetes by dark-field microscopy in a fresh specimen obtained by sampling a suspected lesion is diagnostic of syphilis. Most primary lesions in the female occur on the cervix or posterior fornix and are not seen by the subject. Therefore, screening for syphilis is based on a combination of nonspecific and specific serologic testing. Nonspecific antibody tests include the Venereal Disease Research Laboratory (VDRL) and the rapid plasma reagent (RPR) tests. These tests detect antibodies to cardiolipin produced by the spirochete.[5] They have a sensitivity ranging from 78% to 100% depending on the stage of syphilis.[4] A reactive (positive) VDRL or RPR result must be confirmed by *T. pallidum*–specific tests, which include the *T. pallidum* immobilization (TPI) test, the fluorescent treponemal antibody absorption (FTA-ABS) test, and the microhemagglutination test for *T. pallidum* (MHA-TP).[10]

What are the implications of testing?

What does an abnormal test result mean? Asymptomatic individuals with reactive nonspecific antibody tests confirmed by reactive specific antitreponemal-specific antibody tests are considered to have latent syphilis. Persons known to have had a nonreactive test within the previous year are classified as having early latent syphilis, whereas those whose previous serology is unknown are classified as having late latent syphilis and must be evaluated for tertiary syphilis. Women with a positive dark-field examination or a positive VDRL/RPR test result plus a specific confirmatory test have infectious syphilis. Successful maternal treatment ends the risks of spread and long-term sequelae. It does not necessarily cure the infected fetus.

False-positive, nonspecific antibody test results may occur in women with connective tissue or autoimmune diseases, other infectious diseases, drug addiction, and pregnancy.[4] Generally, these conditions yield borderline or weakly positive results (VDRL titers < 1:8). False-positive antitreponemal antibody–specific tests occur in 1% of the population. They are usually transient, of unknown etiology, and may be associated with systemic lupus erythematosus or Lyme disease.[5]

In the newborn, positive serologic tests can represent either active disease or passively transferred antibodies from the mother. In the latter instance, antibody titers will progressively decrease and disappear by three to four months of age.[11]

The US Centers for Disease Control and Prevention (CDC) has outlined their current recommendations for the treatment of syphilis.[12] Penicillin remains the drug of choice. A single injection of penicillin for early infection during pregnancy has a 98% success rate in preventing congenital syphilis.[13] Alternatives for nonpregnant subjects include tetracycline, ceftriaxone, and azithromycin, although the data to support these alternative medications are limited. Pregnant women with a history of penicillin allergy should be skin tested with dilute solutions of penicillin.[12] If allergic, they should be desensitized in a monitored setting and then receive treatment with penicillin.

Approximately 10% to 25% of individuals (and 45% of pregnant women) treated with penicillin develop the Jarisch-Herxheimer reaction.[14,15] The associated symptoms include fever, chills, myalgias, hyperventilation, tachycardia, and headache. Symptoms resolve in 12 to 14 hours.[16]

What does a normal test result mean? Women with negative serologic testing do not have syphilis. The results from both the nonspecific antibody tests (VDRL or RPR) and the treponemal-specific tests (FTA-ABS or MHA-TP) may be nonreactive when the syphilitic chancre first appears.[10] Clinical judgment may dictate repeated testing in individuals at risk because it may take 4 weeks after the initial exposure for the serum tests to become positive. The CDC recommends that all women be screened at the time they initiate antenatal care. In areas with a high prevalence of syphilis, the CDC recommends testing at 28 weeks' gestation and at delivery.[12]

What is the cost of testing?

The typical cost for screening serology is approximately $40. The cost increases to $100 if specific antibody testing is required. Although it is likely that routine screening in low-prevalence areas is strictly speaking not cost-effective, congenital syphilis is a preventable disease with major sequelae to the offspring and costs to society if undetected. The CDC recommends active surveillance for congenital syphilis in hospitals in any area with a prevalence of five or more women with early infectious syphilis per 100,000 population.[17] This includes testing blood samples from the umbilical cord. The CDC recommendations for syphilis screening include testing all pregnant women, all sexual contacts of women with infectious syphilis, and other high-risk groups. Others support these recommendations.[18,19] Efficient screening prevents the spread of disease, allows for early treatment, and, in the pregnant woman, helps prevent the devastating effects of syphilis infection on the fetus.

■ Conclusions and Recommendations

Because primary lesions are usually asymptomatic in women, serologic testing assumes a prominent role in diagnosing syphilis. Authorities now recommend routine serologic testing in both the first and third trimesters.[12] Although it is likely that routine screening in low prevalence areas is not strictly speaking cost-effective, congenital syphilis is a preventable disease with major sequelae to the offspring and costs to society if undetected. Detection and adequate treatment of pregnant women is essential.

Infected individuals should be educated about syphilis, its sequelae, mode of transmission, and association with other sexually transmitted diseases. Because of the association between ulcerative diseases such as syphilis and concurrent HIV infection, counseling and testing for HIV are essential. It is crucial that any recent sexual contacts be concomitantly treated to avoid reinfection.

■ Summary

1 ■ What Is the Problem that Requires Screening?

Infectious and congenital syphilis.

a. What is the incidence/prevalence of the target condition?

The current prevalence of infectious syphilis in the United States is 2.4/100,000 population. The rate of congenital syphilis has been decreasing primarily due to an intensive preventive campaign. More than one fourth of congenital syphilis cases occur among women receiving no antenatal care.

Continued

■ **Summary—cont'd**

b. ***What are the sequelae of the condition that are of interest in clinical medicine?***
The clinical sequelae include primary, secondary, latent, and tertiary stages of syphilis. If treatment is not provided, 25% to 30% of patients develop tertiary syphilis. Syphilis may infect the fetus at any gestational age. Untreated primary or secondary syphilis is associated with a 50% probability of congenital syphilis and perinatal death.

2 ■ **The Tests**

a. ***What is the purpose of the tests?***
To identify women with infectious syphilis.

b. ***What is the nature of the tests?***
Screening for syphilis is based on nonspecific (VDRL or RPR) and specific serologic testing (FTA-ABS or MHA-TP). Identification of spirochetes by dark-field microscopy is diagnostic of syphilis.

c. ***What are the implications of testing?***
1. What does an abnormal test result mean?
   Asymptomatic persons with reactive nonspecific antibody tests confirmed by a reactive antitreponemal-specific antibody tests are considered to have latent syphilis. Visualization of spirochetes by dark-field microscopy is diagnostic of primary syphilis.
   False-positive, nonspecific antibody tests may occur in women with connective tissue or autoimmune diseases, other infectious diseases, drug addiction, and pregnancy. Generally, these conditions yield borderline or weakly positive results. False-positive antitreponemal antibody tests occur in 1% of the population. They are usually transient, of unknown etiology, and may be associated with systemic lupus erythematosus or Lyme disease.
   In the newborn, positive serologic test results represent either active disease or passively transferred antibodies from the mother. In the latter, antibody titers progressively decrease and disappear by 3 to 4 months of age.

Penicillin remains the drug of choice. A single injection in mothers with early infection produces a 98% success rate in preventing congenital syphilis. Approximately 10% to 45% of patients treated with penicillin develop Jarisch-Herxheimer reaction.

2. What does a normal test result mean?

Women with negative serologic testing do not have syphilis. However, the results from both the nonspecific antibody tests and the treponemal-specific tests may be nonreactive when the syphilitic chancre first appears. Clinical judgment may dictate repeated testing in individuals at risk because it may take 4 weeks after the initial exposure for the serum tests to become positive.

d. *What is the cost of testing?*

Standard charges for screening serology are approximately $40, with specific antibody testing being approximately $70.

3 ■ Conclusions and Recommendations

Because primary lesions are usually asymptomatic in women, identification requires serologic screening. In pregnant women at risk, authorities are now recommending serologic testing in both the first and third trimesters. To avoid reinfection, it is crucial that any recent sexual contacts be concomitantly treated.

References

1. Groseclose SL, Brathwaite WS, Hall PA, et al. Summary of notifiable diseases—United States, 2002. *MMWR Recomm Rep* 2004;51:53–84.
2. Centers for Disease Control and Prevention. Primary and secondary syphilis—United States, 2002. *MMWR Recomm Rep* 2003;52:1117–1120.
3. Anonymous. Congenital syphilis—United States, 2000. *MMWR Recomm Rep* 2001;50:2773–2777.
4. Golden MR, Marra CM, Holmes KK. Update on syphilis: resurgence of an old problem. *JAMA* 2003;290:1510–1514.
5. Brown DL, Frank JE. Diagnosis and management of syphilis. *Am Fam Physician* 2003;68:283–290.
6. Harter C, Benirschke K. Fetal syphilis in the first trimester. *Am J Obstet Gynecol* 1976;124:705–711.
7. Pao D, Goh BT, Bingham JS. Management issues in syphilis. *Drugs* 2002;62:10447–1461.
8. Fiumara NJ, Fleming WL, Downing JG, Good FL. The incidence of prenatal syphilis at the Boston City Hospital. *N Engl J Med* 1952;247:48–52.

9. Gust DA, Levine WC, St Louis ME, et al. Mortality associated with congenital syphilis in the United States, 1992–1998. *Pediatrics* 2002;109:E79.

10. Jaffe HW. The laboratory diagnosis of syphilis: new concepts. *Ann Int Med* 1975;83:646–650.

11. Ikeda MK, Jenson HB. Evaluation and treatment of congenital syphilis. *J Pediatr* 1990;117:643–652.

12. Anonymous. Sexually transmitted treatment guidelines 2002: Centers for Disease Control and Prevention. *MMWR Recomm Rep* 2002;51:1–78.

13. Alexander JM, Sheffield JS, Sanchez PJ, et al. Efficacy of treatment for syphilis in pregnancy. *Obstet Gynecol* 1999;93:1–8.

14. Sheffield JS, Sanchez PJ, Morris G, et al. Congenital syphilis after maternal treatment for syphilis during pregnancy. *Am J Obstet Gynecol* 2002;186:369–373.

15. Myles TD, Elam G, Park-Hwang E, et al. The Jarisch-Herxheimer reaction and fetal monitoring changes in pregnant women treated for syphilis. *Obstet Gynecol* 1998;92:559–564.

16. Hollier LM, Workowski K. Treatment of sexually transmitted diseases in women. *Obstet Gynecol Clin North Am* 2003;30:451–475.

17. Anonymous. Guidelines for the prevention and control of congenital syphilis. *MMWR Recomm Rep* 1988;37[Suppl 1]:1–13.

18. Kiss H, Widhalm A, Geusau A, et al. Universal antenatal screening for syphilis: is it still justified economically? A 10-year retrospective analysis. *Eur J Obstet Gynecol Reprod Biol* 2004;112:24–28.

19. Schmid G. Economic and programmatic aspects of congenital syphilis prevention. *Bull World Health Organ* 2004;82:402–409.

12

Gonorrhea

R. Phillip Heine

Michael J. Paglia

■ What Is the Problem that Requires Screening?

Infectious anogenital gonorrhea.

What is the incidence/prevalence of the target condition?

Neisseria gonorrhea continues to be a major public health issue worldwide. This remains true in the United States despite a decline in the number of reported cases since 1981.[1] In the United States, the annual rate of reported cases is 125 cases per 100,000 population. Non-Hispanic black women in the United States aged 15 to 19 years have the highest rate of any racial/age group (3.3/100,000).[2] The highest rates of disease occur in women aged 15 to 19 years who are poor, of minority race,[3,4] unmarried, promiscuous, and exposed to other sexually transmitted diseases (STDs).

The prevalence of positive cultures for *N. gonorrhea* varies with the population screened. During pregnancy, the prevalence of gonorrhea ranges from 0% to 10%.[5] In the STD clinics of major cities, 9% of patients test positive for gonorrhea.[6] In contrast, the prevalence among US adults is 0.4%[4]

What are the sequelae of the condition that are of interest in clinical medicine?

Infertility, sepsis, pelvic inflammatory disease, ectopic pregnancies, chronic pelvic pain, and perinatal complications including preterm rupture of the membranes and neonatal conjunctivitis all may result from a gonorrhea infection.[1] Gonorrhea is transmitted almost entirely by sexual contact. In the female, the primary site is the columnar epithelium of the endocervical canal. Ten to seventy percent of women with acute salpingitis have *N. gonorrhea* isolated from their cervices.[7] Half of the women with gonococcal cervicitis develop rectal infection with or without a history of penile–anal contact.[8] Disseminated gonococcal infection develops in 0.2% to 1.9% of women with mucosal infection.[9] Disseminated gonococcal infection typically occurs during menstruation and late pregnancy and commonly manifests as a dermatitis–tenosynovitis syndrome or a septic arthritis syndrome. Gonococcal endocarditis, meningitis, and osteomyelitis are each rare manifestations of disseminated gonococcal infection. Several investigators have identified an association between untreated maternal endocervical gonorrhea and perinatal complications, including an increased risk of preterm rupture of the membranes, preterm delivery, chorioamnionitis, neonatal conjunctivitis and sepsis, and maternal postpartum infection.[10,11]

■ The Tests

Culture of *N. gonorrhea* from potentially infected sites remains the gold standard for diagnosis. Specimens for culture should be collected from the endocervix and the urethra. The rectum and pharynx should also be cultured when a sexual history suggests it is appropriate. In the United States, the Centers for Disease Control and Prevention (CDC) recommends culture as the primary test due to its low cost and the ability to monitor for antimicrobial resistance.[12]

What is the purpose of the tests?

To detect women with *N. Gonorrhea* infection who are thus potential transmitters of the disease and at risk of the previously noted medical complications. Because most nonpregnant and pregnant women are asymptomatic,[4] obstetric, gynecologic and family planning clinics with high-prevalence populations culture routinely. Where routine screening is not practiced, high-risk women should be screened. Women at high risk of infection with *N. gonorrhea* include drug users, women with prior STDs or multiple sexual partners, and women who exchange sex for money or drugs. High-risk pregnant women should be screened at their initial visit and periodically thereafter.[1] Because co-infection rates are as high as 70%, women positive for *N. gonorrhea* should also be screened for other STDs including *Chlamydia trachomatis*.[4,6]

What is the nature of the tests?

Methods for the diagnosis of *N. gonorrhea* include culture in Thayer-Martin media, Gram stain, detection of the gonococcal antigen by enzyme-linked immune assays (EIAs), nucleic acid hybridization (GEN-PROBE), and nucleic acid amplification tests. Thayer-Martin broth consists of a medium base supplemented with bovine erythrocytes and contains vancomycin, colistin, and nystatin. Gram stain is not recommended for testing.[12] Although EIA is highly specific (97%) for the detection of gonococcal antigen, it is only 60% sensitive.[12] Nucleic acid hybridization has excellent sensitivity and specificity,[13] but is more costly and no more accurate than culture. Therefore, the laboratory diagnosis of *N. gonorrhea* is best accomplished by isolating the organism on a selective medium such as Thayer-Martin broth. Because a small percentage of

N. gonorrhea is sensitive to vancomycin, simultaneous use of a nonselective media such as chocolate blood agar with Thayer-Martin increases the yield.

Nucleic acid amplification tests can be performed on a urine sample or an endocervical sample. This test amplifies nucleic acid sequences specific for the organism being tested. The sensitivity of this test is estimated to be 97%,[14] although sensitivities are lower in urine than endocervical samples. Most CDC consultants believe that nonnucleic acid amplification tests are substantially less sensitive than nucleic acid amplification tests on urine samples.[12] This test does not require the presence of live organisms and for accurate test results requires only a small number of organisms. In addition, this test can be easily performed in places where obtaining cervical samples is not possible.[1] A drawback of this test is the inability to determine antibiotic sensitivities of the organism and its cost.

What are the implications of testing?

What does an abnormal test result mean? A positive culture for *N. gonorrhea* is diagnostic of infection and mandates treatment. The CDC recommends treatment for women diagnosed with *N. gonorrhea* and their sexual partners from the past 60 days.[14] Intercourse should be avoided for 7 days after treatment. The CDC recommends that all subjects treated for gonorrhea should also be treated for *C. trachomatis* as well.[14] The β-lactamase–resistant antimicrobial agents are now the preferred treatment with the emergence of resistant strains of *N. gonorrhea*. Ceftriaxone, an extended-spectrum cephalosporin with a long serum half-life and high bactericidal blood levels, provides a cure rate of 99% for treatment of uncomplicated urogenital and anogenital gonorrhea.[15] Presumptive treatment for chlamydial infection is indicated. The fluoroquinolones may also be used for a single-dose treatment, but are generally considered contraindicated in pregnancy.[1] Decreased susceptibility to fluoroquinolone antibiotics is reported in some regions.[2] Treatment reduces the risk of long-term complications.

What does a normal test result mean? Although no test is a 100% sensitive or specific, a negative culture for *N. gonorrhea* or a negative antigen test effectively excludes the diagnosis.

What is the cost of testing?

Culture is inexpensive to perform with laboratory materials costing less than $0.25 per test. Personnel time to read the culture and characterize the organism is the most expensive aspects of culture. Subject charges vary depending on location and range from free at health departments to approximately $30 (many university student health services). Total charges for antigen detection and nucleic acid detection are consistently higher than culture.

■ Conclusions and Recommendations

All high-risk women should be screened for *N. gonorrhea* because its identification and treatment reduce medical complications and is cost-effective. Those patients testing positive as well as any recent sexual contacts should be treated for *N. gonorrhea* and presumptive chlamydial infection. In addition, patients with gonorrhea should have serologic testing for syphilis as well as human immunodeficiency virus (HIV) infection, subject to appropriate counseling.

■ Summary

1 ■ What Is the Problem that Requires Screening?

Infectious anogenital gonorrhea

a. *What is the incidence/prevalence of the target condition?*

The prevalence of reported cases is 125 cases per 100,000 population. In pregnancy, the prevalence of gonorrhea ranges from 0.5% to 5% depending on the populations screened.

b. *What are the sequelae of the condition that are of interest in clinical medicine?*

In 10% to 20% of infected women, failure to seek treatment or inadequate treatment of an initial gonococcal infection results in ascending infection of the upper reproductive tract. Several investigators have identified an association between untreated maternal endocervical gonorrhea and poor pregnancy outcome, including preterm birth, neonatal conjunctivitis and sepsis, and maternal postpartum infection.

2 ■ The Tests

Culture of *N. gonorrhea* from potentially infected sites is the gold standard for diagnosis.

a. *What is the purpose of the tests?*

To detect women with *N. gonorrhea* infection.

b. What is the nature of the tests?

Methods for the diagnosis of *N. gonorrhea* include Gram stain, detection of the gonococcal antigen by EIA, nucleic acid hybridization, and culture in Thayer-Martin media.

c. What are the implications of testing?

1. What does an abnormal test result mean?

   A positive culture for *N. gonorrhea is* diagnostic of infection and mandates treatment of the infected individual and her recent sexual contacts. Treatment reduces the risk of sequelae.

2. What does a normal test result mean?

   A negative culture for *N. gonorrhea* excludes the diagnosis.

d. What is the cost of testing?

Testing for gonorrhea is inexpensive.

3 ■ Conclusions and Recommendations

All high-risk women should be screened for *N. gonorrhea* during pregnancy. If the prevalence of gonorrhea exceeds 1%, screening during pregnancy is cost-effective and should be performed.

References

1. Campos-Outcalt D. Sexually transmitted disease: easier screening tests, single-dose therapies. *J Fam Pract* 2003;52:965–969.
2. Groseclose SL, Brathwaite WS, Hall PA, et al. Summary of notifiable diseases—United States, 2002. *MMWR Recomm Rep* 2004;51:53–84.
3. Anonymous. Gonorrhea—United States, 1998. *MMWR Recomm Rep* 2000;49:538–542.
4. Miller WC, Ford CA, Morris M, et al. Prevalence of chlamydial and gonococcal infections among young adults in the United States. *JAMA* 2004;291:2229–2236.
5. Miller JM, Jr., Maupin RT, Mestad RE, et al. Initial and repeated screening for gonorrhea during pregnancy. *Sex Transm Dis* 2003;30:928–930.
6. Lyss SB, Kamb ML, Peterman TA, et al. Chlamydia trachomatis among patients infected with and treated for *Neisseria gonorrhoeae* in sexually transmitted disease clinics in the United States [see comment]. *Ann Intern Med* 2003;139:378–385.
7. Holmes KK, Eschenbach DA, Knapp JS. Salpingitis: overview of etiology and epidemiology. *Am J Obstet Gynecol* 1980;138:893–900.
8. Dans PE. Gonococcal anogenital infection. *Clin Obstet Gynecol* 1975;18:103–119.
9. Ross JD. Systemic gonococcal infection. *Genitourin Med* 1996;72:604–607.
10. Edwards LE, Barrada MI, Hamann AA, et al. Gonorrhea in pregnancy. *Am J Obstet Gynecol* 1978;132:637–641.

11. Amstey MS, Steadman KT. Asymptomatic gonorrhea and pregnancy. *J Am Vener Dis Assoc* 1976;3:14–16.
12. Johnson RE, Newhall WJ, Papp JR, et al. Screening tests to detect *Chlamydia trachomatis* and *Neisseria gonorrhoeae* infections—2002. *MMWR Recomm Rep* 2002;51:1–38.
13. Hosein IK, Kaunitz AM, Craft SJ. Detection of cervical *Chlamydia trachomatis* and *Neisseria gonorrhoeae* with deoxyribonucleic acid probe assays in obstetric patients. *Am J Obstet Gynecol* 1992;167:388–391.
14. Anonymous. Sexually transmitted treatment guidelines 2002: Centers for Disease Control and Prevention. *MMWR Recomm Rep* 2002;51:1–78.
15. Moran JS, Levine WC. Drugs of choice for the treatment of uncomplicated gonococcal infections. *Clin Infect Dis* 1995;20:S47–65.

13

Chlamydial Infection

R. Phillip Heine

Michael J. Paglia

■ What Is the Problem that Requires Screening?

Urogenital tract chlamydial infection.

What is the incidence/prevalence of the target condition?

Urogenital tract chlamydial infection is the most common bacterial sexually transmitted disease in the United States.[1] The rate of chlamydial infection is double that of gonorrhea.[2] The reported rates of *Chlamydia trachomatis* are rising.[3] A recent nationwide study of young adults found a 4.7% prevalence of *C. trachomatis* among women. The rate was two times higher in the Southern United States than in the Northeast.[4] The prevalence of chlamydial infection varies with the population tested. Among US female college students, the chlamydial rate ranged from 2% to 7%. Rates ranging between 6% and 20% are reported among men and women attending sexually transmitted disease (STD) clinics or entering a correctional facility.[5,6] More than 834,000 US cases of *C. trachomatis* were reported in 2002.[2] Chlamydial infection among women is higher in the young (<25 years, and especially <20 years), the poor, the unmarried, black race, those who had first intercourse at an early age, oral contraceptive users, and women with multiple sex partners.[7] Among race groups, young adult black women have the highest prevalence (14%) compared with white women, who have the lowest prevalence (3%).[4]

The single factor most strongly associated with infection is young age.[8] Younger women have a higher level of sexual activity and have a larger cervical target area for infection.[9] A recent report from five public STD clinics found that 42% of women with laboratory-confirmed *Neisseriae gonorrhea* also had *C. trachomatis*.[10] Even higher rates of co-infection were found in one national cohort study.[4]

The prevalence of chlamydial infection of the endocervix in pregnant women ranges from 2% to 37%.[11–13] A recent screening program among pregnant women from Mississippi found a 5% rate.[14]

What are the sequelae of the condition that are of interest in clinical medicine?

Numerous clinical conditions are attributed to C. *trachomatis*. They include acute urethral syndrome, urethritis, mucopurulent endocervicitis, salpingitis, bartholinitis, perihepatitis (Fitz-Hugh-Curtis syndrome), endometritis, reactive arthritis, and antenatal infection.[15] The endocervix is the organ most commonly infected in the female.

In the 1970s, Swedish investigators began the laparoscopic biopsy of the fallopian tubes in women with presumed pelvic inflammatory disease (PID). Their results suggested that C. *trachomatis* caused up to a third of all PID cases.[16] In the United States, rigorous studies using endometrial biopsy, laparoscopy, and fallopian tube plus endocervical cultures yielded similar conclusions.[17] Acute PID increases the risk of chronic pelvic pain, infertility, and ectopic pregnancy.[18,19] Up to one third of cases of ectopic pregnancy may be due to chlamydial infection.[20] Many experts believe that C. *trachomatis* is the most important organism involved in tubal scarring, because it appears to cause a mild form of PID associated with delayed diagnosis and treatment.[21]

C. *trachomatis* infection during pregnancy increases the risk of preterm labor, premature rupture of membranes, neonatal death, low birth weight, and postpartum endometritis.[22,23] Treatment of infected women may improve their obstetric outcome.[24,25] An infant can become infected with C. *trachomatis* during delivery.[26] Up to 75% of newborns delivered vaginally to infected women acquire C. *trachomatis* at some anatomic site. Conjunctivitis occurs within the first 2 weeks of life in 30% to 50% of exposed infants; pneumonia occurs within 3 to 4 months in 10% to 20% of exposed infants.[5,13]

■ The Tests

What is the purpose of the tests?

The detection of urogenital chlamydial infection in asymptomatic and symptomatic women.

What is the nature of the tests?

Methods used for the detection of chlamydial infection include tissue culture isolation of the organism (the gold standard), direct fluorescent antibody (DFA) test, enzyme-linked immune assay (EIA) test, nucleic acid hybridization (GEN-PROBE), and amplification techniques, including nucleic acid amplification tests, such as polymerase chain reaction (PCR), ligase chain reaction (LCR), and transcription-mediated amplification of RNA.

The currently accepted standard laboratory test for the detection of C. *trachomatis* is culture in mammalian cell lines. Centrifugation and sensitization of cell monolayers to the polycation diethylaminoethyl (DEAE) before inoculation improve the yield. In addition to proper technique, special precautions must be taken to properly collect and transport clinical specimens.

Wooden swabs containing chemicals toxic to cell cultures must be avoided; the tips of the swabs should be constructed of Dacron. Because *C. trachomatis* is sensitive to temperature and looses viability rapidly at room temperature, specimens should be refrigerated at 4°C (39.2°F). The specimen should then either be transported to the laboratory within 24 hours or frozen at −70°C (−158°F) and shipped on dry ice. These requirements make tissue culture isolation of *C. trachomatis* cumbersome, difficult to standardize, and expensive.[3]

The nonculture diagnostic tests commonly used for the detection of *C. trachomatis* include antigen detection tests such as EIA and DFA, nucleic acid hybridization (e.g., GEN-PROBE), and amplification techniques such as PCR or LCR. EIA detects specific chlamydial antigens. DFA uses fluorescein-conjugated monoclonal antibodies, which bind specifically to bacterial antigens in smears. The sensitivity of this test ranges from 68% to 100%, although its specificity is more than 95%.[31,32] DFA has the advantages of no special storage or transportation techniques, a rapid result, and lower costs compared with culture. Its disadvantages include a higher false-positive rate and the need for an experienced microscopist.[3]

Enzyme immunoassays are often used to detect *C. trachomatis* antigens. The sensitivity of EIA ranges from 64% to 100%, whereas its specificity ranges from 89% to 100%.[31] Cross-reactivity with antigenic components of gram-negative organisms is reported.[3] EIA test results are available within 4 hours, are objectively interpreted, and require less expertise than DFA or cell culture. In addition, the specimens can be stored for more than 7 days before running the test.[3]

Nucleic acid probes are also available for the detection of *C. trachomatis*. A study comparing two such probes, the MicroTrak EIA and the GEN-PROBE Pace 2 with cell culture revealed that both assays were less sensitive than culture.[33] The sensitivity (with culture as the gold standard) for the GEN-PROBE ranges from 80% to 95%, whereas the specificity is more than 95%.[33] The positive and negative predictive values are 90% to 94%.

Nucleic acid amplification tests are designed to amplify nucleic acid sequences that are specific for the organism to be detected. These tests do not require viable organisms. A positive signal can be produced from as little as a single copy of target DNA or RNA, which increases the sensitivity of these tests. Nucleic acid amplification tests can detect *C. trachomatis* from endocervical swabs and from urine. Nucleic acid amplification tests are thought to be considerably more sensitive on urine than non–nucleic acid amplification tests.[3] The sensitivity of PCR approaches 100% compared with that of cell culture.[34] PCR is easily performed and can be analyzed within 1 day. Detection of infection by amplification techniques on urine specimens is noninvasive. The main disadvantages of amplification techniques is the need for a suitable laboratory and the relatively high cost of the tests.[3]

The US Centers for Disease Control and Prevention (CDC) recommends that a nucleic acid amplification test performed on an endocervical swab (if a pelvic examination is required) be used as a first-line test to screen women for chlamydial infection because it provides the highest sensitivity; otherwise, a Nucleic acid amplification test can be performed on urine, which allows for testing in places where pelvic examinations are not performed. EIAs and DFAs performed on an endocervical swab are acceptable screens, although they are less sensitive. The CDC states that culture too is suitable for screening, but it does not have as high a sensitivity as nucleic acid amplification tests and can be a difficult to perform well.[3]

Swabs of the vaginal introitus have shown a higher sensitivity (92%) for the detection of *C. trachomatis* using PCR then swabs of the cervix or urethra. The sensitivity of PCR on urine samples is 73%. Patient self-collection of introital specimens may present an even better and less-invasive opportunity to collect a sensitive specimen to screen for *C. trachomatis*.[35]

Most chlamydial infections (>85%) are asymptomatic.[27] Detection requires screening at the time of a pelvic examination. More than 50% of endocervical chlamydial infections are unassociated with a clinically detectable inflammatory response.[28] Brunham et al.[29] noted that a yellow discharge on a swab and/or ten or more white blood cells per oil immersion field on a Gram-stained smear of endocervical secretions strongly correlates with chlamydial cervical infection. These observations apply to pregnant women, although the predictive value of clinical cervicitis for chlamydial infection during pregnancy appears lower than in nonpregnant women.[30]

What are the implications of testing?

What does an abnormal test result mean? The woman has been infected with *C. trachomatis*. She should be counseled and appropriately treated as should any recent sex partners to prevent reinfection. The recommended treatment for uncomplicated urethral, endocervical or rectal chlamydial infection in the non-pregnant patient is doxycycline, 100 mg orally twice daily for 7 days, or azithromycin, 1 g orally in a single dose. The results of a randomized trial demonstrated equal efficacy with cure rates greater than 95%.[36] Women should not resume intercourse until either the completion of the 7-day course or 7 days after the one-time dose.[1] During pregnancy the following can be used: either erythromycin base, 500 mg orally four times daily for 7 days; amoxicillin, 500 mg orally three times daily for 7 to 10 days, or, azithromycin 1 g orally. Azithromycin has a cure rate similar to the other treatments.[37,38]

The patient should be tested for other sexually transmitted diseases including syphilis, gonorrhea, and human immunodeficiency virus (HIV), subject to appropriate counseling. A "test of cure" is not necessary after treatment unless a patient presents with symptoms, reinfection is suspected, or there is doubt about patient treatment compliance. Pregnant women are an exception to this rule.[1,3]

What does a normal test result mean? The woman is not infected with *C. trachomatis*.

What is the cost of testing?

The total cost (direct and indirect) of female urogenital chlamydial infection is estimated to exceed $2 billion per year.[39,40] Women who are culture-positive for *C. trachomatis* frequently have other sexually transmitted diseases.

In low-prevalence populations, several investigators have shown that targeted screening based on risk factors is less costly than routine screening and would detect more than 90% of cases.[41,42] These risk factors include cervical friability, a suspicious discharge, urinary frequency, intermenstrual bleeding, and a new sex partner within the past year. A study reporting a high rate of *C. trachomatis* (24.1%) in young, inner-city women was the basis for the recommendation that young, sexually active women be screened every 6 months.[43]

In a recent study, sensitivity analyses were performed to determine the robustness of incremental cost-effectiveness ratios to changes in the incidence of long-term sequelae and costs.[44] The prevalence of infection was determined by nucleic acid amplification of urine samples or endocervical swabs. Knowledge of chlamydial infection and women's views of screening were determined using structured questionnaires. The estimated cost of screening 250 women in each age group in each of the four sample populations (total population of 3,750) is £49,367 sterling, while preventing 64 major sequelae. This represents a net cost of £771.36 in preventing one major sequela. Targeted screening of all women younger than 20 years and all women attending abortion clinics were shown to be the most cost-effective strategies. These results were relatively insensitive to changes in estimated parameters, such as uptake rate, probabilities, and unit costs of all major sequelae averted.

■ Conclusions and Recommendations

C. trachomatis is the cause of several, common sexually transmitted disease syndromes, including mucopurulent cervicitis, urethritis, and pelvic inflammatory disease. There is strong evidence that *C. trachomatis* is a cause of obstructive infertility and ectopic pregnancy and that these complications reflect chronic inflammation and secondary scarring elicited by long-term, relatively asymptomatic infection. The total cost of disease is high. Because treatment with tetracycline, erythromycin, or azithromycin is simple, effective, and inexpensive, major efforts should be made to identify infected but asymptomatic women. High-risk categories include sexually active young women, black women, and women with multiple sex partners. Selective screening based on risk factors is effective even in low-prevalence settings. Male sex partners of infected women must also be treated, and these women should be screened for other sexually transmitted diseases, subject to appropriate counseling.

■ **Summary**

1 ■ **What Is the problem that requires screening?**

Chlamydial infection

a. *What is the incidence/prevalence of the target condition?*
Chlamydial infection is the most common sexually transmitted disease in the United States. Risks of chlamydial infection include age, socioeconomic status, number of sex partners, and use of nonbarrier contraception. Up to 70% of infants delivered vaginally to women with chlamydial infection acquire the infection.

b. *What are the sequelae of the condition that are of interest in clinical medicine?*
Acute urethral syndrome, urethritis, mucopurulent endocervicitis, salpingitis, endometritis, and prenatal infections are attributed to *C. trachomatis*. Most chlamydial infections are asymptomatic.

2 ■ **The Tests**

a. *What is the purpose of the tests?*
To detect urogenital chlamydial infection.

b. *What is the nature of the tests?*
The CDC recommends a nucleic acid amplification test as a first-line test, either using an endocervical specimen or the woman's urine. Other approved tests include EIAs and DFAs. Although culture is suitable for screening, it can be a difficult test to perform and should not be frontline.

c. *What are the implications of testing?*
1. What does an abnormal test result mean?
   The woman has an infection with *C. trachomatis*.
2. What does a normal test result mean?
   The woman is not infected with *C. trachomatis*.

d. *What is the cost of testing?*
The total cost of chlamydial infection in women has been projected at over $2 billion per year.

3 ■ Conclusions and Recommendations

C. trachomatis causes a number of common sexually transmitted disease syndromes, including mucopurulent cervicitis, urethritis, and pelvic inflammatory disease. High-risk categories include sexually active young women, older women who are not monogamous, and unmarried pregnant women. Male sex partners of infected women must also be treated to prevent reinfection, and infected women should be screened for other sexually transmitted diseases, subject to appropriate counseling.

References

1. Anonymous. Sexually tranmitted treatment guidelines 2002: Centers for Disease Control and Prevention. *MMWR Recomm Rep* 2002;51[RR-6]:1–78.
2. Anonymous. STD Surveillance 2002: Centers for Disease Prevention. 2002.
3. Johnson RE, Newhall WJ, Papp JR, et al. Screening tests to detect *Chlamydia trachomatis* and *Neisseria gonorrhoeae* infections: 2002. *MMWR Recomm Rep* 2002;51:1–38.
4. Miller WC, Ford CA, Morris M, et al. Prevalence of chlamydial and gonococcal infections among young adults in the United States. *JAMA* 2004;291:2229–2236.
5. Holmes KK, Mardh PA, Sparling PF, eds. *Sexually Transmitted Diseases*, 3rd edition. New York: McGraw-Hill, 1999.
6. Hardick J, Hsieh YH, Tulloch S, et al. Surveillance of *Chlamydia trachomatis* and *Neisseria gonorrhoeae* infections in women in detention in Baltimore, Maryland. *Sex Transm Dis* 2003;30:64–70.
7. Gaydos CA, Howell MR, Pare B, et al. *Chlamydia trachomatis* infections in female military recruits. *N Engl J Med* 1998;339:739–744.
8. Gaydos CA, Howell MR, Quinn TC, et al. Sustained high prevalence of *Chlamydia trachomatis* infections in female army recruits. *Sex Transm Dis* 2003;30:539–544.
9. Faro S, Soper DE, eds. *Infectious Diseases in Women*. Philadelphia: WB Saunders, 2001.
10. Lyss SB, Kamb ML, Peterman TA, et al. *Chlamydia trachomatis* among patients infected with and treated for *Neisseria gonorrhoeae* in sexually transmitted disease clinics in the United States. *Ann Int Med* 2003;139:378–385.
11. FitzSimmons J, Callahan C, Shanahan B, et al. Chlamydial infections in pregnancy. *J Reprod Med* 1986;31:19–22.
12. Sweet RL, Landers DV, Walker C, et al. *Chlamydia trachomatis* infection and pregnancy outcome. *Am J Obstet Gynecol* 1987;156:424–433.
13. Schachter J, Grossman M, Sweet RL, et al. Prospective study of perinatal transmission of *Chlamydia trachomatis*. *JAMA* 1986;255:3374–3377.
14. Rivlin ME, Morrison JC, Grossman JH III. Comparison of pregnancy outcome between treated and untreated women with chlamydial cervicitis. *J Miss State Med Assoc* 1997;38:404–407.
15. Peipert JF. Genital chlamydial infections. *N Engl J Med* 2003;349:2424–2430.
16. Mardh PA, Ripa T, Svensson L, et al. *Chlamydia trachomatis* infection in patients with acute salpingitis. *N Engl J Med* 1977;296:1377–1379.
17. Wasserheit JN, Bell TA, Kiviat NB, et al. Microbial causes of proven pelvic inflammatory disease and efficacy of clindamycin and tobramycin. *Ann Intern Med* 1986;104:287–293.
18. Svensson L, Mardh PA, Westrom L. Infertility after acute salpingitis with special reference to *Chlamydia trachomatis*. *Fertil Steril* 1983;40:322–329.
19. Westrom L. Incidence, prevalence, and trends of acute pelvic inflammatory disease and its consequences in industrialized countries. *Am J Obstet Gynecol* 1980;138:880–892.

20. Paavonen J, Eggert-Kruse W. *Chlamydia trachomatis*: impact on human reproduction. *Hum Reprod Update* 1999;5:433–447.

21. Svensson L, Westrom L, Ripa KT, et al. Differences in some clinical and laboratory parameters in acute salpingitis related to culture and serologic findings. *Am J Obstet Gynecol* 1980;138: 1017–1021.

22. Mardh PA. Influence of infection with *Chlamydia trachomatis* on pregnancy outcome, infant health and life-long sequelae in infected offspring. *Best Pract Res Clin Obstet Gynaecol* 2002;16:647–664.

23. Andrews WW, Goldenberg RL, Mercer B, et al. The Preterm Prediction Study: association of second-trimester genitourinary chlamydia infection with subsequent spontaneous preterm birth. *Am J Obstet Gynecol* 2000;183:662–668.

24. Ryan GM, Jr., Abdella TN, McNeeley SG, et al. *Chlamydia trachomatis* infection in pregnancy and effect of treatment on outcome. *Am J Obstet Gynecol* 1990;162:34–39.

25. Cohen I, Veille JC, Calkins BM. Improved pregnancy outcome following successful treatment of chlamydial infection. *JAMA* 1990;263:3160–3163.

26. Jain S. Perinatally acquired *Chlamydia trachomatis* associated morbidity in young infants. *J Matern Fetal Med* 1999;8:130–133.

27. Cecil JA, Howell MR, Tawes JJ, et al. Features of *Chlamydia trachomatis* and *Neisseria gonorrhoeae* infection in male Army recruits. *J Infect Dis* 2001;184:1216–1219.

28. Harrison HR, Costin M, Meder JB, et al. Cervical *Chlamydia trachomatis* infection in university women: relationship to history, contraception, ectopy, and cervicitis. *Am J Obstet Gynecol* 1985;153:244–251.

29. Brunham RC, Paavonen J, Stevens CE, et al. Mucopurulent cervicitis: the ignored counterpart in women of urethritis in men. *N Engl J Med* 1984;311:1–6.

30. Kiviat NB, Paavonen JA, Brockway J, et al. Cytologic manifestations of cervical and vaginal infections, I: epithelial and inflammatory cellular changes. *JAMA* 1985;253:989–996.

31. Taylor-Robinson D, Thomas BJ. Laboratory techniques for the diagnosis of chlamydial infections. *Genitourin Med* 1991;67:256–266.

32. Barnes RC. Laboratory diagnosis of human chlamydial infections. *Clin Microbiol Rev* 1989;2:219–236.

33. Clarke LM, Sierra MF, Daidone BJ, et al. Comparison of the Syva MicroTrak enzyme immunoassay and Gen-Probe PACE 2 with cell culture for diagnosis of cervical *Chlamydia trachomatis* infection in a high-prevalence female population. *J Clin Microbiol* 1993;31:968–971.

34. Ostergaard L, Birkelund S, Christiansen G. Use of polymerase chain reaction for detection of *Chlamydia trachomatis*. *J Clin Microbiol* 1990;28:1254–1260.

35. Wiesenfeld HC, Heine RP, Rideout A, et al. The vaginal introitus: a novel site for *Chlamydia trachomatis* testing in women. *Am J Obstet Gynecol* 1996;174:1542–1546.

36. Martin DH, Mroczkowski TF, Dalu ZA, et al. A controlled trial of a single dose of azithromycin for the treatment of chlamydial urethritis and cervicitis: the Azithromycin for Chlamydial Infections Study Group. *N Engl J Med* 1992;327:921–925.

37. Jacobson GF, Autry AM, Kirby RS, et al. A randomized controlled trial comparing amoxicillin and azithromycin for the treatment of *Chlamydia trachomatis* in pregnancy. *Am J Obstet Gynecol* 2001;184:1352–1354.

38. Kacmar J, Cheh E, Montango A, et al. A randomized trial of azithromycin versus amoxicillin for the treatment of *Chlamydia trachomatis* in pregnancy. *Infect Dis Obstet Gynecol* 2001;9:197–202.

39. Eng TR, Butler WT. *The Hidden Epidemic: Confronting Sexually Transmitted Diseases*. Washington, DC: National Academy Press, 1997.

40. Washington AE, Johnson RE, Sanders LL, Jr. *Chlamydia trachomatis* infections in the United States. What are they costing us? *JAMA* 1987;257:1070–1072.

41. Phillips RS, Aronson MD, Taylor WC, et al. Should tests for *Chlamydia trachomatis* cervical infection be done during routine gynecologic visits? An analysis of the costs of alternative strategies. *Ann Int Med* 1987;107:288–294.

42. Sellors JW, Pickard L, Gafni A, et al. Effectiveness and efficiency of selective vs universal screening for chlamydial infection in sexually active young women. *Arch Int Med* 1992;152:1837–1844.

43. Burstein GR, Gaydos CA, Diener-West M, et al. Incident *Chlamydia trachomatis* infections among inner-city adolescent females. *JAMA* 1998;280:621–626.
44. Norman JE, Wu O, Twaddle S, et al. An evaluation of economics and acceptability of screening for *Chlamydia trachomatis* infection, in women attending antenatal, abortion, colposcopy and family planning clinics in Scotland. *Br J Obstet Gynaecol* 2004;111:1261–1268.

14

HIV Infection

R. Phillip Heine

Michael J. Paglia

■ What Is the Problem that Requires Screening?

Adult and perinatal transmission of human immunodeficiency virus (HIV).

What is the incidence/prevalence of the target condition?

At the end of 2002, an estimated 384,906 persons were known to be living with acquired immunodeficiency syndrome (AIDS)[1] and an additional 143,904 living with HIV infection.[2] The prevalence rate of HIV infection among adults was 126/100,000, and for children, it was 6/100,000. The prevalence AIDS rate is higher in men (23/100,000) than it is in women (8/100,000). It varies significantly with age group. It is 1.2/100,000 in children younger than 1 year, 4.7/100,000 for people 15 to 24 years old, and 32/100,000 for people 25 to 39 years old.[1] There is a large racial discrepancy in the rate of AIDS between blacks and whites. The rate of AIDS among blacks is 63/100,000, whereas in whites, it is 7/100,000.[2] Thirty-five percent of all new HIV cases result from heterosexual sex, 64% of these cases occur in women.[3] Seventy percent of HIV/AIDS in women result from heterosexual contact. The second major route of transmission is intravenous drug use.[2] The prevalence of AIDS in the United States has gradually declined over the years,[2] peaking in 1993 at 40/100,000; it was 15/100,000 in 2002.

The US Centers for Disease Control and Prevention (CDC) estimates that there are 280 to 370 cases of perinatal HIV transmission in the United States annually. Maternal to fetal transmission rates are 25% to 35% when there is no treatment during pregnancy.[4–6] The rate of transmission to infants by infected mothers increases with the clinical severity of maternal disease and is inversely proportional to the maternal CD4 cell count.[7] Disease progression in infants varies directly with the disease severity in the mother at the time of delivery.[8] Factors that may increase the perinatal transmission of HIV include CD4 cell counts of less than 400/mm[7] and advanced maternal AIDS-defining illnesses.[9] Perinatal transmission is greatly reduced by antepartum antiretroviral treatment and intrapartum treatment of previously untreated women.[10]

What are the sequelae of the condition that are of interest in clinical medicine?

The spread of infection to sexual partners and offspring. HIV infection leads to a progressive debilitation of the immune system. An HIV-infected patient is diagnosed as having AIDS when there is one of several specific opportunistic infections or neoplasias such as cervical cancer, pulmonary tuberculosis, recurrent bacterial pneumonia, dementia and encephalopathy, wasting syndrome, or CD4 cell counts of less than 200/uL.[11]

Forty to ninety percent of subjects with primary HIV infection experience acute retroviral syndrome. Symptoms typically occur 2 to 6 weeks after exposure and may include night sweats, fever, weight loss, headaches, nausea, and diarrhea.[12,13] Subjects may present with a rash, mucosal ulcers, and lymphadenopathy. Laboratory tests may show thrombocytopenia, mild elevation in transaminases, and leukopenia. One study noted that one fourth of individuals with these symptoms were correctly diagnosed.[13] There is considerable debate as to whether a patient with primary HIV infection should start on antiretroviral therapy. It is important for the clinician to initiate counseling and education for prevention of further HIV transmission. It is optimal at this time to offer testing to any recent sexual partners.[14]

Early clinical manifestations of HIV infection in women may center on the genital tract. They include vulvovaginal candidiasis, pelvic inflammatory disease (PID), and cervical dysplasia.[15–17] The medical management of vaginal candidiasis is unaltered by HIV serologic status, and cure rates are similar to those of seronegative women.[18] PID may follow a more aggressive course in HIV-infected women. Studies have shown that the symptoms and the response to antibiotics are similar between HIV-positive and HIV-negative patients. It is still unknown whether HIV-positive women need more aggressive treatment for PID.[18] The risks of HPV infection and cervical dysplasia are higher in HIV-infected women.[19]

▓ The Tests

What is the purpose of the tests?

To detect HIV-Infected individuals.

What is the nature of the tests?

There are three screening assays for the identification of HIV infection: enzyme-linked immunosorbent assay (ELISA), the rapid latex agglutination assay, and the dot-blot immunobinding assay (HIV CHEK). The three known confirmatory assays for HIV are Western blot (WB), radioimmunoprecipitation assay (RIPA), and indirect immunofluorescence assay (IFA). The use of the ELISA screening test followed by the Western blot confirmatory test is standard for making the diagnosis of HIV in the United States.[20]

The ELISA detects HIV-specific antibodies in the serum. This test is usually negative in patients who present with acute infection. A similar technique, called a capture ELISA, is used to measure the core antigen (p24) of HIV in the plasma of infected individuals. This test is licensed for earlier detection of HIV and is positive before the development of HIV antibodies.[12] To screen for early infection, a plasma HIV viral load can be performed. Patients with acute infection typically have a high viral load, often exceeding 1 million copies per milliliter.[22]

Evidence shows that an increased maternal viral burden, as measured by either PCR or p24 antigenemia, is associated with an increased perinatal transmission risk.[23–26]

Data submitted by the manufacturers indicate that the sensitivities and specificities of the immunoassay tests currently marketed in the United States are all more than 99%.[20] Repeating each initial reactive test increases the validity of the test by decreasing the likelihood of a laboratory error. An ELISA test specificity of 99% has consistently been reported by several laboratories across the United States.[20] The use of the ELISA screening assay along with the Western blot confirmatory test for determining infection with HIV has a positive predictive value of 99.5% in both low-risk and high-risk populations. The combined use of these tests for the diagnosis for HIV yields a false-positive rate of less than one per 1,000 individuals tested.[27]

A reactive Western blot confirmatory test in individuals with two sequentially positive ELISA screening tests requires at least two of three major bands be present: gp160 or gp120, gp41, and p24.[20] The absence of any bands indicates a false-positive result, whereas the presence of a single HIV-1–related band means an indeterminate test.

The CDC recommends that all reproductive-age women at risk of HIV infection, which includes essentially any sexually active woman, be counseled and tested for HIV. Since 1995, the US Public Health Service has recommended universal antenatal HIV counseling and testing for all pregnant women.[28] Risk factors for acquiring HIV infection are listed in Table 14–1.

There are now screening tests that return a result in less than 1 hour. These tests can be used in the labor and delivery unit to screen previously untested women.

Table 14–1   **Risk factors for human immunodeficiency virus**
(a) Multiple sex partners
(b) Illicit drug use
(c) Bisexual activity
(d) History or current sexually transmitted diseases (ulcerative and nonulcerative)
(e) Transfusion of blood or blood products.

What are the implications of testing?

What does an abnormal test result mean? The CDC strongly recommends confirmatory testing on all reactive rapid HIV tests.[21] The woman is infected with HIV when confirmatory testing is positive. She should be counseled and treated with antiretrovirals before delivery to reduce the transmission rate.[20]

An individual with newly diagnosed HIV infection requires specific and extensive counseling at the time the results become known (Table 14–2). It is essential the pregnant woman also receives information on the risk of perinatal transmission and the possible effects of pregnancy on the progression of her disease. Pregnant women with HIV should be offered antiretroviral therapy during the course of the pregnancy. The goal is to reduce their viral load to an undetectable level. The administration of antiretrovirals to the mother during pregnancy, labor, and delivery, and to the newborn for 6 weeks after delivery markedly reduces the risk of perinatal transmission of HIV.[10] Treatment during pregnancy reduces the rate of transmission to less than 2%, compared with a 12% to 13% risk of transmission when treated during labor. Women who receive no preventive treatment have a 25% risk of transmission to their babies.[10]

Data from two prospective cohort studies, a meta-analysis from 15 prospective studies, and an international randomized trial, found a statistically significant relationship between the mode of delivery and transmission of HIV.[29–32] The results of these studies reveal that a scheduled cesarean delivery reduces the likelihood of vertical transmission. The American College of Obstetricians and Gynecologists recommends that all women with a HIV viral load greater than 1,000 copies per milliliter be counseled and advised to undergo a scheduled cesarean delivery. The delivery should be scheduled before 39 weeks' gestation to minimize the risks prior to delivery of labor onset or rupture of membranes. An amniocentesis to check for fetal lung maturity should be avoided.[33] Intravenous zidovudine should be commenced 3 hours prior to surgery. Other antiretroviral agents that the woman has taken for the duration of the pregnancy are also continued.[34] It is uncertain how long the benefit of a cesarean delivery lasts after spontaneous rupture of membranes. Furthermore, it is uncertain whether a scheduled cesarean delivery further reduces the risk of vertical transmission in women with viral loads less than 1,000 copies per milliliter.[33]

Table 14–2 **Contents of human immunodeficiency virus counseling**
(a) Discussion of the early manifestations of HIV infection
(b) Natural history and prognosis of HIV infection
(c) Institution of immediate medical care
(d) Emphasis on responsible sexual behavior and the notification of sex partners as well as avoidance of sharing needles
(e) Prohibition from donating blood
(f) Notification of health care workers concerning the individual's HIV status.

HIV, human immunodeficiency virus.

Long-term follow-up for women with HIV infection should incorporate the medical, gynecological, psychological, and social implications of HIV infection. The CDC recommends Pap smear screening of HIV-infected women at their initial evaluation and 6 months later. Women with two normal pap smears should thereafter have an annual Pap smear. Women with abnormal Pap smears should be treated in the routine fashion.[18] Other needs include appropriate vaccination, antiviral therapy, and prophylactic antibiotic therapy when needed; ongoing counseling about HIV infection; and referral for psychotherapy or peer support group therapy. Issues concerning physical well-being and loss of function, childcare, and custody arrangements, and death and dying should be discussed in patients with advanced HIV disease.[35]

What does a normal test result mean? HIV infection is unlikely, but a negative test result does not exclude infection, as there is a 6- to 12-week window during incubation when a recent infection cannot be detected.[36] Information concerning the risk of a false-negative test should be provided to women with negative test results. The woman should be retested within 6 months if she engages in at-risk behaviors. A discussion of the importance of HIV counseling and testing of her sexual partners is also essential.

Repeated testing is offered to individuals whose test results are inconclusive due to the lack of sufficient criteria for serologic diagnosis. These women will also require counseling and reassurance during this additional waiting period.

What is the cost of testing?

Screening and institution of zidovudine during pregnancy and labor and delivery are cost-beneficial if one takes into account the enormous cost, both economical and social, of newborn and infant morbidity and mortality from perinatal transmission.

■ Conclusions and Recommendations

The rate of HIV infection and AIDS is increasing in reproductive-age women and their children. For this reason, the obstetrician/gynecologist is increasingly assuming a central role in the testing and counseling of women at risk of HIV infection. Standard testing in the United States includes an initial ELISA screen, which should be repeated if positive. No antibody test result is considered a correct positive until a Western blot confirmatory assay has been performed and is reactive.

The counseling of the HIV-infected subject must be comprehensive, including the medical and psychosocial aspects of coping with the disease. Women who test negative for HIV but continue to engage in high-risk behaviors should be offered repeated testing for themselves and their sexual partners within 6 months. There should be an emphasis during their post-test counseling session on the need for responsible sexual behavior and the avoidance of sharing needles.

■ Summary

1 ■ What Is the Problem that Requires Screening?

Adult and perinatal transmission of HIV.

a. What is the incidence/prevalence of the target condition?

Women account for approximately 21% of all reported cases of AIDS. The prevalence of AIDS in the United States is 15/100,000 (2002). Studies show relatively uniform maternal to fetal transmission rates of 25% to 35% when the woman is not treated during pregnancy or during labor.

b. What are the sequelae of the condition that are of interest in clinical medicine?

HIV infection causes progressive debilitation of the immune system. An HIV-infected patient with one of several specific opportunistic infections or neoplasias (such as cervical cancer, tuberculosis, recurrent bacterial pneumonia, dementia, encephalopathy, wasting syndrome or CD4 cell counts of less than 200 mm³ is diagnosed as having AIDS. Early clinical manifestations of HIV infection in women may center on the genital tract. These include vulvovaginal candidiasis, PID, and cervical dysplasia.

2 ■ The Tests

a. What is the purpose of the tests?

To detect individuals infected with HIV.

b. What is the nature of the tests?

The ELISA detects HIV-specific antibodies in the serum of individuals who are tested. An ELISA screening assay coupled to a Western blot test has a positive predictive value of 99.5% in both low-risk and high-risk populations.

c. What are the implications of testing?

1. What does an abnormal test result mean?
   The woman is infected with HIV when confirmatory testing is positive. The diagnosis requires specific and extensive counseling and treatment when the results become known. Long-term follow-up for women with HIV infection should

Continued

■ **Summary—cont'd**

incorporate the medical, gynecological, psychological, and social implications of HIV infection.

2. What does a normal test result mean?
HIV infection is unlikely, but a negative test result does not exclude infection. Repeated testing should be offered to women whose tests are inconclusive. Information concerning false-negative tests should be provided to women whose results are negative.

d. What is the cost of testing?

Screening and institution of zidovudine during pregnancy and labor and delivery is cost-beneficial if one takes into account the enormous cost, both economic and social, of newborn and infant morbidity and mortality from perinatal transmission.

3 ■ Conclusions and Recommendations

The rate of HIV infection and AIDS is increasing in reproductive-age women and their children. Standard testing in the United States includes an initial ELISA screen, which should be repeated if positive. No antibody test result should be considered a correct positive unless a Western blot confirmatory assay has been performed and is reactive. Antiretroviral drugs dramatically reduce the risk of perinatal transmission. All pregnant women should be offered a screening test for HIV, subject to appropriate counseling.

References

1. Groseclose SL, Brathwaite WS, Hall PA, et al. Summary of notifiable diseases–United States, 2002. *MMWR Recomm Rep* 2004;51:531–584.
2. Anonymous. HIV/AIDS Surveillance Report 2002: Centers for Disease Control and Prevention. 2002;14:1–48.
3. Centers for Disease Control and Prevention. Heterosexual transmission of HIV—29 states, 1999–2002. *MMWR Recomm Rep* 2004;53:125–129.
4. Anonymous. Mother-to-child transmission of HIV infection: the European Collaborative Study. *Lancet* 1988;2:1039–1043.
5. Anonymous. Epidemiology, clinical features, and prognostic factors of paediatric HIV infection: Italian Multicentre Study. *Lancet* 1988;2:1043–1046.
6. Cowan MJ, Walker C, Culver K, et al. Maternally transmitted HIV infection in children. *AIDS* 1988;2:437–441.
7. Anonymous. National HIV serosurveillance summary: results through 1990. Atlanta GA; 1991.

8. Blanche S, Mayaux MJ, Rouzioux C, et al. Relation of the course of HIV infection in children to the severity of the disease in their mothers at delivery. *N Engl J Med* 1994;330:308–312.

9. Blanche S, Rouzioux C, Moscato ML, et al. A prospective study of infants born to women seropositive for human immunodeficiency virus type 1: HIV Infection in Newborns French Collaborative Study Group. *N Engl J Med* 1989;320:1643–1648.

10. Anonymous. HIV testing among pregnant women—United States and Canada, 1998–2001. *MMWR Recomm Rep* 2002;51:1013–1016.

11. Anonymous. 1993 revised classification system for HIV infection and expanded surveillance case definition for AIDS among adolescents and adults. *MMWR Recomm Rep* 1992;41:1–19.

12. Kahn JO, Walker BD. Acute human immunodeficiency virus type 1 infection. *N Engl J Med* 1998;339:133–139.

13. Schacker T, Collier AC, Hughes J, et al. Clinical and epidemiologic features of primary HIV infection. *Ann Int Med* 1996;125:257–264.

14. Kassuto S, Rosenberg ES. Primary HIV type 1 Infection. *Clin Infect Dis* 2004;38:1447–1453.

15. Witkin SS. Immunologic factors influencing susceptibility to recurrent candidal vaginitis. *Clin Obst Gynecol* 1991;34:2662–2668.

16. Korn AP, Landers DV, Green JR, et al. Pelvic inflammatory disease in human immunodeficiency virus-infected women. *Obstet Gynecol* 1993;82:765–768.

17. Maiman M, Fruchter RG, Serur E, et al. Human immunodeficiency virus infection and cervical neoplasia. *Gynecol Oncol* 1990;38:377–382.

18. Anonymous. Sexually transmitted treatment guidelines 2002: Centers for Disease Control and Prevention. *MMWR Recomm Rep* 2002;51:1–78.

19. Jay N, Moscicki AB. Human papillomavirus infections in women with HIV disease: prevalence, risk, and management. *AIDS Reader* 2000;10:659–668.

20. Anonymous. Update: serologic testing for antibody to human immunodeficiency virus. *MMWR Recomm Rep* 1988;36:833–840, 845.

21. Anonymous. Notice to readers: protocols for confirmation of reactive rapid HIV tests. *MMWR Recomm Rep* 2004;53:10221–10222.

22. Rosenberg ES, Altfeld M, Poon SH, et al. Immune control of HIV-1 after early treatment of acute infection. *Nature* 2000;407:523–526.

23. Shaffer N, Chuachoowong R, Mock PA, et al. Short-course zidovudine for perinatal HIV-1 transmission in Bangkok, Thailand: a randomised controlled trial. Bangkok Collaborative Perinatal HIV Transmission Study Group. *Lancet* 1999;353:773–780.

24. Mofenson LM, Lambert JS, Stiehm ER, et al. Risk factors for perinatal transmission of human immunodeficiency virus type 1 in women treated with zidovudine. Pediatric AIDS Clinical Trials Group Study 185 Team. *N Engl J Med* 1999;341:6385–6393.

25. Garcia PM, Kalish LA, Pitt J, et al. Maternal levels of plasma human immunodeficiency virus type 1 RNA and the risk of perinatal transmission: Women and Infants Transmission Study Group. *N Engl J Med* 1999;341:394–402.

26. Anonymous. Maternal viral load and vertical transmission of HIV-1: an important factor but not the only one: the European Collaborative Study. *AIDS* 1999;13:1377–1385.

27. Schwartz JS, Dans PE, Kinosian BP. Human immunodeficiency virus test evaluation, performance, and use: proposals to make good tests better. *JAMA* 1988;259:2574–2579.

28. Anonymous. U.S. Public Health Service recommendations for human immunodeficiency virus counseling and voluntary testing for pregnant women. *MMWR Recomm Rep* 1995;44:1–15.

29. Kind C, Rudin C, Siegrist CA, et al. Prevention of vertical HIV transmission: additive protective effect of elective Cesarean section and zidovudine prophylaxis: Swiss Neonatal HIV Study Group. *AIDS* 1998;12:205–210.

30. Mandelbrot L, Le Chenadec J, Berrebi A, et al. Perinatal HIV-1 transmission: interaction between zidovudine prophylaxis and mode of delivery in the French Perinatal Cohort. *JAMA* 1998;280:155–160.

31. Anonymous. Elective caesarean-section versus vaginal delivery in prevention of vertical HIV-1 transmission: a randomised clinical trial. The European Mode of Delivery Collaboration. *Lancet* 1999;353:1035–1039.

32. Anonymous. The mode of delivery and the risk of vertical transmission of human immunodeficiency virus type 1—a meta-analysis of 15 prospective cohort studies. The International Perinatal HIV Group. *N Engl J Med* 1999;340:977–987.

33. Committee on Obstetric P. ACOG committee opinion scheduled Cesarean delivery and the prevention of vertical transmission of HIV infection. Number 234, May 2000 (replaces number 219, August 1999). *Int J Gynaecol Obstet* 2001;73:279–281.

34. Anonymous. Recommendations of the U.S. Public Health Service Task Force on the use of zidovudine to reduce perinatal transmission of human immunodeficiency virus. *MMWR Recomm Rep* 1994;43:1–20.

35. Ybarra L. Women and AIDS: implications for counseling. *J Counsel Dev* 1991;69:285–287.

36. Anonymous. Public Health Services guidelines for counseling and antibody testing to prevent HIV infection and AIDS. *MMWR Recomm Rep* 1987;36:509–515.

15

Screening for Cystic Fibrosis Carrier Status

Darren A. Shickle

Adrienne R. Hunt

■ What Is the Problem that Requires Screening?

Cystic fibrosis (including carrier status).

What is the incidence/prevalence of the target condition?

Cystic fibrosis (CF) is the most common autosomal recessive disorder among whites, occurring in 1/2,500 live births in the United Kingdom[1] About one in 25 whites is a carrier of a CF mutation. The disease is much rarer among non-whites—one in 14,000 live births among American blacks, one in 25,500 among Asians, and one in 11,500 Hispanics.[2] There are approximately 7,000 individuals affected by the disease in the United Kingdom, 30,000 in the United States, and at least 60,000 worldwide.[3]

What are the sequelae of the condition that are of interest in clinical medicine?

The mutant gene responsible for CF is located on the long arm of chromosome 7.[4] More than 1,300 mutations are known, the frequency of which varies among populations.[5] The gene product is a 1,480–amino acid membrane protein (cystic fibrosis transmembrane regulator, CFTR), which acts as a cyclic adenosine monophosphate (cAMP)–regulated chloride channel.[6] Patients with classic cystic fibrosis have defects of exocrine secretion characterized by low water content and thus a high concentration of electrolytes (e.g., diagnostically high sodium and chloride levels in sweat) and protein, which leads to increased secretion viscosity and blockage of ducts. There is also an increased electrical potential difference across epithelial surfaces.

Multiple organs are affected by mutations in this gene. There is a wide spectrum of clinical variability resulting from these mutations ranging from infertility or mild pulmonary symptoms in otherwise healthy individuals to life-threatening bowel obstruction or severe lung damage from recurrent lung infections in others.[7]

Lungs: Bronchial and bronchiolar obstruction by viscid secretions leads to recurrent distal infection and ultimately to right-sided heart failure (cor pulmonale). Respiratory symptoms are the dominant symptoms at the time of diagnosis in 45% of patients.[2]

Pancreas: Inspissated pancreatic secretions lead to destruction of secretory tissue in 85% to 90%; pancreatic insufficiency with diabetes mellitus, gastrointestinal malabsorption, and slow weight gain occurs in 10% to 12% of affected individuals. Ketoacidosis is rare.

Gut: Meconium ileus leads to intestinal obstruction in 10% to 20% of affected neonates. Rectal prolapse occurs in 20% of affected children.

Liver: Bile duct blockage can cause prolonged obstructive neonatal jaundice. Symptomatic biliary cirrhosis occurs relatively rarely in up to 5% of cases. Those with meconium ileus may have a higher risk of liver complications.

Testes: Spermatogenesis is normal, but blockage of the vas deferens and epididymis leads to azoospermia. Fertility is also reduced in females.

These pathophysiologic alterations allow the early diagnosis of affected individuals. The "sweat test" involves the analysis of sweat produced by pilocarpine iontophoresis. An abnormal sweat sodium or chloride value (usually in the range of 50–70 mmol/L) indicates CF. The sweat test is the diagnostic tool nearest to a "gold standard" for the detection of homozygotes in the absence of a complete library of gene probes.[6,8] However, sweat tests are difficult to perform in the newborn because 100 mg of sweat is required. Affected newborns also have raised blood levels of pancreatic trypsin due to leakage from the obstructed pancreas. Immunoreactive trypsinogen (IRT) can be measured in the dried blood spot obtained from neonates for phenylketonuria, hypothyroidism, and galactosemia testing in many countries. If the value is above the 99 percentile for the normal population, the positive predictive value of this test is 3%.[9] These children should undergo a sweat test at a later date.

Additional diagnostic methods complementary to the sweat test have been suggested.[7] These include mutation analysis, measurements of the transepithelial bioelectric properties, and measurement of the nasal potential difference. Individuals with CF have a greater negative potential difference across the nasal respiratory epithelia (mean value 46 mV in affected individuals compared to 19 mV in unaffected individuals).

Mortality rates from CF are highest during the first year of life and are related to respiratory insufficiency in 90%.[7] Mortality in the first month of life is higher when a meconium ileus is present. Thereafter, the clinical course is similar regardless of whether meconium ileus was present.[10]

In 1993 the median survival from birth was quoted as 24 years for females and 25 years for males, excluding recipients of lung, heart, and pancreas transplants.[11] The present life expectancy of affected individuals has increased to a median of 30 years.[7] Birth cohort analysis suggests that survival has continued to improve—perhaps due to a combination of earlier detection and improved treatment. Although life expectancy of CF sufferers has increased, the long-term sequelae of the disease, such as osteoporosis[12,13] and digestive tract cancer[14] have increasingly been reported.

Additional medical advances are on the horizon, such as gene therapy to correct the fundamental genetic defect using a helper virus to insert the normal gene.[15] However, the consequences of unregulated expression of the *CFTR* gene, the minimum amount of CFTR mRNA required for normal cell function, the effects of long-term repeated administration, and vector-induced inflammatory response are issues yet to be addressed.[16]

A recent study investigating the social and demographic features of adults with cystic fibrosis found that their employment rates are lower than those for the general population at all ages except those over 50.[17] In particular, between 25 and 49 years, the employment rate for men was 88% of the general population and for women it was 71% of the general population. In a comparable study conducted in 1990, the proportion employed had fallen. However, the proportion of those not working due to ill health had also fallen.[18]

■ The Tests

What is the purpose of the tests?

The purpose of CF carrier screening is to identify couples at high risk of having a child with CF. Couples are considered to be at high risk if both are carriers of a detectable *CFTR* gene mutation.

What is the nature of the tests?

Genetic testing for the CF gene mutations. The *CFTR* gene was first cloned in 1989.[4,19,20] Over 1,300 different *CFTR* mutations have been described.[5] The relationship between genotype and phenotype is variable with many genotypes being difficult to interpret clinically due to variable penetrance.[21,22]

The ΔF508 mutation accounts for 70% to 80% of all *CFTR* mutations among whites, whereas the next mutation, G542X, has an allelic frequency of 2%.[23] The variety and frequency of mutations vary by ethnic group. For example, ΔF508 accounts for 70% and 55% of mutations detected in North and South European populations, respectively, and 28% and 18% of Middle East and North African (Arabic) populations, respectively.[5]

The subject's DNA is extracted from cells collected from mouthwashes or EDTA blood samples and analyzed by polymerase chain reaction (PCR) assays. Only a limited number of the common mutations are tested for during screening. Testing centers must select the mutations tested on the basis of their target population. It is generally feasible to test for at least 85% of the known mutations, permitting detection of at least 70% (0.85 × 0.85) of carrier couples. Haddow et al.[24] reviewed 19 published reports of antenatal CF screening trials, finding that nearly all had chosen to use forward dot-blot, reverse dot-blot, or ARMS (amplification refractory mutation systems, Astra Zeneca Diagnostics) technologies.

The absence of practice guidelines has led to a proliferation of test panels (a set of mutations used in mutation analysis), which vary widely in the number and selection of mutations.[25,26] The American College of Obstetricians and Gynecologists, in partnership with the American College of Medical Genetics, recently recommended a pan-ethnic core panel of 25 mutations as a standard.[27] This panel includes all CF-causing mutations with an allele frequency of 0.1% or higher in the general US population. The recommended panel can detect 97%, 80%, and 69% of carriers for Ashkenazi Jews, European whites and African Americans, respectively. The carrier risk before testing and the residual risk after a negative test result is estimated to decline from one in 29 to one in 930 for Ashkenazi Jews, one in 29 to one in 140 for European whites and one in 65 to one in 207 for African Americans.[27] The 1999 UK Health Technology Assessment reported three commercially available tests that detect 85% of carriers in Scotland, Wales, and the North of England or 80% elsewhere, 35% of Asians, and 41% of blacks.[16]

There are two principle models for genetic carrier testing: "inwards-out" (also known as cascade screening) and "outwards-in."[28] The first approach involves identification of an index case homozygous or compound heterozygous for the *CFTR* mutation and then offering testing to immediate relatives and their family members if found to be carriers. The alternative outwards-in model involves screening individuals in an at-risk population as part of a population genetics screening program (sometimes called community genetics or primary care genetics). Holloway and Brock[29] estimated that inwards-out screening would identify a high ratio of carriers to people tested (one in three compared with one in 25 for general population screening). A recent report concluded that, for CF (carrier frequency of 4%), testing all the siblings and first cousins of all identified carriers would require locating and testing 1.9% of the whole population, but detect only 15% of all new cases.[30] In contrast to the inwards-out model, outwards-in CF screening programs[31–33] detect at least 50% of carrier couples and can be applied any time during life. In his recent editorial, Morris[30] concluded that although a case may be made for cascade screening of autosomal dominant and X-linked disorders, cascade screening of autosomal recessive disorders, such as CF, is not worthwhile.

Murray et al.[16] conducted a comprehensive review of 20 prospective neonatal screening programs. Eight states in the United States have added CF screening to their newborn screening programs[7] and neonatal screening is already routine in Australia.[34] In the United Kingdom, 20% of newborns are currently enrolled in CF newborn screening programs with national roll-out of the program expected in 2007.[35]

Neonatal screening usually involves IRT testing to detect homozygotes (rather than carriers) for the purpose of early treatment. However, one fourth of the 24 protocols used in the 20 programs reviewed by Murray et al.[16] involved a DNA test. Infant carrier status can be determined with DNA tests. This suggests that the levels of genetic counseling required may be increased beyond that required for parents of affected children alone.[36]

Pilot programs of preconceptual carrier screening within primary care have been conducted.[37,38] Clayton et al.[39] observed a general lack of interest by non-pregnant couples in population-based CF carrier screening. This trend was also observed in the early trials where the stated interest in testing was greater than utilized when screening was offered as part of the routine antenatal care.[23]

Two UK studies suggest there is considerable support among primary health care professionals for CF screening carried out in local practices[40–42] Mennie et al.[42] surveyed 334 general practitioners working in an area with an established antenatal screening program. They found that 295 (88%) of the 334 surveyed considered it appropriate to offer screening to those with a family history, although only 44 (13%) thought it appropriate to offer screening to individuals without a family history.

Mennie et al.[42] also observed that many general practitioners would like to be involved in offering screening, giving information before a test, and disclosing negative results. However, they were less enthusiastic about the prospect of disclosing positive results and for counseling. The respondents claimed support would be necessary for both activities. Although preconceptual screening maximizes reproductive autonomy, it will not be desirable until these training and support issues are addressed. The advantages and disadvantages of the main strategies are outlined in Table 15–1.

Antenatal CF carrier screening seeks to identify during pregnancy couples who both have a *CFTR* mutation. The antenatal diagnosis is based on fetal DNA obtained by chorionic villus sampling (CVS) in the first trimester or by amniocentesis in the second or third trimester.[7] This allows the couple the opportunity to make an informed choice on the outcome of the pregnancy. However, both techniques carry a risk of a pregnancy loss.

In vitro fertilization (IVF) with preimplantation diagnosis (PGD) has been performed to increase the reproductive choices of a high-risk couple.[43] Gene chip technology may be the future of semi-automated genetic testing for both PGD and antenatal diagnosis, providing a rapid diagnosis.[44] However, this technology remains to be refined.

What are the implications of testing?

What does an abnormal test result mean? A positive result indicates the tested individual is a carrier for one of the *CFTR* mutations. There are two general approaches to screening: two-step and couple (Figure 15–1). The woman is tested first in the two-step approach. The partners of carrier women are subsequently tested after appropriate counseling. In contrast, both the man and woman are sampled simultaneously in couple screening. One specimen is tested first, and the second tested only if the first is positive. The couple is usually told their carrier status only if both partners are positive and should otherwise assume they are at low risk unless contacted.[32]

There are generally more ethical concerns about couple screening because the pair are given a combined-risk result, rather than their individual gene status. Some pilot projects, for example in Edinburgh, United Kingdom, disclose

Table 15–1   Comparison of screening strategies at different times in life cycle

	Advantages	Disadvantages
Neonatal screening	Mechanisms already exist for collection of blood samples Community midwife/health visitors provide counseling Early treatment possible	Autonomy increased in subsequent pregnancies only Parents give consent on behalf of the child Knowledge that child not "perfect" can affect parent/baby relationship Knowledge of carrier status only of importance for the next generation Information may be lost/misunderstood before child reaches reproductive age Problem of detection of non-paternity or sex chromosome abnormalities
Antenatal screening	Easy to organize Most pregnant women attend antenatal clinic Performed along with other antenatal tests Only offered to people of reproductive age More receptive to issues affecting their children	Consent may not be fully informed Availability of partner may be a problem Limited period to perform counseling, etc. Anxiety about pregnancy may make counseling more difficult Termination may not be an acceptable option
Childhood (teenager) screening	Aware of being a carrier before long term relationship formed Could choose to avoid having children with another known carrier	Consent a problem Adolescence already a time of sexual confusion Stigmatization
Young adults of reproductive age	Maximizes autonomy and reproductive choice Informed choice easiest to obtain	Primary care staff may not have skills or time to devote to counseling Many young adults do not visit their primary care giver Many pregnancies not planned May be a middle-class bias if individuals have to request screening

carrier status if the woman is found to be a carrier even if the father is not.[45] This practice is not routine, and women ordinarily receive information about individual carrier status only if they specifically request it.[46] Concerns about nondisclosure arise because the residual risk may be as high as one in 667 for couples where one member is a confirmed carrier, a risk higher than background (1/2,500). In addition, carriers whose partners do not have a *CFTR* gene mutation may be falsely reassured that they cannot have an affected child even if they change partners. Therefore, counseling should include the residual risk and the need for retesting if the couple forms new relationships. Couple screening does not eliminate the need for counseling; it only changes the timing—

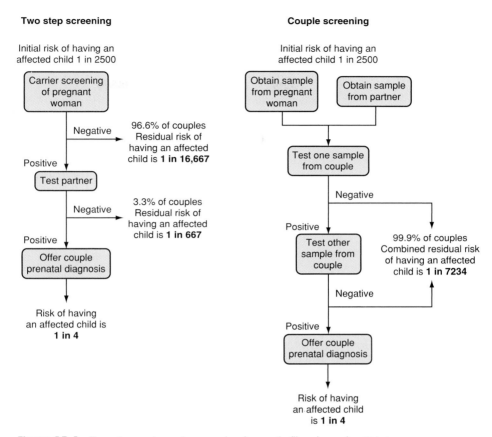

Figure 15-1   Two-step and couple screening for cystic fibrosis carrier status.

pretest counseling is particularly important. The advantages of couple screening are that women found to be carriers do not experience anxiety while they wait for their partner to be tested, less counseling is required where only test-positive couples are informed of carrier status, and there is decreased stigmatization and the fostering of a feeling of unity between partners.[46]

A major disadvantage of antenatal screening is the limited time available to provide counseling and testing before a decision on pregnancy termination is required. It is desirable for women to book earlier or for the screening itself to be conducted within primary care. Primary care–based antenatal screening has been successfully piloted[41,47–50] (all referenced in Haddow et al.[24]), although the knowledge base of primary care staff remains an issue.

Haddow et al.[24] reviewed 19 published antenatal CF screening trials conducted in the United States and in Europe. The couple model was used by four sites in the United Kingdom and one site in the United States to screen 37,178 couples. The two-step model was used by four sites in the United Kingdom and the United States and three sites elsewhere in Europe to screen 35,469 couples.

They observed that the uptake rates were high using either model in both the United States (average, 69%; range, 57%–78%) and in the European trials (average, 78%; range, 62%–99%). Ninety-three percent of couples with a positive screening result chose to have counseling and antenatal diagnosis. Subsequently, 21 of 24 couples who had a fetus diagnosed as homozygous for CF chose to terminate the pregnancy (100% in Europe and 63% in the United States). The authors point out that the reviewed trials may not be representative of decision making in other racial/ethnic groups.

Two of the reviewed intervention trials that used the two-step model showed initial increases in anxiety levels in carrier woman that later declined when the partner's negative result was reported[31,51] (quoted in Haddow et al.[24]). However, two other two-step model trials did not find this initial increase[52,53] (quoted in Haddow et al.[24]).

Miedzybrodzka et al.[54] found that many screen-negative women did not fully appreciate they could either still be carriers (21% two-step and 13% couple screening) or could have a child with cystic fibrosis (19% and 17%, respectively). Twenty-one percent of women in the couple-screening group had forgotten that repeated testing was indicated should there be a future pregnancy with a new partner.

The American College of Obstetricians and Gynecologists, in partnership with the American College of Medical Genetics, has developed and released recommendations for how antenatal screening should be conducted in the United States.[27,55] They endorsed the two-step (sequential) model and a core pan-ethnic panel of 25 mutations. They recommended against use of the couple model unless in a modified format. In the modified couple model, notification is made when a mutation is found in either partner, and counseling is provided. It is hoped that this method overcomes ethical questions surrounding nondisclosure of test results to both individuals (as described in previous paragraphs). In addition, the method provides a positive member of the positive-negative couple the opportunity of informing his or her relatives of their risk, thus optimizing the chances of inwards-out screening within a family.

The guidelines are the basis of a new standard practice in which all white couples contemplating pregnancy, those already pregnant, or those with a family history are routinely offered screening. Screening is also available on request to other lower risk ethnic groups.

Recently, implementation failures were highlighted, raising concerns over consistency of screening service delivery in the United States.[46] Some problems have also occurred with the two-step model, for example, difficulties obtaining samples from partners of test-positive women. This is due to a number of different reasons, for example, the partner is unavailable or unwilling to be tested or samples are sent to a different laboratory either because they are processed through a different physician or they are rerouted due to constraints imposed by insurance coverage. Haddow[46] expressed concern that such discontinuity will lead to errors in the final, combined interpretation of the partners' results. Furthermore, he warned that some CF laboratories have failed to implement programmatic components that include the couple or two-step model. In the absence of either model, the laboratory may be unaware whether samples have been submitted for antenatal testing, carrier testing, or diagnostic purposes. Although legally the laboratory is only responsible for providing a report indicating whether or not a CF mutation is present, this trend raises ethical considerations as to who should be responsible for providing the couple with a complete and accurate screening interpretation.

The experience of the United States may influence the practice in those countries yet to establish antenatal screening programs. For example, a 1999 UK Health Technology Assessment[16] recommended that antenatal screening should be offered routinely. The UK National Screening Committee policy, however, concluded that screening should not be offered routinely.[56] This position is scheduled for review in the near future.

Figure 15–2 illustrates the various outcomes of screening a population of 1 million couples where the panel of mutations used would detect 85% of mutations in the population (Tables 15–2 and 15–3). Ninety-six percent will be homozygous normal with a negative test result (true negatives). However, 15% of carriers with one of the less common mutations will also have a negative result (false negative). Of the 3.4% of carriers correctly identified, 4% will have a partner who is also a carrier (although 15% of these mutations will also be missed). Thus, 0.12% of couples (1,156/1,000,000) will be diagnosed as "high risk'" (correctly identified positives) whereas 0.04% (444/1,000,000) will be incorrectly described as "low risk" (false negatives). Those couples with a negative result have only a 0.04% chance of actually being positive (444/998,844). There is a one in four chance of an "at-risk" couple having an affected child in any given pregnancy. At best, 289 of 400 CF fetuses (1/2,500 births) will be detected. In practice, the number detected will be lower because the uptake of screening is less than 100%. The assumed false-negative rate above (15%) will decrease as detection techniques improve, for example through the use of gene chip technology whereby many mutations can be screened.

What does a normal test result mean? Couples who test negative for a known *CFTR* mutation are at low risk of having a child with CF. Some risk remains because not all mutations are yet detectable, and it is not feasible to screen for all known mutations.

Table 15–2	**Validity of individual's test results**		
Individual's Test result	**CF Gene**	**Status**	
	CF carrier	**Normal**	
Positive	34,000	0	34,000
Negative	6,000	960,000	966,000
	40,000	960,000	1,000,000

Sensitivity, 34,000/40,000 = 85%; specificity = 960,000/960,000 = 100%.

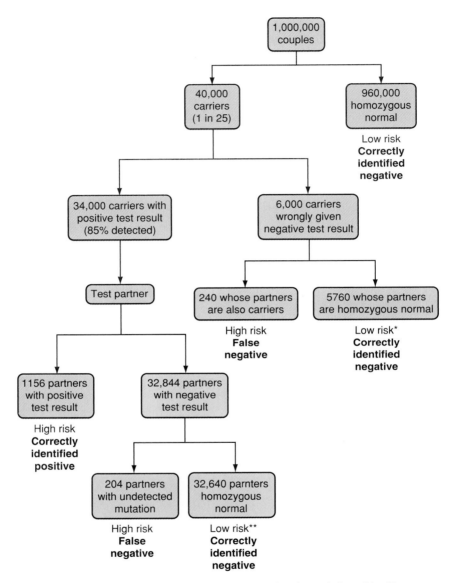

Figure 15-2   Flowchart of screening outcomes in a notational population of 1 million women and their partners. Single asterisk identifies couples correctly described as low risk, even though the mutation was missed, because the partners were homozygous normal. Double-asterisk: couples correctly described as low risk. Carrier females screened by the two-step approach may experience anxiety until their partners are shown to be normal. This problem does not arise with couple screening because the couple are not given the diagnosis.

Table 15-3	**Validity of couple's test results**		
Couple's Test result	**CF Gene**	**Status**	
	Both partners carriers	**Zero or one partner carrier**	
Positive	1,156	0	1,156
Negative	444	998,400	998,844
	1,600	998,400	1,000,000

Sensitivity, 1,156/1,600 = 72.3%; specificity, 998,400/998,400 = 100%.

What is the cost of testing?

Cost of testing incorporates several components including providing education and information, obtaining informed consent, collecting and transporting samples, performing/interpreting the DNA test, reporting results/counseling, performing diagnostic testing, and performing selective terminations of affected pregnancies where that option is chosen.[24,57]

A 1999 Working Conference on prenatal screening for CF considered two economic analyses.[24] The first, by Rowley et al.[58] reported costs based on a single program's experience and calculated the cost for each case voluntarily averted. In addition, they performed a quality of life analysis. The second study, by Loader et al.[52] (quoted by Haddow et al.[24]) reported the cost for each case detected and based calculations on summary estimates of participation rates and choices that couples made at each step of the screening process (based on previously published trials from both the United Kingdom and the United States).

A range of program parameters was also used (e.g., uptake rate and amniocentesis acceptance rate). The cost saving primarily results from the lifetime medical costs directly associated with treatment. Most studies conducted in the early 1990s suggested that the annual direct medical care costs for an average individual with cystic fibrosis were $15,000 to $20,000 in 1996 dollars.[57] Taking into account realistic life expectancy and recommended discounting rates, the report edited by Haddow and Palomaki[57] estimated from these figures that the lifetime medical care costs for an average individual with cystic fibrosis was between $300,000 and $500,000.

The cost per CF case antenatally identified is estimated to be between $300,000 and $500,000 (although individual studies reported a wider range influenced significantly by the cost of the DNA test).[24] Estimates did not appear to be influenced by the screening model used (couple or two-step). Haddow et al.[24] notes that these estimates are sensitive to screening uptake, partner participation, and amniocentesis acceptance rates.

Estimates are also sensitive to the laboratory component, which in turn depends on other factors such as the number of mutations tested and discounts for bulk orders. Estimates have ranged from $29 (for an unstated number of mutations[16]) to an upper cost of $150 for 70 mutations commercially tested.[58]

The report edited by Haddow and Palomaki[57] reviewed and standardized costing literature of antenatal screening programs conducted from 1994 to 2001 to a testing population of 100,000 couples. They reported cost per woman screened and per CF case identified from 1 year of screening. The three United Kingdom reports ranged from $54 to $77 and $189,166 to $266,031 respectively[59–61] (quoted in Haddow and Palomaki[57]). The four US studies ranged from $116 to $195 and $500,647 to $991,782, respectively.[58,62,63]

Are women willing to bear the cost of screening? Murray et al.[16] report that Zeneca Diagnostics would supply their Amplification Refractory Mutation System (ARMS) kit, Elucigene, for £12 per test (including royalties and licenses), if the purchaser can commit to buying at least 5,000 kits per annum.[16] Furthermore, they considered the increased cost, taking into account reagents, labor to collect and perform the test, and administration. The adjusted cost of £18, although notably at the lower end of the costing range, compares with a stated willingness of women undergoing antenatal CF carrier screening to pay up to £22 for the test.[64] Rowley et al.[58] surveyed more than 2,000 women and found that the modal response was that 77% would be prepared to pay up to $25 for a test. Ninety-four percent of the group was prepared to pay up to $50 for the test. Both surveys noted problems with such estimates: Patients asked hypothetical questions may not give valid responses due to lack of familiarity with the disease and the lack of a frame of reference given that many people do not receive bills for laboratory tests.[58]

■ Conclusions and Recommendations

Cystic fibrosis carrier screening provides a means of increasing a couple's reproductive autonomy when conducted in the preconceptual or antenatal setting. The focus is now moving from questioning the feasibility and necessity of CF screening to implementation and delivery strategies. Early carrier screening programs are focusing on couples who are pregnant or contemplating pregnancy and are at risk due to ethnic group and/or family history.

The two-step screening model has the advantage that all women receive their individual screen result, as do any men subsequently screened. Some but not all studies observed increased levels of anxiety in women found to be carriers while waiting for their partner's result. The couple model has the advantage that the couple is viewed as a unit, ensuring participation of both partners from the offset. The classic couple model has the disadvantage that couples are given a combined screen result that may, if negative, not reflect the increase in risk the couple faces if one partner is test positive. Several trial sites have aimed to avoid this situation by providing individual test results within the context of the couple model.

Economic evaluations have been performed. These evaluations are sensitive to a number of factors including the cost of the test, uptake of screening, and the proportion of affected fetuses terminated. Factors affecting the economic feasibility of antenatal screening are being confronted as new screening programs are implemented. Experience in the United States revealed problems of sample collection for the two-step model if the partner is unwilling or unavailable to provide a sample. Further problems have arisen with respect to joint test interpretation and counseling.

There are several points to consider when establishing new programs, for example which model should be established and should screening be offered universally or targeted to specific ethnic groups? Within this framework, there should be standardization of the size and composition of the core mutation panel, training and support of physicians, standardization of test reporting, and counseling and encouragement of early testing to permit couples time to fully consider treatment options. Expertise in the area of genotype interpretation is also necessary as variable penetrance of genotypes result in difficulties in providing a clinical interpretation.

■ Summary

1 ■ What Is the Problem that Requires Screening?

Cystic fibrosis.

a. *What is the incidence/prevalence of the target condition?*

Cystic fibrosis (CF) is the most common autosomal recessive disorder affecting whites, with a frequency of one in 2,500 live births. About one in 25 whites is a carrier of a CF mutation

b. *What are the sequelae of the condition that are of interest in clinical medicine?*

Patients with CF have defects of exocrine secretions characterized by low water content and thus high concentrations of electrolytes (notably the diagnostically high sodium and chloride levels in sweat) and protein (leading to increased secretion viscosity and blockage of ducts). Multiple organs are affected by mutations in the *CFTR* gene.

2 ■ The Tests

a. *What is the purpose of the tests?*

To identify couples at high risk of having a child with CF.

Continued

■ **Summary—cont'd**

b. ***What is the nature of the tests?***
Genetic testing (usually by PCR) for the CF gene mutations.

c. ***What are the implications of testing?***
1. What does an abnormal test result mean?
There are two general approaches to screening: two-step and couple (see Figure 15–1). In a two-step approach, the woman is tested first and her partner tested subsequently only if she is shown to be a carrier. Both the man and woman are sampled simultaneously in couple screening. One specimen is tested, the other examined only if the first is positive. The couple is usually told to assume they are at low risk unless they are contacted. Traditionally the couple is not told their individual results unless specifically requested. However, recent programs have included full disclosure to both couples due to the ethical considerations associated with not fully informing couples of residual risk. A major disadvantage of antenatal screening is the limited time available to provide counseling and testing before a decision on pregnancy termination is required. It would be desirable either for women to book earlier or for the screening itself to be conducted within primary care. Primary care–based antenatal screening has been successfully piloted, although the knowledge base of primary care staff remains an issue.
2. What does a normal test result mean?
Couples who test negative for a known CF mutation are at low risk of having a child with CF. Some risk remains for low-risk pregnancies screened by either method because not all mutations are detectable, and it is not feasible to screen for all known mutations.

d. ***What is the cost of testing?***
Estimates range from $189,166 to $991,782 per CF child identified depending on the assumptions made regarding screen acceptance, partner participation, sensitivity and cost of DNA test, and amniocentesis or chorionic villus sampling acceptance rates.

3 ■ Conclusions and Recommendations

Recent recommendations have promoted CF carrier screening as a new standard practice in the United States in which all white couples contemplating pregnancy, those already pregnant, or those with a family history are routinely offered screening. Screening is also available on request to other lower risk ethnic groups, although sensitivity of testing in certain ethnic groups remains low.

Future programs will have to take into consideration standardization of the size and composition of a core mutation panel, training and support of physicians, standardization of test reporting, counseling, and encouragement of early testing to permit couples time to fully consider treatment options.

References

1. Dodge JA. Cystic fibrosis in the United Kingdom 1977-85: an improving picture. *BMJ* 1988;97:1599–1602.
2. FitzSimmons SC. The changing epidemiology of cystic fibrosis. *J Pediatr* 1993;122:1–9.
3. Tanne J. News: US trial of gene therapy for cystic fibrosis. *BMJ* 1999;318:1096.
4. Rommens JM, Iannuzzi MC, Kerem B, et al. Identification of the cystic fibrosis gene: chromosome walking and jumping. *Science* 1989;245:1059–1065.
5. Cystic Fibrosis Genetic Analysis Consortium. 2004 Cystic fibrosis mutation database. statistics. Available at http://www.genet.sickkids.on.ca/cftr.
6. Bye MR, Ewig JM, Quittell LM. Cystic fibrosis. *Lung* 1994;172:251–270.
7. Lyon E, Miller C. Current challenges in cystic fibrosis screening. *Arch Pathol Lab Med* 2003;127:1133–1139.
8. Webb AK, David TJ. Clinical management of children and adults with cystic fibrosis. *BMJ* 1994;308:459–462.
9. Ranieri E, Lewis BD, Gerace RL, et al. Neonatal screening for cystic fibrosis using immunoreactive trypsinogen and direct gene analysis: four years' experience. *BMJ* 1994;308: 1469–1472.
10. Coutts JAP, Docherty JG, Carachi R, et al. Clinical course of patients with cystic fibrosis presenting with meconium ileus. *Br J Surg* 1997;84:555.
11. Dodge JA, Morison S, Lewis PA, et al. Cystic fibrosis in the United Kingdom, 1968-1988: incidence, population and survival. *Paed Perinat Epidemiol* 1993;7:157–166.
12. Aris RM, Renner JB, Winders AD, et al. Increased rate of fractures and severe kyphosis: sequelae of living into adulthood with cystic fibrosis. *Ann Intern Med* 1998;128:186–193.
13. Brenckmann C, Papaioannou A, Freitag A, et al. Osteoporosis in Canadian adult cystic fibrosis patients: a descriptive study. *BMC Musculoskelet Disord* 2003;4:1–13.
14. Maisonneuve P, FitzSimmons SC, Neglia JP, et al. Cancer risk in nontransplanted and transplanted cystic fibrosis patients: a 10 year study. *J Natl Cancer Inst* 2003;95:381–387.
15. Boucher RC. Perspective: status of gene therapy for cystic fibrosis lung disease. *J Clin Invest* 1999;103:441–445.
16. Murray J, Cuckle H, Taylor G, et al. Screening for cystic fibrosis. *Health Technol Assess* 1999;3:1–104.

17. Walters S, Warren R. Cystic fibrosis adults: Millenium survey: a survey of social and demographic characteristics of adults with cystic fibrosis in the United Kingdom, their medical care and quality of life in the year 2000. Issued to the Cystic Fibrosis Trust, 2001. Available at http://www.cfstudy.com/sarah/Report2000_2.pdf.
18. Walters S, Britton J, Hodson ME. Demographic and social characteristics of adults with cystic fibrosis in the United Kingdom. *BMJ* 1993;306:549–552.
19. Kerem B, Rommens JM, Buchanan JA, et al. Identification of the cystic fibrosis gene: genetic analysis. *Science* 1989;345:1073–1080.
20. Riordan JR, Rommens JM, Kerem B, et al. Identification of the cystic fibrosis gene: cloning and characterization of complementary DNA. *Science* 1989;245:1066–1073.
21. Groman JD, Hefferon TW, Casals T, et al. Variation in a repeat sequence determines whether a common variant of the cystic fibrosis transmembrane conductance regulator gene is pathogenic or benign. *Am J Hum Genet* 2004;74:176–179.
22. McKone EF, Emerson SS, Edwards KL, et al. Effect of genotype on phenotype and mortality in cystic fibrosis: a retrospective cohort study. *Lancet* 2003;36:1671–1676.
23. Grody WW. Cystic fibrosis: molecular diagnosis, population screening, and public policy. *Arch Pathol Lab Med* 1999;123:1041–1046.
24. Haddow JE, Bradley LA, Palomaki GE, et al. Issues in implementing prenatal screening for cystic fibrosis: results of a working conference. *J Med Screen* 1999;6:60–66.
25. Grody WW, Desnick RJ, Carpenter NJ, et al. Diversity of cystic fibrosis mutation screening practices [letter]. *Am J Hum Genet* 1998;62:1252–1254.
26. Grody WW, Desnick RJ. Cystic fibrosis population carrier screening: here at last—are we ready? [editorial] *Genet Med* 2001;3:87–90.
27. Grody WW, Cutting GR, Klinger KW, et al. Laboratory standards and guidelines for population-based cystic fibrosis carrier screening. *Genet Med* 2001;3:149–154.
28. Shickle D, Harvey I. "Inside-out," back-to-front: a model for clinical population genetic screening. *J Med Genet* 1993;30:580–582.
29. Holloway S, Brock DJH. Cascade testing for the identification of carriers of cystic fibrosis. *J Med Screen* 1994;1:159–164.
30. Morris JK. Is cascade testing a sensible method of population screening [editorial]? *J Med Screen* 2004;11:57–59.
31. Mennie ME, Gilfillan A, Compton M, et al. Prenatal screening for cystic fibrosis. *Lancet* 1992;340:214–216.
32. Livingstone J, Axton RA, Gilfillan A, et al. Antenatal screening for cystic fibrosis: a trial of the couple model. *BMJ* 1994;308:1459–1462.
33. Wald NJ, George LM, Wald NM. Couple screening for cystic fibrosis. *Lancet* 1992;342:1307–1308.
34. Williamson R. The balance between privacy, safety and community health [editorial comment]. *J Paediatr Child Health* 2003;39:507.
35. National Screening Committee (March 2004a). Cystic fibrosis: National Screening Committee Policy Position (Neonatal). Available at http://www.nelh.nhs.uk/screening/child_pps/cystic fibrosis_neonatal.html.
36. Dankert-Roelse JE, Meerman GJ. Screening for cystic fibrosis—time to change our position? *N Engl J Med* 1997;337:997–998.
37. Watson EK, Mayall E, Chapple J, et al. Screening for carriers of cystic fibrosis through the primary care services. *BMJ* 1991;303:504–507.
38. Bekker H, Modell M, Denniss G, et al. Uptake of cystic fibrosis testing in primary care: supply push or demand pull? *BMJ* 1993;306:1584–1586.
39. Clayton EW, Hannig VL, Pfotenhauer JP, et al. Lack of interest by nonpregnant couples in population-based cystic fibrosis carrier screening. *Am J Hum Genet* 1996;58:617–627.
40. Boulton M, Cummings C, Williamson R. The views of general practitioners on community carrier screening for cystic fibrosis. *Br J Gen Pract* 1996;46:299–301.
41. Harris H, Wallace A, Scotcher D, et al. Pilot study of the acceptability of cystic fibrosis carrier testing during routine antenatal consultations in general practice. *Br J Gen Pract* 1996;46:225–227.

42. Mennie M, Campbell H, Liston WA, et al. Attitudes of general practitioners to screening for cystic fibrosis. *J Med Screen* 1998;5:11–15.
43. Ao A, Handyside A, Winston RML. Preimplantation genetic diagnosis of cystic fibrosis (ΔF508). *Eur J Obstet Gynecol Reprod Biol* 1996;65:7–10.
44. Ryan C. Gene tests "improves embryo checks." BBCNews (UK Edition); June 29, 2004. Available at http://news.bbc.co.uk/1/hi/health/3847815.stm.
45. Antenatal Screening for Cystic Fibrosis (UK): Workshop (December 3rd 2002) Available Online at URL: http://www.nelh.nhs.uk/screening/antenatal_pps/cystic_fibrosis.html.
46. Haddow JE. Prenatal screening for cystic fibrosis in the United States—time to re-evaluate implementation policies. *J Med Screen* 2003;10:105–106.
47. Harris H, Scotcher D, Hartley N, et al. Cystic fibrosis carrier testing in early pregnancy by general practitioners. *BMJ* 1993;306:1580–1583.
48. Hartley NE, Scotcher D, Harris H et al. The uptake and acceptability to patients of cystic fibrosis carrier testing offered in pregnancy by the GP. *J Med Genet* 1997;34:459–464.
49. Doherty RA, Palomaki GE, Kloza EM, et al. Couple-based prenatal screening for cystic fibrosis in primary care settings. *Prenat Diagn* 1996;16:397–404.
50. Bradley LA, Johnson DD, Doherty RA, et al. Routine prenatal cystic fibrosis screening in primary care offices. *Am J Hum Genet* 1998;63:A13.
51. Grody WW, Dunkle-Schetter C, Tatsugawa ZH, et al. PCR-based screening for cystic fibrosis carrier mutations in an ethnically diverse pregnant population. *Am J Hum Genet* 1997;60:935–947.
52. Loader S, Caldwell P, Kozyra A, et al. Cystic fibrosis carrier population screening in the primary care setting. *Am J Hum Genet* 1996;59:234–247.
53. Witt DR, Schaefer C, Hallam P, et al. Cystic fibrosis heterozygote screening in 5161 pregnant women. *Am J Hum Genet* 1996;58:823–835.
54. Miedzybrodzka Z, Hall MH, Mollison J, et al. Antenatal screening for carriers of cystic fibrosis: randomisation trial of stepwise v couple screening. *BMJ* 1995;310:353–357.
55. National Institute of Health. Consensus Development Conference Statement: Genetic testing for cystic fibrosis. April 14–16, 1997. *Arch Intern Med* 1999;159:1529–1539.
56. National Screening Committee. Cystic fibrosis: National Screening Committee Policy Position (Antenatal) March 2004. Available at http://www.nelh.nhs.uk/screening/antenatal_pps/cystic_fibrosis.html.
57. Haddow JE, Palomaki GE. Population-based prenatal screening for cystic fibrosis via carrier testing: ACCE review, 2002. Available at http://www.cdc.gov/genomics/info/reports/research/FBR/ACCE.htm.
58. Rowley PT, Loader S, Kaplan RM. Prenatal screening for cystic fibrosis carriers: an economic evaluation. *Am J Hum Genet* 1998;63:1160–1174.
59. Beech R, Bekker H. Planning the development of cystic fibrosis gene carrier screening. *J Health Serv Res Policy* 1996;1:81–92.
60. Cuckle HS, Richardson GA, Sheldon TA, et al. Cost effectiveness of antenatal screening for cystic fibrosis. *BMJ* 1994;311:1460–1464.
61. Morris JK, Oppenheimer PM. Cost comparison of different methods of screening for cystic fibrosis. *J Med Screen* 1995;2:22–27.
62. Vintzileos AM, Ananth CV, Smulian JC, et al. A cost-effectiveness analysis of prenatal carrier screening for cystic fibrosis. *Obstet Gynecol* 1998;91:529–534.
63. Lieu TA, Ray GT, Farmer G, Shay GF. The cost of medical care for patients with cystic fibrosis in a health maintenance organization. *Pediatrics* 1999;103:E72–76.
64. Miedzybrodzka Z, Shackley P, Donaldson C, Counting the benefits of screening: a pilot study of willingness to pay for cystic fibrosis carrier screening. *J Med Screen* 1994;1:82–83.

16

Screening for Hemoglobinopathies

Joan S. Henthorn

Sally C. Davies

■ What Is the Problem that Requires Screening?

Clinically relevant hemoglobinopathies.

The hemoglobinopathies are a family of inherited disorders of the hemoglobin oxygen transporting protein in red blood cells. They are inherited in a Mendelian-recessive manner so that two parents carrying a hemoglobinopathy trait have a 1:4 risk of producing a child with clinically significant disease (homozygote or compound heterozygote), a 1:2 chance of the child inheriting the hemoglobinopathy trait and only a 1:4 chance of inheriting normal adult hemoglobin.

Hemoglobin is made up of two pairs of globin chains, which in normal, healthy adults are alpha, beta, delta, and gamma. These pairs combine to produce one major hemoglobin, Hb A (two alpha, two beta) and two minor ones: Hb A_2 (two alpha, two delta) and HbF (two alpha, two gamma). Over 1,000 different mutations that affect the genes producing hemoglobin are recognized.

Some, the thalassemia mutations, affect the quantity of hemoglobin synthesized;[1] others produce a variant hemoglobin by substituting or deleting one or more amino acids that make up the globin chains. Most of these variant hemoglobins have no clinical significance in the heterozygote, but certain common variants, such as sickle hemoglobin, produce severe clinical disease in the homozygous or compound heterozygous form.[2] The hemoglobins generally regarded as most important clinically are shown in Table 16–1 (see also Chapter 17).

What is the incidence/prevalence of the target condition?

The hemoglobinopathy gene mutations generally confer some survival advantage against malaria in the carrier state. This is particularly well documented for sickle hemoglobin. As a consequence, most hemoglobinopathies are found among peoples originating in parts of the world where malaria is or was

Table 16–1   Clinically significant hemoglobinopathies

Notation	Synonyms	Severity	
SS	Sickle cell anemia	Severe, variable	
SD-Punjab	Sickle Hb D disease, Hb SD disease	Severe, variable	
S-β Thal	Sickle beta thalassemia	Severe, variable	
S-Lepore	Sickle Hb Lepore disease	Severe, variable	
SC	Sickle Hb C disease, Hb SC disease	Moderate, variable	Sickle Cell Diseases
SO-Arab	Sickle Hb O-Arab disease	Moderate, variable	
SE	Sickle Hb E disease	Mild	
β Thal major	Beta thalassemia major	Severe	
Δ/β Thal major	Delta/beta thalassemia major	Severe	
Lepore	Homozygous Lepore	Severe, variable	
E-β Thal	Hb E beta thalassemia	Severe, variable	
β Thal intermedia	β Thalassemia intermedia	Variable	
CC	Hb C disease	Mild	
C-β Thal	Hb C thalassemia	Mild	
Hb H disease		Mild to moderate	
α Thal major	Bart hydrops fetalis	Fatal	

SD, sickle cell disease.

endemic including the sub-Saharan African nations, the Middle East, the Mediterranean, India and Asia. Migration brought the hemoglobinopathies to Northern Europe and Northern America, while occasional mutations in the autochthonous populations of Northern Europe and intermarriage have made it impossible to screen by personal appearance. Carrier rates and estimates for affected fetuses by ethnic group are shown in Table 16–2.

Census data and calculations based on gene frequencies suggest there are more than 60,000 black American sufferers of sickle cell disease, 15,000 in England, and a similar number of sufferers in France and the Mediterranean countries, and some 1,000 patients with β thalassemia major in the United States,

Table 16–2   Prevalence of Hbs S, C, and beta thalassemia by ethnic group

Ethnic group	Carrier rate S	Carrier rate C	Carrier rate β thalassemia	Affected fetuses/1,000
White			0.001	0.0003
Black Caribbean	0.11	0.04	0.009	5.6
Black African	0.20	0.03	0.009	14.7
Indian	0.01		0.035	0.4
Pakistani			0.045	1.0
Bangladeshi			0.03	0.8
Chinese			0.03	0.2
Cypriot	0.0075		0.16	5.6
Other Asian			0.03	0.2
All other			0.001	0.0003

with 600 in England, mainly of Greek, Italian, Turkish, and Pakistani or Indian origins.[3] These patients generally have a shorter lifespan and are transfusion dependent. α thalassemia carrier rates vary between 5% and 15% in the affected populations of China, South East Asia, Turkey, and Greece.[4]

What are the sequelae of the condition that are of interest in clinical medicine?

The hallmarks of sickle cell disease, including the homozygous sickle cell anemia and the compound heterozygotes, are the painful vaso-occlusive crises, infection, acute chest syndrome, and chronic organ damage. The clinical course can vary from mild to severe, but the median age of survival for sickle cell anemia is the fifth decade.[5,6]

Patients with β thalassemia major, also termed Cooley anemia, suffer severe anemia and without regular red cell transfusions every 3 to 4 weeks will die in infancy or childhood. Regular transfusions maintain growth and quality of life, but in turn lead to toxicity from accumulated iron. Iron chelation therapy is therefore essential and is generally given parenterally—an arduous, expensive, and on occasion toxic regime.[7]

■ The Tests

What is the purpose of the tests?

Screening is performed to identify carrier status or to make the diagnosis of an affected individual. Ideally, at-risk subjects are screened before their reproductive years, although this is often the exception.

The aim of antenatal screening is twofold: to detect women with significant hemoglobinopathies who may require special care and to offer fetal diagnosis. All women at risk of producing a child of the conditions noted in Table 16–1 can be asked to bring their partner for screening early enough in pregnancy to offer either preimplantation or antenatal diagnosis if desired. Antenatal diagnosis can be accomplished early by chorionic villus sampling, or later by either amniocentesis or fetal blood sampling. The couples will need support and nondirective genetic counseling. In the case of hemoglobin S, a rapid "sickle-screening test" is often requested before the administration of a general anesthetic because conditions of anoxia favor in vivo sickling even in the heterozygous state. This practice is of doubtful value with modern-day anesthesia, but the test itself is valuable in confirming the presence of Hb S detected in a screening program.

What is the nature of the tests?

Screening methods for structural hemoglobin variants exploit differences in electrical charge. They include alkaline electrophoresis and more sophisticated methods such as iso-electric focusing (IEF) and high-performance liquid chromatography (HPLC). The sample required for laboratory screening is EDTA-anticoagulated blood.

Screening can be universal or targeted. Although screening can begin with an ethnic question, it needs to relate not only to the patient, but also to her partner and their ancestors. Testing should follow if either partner is of non–Northern European origin. All populations show sporadic incidence of hemoglobinopathies, so that in many areas it is best not to rely on ethnic origin questions because of intermarriage, but rather to use a universal blood screening policy. In nonemergency situations the sickle cell solubility test is not recommended as a screening test, as it is not 100% reliable.

Lower prevalence areas using an ethnic question to determine who should be offered screening may need to choose among several methods targeted to the workload or consider collaborating with other laboratories to form a larger unit. More specialized laboratories may be required for the less common studies. DNA analysis is still expensive and time-consuming. It should only be performed according to strict guidelines (e.g., in confirming the exact mutation in β thalassemia and in confirming β thalassemia).

The diagnosis of thalassemia. Thalassemia is the absence of synthesis or, in some cases, the underproduction of a particular hemoglobin chain. Screening begins with the full blood count and applying a cutoff mean corpuscular hemoglobin (MCH) below 27 pg to trigger further investigations such as HPLC.[8] Carriers of β thalassemia are diagnosed by their reduced MCH level and raised Hb A_2 levels. Hb A_2 is a normal, but very minor hemoglobin fraction in adults (about 2%–3%). Carriers may have a slightly raised Hb F, which in healthy adults is typically below 1%. Pregnant women often have slightly raised Hb F (up to 5%); levels below this are rarely significant.

Acquired disorders that increase the red cell indices, such as vitamin B_{12} or folate deficiencies, may mask the appearance of β thalassemia trait, so that if an Hb A_2 measurement is not performed, there is a risk some carriers will be missed. Iron deficiency reduces the Hb A_2 level, so sometimes it may not be possible to diagnose thalassemia until the patient is iron replete. This should not delay partner testing, as a normal finding in the partner rules out the risk of a major thalassemia syndrome in the infant in most cases. Rare cases of silent β carriers will be missed using routine laboratory methods.

Carriers of α thalassemia trait have a normal or reduced MCH and a normal or slightly reduced Hb A_2. Four genes govern the production of the α chains, so the effects on the MCH depend on how many genes are deleted, or, in rare cases, nonfunctional. Table 16–3 illustrates the more common gene arrangements and the corresponding findings. Although the diagnosis of $α^+$ and $α^0$ may be suspected from the MCH and Hb A_2 levels, the definitive diagnosis can only be made by examining DNA. However, the important genotype to detect

Table 16-3	**Alpha gene phenotypes**	
Genotype	**Phenotype**	**Significance**
αα/αα	Normal	Normal
−α/αα	Alpha⁺ thalassemia trait	None for carrier, risk of H disease if partner carries —/αα or —/−α
−α/−α	Alpha⁰ thalassemia trait	None for carrier, risk of H disease if partner carries —/αα or —/−α
—/αα	Alpha⁰ thalassemia trait	None for carrier, risk of H disease if partner carries −α/αα, −α/−α, or —/−α; or hydrops if partner carries —/αα or —/−α
—/−α	Hb H disease	Mild to moderate anemia
—/—	Bart hydrops fetalis	Severe disease
ααα/αα	Triplicated alpha	Interactions with β thal trait

Thal, thalassemia.

(—/αα) occurs predominantly in South East Asia and to a lesser extent around the Mediterranean; only very infrequently does it occur in other population groups. It is important to identify couples at risk of the most severe from of α thalassemia, hydrops fetalis, which is usually due to deletion of all four α-chain genes. The affected fetus has red blood cells containing only Hb Barts, a tetramer composed of λ chains, a condition that is inevitably fatal. In addition, mothers of α thalassemia major fetuses are at increased risk of severe early onset pre-eclampsia. α thalassemia major may be associated with an increased prevalence of other fetal anomalies.

Hb H disease (α–/—) is a mild to moderate disorder that does not require regular intervention.

The converse of α thalassemia trait is the possession of a triplicated α gene (ααα/αα), which makes the chain imbalance more severe.

Interactions between α and β thalassemia also present diagnostic difficulties in an individual as although the Hb A$_2$ remains raised, the indices are normalized and using an MCH cut off may cause these to be missed. The combination of α thalassemia trait in one partner and β thalassemia trait in the other is of no significance.

The diagnosis of hemoglobin variants. Screening methods for structural hemoglobin variants exploit the difference in electrical charge between normal Hb A and the variant hemoglobins. They include alkaline electrophoresis and more sophisticated methods such as iso-electric focusing (IEF) and HPLC. Confirmation of the identity of any variant found will require at least one other method to be performed. Many variants are found by these methods, and while most of them of little clinical significance, they all need careful scrutiny. The important structural variants to detect and which require partner screening are Hbs S, C, D, E, O-Arab and Lepore.[8]

What are the implications of testing?

What does an abnormal test result mean? A woman with a positive screening test may either have a hemoglobinopathy or be a carrier, and definitive testing is required. The presence or absence of sickle hemoglobin should be noted in the medical record in case of general anesthetic. A woman with a clinically significant hemoglobinopathy may benefit from consultation with a specialist in hematology and treated where indicated. When the mother has a hemoglobinopathy trait, she should be counseled and encouraged to ensure her partner is tested. If the fetus is at risk of inheriting a clinically important hemoglobinopathy, antenatal diagnosis should be offered in the context of nondirective genetic counseling and if affected, pregnancy termination made available.

What does a normal test result mean? Individuals with a normal screening test can be reassured for the most part that they do not have a hemoglobinopathy.

What is the cost of testing?

The full blood count is performed routinely at the woman's initial prenatal visit and therefore is not an additional cost. As with most laboratory tests, the cost per test is closely related to the throughput volume; thus, screening by HPLC can be very cost-effective. This is a highly automated procedure and even in the high-prevalence areas, most test results will be normal and will need no further work, and validity and reproducibility of abnormal results are generally improved with greater experience.

We have demonstrated in our North London program that universal antenatal screening of women with proactive nurse counseling averts 10% of sickle cell disease and 95% of β thalassemia major fetuses. At 1994/1995 prices, the laboratory identification per woman with an abnormal hemoglobin cost £209. Significant savings in health sector costs arise when the overall hemoglobinopathy prevalence is quite low (1%) particularly if 75% are β thalassemia as shown in Table 16–4.[9] Clearly, the cost per case identified rises as the ethnic minority population falls.

■ Conclusions and Recommendations

There is only a need to screen and test people once in their adult life assuming high laboratory standards and good medical record keeping. This cost-effective outcome is rarely achieved. The ideal time to screen a subject for their hemoglobin status is before their reproductive lives begin, perhaps in family planning clinics. Certainly, women found to carry a relevant hemoglobinopathy trait should be informed, counseled accordingly, and encouraged to bring their partners for testing early in their relationship or pregnancy. This is also important for carrier women undergoing fertility treatment. Many clinics using sperm donors have not yet instituted the necessary checks for hemoglobinopathies.

Table 16–4	**Estimated annual NHS savings of universal screening in £ at 1994/1995 prices at different combinations of prevalence and proportions of carriers for beta thalassemia (2,101 women)**			
	% Overall prevalence (all carriers sickle and thalassemia)			
% β Thalassemia				
	7.5	5.0	2.5	1.0
25	61,100	37,100	13,100	(1350)
50	142,000	91,000	40,000	9500
100	305,000	199,100	95,000	31,000

NHS, National Health Service.

Each woman from an area whose prevalence exceeds 1% should be considered for hemoglobin screening at presentation if not previously screened to ensure timely and appropriate counseling respecting abnormal results. In this way women and couples will be able to exercise genetic choice relating to their outcomes. Zeuner et al.[10] have suggested

The use of economic criteria alone to determine whether a local screening policy should be universal or selective is not equitable: ethnic minority mothers and infants in lower-prevalence areas would receive a lower-coverage screening service than would be available to them in a high-prevalence area.

■ **Summary**

1 ■ **What Is the Problem that Requires Screening?**

Clinically relevant hemoglobinopathies.

a. *What is the incidence/prevalence of the target condition?*
Varies with the ethnic make-up of the population from 3/10,000 to 150/10,000 (see Table 16–2)

b. *What are the sequelae of the condition that are of interest in clinical medicine?*
Sickle cell disease: severe life-threatening crises
β Thalassemia: life-long transfusion support.

2 ■ The Tests

a. What is the purpose of the tests?

To identify carriers (and those with the disease) to offer counseling and antenatal diagnosis for couples at risk of an affected fetus

b. What is the nature of the tests?

Screening methods begin with a blood film and full blood count when sickle cell disease or thalassemia is suspected. Using tests that exploit differences in electrical charge, abnormal results trigger confirmation. These include cellulose acetate electrophoresis, iso-electric focusing, and HPLC. In thalassemia, the definitive diagnosis can only be made by examining DNA. In nonemergency situations the sickle cell solubility test is not recommended as a screening test, as it is not 100% reliable.

c. What are the implications of testing?

1. What does an abnormal test result mean?

   A woman with a positive screening test may either have a hemoglobinopathy or be a carrier, and definitive testing is required. A woman with a clinically significant hemoglobinopathy may benefit from consultation with a specialist in hematology and treated where indicated. When the mother has a hemoglobinopathy trait, she should be counseled and encouraged to ensure her partner is tested. Antenatal invasive diagnosis should be offered, where indicated

2. What does a normal test result mean?

   No risk of hemoglobinopathy in the infant

d. What is the cost of testing?

£15 including counseling but not antenatal diagnosis.

3 ■ Conclusions and Recommendations

All women from areas with a prevalence above 1% should be considered for hemoglobinopathy screening.

References

1. Weatherall DJ, Clegg JB. *The Thalassaemia Syndromes*. Malden, MA: Blackwell Science, 2001.
2. Bain BJ. *Haemoglobinopathy Diagnosis*. Malden, MA: Blackwell Science, 2001.
3. Hickman M, Modell B, Greengross P, et al. Mapping the prevalence of sickle cell and beta thalassaemia in England: estimating and validating ethnic-specific rates. *Br J Haematol* 1999;104:860–867.
4. Lau YL, Chan LC, Chan YYA, et al. Prevalence and genotypes of α and β thalassemia carriers in Hong Kong: implications for population screening. *N Engl J Med* 1997;336:1298–1301.
5. Davies SC, Oni L. Fortnightly review: management of patients with sickle cell disease. *BMJ* 1997;315:656–660.
6. Serjeant GR, Serjeant BE. *Sickle Cell Disease*, 3rd edition. Oxford: Oxford University Press, 2001.
7. Cunningham MJ, Macklin EA, Neufeld EJ, et al. Complications of beta-thalassemia major in North America. *Blood.* 2004;104:34–39.
8. Guidelines on the laboratory diagnosis of haemoglobinopathies. *Br J Haematol* 1998;101:783–792.
9. Davies SC, Cronin E, Gill M, et al. Screening for sickle cell disease and thalassaemia: a systematic review with supplementary research. *Health Technol Assess* 2000;4:1–99.
10. Zeuner D, Ades AE, Karnon J, et al. Antenatal and Neonatal haemoglobinopathy screening in the UK: review and economic analysis. *Health Technol Assess* 1999;3:1–183.
    Further information on antenatal hemoglobin screening in England may be obtained from: www.kcl-phs.org.uk/haemscreenig/.

17

Early-onset Genetic Diseases

Grazia M. S. Mancini

■ What Is the Problem that Requires Screening?

Early-onset genetic diseases.

Early-onset genetic diseases, particularly those affecting the nervous system, are usually not treatable and constitute a heavy burden for both the family and the community. Some manifest early with severe deterioration causing great emotional impact on the family, whereas others are associated with prolonged survival and need life-long support, causing high costs to the community. Most early-onset genetic disorders are rare and typically inherited as recessive (autosomal or X-linked) traits. The prevalence is higher in consanguineous marriages than in the general population. However, the prevalence is higher in some communities even in apparently nonconsanguineous marriages. Factors that contribute to this high prevalence include geographic isolation, religious/cultural background favoring isolation and inbreeding (i.e., founder effects and genetic drift), and selective carrier advantage driven by environmental factors (e.g., thalassemic trait offering resistance against malaria[1,2] and cystic fibrosis heterozygosity conveying protection from cholera.[3]

We focus in this chapter on early-onset disorders that meet the general screening criteria and for which (DNA) tests are available to easily identify healthy carriers who can then be counseled. Examples of ethnic groups to whom carrier testing has been validated and is presently offered include the Jews of East-European (Ashkenazi) descent,[4] the Mediterranean (Italian/Greek/Cypriots) populations, the African blacks, the Southeastern Asians and Chinese,[5–7] and the North-European whites for cystic fibrosis (carrier frequency 1:25/30, disease prevalence 1:2,500) (reviewed in Chapter 15).

Disorders with high prevalence in the Jewish community are listed in Table 17–1. These disorders constitute the screening program, with the exception of congenital deafness and the addition of cystic fibrosis, that is recommended by the American College of Obstetricians and Gynecologists for individuals of

Table 17–1	**Disorders of early onset**

Disorders with high prevalence in the Jewish community:
Tay-Sachs disease (early infantile GM2 gangliosidosis)
Gaucher disease (glucosylceramidose)
Niemann-Pick disease type A and B (sphingomyelinosis)
Canavan disease (N-acetyl aspartate acylase deficiency)
Riley-Day disease (familial dysautonomia, HSAN-III)
Fanconi anemia (pancytopenia)
Bloom syndrome
Nonsyndromic hearing loss (autosomal recessive congenital deafness)

Diseases with high prevalence in the Mediterranean (Continental Italians/Sardinians/Greeks/Cypriots) populations include hemoglobinopathies:
Beta-thalassemia
Alpha-thalassemia
Sickle cell anemia

Eastern European Jewish ancestry as part of obstetric care.[8] Screening for one cause of congenital nonsyndromic hearing loss (DFNB1 caused by mutations in the *GJB2* connexin 26 gene) should also be offered to this community (www.jewishgeneticscenter.org). Some screening programs also include mucolipidosis IV (ML-IV), a rare lysosomal storage disease. With a carrier frequency of 1:120, ML-IV is not among the most common disorders in Ashkenazi Jews. Late-onset/ milder disorders frequent in the Ashkenazi for which antenatal testing is being offered also include nonclassical congenital adrenal hyperplasia (21-beta-hydroxylase mutations), torsion dystonia (*DYT1* gene mutations), and factor XI deficiency (hemophilia C, plasma thromboplastin antecedent [PTA] deficiency) (see: www.jewishgeneticscenter.org).

Diseases with a high prevalence in the Mediterranean (Continental Italians/Sardinians/Greeks/Cypriots) populations are listed in Table 17–1. Hemoglobinopathy screening is also offered to Pakistanis and Cypriots in the United Kingdom (see Chapter 16).[9–11] Screening programs are also being developed in Southeast Asia, India, and China.

Other early-onset diseases with high prevalence in North-European whites that are amenable to prenatal screening include spinal muscular atrophy (SMA), fragile-X syndrome (see Chapter 18), and cystic fibrosis (see Chapter 15). No screening for SMA has been implemented yet (affecting 1/10,000 live births, with a carrier prevalence of 1/50), due partially to technical limitation of the available tests requiring appropriate pretest counseling.[12] Carrier screening for fragile-X syndrome was implemented in an Israeli pilot study.[13]

What is the incidence/prevalence of the target condition?

The relevant prevalences are listed in Table 17–2. TSD (OMIM 272800), also known as infantile GM2 gangliosidosis (obsolete name: infantile amaurotic idiocy), is a severe neurodegenerative lysosomal storage disease that, beginning at 3 months of age, causes psychomotor regression, macrocephaly,

Table 17–2.   Prevalence of common disorders of early onset

Disorders with high prevalence in the Ashkenazi Jewish community

	Carrier prevalence	Disease prevalence
Tay-Sachs disease[1]	1:25	1:2500
Gaucher disease	1:13	1:676
Familial dysautonomia	1:25-1:36	1:4096
Canavan disease	1:40-1:57	1:6724
Niemann-Pick disease	1:80	1:25600
Fanconi anemia	1:80	1:25600
Bloom syndrome	1:107	1: 45726
Nonsyndromic deafness	1:25	1:1700

Disorders with high prevalence in the Mediterranean and Asian population: Hemo-globinopathies:

	Carrier prevalence	Disease prevalence
Beta-Thalassemia	1:38 (average Mediterranean)	
	1:8 (Sardinian/South Italians)	1:250 (before screening)
Alpha-thalassemia (Southeastern Asians, Indians, Chinese, Sardinians)	1:20	1:2500
Sickle cell anemia (Black Africans and African-Americans)	1:12	1:400-1:600

[1]The carrier prevalence of Tay-Sachs disease is 10 times lower (1:250-1:300) in Caucasians and Sephardic Jews. Certain populations that are relatively isolated genetically, such as the French Canadians of the eastern St. Lawrence River Valley area of Quebec, the Cajuns from Louisiana and the Old Order Amish in Pennsylvania carry Tay-Sachs gene mutations with frequencies comparable to or even greater than those observed in Ashkenazi Jews.

epilepsy, and blindness from macular degeneration. Death usually occurs within the first few years of life. TSD is caused by recessively inherited mutations of the *HEXA* gene, which encodes for the alpha subunit of lysosomal beta-hexosaminidase (HEXA), a soluble glycohydrolase-degrading terminal N-acetylgalactosamine sugar from oligosaccharides and GM2 ganglioside. The enzyme consists of two dimeric isoforms: a heterodimer of one alpha subunit and one beta subunit ($\alpha\beta$, HEXA catalytic activity) and a homodimer of two beta-subunits ($\beta\beta$, HEXB catalytic activity). *HEXA* gene mutations on chromosome 15q23-q24 lead to Tay-Sachs disease. Mutations in the beta subunit gene *HEXB* cause total hexosaminidase deficiency, leading to Sandhoff disease (OMIM 268800).

Gaucher disease. Gaucher disease is another lysosomal storage disease caused by defective degradation of the sphingolipid glucosylceramide by the lysosomal membrane enzyme glucosylceramidase (glucocerebrosidase, beta-glucosidase,

OMIM 606463). There are three clinical forms, all autosomal recessive and caused by mutations in the glucosylceramidase gene on chromosome 1q21. The symptoms involve either the reticuloendothelial system with progressive hepatosplenomegaly and skeletal infiltration but no neurologic signs (type I) or predominantly the central nervous system with spasticity, cranial nerve paresis, mental retardation, and hepatosplenomegaly with early-onset (type II) or neurologic signs and splenomegaly over a prolonged period (type III). Lethal perinatal forms and distinctive cardiovascular forms are also described. The correlation of genotype to phenotype is not perfect. In Ashkenazi, the most prevalent mutation is N370S leading to type I (if homozygous) or to type II. The very high prevalence seems justified by the fact that homozygous N370S individuals can be asymptomatic. Enzyme replacement therapy is possible with a synthesized enzyme (Ceradase; Genzyme, Cambridge, MA) as well as substrate reduction therapy using miglustat. A regimen incorporating both approaches seems promising in the nonneuronopathic forms.[14,15]

Niemann-Pick disease. Niemann-Pick disease is an autosomal recessive disorder caused by mutations in the gene *SMPD1* encoding for the enzyme acid sphingomyelinase and presents clinically as one of two main phenotypes. Type A is characterized by an early-onset hepatosplenomegaly, foamy cells in bone marrow, neurologic regression, and early death. Type B presents with milder symptoms, no neurologic deterioration, and prolonged course (OMIM 257200 and 607616). Niemann-Pick disease type C is caused by mutations in other genes and is not common in the Jewish population. The prevalence of Niemann-Pick disease type A is highest among Ashkenazi Jews. Type B is more common in non-Jews but has been reported in Ashkenazi Jews. Different mutations in *SMPD1* presumably explain the different Niemann-Pick disease phenotypes.[16] Therapeutic trials with allogenic bone marrow transplantation have been reported.[17]

Canavan disease. The enzyme aspartoacylase (aminoacylase-2) responsible for degradation of N-acetyl aspartic acid to aspartate and acetate is deficient in Canavan disease as a result of autosomal recessive mutations in the *ASPA* gene on chromosome 17p (OMIM 271900 and 608034). This early-onset (3 months of age) leukoencephalopathy includes spasticity, progressive macrocephaly, blindness, and epilepsy, culminating in an early childhood death. The disease is easily diagnosed by brain imaging with magnetic resonance imaging (MRI) combined with 1H-MRS, showing high brain N-acetyl-aspartate peak.

Riley-Day disease (familial dysautonomia, hereditary sensory autonomic neuropathy-III). The autosomal recessive familial dysautonomia (FD, OMIM 223900) results from mutations of the *IKBKAP* gene on chromosome 9q31. It affects sympathetic and parasympathetic neurons causing severe symptoms in infancy characterized by progressive neuronal degeneration. This gene encodes for a scaffold protein that normally promotes phosphorylation and degradation of transcription factor nuclear factor-kappa B (NF-κB), which coordinates the activation of numerous genes in response to pathogens and proinflammatory cytokines.[18,19] In FD, gastrointestinal symptoms with vomiting and pseudo-obstruction, decreased sensitivity to pain and temperature, decreased tear production, cardiovascular instability, and decreased tendon reflexes with motor impairment are all severe and progressive. Although survival is shortened, patients with FD can reach adult age and eventually reproduce with appropriate support.[20]

Fanconi anemia/pancytopenia. Fanconi anemia (FA, OMIM 227645) is characterized by physical abnormalities (in 60% to 75%), bone marrow failure, and an increased risk of malignancy. The physical abnormalities include short stature, abnormal skin pigmentation, and malformations of the thumbs, forearms, skeletal system, eyes, kidneys, urinary tract, ear, heart, gastrointestinal system, oral cavity, and central nervous system. Hearing loss, hypogonadism, and developmental delay are also observed. Progressive bone marrow failure with pancytopenia typically presents during the first decade, often with thrombocytopenia or leukopenia. The estimated cumulative incidence of bone marrow failure by age 40 to 48 years is 90%; of hematologic malignancies (primarily acute myeloid leukemia), 10% to 33%; and of nonhematologic malignancies (solid tumors, particularly of the head and neck, skin, gastrointestinal tract, and genital tract), 28% to 29%. The diagnosis of FA is dependent on the detection of chromosomal aberrations (breaks, rearrangements, radials, exchanges) in cells after culture in the presence of a DNA interstrand cross-linking agent such as diepoxybutane or mitomycin C.

Genetically, FA is a heterogeneous disorder caused by mutations in at least 11 different genes, as revealed by genetic complementation experiments (complementation groups A, B, C, D1 [*BRCA2*], D2, E, F, G, I, J, and L). Only eight of these genes are known. In the Ashkenazi Jews, a common mutation in the *FANCC* gene (Fanconi anemia complementation group C) is seen and carriers are asymptomatic. It is not known whether FA heterozygotes have, like *BRCA2* heterozygotes, an increased risk of developing malignancies.[21]

Bloom syndrome. Bloom syndrome (OMIM 210900) is an autosomal recessive disorder characterized by proportionate pre- and postnatal growth deficiency; sun-sensitive, telangiectatic, hypo- and hyperpigmented skin; a predisposition to malignancy; and chromosomal instability. Immunologic markers include an immunoglobulin deficiency (immunoglobin A [IgA], IgG, IgM) and an impaired lymphocyte proliferation response to malignancy. Other laboratory abnormalities are high sister chromatid exchange (SCE) rate and increased chromosomal breakage. Bloom syndrome is caused by mutations in the RecQ protein–like 3 gene on chromosome 15q26 (*RECQL3*). RecQ is an *Escherichia coli* gene that is a member of the RecF recombination pathway, a pathway of genes in which mutations abolish the conjugational "recombination proficiency" and ultraviolet resistance of a mutant strain. The absence of the *RECQL3* gene product probably destabilizes other enzymes that participate in DNA replication and repair, perhaps through direct inter-action and more general responses to DNA damage.[22] The common Ashke-nazi mutation consists of a 6–base pair (bp) deletion and a 7-bp insertion at nucleotide 2281.[23]

Nonsyndromic hearing loss. One of the first loci to be identified for autosomal recessive early-onset nonsyndromic deafness (ARNSD) was the DFNB1 locus on chromosome 13q12-13 (OMIM 220290). The gene is identified as *GJB2*, which encodes for a transmembrane protein called connexin 26 (Cx26). Con-nexin 26 oligomerizes with five other connexins to form a connexon, the con-stituent component of gap junctions.[24] Mutations in *Cx26* gene account for about 50% of the cases of severe/profound congenital ARNSD in several pop-ulations. However, the degree of deafness as a result of the *Cx26* mutation varies among individuals.

The carrier frequency of *GJB2* mutations in the Ashkenazi Jews is 1/20–25, with a disease incidence of 1/1,700, whereas in the white US population, the carrier frequency is estimated to be 1/35 and the disease frequency of 1:7,000. In the Ashkenazi Jewish population, the 167delT is the most common variant. In whites, the most common variant in the *Cx26* gene is the 35delG mutation. One research study observed a carrier rate in the Ashkenazi Jewish population of 1/130 for 35delG and 1/25 for 167delT.[47]

β thalassemia. Mutations in the hemoglobin beta-chain (*HBB* gene) cause β thalassemia. It consists of a quite variable microcytic hypochromic anemia, an abnormal peripheral blood smear with nucleated red blood cells, and reduced amounts of hemoglobin A (Hb A) on hemoglobin electrophoresis. Clinically, β thalassemia may present as (a) *thalassemia trait (thalassemia minor)*, character-ized by mostly asymptomatic hematologic changes with microcythemia, an increased red blood cell (RBC) count, and heterozygous beta-globin gene mutations; (b) *intermediate thalassemia*, characterized by mild to moderate decreased RBC resistance to hemolysis, jaundice, hepatosplenomegaly, and mild skeletal changes; or (c) *thalassemia major* (Cooley anemia), a full-blown hemolytic anemia requiring maintenance transfusion therapy from infancy leading to signs of iron overload in spleen, liver, heart, and skeleton if not aggressively treated with chelating agents. Homozygosity for β thalassemia usually results in transfusion-dependent thalassemia major and, rarely, in mild nontransfusion-dependent conditions. Double heterozygotes for alpha-chain and beta-chain gene variants can also lead to *thalassemia major* or *inter-mediate thalassemia*.

β thalassemia is highly heterogeneous at the molecular level, with more than 150 different molecular defects identified. Despite this heterogeneity, each at-risk population has its own spectrum of common mutations, usually from five to 15, a finding that simplifies mutation analysis and population screening.[13,25] Successful genetic screening programs for high school students in the Montreal population,[26] for the Italian population (www.anmi-microcitemie-roma.it/centro.htm), and for women of child-bearing age have been implemented.[12] A 20-year Sardinian screening program has reduced the birth rate of thalassemia major from 1/250 live births to 1/4,000.[12]

α thalassemia. α Thalassemia results from mutations in the alpha chain of hemoglobin. Full-blown α thalassemia presents with severe infantile or antenatal hemolytic anemia causing hydrops fetalis (Bart hydrops). However, the type of mutations determines the disease phenotype. The globin alpha-chain gene on chromosome 16p is duplicated, containing two identical genes on each chromosome. The four alpha-chain genes encode for four alpha-chains in a healthy individual. Three normal alpha genes result in a silent carrier state. Two normal alpha genes result in microcytosis (so-called heterozygous α thalassemia). One normal alpha gene results in microcytosis and hemolysis (so-called Hb H disease). No normal alpha gene results in "homozygous α thalassemia" manifested as fatal hydrops fetalis. Recent analysis of thalassemia carriers in Sardinia has shown that α thalassemia heterozygosity is very common in the Sardinians, as well as in other Mediterranean communities.[27] This means that carrier screening in this population must include both alpha- and beta-chain globin genes. In total, a gene frequency of 11.7% for alpha-chain versus a 3.87% for the beta-chain was calculated in a Chinese community, indicating high prevalence in this population.[28] Screening for α thalassemia, is highly recommended by the World Health Organization (WHO) in a Southeastern Asian population as illustrated by recent epidemiologic studies.[10,29,30]

Sickle cell anemia. The most common Mendelian disorder in black Americans (about 1/ 400), sickle cell anemia is an autosomal recessive disorder caused by a mutation in the sixth codon of the *HBB* gene. A single nucleotide substitution (GAG to GTG) leads to the transcription of valine instead of glutamic acid, resulting in an abnormal Hb molecule (Hb S).

The prevalence of *HBB* alleles associated with sickle cell disease is even higher in other parts of the world—as high as 25% to 30% in West Africa, resulting in the annual birth in Africa of 120,000 babies with sickle cell disease. The clinical manifestations of sickle cell disease reflect variable degrees of hemolysis and intermittent episodes of vascular occlusion resulting in tissue ischemia and acute and chronic organ dysfunction (most often in the spleen, brain, lungs, and kidneys). Consequences of hemolysis include chronic anemia, jaundice, predisposition to aplastic crisis, cholelithiasis, and delayed growth and sexual maturation. Vascular occlusion and tissue ischemia can cause acute and chronic injury to virtually every organ of the body.[31] In addition to carrier screening, newborn screening for sickle cell anemia has been implemented in the some states in the United States. It is recommended prophylactic antibiotics be given to those affected to decrease the incidence of infection, which provokes sickle cell crisis[32] (www-phm.umds.ac.uk/haem-screening).

■ The Tests

What is the purpose of the tests?

The purpose of screening is to identify carriers of rare early-onset genetic diseases in populations with a high gene frequency, and to provide an opportunity of review and reproductive choice in carriers. Carrier couples can be offered antenatal diagnosis by biochemical or DNA analysis. Preimplantation diagnosis or stem cell transplants may become alternatives to termination of affected pregnancies. Another purpose of testing is to extend the screening to the families of carriers with the goal of prevention by genetic counseling.

What is the nature of the tests?

Tay-Sachs disease. The measurement of HEXA enzymatic activity in serum or leukocytes using synthetic substrates provides a simple, inexpensive, and highly accurate method for heterozygote identification. More than 90 disease-causing mutations have been identified in the *HEXA* gene. Screening panels have been developed for the different ethnic groups to reflect the different founder mutations observed in different populations. Serum may be used for testing all males and those women who are not pregnant and not using oral contraceptives. Leukocytes are used to test women who are pregnant or who are using oral contraceptives and for any individual whose serum HEXA enzymatic activity is in an inconclusive range. When the enzymatic test is abnormal, the mutation is confirmed by mutation analysis. The detection rate is 98%.

Six most common mutations have been identified in the Ashkenazi Jews. The panel of six mutations comprises (a) three mutations leading to no protein activity (null allele) (+TATC1278, +1IVC12, +1IVS9), in which either the homozygous state or compound heterozygosity are associated with Tay-Sachs disease; (b) the G269S allele, which is associated with an adult-onset form of hexosaminidase A deficiency in the homozygous state or in the compound heterozygote with a null allele; and (c) the two *pseudodeficiency* alleles (R247W and R249W), which are not associated with neurologic disease, but are associated with reduced degradation of synthetic substrate used when the HEXA enzymatic activity is determined. The presence of one pseudodeficiency allele reduces HEXA enzymatic activity toward synthetic substrates, but does not reduce enzymatic activity with the natural substrate, GM2 ganglioside (not commercially available as substrate). Thus, a potential problem exists distinguishing between a disease-causing allele, which decreases HEXA enzymatic activity toward both artificial and natural substrate, and a pseudodeficiency allele, which decreases HEXA enzymatic activity to artificial substrate *only*. This problem is avoided by using a DNA-based assay that includes testing of pseudodeficiency alleles when the enzyme assay shows abnormal HEXA activity. About 35% of non-Jewish individuals identified as heterozygotes by HEXA enzyme–based testing are carriers of a pseudodeficiency mutation. In contrast, only about 2% of Jewish individuals with reduced HEXA enzymatic activity are heterozygotes for the pseudodeficiency allele R247W.[33] This panel identifies about 92% of carriers of Jewish ancestry and 23% of non-Jewish carriers. The American College of Obstetrics and Gynecology recommends offering testing of Tay-Sachs enzymatic activity to both members of a couple in which one member is of Ashkenazi Jewish heritage.

The +IVS9 mutation is not common in Jews, and therefore is not included in screening programs for this population. However, this mutation is frequent among other ethnic groups like individuals of Celtic, French, Cajun, or Pennsylvania-Dutch ancestry and is included in most screening panels. In Quebec, a 7.6-kilobase (kb) deletion is the most common allele associated with Tay-Sachs disease. Therefore this mutation is included in the screening panel for French-Canadians[34] (www.genetests.org).

Gaucher disease. DNA analysis of the glucocerebrosidase gene is used for carrier screening. A panel of four mutations (N370S, L444P, 84GG, IVS2+1) detects up to 97% of healthy Ashkenazi carriers and up to 60% of non-Ashkenazi Jewish carriers.[7,35] The biochemical assay of glucocerebrosidase is not sensitive enough to detect carriers.

Niemann-Pick disease. Three mutations are account for more than 95% of all cases of type A Niemann-Pick disease (NPD) among Ashkenazi Jews (L302P, R496L, fsP330). Less is known about mutations responsible for type B NPD, although one mutation (δR608) has been identified in both Ashkenazi Jews and non-Jews. Screening of the Ashkenazi Jewish population will detect more than 95% of NPD carriers using a four-mutation panel that includes L302P, R496L, fsP330, and δR608, the three predominant type A mutations and one recurrent type B mutation.[19] As for Gaucher disease, the sphingomyelinase biochemical assay is not sensitive enough to detect carriers.

Canavan disease. A panel of four mutations in the *ASPA* gene is used for carrier screening test of people of Ashkenazi Jewish descent: Y231X, E285A and 305E. The carrier detection rate with this panel is 98%.[36] The enzymatic test of *N*-acetyl-aspartate acylase is not sensitive enough for carrier screening.

Familial dysautonomia. The genetic diagnosis of familial dysautonomia is established by analysis of the *IKBKAP* gene. Two mutations account for more than 99% of mutant alleles in individuals of Ashkenazi Jewish descent affected with FD: IVS20(+6T→C), the major founder mutation, which is responsible for virtually all occurrences of FD among the Ashkenazim, and the rarely identified R696P mutation.[37]

Fanconi anemia. Three common mutations in the *FANCC* gene are identified (IVS4 +4 A to T; R548X, and 322delG),[38] as well as several rare mutations (Q13X, R185X, and L554P). The mutation prevalent in Ashkenazi Jews is IVS4 +4 A to

T, and carrier screening for FA in this population is based on testing for this single mutation with a detection rate of 99% (www.fanconi.org).

Bloom syndrome. Screening of Ashkenazi Jews is performed by DNA testing for the common Jewish mutation (6-bp deletion and a 7-bp insertion at nucleotide 2281) in the *RECQL3* gene. The detection rate of the test is 97%.

Nonsyndromic hearing loss. Mutations in the *GJB2* gene for Cx26 cause autosomal recessive congenital deafness. The most common mutation in Ashkenazi Jews is 167delT, whereas in whites, it is 35delG (about 2.5% of the population).[39] There is a higher incidence of this particular 35delG mutation in the connexin 26 gene of individuals from Israel, Spain, and Italy who have hearing impairment. However, 10% to 50% of *affected* subjects with GJB2 mutations carry only one mutant allele. Recent studies reveal the genes for connexin 26 and connexin 30 (Cx30) are closely linked and digenic compound heterozygotes for recessive mutations at the two loci are also deaf. This might be responsible for the variable degree of deafness observed in Cx26 mutations.[40] The large truncating mutation often observed in Cx30 is also frequent in Ashkenazi Jews, and a founder effect has been shown in this population. In one large multicenter study, the association of Cx30 with Cx26 mutations explained about 80% to 85% of the apparent Cx26 heterozygotes in Israel, Spain, and France.[41]

Antenatal screening for both 167delT and 35delG mutations in GJB2 is offered to the Ashkenazi Jewish population with a detection rate of 95%[47]. The screening should include the Cx30 deletion. Carrier screening in the white population for the high-prevalence mutations is currently under evaluation.[42] Although GJB2 mutation analysis would detect 50% of the ARNSD, the presence of about 100 genetic causes of nonsyndromic deafness conceivably limits the value of a carrier screening in non-Jewish groups. Furthermore, ethical issues must be addressed when offering antenatal diagnosis for congenital deafness. Rather than antenatal, postnatal screening programs for hereditary deafness (early hearing detection and intervention [EHDI] programs), which accounts for 50% of congenital deafness, are being exploited.[43,44]

β thalassemia. Carrier screening for thalassemias has been implemented in about 13 countries. Carrier screening is performed by hematologic tests and mutation analysis of the beta-globin gene (HBB gene). Carriers show a hematologic profile characterized by a reduced mean corpuscular volume (MCV), mean corpuscular hemoglobin (MCH), and RBC morphologic changes that are less severe than in affected individuals. No erythroblastosis is present. If the hematologic analysis is abnormal, hemoglobin electrophoresis is performed and the presence of a mildly increased Hb F (0.5%–4%) and Hb A2 (>3.5%) with a corresponding reduction of Hb A (92%–95%) suggests carrier diagnosis.[45] At this point, mutation panels are tested according to the ethnic origin of the subject.[46] Since the introduction of polymerase chain reaction (PCR)–

based sequence analysis, screening for β thalassemia variants and sickle-cell mutations are performed in the same test. Often the screening panel includes the sequencing of the alpha-chain, as it is in the Sardinian population.[30] Some communities have combined β thalassemia screening with Tay-Sachs screening.[29]

α thalassemia. Several screening programs are being evaluated in Southeast Asia and China using cost-effective hematologic and molecular tests for α thalassemia in combination with β thalassemia.[9,10,31,50] In Sardinians, the screening for thalassemias includes PCR-based analysis of alpha- and beta-chain genes.[30]

Sickle cell anemia. The beta-globin gene *HBB* (OMIM 141900) contains a mutation that causes sickling of hemoglobin rather than reducing the amount of beta globin as in β thalassemia. The most common cause of sickle cell anemia is Hb S, with Sickle cell disease being most prevalent in blacks. The other forms of sickle cell disease result from co-inheritance of Hb S with other abnormal beta chain variants, the most common forms being sickle-hemoglobin C disease (Hb SC) and two types of sickle ß-thalassemia (Hb Sß(+)-thalassemia and Hb Sß°-thalassemia). Other globin beta chain variants such as D-Punjab and O-Arab also cause sickle cell disease when co-inherited with Hb S. Carrier screening uses a DNA test that targets the four variants (Hb S, Hb C, Hb D, Hb O) and is usually combined with the α and β thalassemia screening (www.genetests.org).

What are the implications of testing?

What does an abnormal test result mean? All the tests described here seek the identification of carriers of autosomal-recessive diseases. Carrier identification by enzymatic tests is subject to pitfalls, as in the case of Tay-Sachs disease and pseudodeficiency allele. In Tay-Sachs disease, carriers are individuals with a disease causing DNA mutation or carrier level enzyme analysis result on both serum and leukocyte testing with no detectable mutation and no pseudodeficiency alleles. If both partners are found to be carriers, they should be counseled they have a 25% risk of having an affected child with each pregnancy. Reproductive options available to modify this risk include antenatal diagnosis by amniocentesis or chorionic villus sampling, egg or sperm donation, preimplantation diagnosis, or adoption.

When one individual is identified as a carrier, the partner should also be tested if possible. Particular attention should be paid when one carrier belongs to a high-risk community and the partner comes from a low-risk group. One option is to test the low-risk partner depending on the frequency of the disorder in the general population and on the availability of a test able to significantly screen for mutations in the general population to significantly modify the recurrence risk.[51] For example, the six-mutation *HEXA* panel used for Ashkenazi Jews detects 92% of the Jewish Tay-Sachs carriers but only 23% of the non-Jewish carriers. Because this can lead to risk modification without risk exclusion, informed consent after nondirective counseling is essential.

In the Sardinian β thalassemia carrier-screening program, voluntary screening is offered to prospective parents and to women with an ongoing pregnancy. Education of the population, training of health operators, and use of posters and informative booklets are critical elements in the success of the program. The use of extended family screening magnified the efficacy of the screening program, allowing for the identification of the large majority (>90%) of parents at risk by screening only 11% to 13% of the population at child-bearing age.[12] This approach is particularly cost-effective compared with the financial burden of the screening the entire population, but it does require the education and active participation of the patient (or parents) who act as messengers for family members.[52,53]

What does a normal test result mean? A normal test result generally means the subject is a noncarrier. In the case of Tay-Sachs disease, where part of the test is based on enzymatic activity, noncarriers are individuals with normal enzyme results or carrier range enzyme results *and* a pseudodeficiency allele on DNA mutation analysis. It is important to realize that the diagnosis of noncarrier status is not definitive for any of these disorders, even if the DNA tests are negative. Negative DNA tests usually decreases the residual risk of being a carrier to values below the carrier prevalence for the population. Therefore, they consistently decrease the procreative risk and do not warrant invasive antenatal diagnosis.

What is the cost of the testing?

The costs of genetic screening by biochemical, hematologic, and enzyme analysis are reasonably modest (about 10 to 100 euros; The Netherlands, 2004) compared with the costs of DNA analysis (500–1000 euros per gene; The Netherlands, 2004). However, simple and cost-effective screening panels for contemporary DNA testing of multiple genes are offered by public institutions and private laboratories.[38] To these costs, the eventual costs of genetic counseling and pregnancy termination must be added.

The life-long support costs for individuals with early-onset neurodegenerative diseases and prolonged survival approximates 300,000 euros (The Netherlands, 2004). In the recent Greek experience, the annual cost of treatment of one patient with thalassemia was estimated at $5,000, whereas the total cost of thalassemia prevention in Greece was estimated as equivalent to the cost of treatment of newborn patients for 1 year[28] (www-phm.umds.ac.uk/haemscreening).

While PCR-based DNA analysis of carriers is feasible and cost-effective in Western countries, DNA tests for thalassemia are often not available in developing countries. Simplified and inexpensive screening strategies, based on osmotic fragility and DCIP precipitation for α and β thalassemia and Hb E screening in South-East Asia are being developed.[10]

■ Conclusions and Recommendations

The best validated screening programs for early-onset genetic diseases are those for Tay Sachs disease and thalassemia. A 20-year experience in Montreal screening for Tay-Sachs and β thalassemia has shown reduction in the disease incidence by 90% to 95%.[29] After a similar length of experience in Sardinia, the birth rate of thalassemia major has declined from 1/250 live births to 1/4,000. These results demonstrate effective prevention of severe genetic disorders by screening. However, long-term experience with population-based genetic screening also reveals that the public perception of the biomedical community as advocates for wide-scale testing and screening may be interpreted, in some systems, as conflicts of interest on the part of entrepreneurial scientists, clinicians, and institutions.[54] One drawback might be the long-term psychological effects of genetic testing.[6] Up until 1995 in Sardinia, there was nearly 100% uptake of antenatal diagnosis. But now there are a small proportion of women who refuse antenatal diagnosis or continue with an affected pregnancy, often depending on whether or not they already have affected children or because of the possibility of bone marrow transplants.[28] Although screening programs for early-onset diseases have been effective and well accepted wherever they were applied, the issues of full educational programs, genetic counseling, social environmental factors, and long-term psychological support remain of uppermost importance.

■ Summary

1 ■ What Is the Problem that Requires Screening?

Early-onset genetic disorders.

a. What is the incidence/prevalence of the target condition?

The carrier prevalence varies between 1% and 9%. Disease prevalence ranges from 1/45,000 to 1/700.

b. What are the sequelae of the condition that are of interest in clinical medicine?

Life-long suffering and premature death.

2 ■ The Tests

a. What is the purpose of the tests?

Identify carriers and affected perinates.

Continued

■ **Summary—cont'd**

b. **What is the nature of the tests?**
Depending upon the disorder, the test may be based on the measurement of a metabolite, enzyme activity, or DNA mutation.

c. **What are the implications of testing?**
1. What does an abnormal test result mean?
   The person with an abnormal test is either a carrier or affected with the disorder in question.
2. What does a normal test result mean?
   In general normal test results identify noncarriers.

d. **What is the cost of testing?**
Cost varies according to the nature of the test, but in general tests are considered cost-beneficial especially when part of a population-based program using automated technologies.

3 ■ Conclusions and Recommendations

Screening programs for early-onset diseases have been effective and well accepted wherever they were applied. The issues of full educational programs, genetic counseling, social environmental factors, and long-term psychological support remain of uppermost importance.

Internet resources

www.anmi-microcitemie-roma.it/centro.htm

www.fanconi.org

www.genetests.org

www.jewishgeneticscenter.org/

OMIM (On-line Mendelian Inheritance in Man): www.ncbi.nlm.nih.gov

www-phm.umds.ac.uk/haemscreening

References

1. Hill AV. Molecular epidemiology of the thalassaemias (including haemoglobin E). *Baillieres Clin Haematol* 1992;5:209–238.
2. Karetti M, Yardumian A, Karetti D, et al. Informing carriers of beta-thalassemia: giving the good news. *Genet Test* 2004;8:2109–2113.
3. Bertranpetit J, Calafell F. Genetic and geographical variability in cystic fibrosis: evolutionary considerations. *Ciba Found Symp* 1996;197:97–114; discussion, 114–118.
4. Slatkin, M. A population-genetic test of founder effects and implications for Ashkenazi Jewish diseases. *Am J Hum Genet* 2004;75:282–293.
5. Petrou M, Brugiatelli M, Old J, et al. Alpha thalassaemia hydrops fetalis in the UK: the importance of screening pregnant women of Chinese, other South East Asian and Mediterranean extraction for alpha thalassaemia trait. *Br J Obstet Gynaecol* 1992;99:985–989.
6. Chan K, Wong MS, Chan TK, et al. A thalassaemia array for Southeast Asia. *Br J Haematol* 2004;124:232–239.
7. Fucharoen G, Sanchaisuriya K, Sae-ung N, et al. A simplified screening strategy for thalassaemia and haemoglobin E in rural communities in Southeast Asia. *Bull World Health Organ* 2004;82:364–372.
8. ACOG. Prenatal and preconceptional carrier screening for genetic diseases in individuals of Eastern European Jewish descent. *Obstet Gynecol* 2004;104:2425–2428.
9. Cao A, Rosatelli MC, Galanello R. Control of beta-thalassaemia by carrier screening, genetic counselling and prenatal diagnosis: the Sardinian experience. *Ciba Found Symp* 1996;197:137–151; discussion, 151–155.
10. Cao A, Saba L, Galanello R, et al. Molecular diagnosis and carrier screening for beta thalassemia. *JAMA* 1997;278:1273–1277.
11. Cao A, Galanello R. Effect of consanguinity on screening for thalassemia. *N Engl J Med* 2002;347:1200–1202.
12. Cusco I, Barcelo MJ, Baiget M, et al. Implementation of SMA carrier testing in genetic laboratories: comparison of two methods for quantifying the SMN1 gene. *Hum Mutat* 2002;20:452–459.
13. Toledano-Alhadef H, Basel-Vanagaite L, Magal N, et al. Fragile-X carrier screening and the prevalence of premutation and full-mutation carriers in Israel. *Am J Hum Genet* 2001;69:351–360.
14. Pastores GM, Barnett NL. Substrate reduction therapy: Miglustat as a remedy for symptomatic patients with Gaucher disease type 1. *Expert Opin Investig Drugs* 2003;12:273–281.
15. Pastores GM, Sibille AR, Grabowski GA. Enzyme therapy in Gaucher disease type 1: dosage efficacy and adverse effects in 33 patients treated for 6 to 24 months. *Blood* 1993;82:408–416.
16. Schuchman EH, Miranda SR. Niemann-Pick disease: mutation update, genotype/phenotype correlations, and prospects for genetic testing. *Genet Test* 1997;1:113–119.
17. Victor S, Coulter JB, Besley GT, et al. Niemann-Pick disease: sixteen-year follow-up of allogeneic bone marrow transplantation in a type B variant. *J Inherit Metab Dis* 2003;26:775–785.
18. Cohen L, Henzel WJ, Baeuerle PA. IKAP is a scaffold protein of the I kappaB kinase complex. *Nature* 1998;395:292–296.
19. Anderson SL, Coli R, Daly I, et al. Familial dysautonomia is caused by mutations of the IKAP gene. *Am J Hum Genet* 2001;68:753–758.
20. Slaugenhaupt SA, Gusella JF. Familial dysautonomia. *Curr Opin Genet Dev* 2002;12:307–311.
21. Tischkowitz MD, Hodgson SV. Fanconi anaemia. *J Med Genet* 2003;40:11–20.
22. Ellis NA, Groden J, Ye T-Z, et al. The Bloom's syndrome gene product is homologous to RecQ helicases. *Cell* 1995;83:655–666.
23. Ellis NA, Roe AM, Kozloski J, et al. Linkage disequilibrium between the FES, D15S127, and BLM loci in Ashkenazi Jews with Bloom syndrome. *Am J Hum Genet* 1994;55:453–460.
24. Bruzzone R, White TW, Paul DL. Connections with connexins: the molecular basis of direct intercellular signaling. *Eur J Biochem* 1996;238:11–27.
25. Streetly A. Proceedings of the International Workshop on haemoglobinopathy screening to inform the screenings developments in England, NHS Haemoglobinopathy Screening Pro-

gramme, King's Fund, London, July 2–3 2001. Available at http://www-phm.umds.ac.uk/haemscreening.

26. Mitchell JJ, Capua A, Clow C, et al. Twenty-year outcome analysis of genetic screening programs for Tay-Sachs and beta-thalassemia disease carriers in high schools. *Am J Hum Genet* 1996;59:793–798.

27. Galanello R Sollaino C, Paglietti E, et al. Alpha-Thalassemia carrier identification by DNA analysis in the screening for thalassemia. *Am J Hematol* 1998;59:273–278.

28. Tan JR, Li WJ, Ma JY, et al. Molecular epidemiological study of alpha- and beta-thalassemia in Sihui city. *Di Yi Jun Yi Da Xue Xue Bao* 2003;23:716–719.

29. Sanguansermsri T, Phumyu N, Chomchuen S, et al. Screening for alpha-thalassemia-1 heterozygotes in expecting couples by the combination of a simple erythrocyte osmotic fragility test and a PCR-based method. *Community Genet* 1999;2:126–129.

30. Xu XM, Zhou YQ, Luo GX, et al. The prevalence and spectrum of alpha and beta thalassaemia in Guangdong Province: implications for the future health burden and population screening. *J Clin Pathol* 2004;57:517–522.

31. Vichinsky EP. Comprehensive care in sickle cell disease: its impact on morbidity and mortality. *Semin Hematol* 1991;28:220–226.

32. Gaston MH, Verter JI, Woods G, et al. Prophylaxis with oral penicillin in children with sickle cell anemia: a randomized trial. *N Engl J Med* 1986;314:1593–1599.

33. Kaback M, Lim-Steele J, Dabholkar D, et al. Tay-Sachs disease: carrier screening, prenatal diagnosis, and the molecular era: an international perspective, 1970 to 1993—The International TSD Data Collection Network. *JAMA* 1993;270:2307–2315.

34. Akerman BR, Natowicz MR, Kaback MM, et al. Novel mutations and DNA-based screening in non-Jewish carriers of Tay-Sachs disease. *Am J Hum Genet* 1997;60:1099–2001.

35. Strom CM, Crossley B, Redman JB, et al. Molecular screening for diseases frequent in Ashkenazi Jews: lessons learned from more than 100,000 tests performed in a commercial laboratory. *Genet Med* 2004;6:145–152.

36. Feigenbaum A, Moore R, Clarke J, et al. Canavan disease: carrier-frequency determination in the Ashkenazi Jewish population and development of a novel molecular diagnostic assay. *Am J Med Genet* 2004;124A:2142–2147.

37. Dong J, Edelmann L, Bajwa A, et al. Familial dysautonomia: detection of the IKBKAP IVS20+6T-C and R696P mutations and frequencies among Ashkenazi Jews. *Am J Med Genet* 2002;110:253–257.

38. Whitney MA, Saito H, Jakobs PM, et al. A common mutation in the FACC gene causes Fanconi anaemia in Ashkenazi Jews. *Nat Genet* 1993;4:202–205.

39. Smith RJ. Clinical application of genetic testing for deafness. *Am J Med Genet* 2004;15:18–22.

40. Petit C. Memorial Lecture-Hereditary sensory defects: from gene to pathogenesis. *Am J Med Genet* 2004;130A:3–7.

41. Del Castillo I, Moreno-Pelayo MA, Del Castillo FJ, et al. Prevalence and evolutionary origins of the del(GJB6-D13S1830) mutation in the DFNB1 locus in hearing-impaired subjects: a multicenter study. *Am J Hum Genet* 2003;73:1452–1458.

42. Fitzgerald T, Duva S, Ostrer H, et al. The frequency of GJB2 and GJB6 mutations in the New York State newborn population: feasibility of genetic screening for hearing defects. *Clin Genet* 2004;65:338–342.

43. White KR. Early hearing detection and intervention programs: opportunities for genetic services. *Am J Med Genet* 2004;15:129–136.

44. White KR. The current status of EHDI programs in the United States. *Ment Retard Dev Disabil Res Rev* 2003;9:279–288.

45. Telen MJ, Kaufman RE. The mature erythrocyte. In: Lee GR, et al. (eds.), *Clinical Hematology,* 10th edition. Baltimore: Lippincott Williams & Wilkins, 1999:207.

46. Colosimo A, Guida V, De Luca A, et al. Reliability of DHPLC in mutational screening of beta-globin (HBB) alleles. *Hum Mutat* 2002;19:287–295.

47. Morell RJ, Kim HJ, Hood LJ, et al. Mutations in the connexin 26 gene (GJB2) among Ashkenazi Jews with nonsyndromic recessive deafness. *N Engl J Med* 1998;339:1500–1505.

Screening for Fragile X Syndrome

Anneke Maat-Kievit

Ben A. Oostra

■ What Is the Problem that Requires Screening?

Fragile X syndrome.

What is the incidence/prevalence of the target condition?

The fragile X syndrome (MIM 309550) is the most common form of hereditary cognitive impairment and the second most common cause of mental retardation after Down syndrome, with a frequency of 16–25/100,000 males of European descent, 10–15/100,000 females,[1–3] and 386/100,000 unaffected female mutation carriers.[4] Fragile X syndrome is widespread in human populations, and the frequency of the disease may be higher in some ethnic groups, for instance in Tunisian Jews and perhaps in black Americans.[5,6]

What are the sequelae of the condition that are of interest in clinical medicine?

Delays in language acquisition and/or behavioral problems are often the presenting symptoms. Mental retardation is, in most cases, moderate to severe, with frequent occurrences of autistic-like behaviors, eye gaze avoidance, perseverative speech, and hyperactivity. Suggestive clinical signs, such as mild facial dysmorphia with long face, large protruding ears, high arched palate, prominent jaw, strabismus, joint laxity, and macroorchidism established around puberty, are not sufficiently constant or specific, especially in young children or females, to establish or exclude diagnosis.[7–10] A checklist may help to preselect retarded males for DNA testing.[2,11]

The fragile X syndrome is so-named because of the fragile site found on the long arm of the X chromosome (Xq27.3) of these patients when karyotyped in low folate medium.[12,13] The fragile X mutation is an unstable expansion of a CGG trinucleotide repeat, located in the first exon (non–protein-coding) of the *FMR1* gene (fragile X mental retardation 1).[14–16] The *FMR1* gene is 38 kilobase (kb) in size with 17 exons and a polymorphic CGG repeat in the first 5′ exon.[17,18] The normal CGG repeat has five to about 50 CGGs, interrupted in most cases by one or two AGGs, stabilizing the repeat. Repeats of this size remain stable on transmission.[17]

Two main types of mutations are observed in families, pre- and full mutations, and these are unstable on transmission to the next generation. Both contractions and expansions are seen with the latter being the most prominent.[19]

The full mutation is found in patients with mental retardation (males and females) and corresponds to large expansions of the repeat (from about 200 to >1,000 CGGs), associated with abnormal methylation of the CGG repeat and of neighboring DNA sequences. The full mutation inactivates the expression of the *FMR1* gene, results in loss of FMR1 protein (FMRP), and is associated with mental retardation in 100% of males and in about 60% of heterozygous females, in whom the retardation is usually less severe.[20] In female carriers of the full mutation, variation in the X chromosome inactivation ratio may account for the clinical variability in intellectual capacity.[20] FMRP is found in the cytoplasm of many cell types but is most abundant in neurons.[21]

Premutations are moderate expansions (from about 50 to about 200 CGGs) without interruption of AGG or the presence of only one AGG interruption at the 5′ end of the CCG repeat that are unmethylated with normal FMRP biosynthesis and are found in normal transmitting males and in most clinically normal carrier females.[17,22]

Premutation alleles are unstable during transmission to the next generation, but the transition from premutation to full mutation occurs only through maternal transmission of the abnormal allele (during oogenesis) with a probability that depends on the size of the premutation.[17,23] The smallest premutation repeat size found to expand to a full mutation was 59, a repeat size that is in the gray zone (between 50 and 60 repeats) of expanded alleles with a limited instability, for which the risk of transition to the full mutation in a single generation is very low, about 1% to 3.7%.[23] The risk of expansion to a full mutation is about 17% should the number of repeats be 60 to 69 and about 77% for 70 to 89 repeats. When premutations are longer than 90 CGGs, the probability of transition to a full mutation is about 98% if a mother transmits this allele to her offspring. All mothers of affected children are carriers of a premutation or a full mutation.[17,19] A male carrying a premutation will transmit it without expansion, with contraction, or with small expansion[24,25] to all of his daughters who will thus be carriers, with a high risk of having affected children in the next generation. In contrast, affected males who have a full mutation have a premutation in their sperm and if these males reproduce, which is rare, they will have daughters with a premutation. So, instability occurs after the laying down of the germline cells. The timing of the triplet repeat expansion in this disorder appears early in fetal development (between days 5 and 20), in contrast to Huntington disease, which occurs during gametogenesis. Therefore, fathers, in contrast to mothers, never pass on more than a premutation.[24,26–29]

Premutation carriers do not usually express cognitive impairment, but 20% to 25% of these carriers have prominent ears and mild psychiatric symptoms such as anxiety and social phobia.[30-32] About 20% of the female premutation carriers manifest premature ovarian failure (POF) (younger than the age of 40 years) compared with 1% of the general population,[33,34] and elevated follicle-stimulating hormone levels decrease the efficiency of ovarian stimulation required for preimplantation diagnosis. Women with a paternally inherited premutation might be more prone to POF, whereas women with a maternally inherited premutation are not.[35] Family planning is therefore an important issue for these females.[36]

About 30% of premutation carrier males exhibit a progressive neurodegenerative syndrome, starting at age 50 to 70 years. This syndrome is characterized by intention tremor; cerebellar ataxia; executive function deficits; short-term memory loss; parkinsonian features; peripheral neuropathy; psychiatric symptoms including anxiety, mood liability, and depression; generalized brain atrophy; white matter disease; and intranuclear bodies in neurons and glial cells.[37-40] Penetrance is age-related; symptoms are seen in 17% of males aged 50 to 59 years, in 38% aged 60 to 69 years, in 47% aged 70 to 79 years, and in 75% aged 80 years and older. Recently, some female patients were identified with fragile X–associated tremor/ataxia syndrome (FXTAS), but without dementia.[41] Most females with a premutations however, do not have significant neurologic symptoms.[42,43] Cells of subjects with premutations may be disturbed by a combination of the presence of relatively high levels of an abnormal mRNA, which could trap some CGG binding proteins and decrease the levels of FMRP[44] (Figure 18–1).

About 20% to 40% of patients show a mosaic pattern, a mixture of premutation and full mutation, "size mosaics," caused by the somatic instability of the full mutation in early embryogenesis, which can lead to retraction of the expanded repeat. Another type, "methylation mosaics," is seen with incompletely methylated large expansions in 3% of male patients. In both situations, there is some expression of FMRP1 protein and both are thus associated with milder mental retardation in males.[19,45,46]

■ The Tests

What is the purpose of the tests?

To identify disease and/or carriers of clinically relevant fragile-X mutations.

What is the nature of the tests?

In 1991, the cytogenetic marker, a fragile site at Xq27.3, was replaced by molecular diagnosis after the identification of the *FMR1* gene.[47] The mutation can be tested for by the Southern blot method, which allows determination of both the expansion and the methylation status. Polymerase chain reaction (PCR)–based methods are also useful, especially for precisely sizing premutations or for excluding a diagnosis of fragile X syndrome (when a normal CGG

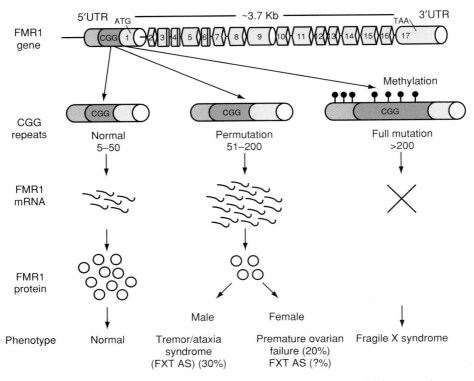

Figure 18-1 Fragile X mental retardation 1 (*FMR1*) gene with the normal CGG repeat, the premutation and the full mutation, and the subsequent amount of mRNA and protein and the phenotype.

repeat allele is found in a male or two normal alleles of different sizes are found in a female).

Monoclonal anti-FMRP antibodies are available that can be used to detect the presence or absence of FMRP in blood smears or hair roots or by Western blot. Thus, they can be used for diagnosing male patients and with a lesser sensitivity, female patients.[56,58] A correlation between FMRP expression and IQ in males with size mosaicism and methylation mosaicism was found.[48] Cognitive functioning in female carriers and males with mosaicism can be predicted by hair root analysis. Human hair roots are of clonal origin and are labeled either positive or negative for FMRP expression depending on which X chromosome is active in the female mutation carrier. A significant correlation was found between cognitive function and the percentage of hair roots expressing FMRP.[49] This technique is important because in contrast to male full-mutation carriers, who are always affected, female full-mutation carriers and male mosaics who can range in affect from moderately retarded to completely unaffected are detectable. The test result might enable parents to choose educational intervention and support at young age.[62]

The fragile X expansion mutation has produced efficient and reliable tools for diagnosis, genetic counseling, and antenatal diagnosis in carriers. Although testing mentally retarded individuals leads to diagnosis and improved support for patients with newly diagnosed fragile X, the yield is rather low (about 1%).[1,2,11,50] After diagnosing a patient as having the fragile X syndrome, all members in a fragile X family should be offered testing, and all women who are carriers of a pre- or full mutation offered genetic counseling before they begin their families to inform them of the risk of transmitting the disease and possible preventive measures. This process is known as "cascade screening." The primary aim is to inform relatives about their risk of carrying a pre- or full mutation, and the secondary aim is to provide information that may influence decisions about childbearing and use of antenatal testing. However, disseminating information after the detection of a new case of the fragile X syndrome can be difficult and ways to improve this are limited.[51] Given the importance and the rather high frequency of the fragile X syndrome, screening of the general population can be considered. There are four options.[52] The first option is population screening of all women of childbearing age. This approach has the advantage of providing women with information about their carrier status and allowing them to make a reproductive choice before pregnancy. There is, however, no natural mechanism of public health policy for conducting such a program, and some of the reproductive choices, like antenatal testing and subsequent pregnancy termination of an affected fetus, are controversial.

The second option is the screening of all pregnant women and offering antenatal testing to all carriers (1/250 being a carrier of a premutation).[49,53,54] This would be less expensive, because it would involve fewer women. However, such a program would require a public health awareness campaign. Women struggling with poverty, who receive little or no prenatal care, may not be reached, and because the women are already pregnant, several reproductive options are no longer available.[49] A practical problem remains with this approach. Although the disorder is serious in males and almost half the females are phenotypically normal, about one fourth are borderline mentally retarded. Screening leads to an irresolvable dilemma if a fragile X genotype is diagnosed in a female fetus.[55] To overcome this dilemma, screening for male fragile X syndrome alone was proposed,[56] identifying male pregnancies by sex determining region Y gene (SRY) PCR in maternal serum during the first trimester, followed by identifying women with male pregnancies who have 59 or more CCG repeats in the *FMR1* gene by PCR of the mother's blood (and if uninformative, Southern blot analysis). Patients with positive results would then be offered chorion villus sampling or amniocentesis and Southern blot analysis to identify male fetuses with 200 or more CCG repeats in the *FMR1* gene. It is recognized that the likelihood of the fragile X premutation expanding to full mutation is significantly lower in individuals ascertained by general prenatal carrier testing than in those with known fragile X families, and this should be taken into account.[57] Other associated problems like inadequate information about the phenotype, receiving test results during pregnancy, and decision making under time pressure because of gestational age should be considered. Antenatal carrier screening has been proposed in the United Kingdom and Finland.[4,58]

The third option is the screening of newborns, an attractive option because a neonatal screening program usually already exists.[49] Screening can be performed by antibody testing (which only detects full mutations and no premutations), offering parents the possibility of anticipating the problems in their child and to make timely informed decisions about further offspring. Early diagnosis, however, may interfere with parent–child bonding, and because there is no cure, there may be little value in an accurate diagnosis beside educational intervention and support, and may lead to stigmatization.[59–61]

The fourth and final screening option is to test at the first sign of delay. This is the least-expensive approach because it limits testing to those children with a documented or suspected developmental delay. Even if all children had access to a pediatrician and were regularly screened for their development and if pediatricians immediately performed fragile X testing when aware of parental concerns, it is still unlikely that a diagnosis would occur before 12 months of age. This eliminates reproductive choice for those families in which a second pregnancy occurs within 12 to 15 months after birth.[49]

Couples at risk who wish to prevent the birth of an affected child can remain childless, use donor oocytes, adopt, opt for a spontaneous pregnancy with prenatal diagnosis and termination of pregnancy if the fetus is affected, or choose preimplantation genetic diagnosis (PGD). The mutation can be detected in chorion villi, amniotic fluid, or umbilical cord blood samples by Southern blotting and PCR of the CCG repeat. Methylation status is unreliable in early chorion villus samples (<12 weeks) because it may differ from the fetal tissue. Methylation status may be informative when based on amniotic cells. The antibody test might also be useful for antenatal diagnosis of at-risk male pregnancies using chorion villi at 12.5 weeks' gestation, uncultured amniotic fluid cells, or fetal blood cells.[57,62] Because unmethylated full mutations result in almost normal amounts of FMRP, the antibody test should be performed on villi obtained after methylation is complete (>12.5 weeks). A major advantage is that the result can be available on the same day. FMRP expression in chorion villi of more than 13 weeks' gestation in full-mutation females shows villi with normal FMRP and villi without FMRP expression due to X inactivation, which occurs in early development before the villi start to proliferate.[63]

Another option for couples at increased risk is PGD.[64] PGD for fragile X syndrome is difficult because females carrying a premutation are at increased risk of both POF and a reduced ovarian response to the stimulation protocols resulting in fewer embryos for biopsy and diagnosis. Furthermore, couples at risk need to be informative for the CCG repeat on their normal alleles, but only 63% of couples have different numbers of repeats.[17] If they are uninformative for the normal repeats, polymorphic linked markers can help.[65] Premutation carrier embryos will be identified only if the number of repeats does not exceed 75. Larger mutations or premutations may not be seen because they are not be amplified by PCR. So, a number of embryos carrying a premutation may be lost for transfer.

There is no reason to test a healthy boy or a healthy girl from a fragile X family because he or she might carry a premutation that will become important only when they have to make decisions about family planning and/or antenatal testing. When children with borderline cognitive deficits are tested, care should be taken that a positive diagnosis, which might avoid unnecessary diagnostic procedures, will be used to improve educational strategies and not to stigmatize them. Also, care should be taken when testing grandparents, as one may suddenly carry the burden of being a transmitter and feel responsible for the disease their grandchildren inherited and they may be at risk of a late-onset debilitating disease (FXTAS) that they do not wish to know of prospectively.

Antenatal testing is an option if an increased risk of the fragile X syndrome in the offspring exists. Women with a family history of fragile X syndrome have a moderately high uptake rate of antenatal testing; most pregnancies of affected male fetuses are terminated, but about one third of affected female fetuses are not,[4,52,55] because their mental capacity cannot be predicted.

What are the implications of testing?

What does an abnormal test result mean? An abnormal test result means the mutation or premutation has been found. A mutation confirms the diagnosis of fragile X syndrome in male or female patients and sometimes can be found in mentally normal women. Premutation confirms carriership of the fragile X syndrome in males or females, with an increased risk of the fragile X syndrome for children and/or grandchildren and for POF, FXTAS, and psychiatric symptoms for themselves.[10,41]

Pregnancy termination is an option for women whose fetus is diagnosed with a full mutation. Pregnancy termination of a fetus with a premutation has not yet been an issue, although premutation carriers are now known to be at risk of late-onset disease like FXTAS, POF, or psychiatric complaints.

What does a normal test result mean? A CCG repeat length of less than 50 repeats is considered normal.[17] A repeat length in this range usually excludes the disease or carriership. In some patients (about 1%), however, a deletion or inactivating point mutation affecting the FMR1 gene can be found manifesting as disease.[66–68]

What is the cost of testing?

The costs of DNA testing vary considerable among laboratories. Antenatal screening detects most carriers and will lead to the highest number of avoided fragile X syndrome patients. The costs per detected carrier are quite similar for all screening programs (around $45,000). All screening strategies have a favorable cost-savings balance ($14 million antenatal screening, $9 million for pre-conceptional screening, and $2 million for school screening).[69] To overcome the dilemma of a fragile X genotype in a female fetus, screening for male fragile X syndrome would cost about £180,000 per male case detected, about three to four times that of antenatal screening for Down syndrome or cystic fibrosis[53] because the disorder is more rare.

■ Conclusions and Recommendations

There is no obstacle to fragile X screening from an economic point of view. The decision to screen or not can (and should) concentrate on the discussion of medical, social, psychological, and ethical considerations. Genetic screening for fragile X appears premature. Its exact prevalence remains unknown. There is overlap between the normal number of CCG repeats and the premutation number of repeats, further complicated by the possibly stabilizing effect of varying numbers of AGG repeats within the CGG repeats. Furthermore, the number of repeats that may be unstable in families with fragile X may be stable in the general population,[54] suggesting that something other than the number of repeats is affecting in these particular families. Fragile X is underdiagnosed, resulting in lack of prevention of new cases. Ideally, the diagnosis should be made when the parents first notice "something wrong," usually at about 1 year of age, followed by cascade screening.

■ Summary

1 ■ What Is the Problem that Requires Screening?

Fragile X syndrome.

a. What is the incidence/prevalence of the target condition?
The frequency is 16–25/100,000 in males, 10–15/100,000 females, and 386/100.000 female carriers.

b. What are the sequelae of the condition that are of interest in clinical medicine?
Delays in language acquisition and/or behavioral problems are often the presenting symptoms. Mental retardation is, in most cases, moderate to severe, with frequent occurrences of autistic-like behaviors, eye gaze avoidance, perseverative speech, and hyperactivity. Suggestive clinical signs, such as mild facial dysmorphia with long face, large protruding ears, high arched palate, prominent jaw, strabismus, joint laxity, and macroorchidism established around puberty are not sufficiently constant or specific, especially in young children or females, to establish or exclude the diagnosis.

2 ■ The Tests

a. What is the purpose of the tests?

Diagnosis of affected patients, carrier screening in females, and antenatal fetal testing in carriers where indicated.

b. What is the nature of the tests?

The mutation can be tested for by the Southern blot method, which allows determination of both the expansion and the methylation status. PCR-based methods are also useful, especially for precisely sizing premutations or for excluding a diagnosis of fragile X syndrome.

c. What are the implications of testing?

1. What does an abnormal test result mean?

   An abnormal test result means the mutation or premutation is present, confirming the diagnosis of fragile X syndrome in male or female patients. It can sometimes can be found in mentally normal women or can confirm carriership in males or females, with an increased risk of the fragile X syndrome for children and/or grandchildren and for POF, FXTAS and psychiatric symptoms for themselves.

2. What does a normal test result mean?

   A repeat length in the normal range usually excludes the disease or carriership. In some patients (about 1%), however, a deletion or inactivating point mutation affecting the *FMR1* gene can be found.

d. What is the cost of testing?

The costs of DNA testing vary considerable among laboratories. The costs per detected carrier are quite similar for all screening programs (around $45,000). All screening strategies have a favorable cost-savings balance.

3 ■ Conclusions and Recommendations

Fragile X is underdiagnosed, resulting in lack of prevention of new cases. Ideally, the diagnosis should be made when the parents first notice "something wrong," usually at about 1 year of age, followed by cascade screening.

References

1. Turner G, Webb T, Wake S, Robinson H. Prevalence of fragile X syndrome. *Am J Med Genet* 1996;64:196–197.
2. De Vries BB, van den Ouweland AM, Mohkamsing S, et al. Screening and diagnosis for the fragile X syndrome among the mentally retarded: an epidemiological and psychological survey. Collaborative Fragile X Study Group. *Am J Hum Genet* 1997;61:660–667.
3. Crawford DC, Acuna JM, Sherman SL. FMR1 and the fragile X syndrome: human genome epidemiology review. *Genet Med* 2001;3:359–371.
4. Murray J, Cuckle H, Taylor G, et al. Screening for fragile X syndrome; information needs for health planners. *J Med Screen* 1997;4:60–94.
5. Falik-Zaccai TC, Shachak E, Yalon M, et al. Predisposition to the fragile X syndrome in Jews of Tunisian descent is due to the absence of AGG interruptions on a rare Mediterranean haplotype. *Am J Hum Genet* 1997;60:103–112.
6. Crawford DC, Meadows KL, Newman JL, et al. Prevalence of the fragile X syndrome in African-Americans. *Am J Med Genet* 2002;110:226–233.
7. Frijns JP. X-Linked mental retardation and the fragile-X syndrome: a clinical approach. In: Davies KE, ed., *The Fragile X Syndrome*. Oxford: Oxford University Press, 1989.
8. Laing, S, Partington M, Robinson H, et al. Clinical screening score for the fragile X (Martin-Bell) syndrome. *Am J Med Genet* 1991;38:256–259.
9. Hagerman RJ. Physical and behavioral phenotype. In: Hagerman RJ, Cronister A, eds., *Fragile X Syndrome: Diagnosis, Treatment and Research*. Baltimore: The Johns Hopkins University Press, 1996.
10. Mandel JL, Biancalana V. Fragile X mental retardation syndrome: from pathogenesis to diagnostic issues. *Growth Horm IGF Res* 2004;14:S158–165.
11. De Vries BBA, Mohkamsing S, van den Ouweland AMW, Collaborative Fragile-X Study Group. Screening for the fragile X syndrome among the mentally retarded: a clinical study. *J Med Genet* 1999;36:467–470.
12. Sutherland GR. Fragile sites on human chromosomes: demonstration of their dependence on the type of tissue culture medium. *Science* 1977;197:265–266.
13. Sherman SL, Morton NE, Jacobs PA, et al. The marker (X) syndrome: a cytogenetic and genetic analysis. *Ann Hum Genet* 1984;48:21–37.
14. Verkerk AJMH, Pieretti M, Sutcliffe JS, et al. Identification of a gene (FMR-1) containing a CGG repeat coincident with a breakpoint cluster region exhibiting length variation in fragile X syndrome. *Cell* 1991;65:905–914.
15. Yu S, Pritchard M, Kremer E, et al. Fragile X genotype characterised by an unstable region of DNA. *Science* 1991;252:1179–1181.
16. Oberle I, Rousseau F, Heitz D, et al. Instability of a 550-base pair DNA segment and abnormal methylation in fragile X syndrome. *Science* 1991;252:1097–1102.
17. Fu YH, Kuhl DP, Pizzuti A, et al. Variation of the CGG repeat at the fragile X site results in genetic instability: resolution of the Sherman paradox. *Cell* 1991;67:1047–1058.
18. Eichler EE, Richards S, Gibbs RA, et al. Fine structure of the human FMR1 gene. *Hum Mol Genet* 1993;2:1147–1153.
19. Rousseau F, Heitz D, Biancalana V, et al. Direct diagnosis by DNA analysis of the fragile X syndrome of mental retardation. *N Engl J Med* 1991;325:1673–1681.
20. De Vries BB, Wiegers AM, Smits AP, et al. Mental status of females with an FMR1 gene full mutation. *Am J Hum Genet* 1996;58:1025–1032.
21. Devys D, Lutz Y, Rouyer N, et al. The FMR-1 protein is cytoplasmic, most abundant in neurons and appears normal in carriers of a fragile X premutation. *Nat Genet* 1993;4:335–340.
22. Eichler EE, Holden JJ, Popovich BW, et al. Length of the uninterrupted CGG repeats determines instability in the FMR1 gene. *Nat Genet* 1994;8:88–94.
23. Nolin SL, Brown WT, Glicksman A, et al. Expansion of the fragile X CGG repeat in females with premutation or intermediate alleles. *Am J Hum Genet* 2003;72:454–464.
24. Reyniers E, Vits L, De Boulle K, et al. The full mutation in the FMR-1 gene of male fragile X patients is absent in their sperm. *Nat Genet* 1993;4:143–148.

25. Nolin SL, Lewis FA 3rd, Ye LL, et al. Familial transmission of the FMR1 CGG repeat. *Am J Hum Genet* 1996;59:1252–1261.
26. Devys D, Biancalana V, Rousseau F, et al. Analysis of full fragile X mutations in fetal tissues and monozygotic twins indicate abnormal methylation and somatic heterogeneity are established early in development. *Am J Med Genet* 1992;43:208–216.
27. Malter HE, Iber JC, Willemsen R, et al. Characterisation of the full fragile X syndrome mutation in fetal gametes. *Nat Genet* 1997;15:165–169.
28. Moutou C, Vincent MC, Biancalana JL, et al. Transition from premutation to full mutation in fragile X syndrome is likely to be prezygotic. *Hum Mol Genet* 1997;6:971–979.
29. Helderman-van den Enden ATJM, Maaswinkel-Mooij PD, Hoogendoorn E, et al. Monozygotic twin brothers with the fragile X syndrome: different CGG repeats and different mental capacities. *J Med Genet* 1999;36:253–257.
30. Sobesky WE. The treatment of emotional and behavioral problems. In: Hagerman RJ, Cronister A, eds., *Fragile X Syndrome: Diagnosis, Treatment, and Research,* 2nd ed. Baltimore: Johns Hopkins University Press, 1996:332–348.
31. Franke P, Leboyer M, Gansicke M, et al. Genotype-phenotype relationship in female carriers of the premutation and full mutation of FMR1. *Psych Res* 1998;80:112–127.
32. Riddle JE, Cheema A, Sobesky WE, et al. Phenotypic involvement in females with the FMR1 gene mutation. *Am J Ment Retard* 1998;102:590–601.
33. Allingham-Hawkins DJ, Babul-Hirji R, Chitayat D, et al. Fragile X premutation is a significant risk factor for premature ovarian failure. The international collaborative POF in fragile X study-preliminary data. *Am J Med Genet* 1999;83:322–325.
34. Sherman SL. Premature ovarian failure in the fragile X syndrome. *Am J Med Genet* 2000;97:189–194.
35. Hundscheid RD, Sistermans EA, Thomas CMG, et al. Imprinting effect in premature ovarian failure confined to paternally inherited fragile X premutations. *Am J Hum Genet* 2000;66:413–418.
36. Murray A, Ennis S, MacSwiney F, et al. Reproductive and menstrual history of females with fragile X expansions. *Eur J Hum Genet* 2000;8:247–252.
37. Hagerman RJ, Leehey M, Heinrichs W, et al. Intention tremor, parkinsonism, and generalized brain atrophy in male carriers of fragile X. *Neurology* 2001;57:127–130.
38. Jacquemont S, Hagerman RJ, Leehey M, et al. Fragile X premutation tremor/ataxia syndrome: molecular, clinical, and neuroimaging correlates. *Am J Hum Genet* 2003;72:869–878.
39. Greco CM, Hagerman RJ, Tassone F, et al. Neuronal intranuclear inclusions in a new cerebellar tremor/ataxia syndrome among fragile X carriers. *Brain* 2002;125:1760–1771.
40. Tassone F, Hagerman RJ, Garcia-Arocena D, et al. Intranuclear inclusions in neural cells with premutation alleles in fragile X associated tremor/ataxia syndrome. *J Med Genet* 2004;41:E43.
41. Hagerman RJ, Leavitt BR, Farzin F, et al. Fragile-X associated tremor/ataxia syndrome (FXTAS) in females with the FMR1 premutation. *Am J Hum Genet* 2004;74:1051–1056.
42. Berry-Kravis E, Lewin F, Wuu J, et al. Tremor and ataxia in fragile X premutation carriers: blinded videotape study. *Ann Neurol* 2003;53:616–623.
43. Jacquemont S, Hagerman RJ, Leehey MA, et al. Penetrance of the fragile-X associated tremor/ataxia syndrome (FXTAS) in a premutation carrier population: initial results from a California family-based study. *JAMA* 2004;291:460–469.
44. Hagerman RJ, Hagerman PJ. The fragile X premutation into the phenotypic fold. *Curr Opin Genet Dev* 2002;12:278–283.
45. Nolin SL, Glicksman A, Houck G Jr. et al. Mosaicism in fragile X affected males. *Am J Med Genet* 1994;51:509–512.
46. Merenstein SA, Sobesky WE, Taylor AK, et al. Molecular-clinical correlations in males with an expanded FMR1 mutation. *Am J Med Genet* 1996;64:388–394.
47. De Vries BBA, Halley DJJ, Oostra BA, et al. The fragile X syndrome. *J Med Genet* 1998;35:579–589.
48. Tassone F, Hagerman RJ, Ikle DN, et al. FMRP expression as a potential prognostic indicator in fragile X syndrome. *Am J Med Genet* 1999;84:250–261.

49. Willemsen R, Smits A, Severijnen L-A, et al. Predictive testing for cognitive functioning in female carriers of the fragile X syndrome using hair root analysis. *J Med Genet* 2003; 40:377–379.

50. Hagerman RJ, Wilson P, Staley LW, et al. Evaluation of school children at high risk for fragile X syndrome utilizing buccal cell FMR-1 testing. *Am J Med Genet* 1994;51:474–481.

51. Van Rijn MA, de Vries BB, Tibben A, et al. DNA testing for fragile X syndrome: implications for parents and family. *J Med Genet* 1997;34:907–911.

52. Bailey DB Jr. Newborn screening for fragile X syndrome. *Ment Ret Dev Dis Res Rev* 2004; 10:3–10.

53. Rousseau F, Rouillard P, Morel ML, et al. Prevalence of carriers of premutation-size alleles of the FMR1 gene - and implications for the population genetics of the fragile X syndrome. *Am J Hum Genet* 1995;57:991–993.

54. Pesso R, Berkenstadt M, Cuckle H, et al. Screening for fragile X syndrome in women of reproductive age. *Prenat Diagn* 2000;20:611–614.

55. Brown WT, Nolin S, Houck Jr G, et al. Prenatal diagnosis and carrier screening for fragile X by PCR. *Am J Med Genet* 1996;64:191–195.

56. Wald NJ, Morris JK. A new approach to antenatal screening for fragile X syndrome. *Prenat Diagn* 2003;23:345–351.

57. Geva E, Yaron Y, Shomrat R, et al. The risk of fragile-X premutation expansion is lower in carriers detected by general prenatal screening than in carriers from known fragile X families. *Genet Testing* 2000;4:289–292.

58. Ryynanen M, Heinonen S, Makkonen M, et al. Feasibility and acceptance of screening for fragile X mutation in low-risk pregnancies. *Eur J Hum Genet* 1999;7:212–216.

59. Willemsen R, Mohkamsing S, de Vries B, et al. Rapid antibody test for fragile X syndrome. *Lancet* 1995;345:1147–1148.

60. Willemsen R, Anar B, De Diego Otero Y, et al. Noninvasive test for fragile X syndrome, using hair root analysis. *Am J Hum Genet* 1999;65:98–103.

61. Godard B, Ten Kate L, Evers-Kieboom G, et al. Population genetic screening programmes: principles, techniques, practices, and policies. *Eur J Hum Genet* 2003;11:549–587.

62. Lambiris N, Peters H, Bollmann R, et al. Rapid FMR1-protein analysis of fetal blood: an enhancement of prenatal diagnostics. *Hum Genet* 1999;105:258–260.

63. Willemsen R, Bontekoe CJ, Severijnen LA, et al. Timing of the absence of FMR1 expression in full mutation chorionic villi. *Hum Genet* 2002;110:601–605.

64. Platteau P, Sermon K, Seneca S, et al. Preimplantation genetic diagnosis for fragile Xa syndrome: difficult but not impossible. *Hum Repr* 2002;17:2807–2812.

65. Apessos A, Abou-Sleiman PM, Harper JC, et al. Preimplantation genetic diagnosis of the fragile X syndrome by use of polymorphic markers. *Prenat Diagn* 2001;21:504–511.

66. Gedeon AK, Baker E, Robinson H, et al. Fragile X syndrome without CCG amplification has an FMR1 deletion. *Mat Genet* 1992;1:341–344.

67. Wohrle D, Kotzot D, Hirst MC, et al. A microdeletion of less than 250 kb, including the proximal part of the FMR-1 gene and the fragile-X site, in a male with the clinical phenotype of fragile-X syndrome. *Am J Hum Genet* 1992;51:299–306.

68. De Boulle K, Verkerk, AJMH, Reyniers E, et al. A point mutation in the FMR-1 gene associated with fragile-X mental retardation. *Nat Genet* 1993;3:31–35.

69. Wildhagen MF, Van Os TA, Polder JJ, et al. Explorative study of costs, effects and savings of screening for female fragile X premutation and full mutation carriers in the general population. *Community Genet* 1998;1:36–47.

19

Screening for Huntington Disease

Anneke Maat-Kievit

■ What Is the Problem that Requires Screening?

Huntington disease (MIM 143100).

What is the incidence/prevalence of the target condition?

The prevalence of Huntington disease is estimated at 3–10/100,000 individuals of European descent,[1] with a lower prevalence in Japan (0.1–0.38/100,000), China (0.37/100,000), Finland (0.5/100,000), and in South African blacks (0.06/100,000),[2–5] and a higher prevalence in Venezuela at Lake Maracaibo (700/100,000),[6] Tasmania (12.1/100,000),[7] and North Sweden (144/100,000).[8] All overt cases of Huntington disease are due to the same mutational mechanism—a CAG repeat expansion—although variable in extent, arising in healthy individuals who carry an intermediate allele, with a repeat number between the normal range and that causing disease. The population prevalence of Huntington disease may relate to the frequency of alleles in the higher normal range, which acts as a source over many generations of still higher repeat number alleles that become unstable and ultimately lead to the repeat number causing clinical Huntington disease.[1]

What are the sequelae of the condition that are of interest in clinical medicine?

Huntington disease is an autosomal dominant, progressive neuropsychiatric disorder usually presenting in adult life. Because the mean age at onset is 45 years (range, 5–80 years), at-risk individuals remain so for a long period of their life. The clinical diagnosis of Huntington disease depends on the recognition of symptoms, given the history and the clinical signs present in the patient and the family history:[1] a family history consistent with autosomal dominant inheritance;[2] progressive motor disability like chorea, bradykinesia, rigidity, gait disturbances, dysarthria, and impaired voluntary motor function; and mental disturbances including cognitive decline, affective disturbances, and/or changes in personality.[3] The diagnosis is based primarily on clinical examination and 85% to 93% are correctly identified using the three noted criteria.[9,10] In 3% to 10% of patients, the onset occurs before age 20 years (so-called juvenile Huntington disease) with presenting features such as mental disturbance, epilepsy, rigidity, and bradykinesia.[1] In 8% to 23%, the onset is over 60 years[11] and the presenting features are predominantly motor with relatively little disability.[12] Atrophy of the caudate nucleus and putamen as visualized on computed tomography (CT) or magnetic resonance imaging (MRI) scan and decreased uptake and metabolism of glucose in the caudate nucleus on positron emission tomography (PET) scan provide additional support for the diagnosis, but their main role is in determining whether other conditions are contributing to the neurologic dysfunction.[13,14] A CAG expansion in the disease range ($\geq$36) in the Huntington disease gene in a symptomatic patient further confirms the diagnosis.[15–17]

Until now, the function of huntingtin, the cognate protein, and the pathophysiologic mechanism leading to disease has not been clearly elucidated, and treatment to alter the natural progression of Huntington disease is still unavailable. Death occurs independent of the age at onset after a mean illness duration of 16 years,[18,19] and ranges between 53.1 and 56.9 years.[20] Secondary complications are typically the proximate cause of death[21,22] and include aspiration pneumonia (33%), cardiovascular disease (24%), choking, nutritional deficiencies, skin ulcers, poisoning, and violence.[21–23] The rate of suicide is four times higher than that of the control population[24,26] and accounts for 1% to 5.7% of deaths from Huntington disease deaths[21,22,24,25] and is unrelated to the age at onset.[26]

The pathology is restricted to the brain and involves neuronal loss and gliosis. The brain shows overall atrophy, which in advanced cases weighs 20% to 30% less than normal. The neostriatum (caudate nucleus and putamen) is particularly affected.[27] Immunohistological analysis of huntingtin in Huntington disease brains shows intranuclear inclusions in the neocortex and neostriatum, consisting of mutated huntingtin and ubiquitin (which may be fatal to the cell) present before symptoms become evident.[28–30]

The Huntington disease gene is on chromosome 4p16.3[31] spanning about 185 kilobase (kb) of DNA in 67 exons. It is expressed as two major mRNA transcripts (13.5 and 10.5 kb) that encode for the same 348-kDa protein named huntingtin (3144 amino acids).[15,32] The Huntington disease CAG repeat is located near the extreme 5' end of the gene in exon 1, 17 codons from the ATG start of translation and, together with two penultimate CAACAG codons, encodes a highly polymorphic segment of glutamines, named polyglutamines. The wild-type allele has six to 35 CAG repeats, while affected subjects have repeats between 36 and 250, but usually less than 100[33–35] (Figure 19–1). The normal repeat segregates as a polymorphic locus, whereas the disease repeat size tends to increase by hairpin-mediated slippage,[36–38] although occasional decreases have been reported in successive generations.[39] An expanded CAG repeat is unstable in transmission. Although small increases may occur in both sexes,

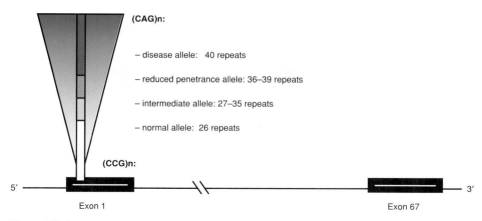

Figure 19-1 Huntington disease gene, with in the first exon the CAG trinucleotide repeat, that has in the normal allele maximal 26 repeats; in the intermediate allele, 27 to 35 repeats; in the Huntington disease allele with reduced penetrance, 36 to 39 repeats; and in the Huntington disease allele, 40 or more repeats. A polymorphic CCG repeat (5–12 repeats) is found downstream of the CAG repeat. The Huntington disease gene has 67 exons (introns and exons not drawn to scale).

large increases are almost exclusively seen in the offspring of males.[40–42] The change in CAG repeat length occurs during gametogenesis.[43] Because of the inverse relation between the number of CAG repeats and the age of symptom onset,[42,44,45] it is not surprising that a preponderance of juvenile cases have an affected father.[46,47] The number of CAG repeats is inversely related to the age at onset and accounts for 50% to 77% of the variation in the age at onset.

Accurate onset and survival curves would be of great value in genetic counseling. The number of years lived before the appearance of Huntington disease symptoms may also be important for predictive test candidates receiving an unfavorable test result. It may also be helpful in clinical trials because a significant extension of the age at onset beyond the median could be an indicator of therapeutic efficacy. However, there was significant differences between the median age of symptom onset in the Dutch and Canadian studies.[42,45] For each repeat size, the Dutch median age at onset was about 10 years later than the Canadian age. This difference remains unexplained. Repeat length is not associated with other clinical features of Huntington disease or rate of progression.[48,49]

■ The Tests

What is the purpose of the tests?

The purpose of the predictive test is to identify healthy individuals at risk of developing Huntington disease long before the disease becomes manifest.

Genetic knowledge of Huntington disease is not the prelude to cure or prevention, but rather it serves to remove uncertainty, enables more informed choices about child bearing, and, more generally, enables the individual to plan the rest of his or her life better.[50] The option of predictive testing necessitates a conscious decision of whether or not to know, and the right not to know is equally important as the right to know.[51] Medical implications such as symptom recognition and options for symptomatic treatment as well as genetic implications such as risk for (future) children are important considerations. Further, psychological implications including the relief of uncertainty and the moral implications relating to family planning, antenatal testing, informing existing children and/or relatives of results that apply to them, confidentiality, informed consent, and freedom of constraint should be considered. Finally, social implications, such as the risk of early medicalization, the uncertain effect of genetic knowledge on behavior, the forming of relationships and motivation, and problems with access to social services and insurance must be considered.

What is the nature of the tests?

The limits of the CAG repeat size in the Huntington disease gene have been redefined[17] on the basis of the total number of normal and symptomatic individuals assessed: normal allele, less than 27 repeats; intermediate allele, 27 to 35 repeats; disease allele with reduced penetrance, 36 to 39 repeats; and disease allele, 40 or more repeats (Figure 19–1).

CAG repeat analysis in the Huntington disease gene is used for diagnosis in symptomatic patients and for predictive and antenatal testing of at-risk individuals/fetuses. In asymptomatic individuals, the size of the CAG repeat, through its natural property of variability in transmission, may in a few percent be of a class, like intermediate- and reduced-penetrance alleles, where a straightforward prediction of the phenotype, future disease, or risk for children is not possible. Predictive and antenatal testing can usually be accurately performed without testing multiple family members as was needed for extensive linkage analysis if Huntington disease was confirmed either by CAG repeat analysis in the Huntington disease gene showing an expanded CAG repeat in an affected family member or if pathologic analysis of the brain of an affected relative clearly shows Huntington disease. In both symptomatic and at-risk individuals (after confirmation of the diagnosis in an affected relative), DNA mutation analysis determines the genetic status with more than 99% accuracy.[15,33] Standardized analysis makes accurate CAG repeat size measurement possible.[34,52,53] Somatic stability is usually found in different analyzed (fetal) tissues and chorion villi samples,[54] probably because the range of expansion in Huntington disease is small.[43] Before 1993, testing was performed by linkage analysis. In case of exclusion (definitive) testing, linkage analysis is still performed.

The diagnosis of Huntington disease has been made using fetal DNA from maternal plasma by quantitative fluorescent polymerase chain reaction (PCR),[55] a noninvasive procedure without a pregnancy risk, unlike chorion villus sampling and amniocentesis, with loss risks of miscarriage ranging from 0.25% to 1%.

Before predictive testing was possible, individuals at risk could only obtain risk estimates based on their current age and prior risk, upon which they had to base their decisions about the future.[56] After localization of the Huntington disease gene,[31] predictive testing became available using linkage analysis. International guidelines were provided for a structured predictive testing procedure,[57] with Huntington disease serving as a paradigm for the predictive testing of hereditary late-onset disorders. When the specific mutation was identified,[15] genetic testing became technically simpler, more reliable, and potentially available to every at-risk individual.

Not surprisingly, the acceptance of testing has been low. Before predictive testing became available, 40% to 84% of at-risk individuals indicated an interest in it.[58–65] Yet the actual uptake was only 2% to 24%.[66–69] The reasons underlying the low uptake include concern for a possible increased risk for existing children, the absence of treatment, the potential loss of health and or life insurance, the financial costs of testing, and the definitive nature of the result. The fear of being unable to cope with the diagnosis of future disease is apparently most important.[56,70–76] Predictive testing for Huntington disease has been described as a "success story"[77] because of the scarcity of adverse effects and catastrophic events, absence of posttest stress, and improvement in psychological health.[78–80] It may be that carriers experience increased distress, however, as they approach the likely moment of onset of their condition.[81]

It is generally agreed that asymptomatic children should not be tested, because it removes their choice, raises the possibility of stigmatization, and could have serious educational, career, and insurance implications.[82,83] Testing should be postponed until they are able to decide for themselves.

Huntington disease has implications for any child born without or after antenatal testing, because parental Huntington disease is inevitable and incurable, the onset unpredictable, and the competence of the affected individual as a participating parent will be steadily lost, increasing the burden on the other partner/parent.[84] Before testing was possible, the only way to prevent Huntington disease was to refrain from having children. A decision to have children (or a nondecision not to prevent it) carried the risk the gene would be passed on and those children would face the same anxieties and uncertainty. Egg or sperm donation is an option, but couples may be denied this method because of their risk of developing Huntington disease. Furthermore, couples who attempt to adopt or foster also face considerable difficulties because of the at-risk status of one of the partners.[85] Reproductive decisions prove very complex and are not solely determined by the rational assumption that an identified Huntington disease carrier will abstain from (further) procreation.[86] Some gene carriers regard prospective children as a source of future support for the other parent.[87]

When genetic linkage testing became available, new choices regarding reproduction emerged for couples at increased risk of having children with Huntington disease[88–90] like predictive and antenatal testing to confirm or exclude their fears (Table 19–1 and Figure 19–2).[91,92] Predictive testing in those who seek testing because of family planning has a significant effect on subsequent reproduction: 39% of carriers have one or more pregnancies versus 69% of the noncarriers. Notwithstanding the desire for children in the pretest period and the presence of family planning as one of the main reasons to have a predictive test, most carriers had no subsequent pregnancy within a follow-up interval of 3 to 7 years. In the total carrier group, antenatal diagnosis is performed in slightly less than two thirds of the pregnancies.[93]

Linkage analysis allows the exclusion of the at-risk chromosome 4 in the fetus if the parent does not wish his or her own status defined. Using this method means that pregnancies not at risk may be terminated, which is not the case in exclusion-definitive testing (Figure 19–2).

When the mutation was identified, direct testing of the fetus without prior testing of the at-risk parent and preimplantation genetic testing (PGD)[94–96] became options, including the option of exclusion and nondisclosure PGD for a 50% at-risk parent who does not wish to know his or her genetic status.

Preconception counseling is preferred, because of the information on the reproductive choices (Table 19–1 and Figure 19–2): The impact of the possible testing outcomes and the decision-making process are quite complex. After pedigree analysis and confirmation of diagnosis, information is given about the testing procedures suitable for the couple and including consequences for the fetus, the "at-risk" parent, and siblings of the (future or existing) children not tested. Also, the consequences of a possible change in decisions about antenatal and/or predictive testing in future is discussed (risk of an "unnecessary" antenatal test and/or termination of pregnancy when a predictive test takes places with a favorable result after antenatal exclusion [definitive] testing; children in the same family with different risks due to prenatal testing not being undertaken in all pregnancies). A very small number of affected pregnancies continue,[97] meaning the continuation of an affected pregnancy, which violates

Table 19–1   Choices regarding reproduction for couples with an increased risk of Huntington disease in the fetus

Choices regarding reproduction	Parent carrier	Parent 50% at risk
Having children	Yes	Yes
Refrain from having children	Yes	Yes
Adoption/fostering	Yes	Yes
Donor sperm insemination/egg donation plus in vitro fertilization	Yes	Yes
Predictive testing of parent	No	Yes
Prenatal diagnosis	Yes	No
Prenatal exclusion testing	No	Yes
Prenatal exclusion–definitive testing	No	Yes
Prenatal mutation testing of fetus alone	No	Yes
Preimplantation genetic diagnosis	Yes	Yes

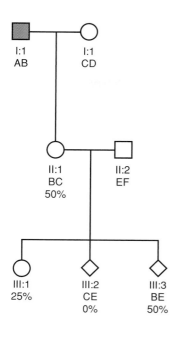

Figure 19-2 Exclusion (definitive) test.
Exclusion test: The grandfather (I.1) is affected with Huntington disease; his daughter (II.1) has a prior risk of 50%; one fetus (III.2) inherits the grandmaternal *C*, 0% risk haplotype and the other fetus (III.3) inherits the grandpaternal *B* 50% risk haplotype. Exclusion– definitive test: If in the fetus (III.3) the mutation is tested after receiving a 50% risk and if the mutation is found, the fetus (III.3) and the mother (II.1) will be carriers and the risk of her daughter (III.1) changes from 25% to 50%. If the mutation is not found, the fetus (III.3), the mother (II.1) and her daughter (III.1) will not be carriers.

the right of the child not to know and might cause increased stress and feelings of responsibility or guilt in the parents or even claims for wrongful life must be discussed.[98]

In several studies surveying attitudes toward antenatal testing for Huntington disease, it was concluded that 32% to 81% of at-risk individuals said they would make use of these tests and 30% to 50% would accept pregnancy termination of an affected fetus.[58,62,99–101] The actual number of antenatal tests remains low (only a few percent) despite the facts that antenatal testing is relatively simple, reliable, accessible, and more acceptable to the public through education. The low uptake may reflect the wish to remain uninformed about one's own genetic status, the fear of being unable to cope with an unfavorable test result, termination or risk of the antenatal test, defense mechanisms like denial and minimalization, ethical reservations about termination of pregnancy for a late-onset disorder, or the hope that a therapy might become available.[102,103] Also, the fact that the test candidates who undergo predictive testing are well in their 30s, already have one or more children, and may have completed their family or choose not to have further children may explain the low uptake.

The uptake of exclusion testing remains low compared with that of direct antenatal testing in most countries except in the United Kingdom, particularly since the mutation test became available. Ethical reservations can be raised regarding pregnancy termination for a fetus that has only a 50% risk of being affected. Furthermore, parents who are found not to be carriers, or after staying asymptomatic into old age, could discover that their fetus was aborted unnecessarily because of the possible 50% risk. Yet, the antenatal exclusion test remains a legitimate choice because it confers benefit upon couples who wish not to know their genetic status and who might otherwise have been deterred from having children.[104]

The antenatal exclusion–definitive test is rarely used especially now that the mutation has been identified and direct mutation analysis of the fetus without prior knowledge of the genetic status of the at-risk parent is possible. If the Huntington disease mutation is found, the at-risk parent simultaneously receives a result, but the risk of disclosure of the parental genetic status is only 25%, which is only half the risk of an exclusion–definitive test.

PGD for couples who do not wish to know their carrier status is possible by nondisclosure testing, selecting embryos with normal repeats without communicating the results to the patient (or by exclusion testing of a single cell by duplex PCR). Nondisclosure PGD might create ethical and practical problems (e.g., the doctor knows the genetic status of the at-risk person and might accidentally disclose it, or that the at-risk person is not a carrier and thus does not need to go through in vitro fertilization [IVF] and PGD cycles [which have risks] and mock transfer if no unaffected embryos were available for transfer). Exclusion PGD, which does not reveal the genetic status of the parent at risk, might then lead to unnecessary IVF and PGD cycles in those who are not carriers, but will not result in termination of unaffected fetuses.

More at-risk female than male subjects applied for predictive (58%) as well as for antenatal (65%) testing.[105] This difference may reflect greater maternal involvement in reproductive decisions or concern for existing children at risk and the fact that men may experience greater difficulty in accepting the implications of being at risk and are less willing or able to deal with the emotions that risk alterations arouse, coping by denial rather than confronting the issue.

Antenatal testing for carriers of intermediate alleles can be considered,[105] and although the exact risks are not yet known, they are considered to be less than 10% for males and very small for females (expansion to a Huntington disease allele has never been described in offspring of females).[1,2,106,107]

What are the implications of testing?

What does an abnormal test result mean? If a disease allele with 40 or more repeats is found, individuals will develop characteristic Huntington symptoms at some point in their lives. A disease allele with reduced penetrance, 36 to 39 repeats, is associated with clinically and pathologically confirmed Huntington disease, although the Huntington disease phenotype is not always penetrant. Penetrance increases with increasing repeat length.[33,34,42,45,108,109] Penetrance of 36 to 39 repeat alleles may be higher in subjects with confirmed Huntington disease ancestry than from those who are collateral branches of new mutations.[103] Reliable empirical penetrance risks are not yet available. If the fetus is affected, termination of pregnancy is an option.

What does a normal test result mean? A normal allele (<27 repeats) confirms the absence of Huntington disease. A normal allele has never been associated with the Huntington disease phenotype nor has it shown instability resulting in a Huntington disease allele in offspring.[17,110]

The intermediate allele, with 27 to 35 repeats, is not associated with a Huntington disease phenotype[33,34] but has demonstrated instability[112] and is found in 1.5%[33,103] to 3.9% of the general population. There is a risk for offspring of an intermediate allele carrier to inherit more than 26 repeats and a small risk that transmission may result in a Huntington disease allele (with reduced penetrance).[15,111–114] The risk of expansion depends on the sex of the transmitting individual, the repeat size, the level of mosaicism in sperm, whether the intermediate allele is on a Huntington disease haplotype or if it is a new mutation family or in the general population, and other, as yet unknown, factors.[115] Risk estimates for expansion of an intermediate allele to 36 or more repeats in the offspring of male carriers vary between 2.25% and 10%. Expansions of intermediate alleles to 36 or more repeats in offspring of female carriers of intermediate alleles are not described, suggesting their risk is much smaller than for male carriers.

Differential diagnostic considerations if a normal CAG repeat is found in the Huntington disease gene of a Huntington disease–like patient include noninherited forms of chorea, like medication-induced dyskinesia, thyrotoxicosis, senile chorea, or Sydenham chorea or inherited forms of chorea, like Huntington disease–like diseases (DL1 and -2),[116,117] dentatorubropallidoluysian atrophy (DRPLA), chorea–acanthocytosis, benign hereditary chorea, paroxysmal hyperkinesias, spinocerebellar ataxia and mitochondrial myoencephalopathies, Gilles de la Tourette, and Hallervorden-Spatz.[118] Thus, confirmation of an expanded CAG repeat in a patient of the family remains a prerequisite before predictive and/or antenatal testing becomes possible.

What is the cost of testing?

The costs of a DNA test vary considerable among laboratories. It is still too early to assess the effect of prenatal diagnosis or of family limitation associated with genetic counseling on prevalence. The prevalence, however, of previously unsuspected cases with onset in old age, together with the transmission of the disorder by individuals with intermediate alleles to their descendents will necessitate a considerable number of individuals already born with the mutation before there is any recognition of the existence of Huntington disease in the kindred.[1] Thus, it will be difficult for screening to reduce the overall prevalence of Huntington disease in the near term.

■ Conclusions and Recommendations

The number of predictive tests performed for Huntington disease far exceeds that for antenatal testing. Nonetheless, it is clearly an important tool for those who use antenatal testing. Although there is debate on whether antenatal testing is ethical for Huntington disease and although the usage of the antenatal test is relatively low, it is essential that at-risk couples be offered genetic counseling and psychological support, including discussion of the nature and consequences of testing, before they decide. Predictive and antenatal testing is probably a mixed blessing: It is both beneficial and burdensome for the minority who use it. The actual benefits and costs of these tests will undoubtedly emerge in time for participants, partners, family members, and friends. Until then, predictive and antenatal testing for Huntington disease should be continued with care. Understanding the nature of the genetic defect may ultimately lead to the development of new treatments. When therapy becomes available for Huntington disease, the context of predictive and antenatal testing is likely to change because of the hope that therapy offers.

■ Summary

1 ■ What Is the Problem that Requires Screening?
Huntington disease.

    a. What is the incidence/prevalence of the target condition?
Three to ten per 100.000 individuals of European descent, with regions or countries with lower or higher prevalence.

    b. What are the sequelae of the condition that are of interest in clinical medicine?
Huntington disease is an autosomal dominant, progressive neuropsychiatric disorder usually presenting in adult life.

2 ■ The Tests
    a. What is the purpose of the tests?
The purpose of the predictive test is to identify healthy individuals at risk of developing Huntington disease long before the disease becomes manifest. The purpose of the antenatal test is to detect fetuses with an increased risk of Huntington disease and to have the option of pregnancy termination. The purpose of the diagnostic test is to confirm the clinical diagnosis of Huntington Disease in patients.

b. *What is the nature of the tests?*

In both symptomatic and at-risk individuals (after confirmation of the diagnosis in an affected relative), DNA mutation analysis determines the genetic status with more than 99% accuracy. Linkage analysis is an option if the parent does not wish his or her risk status defined. Such an approach, however, is not conclusive in terms of diagnosing Huntington disease in the fetus.

c. *What are the implications of testing?*

1. What does an abnormal test result mean?

   If a disease allele with 40 or more repeats is found, individuals will develop characteristic Huntington symptoms at some point in their life. A disease allele with reduced penetrance, 36 to 39 repeats, is associated with clinically and pathologically confirmed Huntington disease, although the Huntington disease phenotype is not always penetrant.

2. What does a normal test result mean?

   A normal allele (<27 repeats) has never been associated with a Huntington disease phenotype nor has it shown instability resulting in a Huntington disease allele in offspring. The intermediate allele, with 27 to 35 repeats, is not associated with a Huntington disease phenotype but has demonstrated instability.

d. *What is the cost of testing?*

The costs of a DNA test vary considerable among laboratories. The effect of screening will not reduce the overall prevalence of Huntington disease in the near term because of expansion of intermediate alleles and non- or late penetrance of expanded repeat sizes.

3 ■ Conclusions and Recommendations

The number of predictive test performed for Huntington disease far exceeds that for antenatal testing. Nonetheless, it is clearly an important tool for those who use antenatal testing. Although there is debate on whether antenatal testing is ethical for Huntington disease and although the usage of the antenatal test is relatively low, it is essential at-risk couples be offered genetic counseling and psychological support including the nature and consequences of testing before they decide.

References

1. Harper PS. Huntington's disease. In: Bates G, Harper PS, Jones L, eds., *Huntington's Disease*, 3rd ed. Oxford: Oxford Medical Publications, 2002.
2. Narabayashi H. Huntington's chorea in Japan: review of the literature. In: *Anonymous Advances in Neurology*. New York: Raven Press, 1973:253–259.
3. Hayden MR, MacGregor JM, Beighton PH. The prevalence of Huntington's chorea in South Africa. *S Afr Med J* 1980;58:193–196.
4. Palo J, Somer H, Ikonen E, et al. Low prevalence of Huntington's disease in Finland. *Lancet* 1987;3:805–806.
5. Leung CM, Chan YW, Chang CM, et al. Huntington's disease in Chinese: a hypothesis of its origin. *J Neurol Neurosurg Psychiat* 1992;55:681–684.
6. Young AB, Shoulson I, Penney JB, et al. Huntington disease in Venezuela: neurologic features and functional decline. *Neurology* 1986;36:244.
7. Pridmore SA. The prevalence of Huntington's disease in Tasmania. *Med J Aust* 1990;153:133–134.
8. Mattsson B. Huntington's chorea in Sweden. *Acta Psychiatr Scand Suppl* 1974;255:221–235.
9. Bird ED. The brain in Huntington's chorea. *Psychol Med* 1978;8:357–360.
10. Folstein SE, Leigh JR, Parhad IM, et al. The diagnosis of Huntington's disease. *Neurology* 1986;36:1279–1283.
11. Myers RH, Sax DS, Schoenfeld M, et al. Late onset of Huntington's disease. *J Neurol Neurosurg Psychiat* 1985;48:530–534.
12. James CM, Houlihan GD, Snell RG, et al. Late-onset Huntington's disease: a clinical and genetic study. *Age and Ageing* 1994;23:445–448.
13. Hayden MR, Marlin WR, Sloessl AJ, et al. Position emission tomography in the early diagnosis of Huntington's disease. *Neurology* 1986;36:888–894.
14. Wardlaw JM, Sellar RJ, Abernethy LJ. Measurement of caudate nucleus area—a more accurate measurement of Huntington's disease. *Neuroradiology* 1991;33:316–319.
15. Huntington's Disease Collaborative Research Group. A novel gene containing a trinucleotide repeat that is expanded in Huntington's disease chromosomes. *Cell* 1993;72:971–983.
16. Hayden M, Kremer B. The metabolic and molecular bases of inherited disease. In: Scriver CR, Beaudet AL, Sly WS, et al., eds., *The Metabolic and Molecular Bases of Inherited Disease*, Vol. III, 27th ed. New York: McGraw-Hill, 1995: 4483–4510.
17. American College of Medical Genetics/American Society of Human Genetics Huntington Disease Genetic Testing Working Group. Laboratory guidelines for Huntington Disease genetic testing. *Am J Hum Genet* 1998;62:1243–1247.
18. Conneally PM. Huntington's disease: genetics and epidemiology. *Am J Hum Genet* 1984;36:506–526.
19. Roos RA, Hermans J, Vegter-van der Vlis M, et al. Duration of illness in Huntington's disease is not related to age at onset. *J Neurol Neurosurg Psychiat* 1993;56:98–100.
20. Hille ETM, Siesling S, Vegter-van der Vlis M, et al. Two centuries of mortality in ten large families with Huntington disease: a rising impact of gene carriership. *Epidemiology* 1999;10:706–710.
21. Lanska DJ, Lanska MJ, Lavine L, et al. Conditions associated with Huntington's disease at death. *Neurology* 1988a;38:769–772.
22. Lanska DJ, Lanska MJ, Lavine L, et al. Conditions associated with Huntington's disease at death. *Arch Neurol* 1988b;45:878–881.
23. Haines JL, Conneally PM. Causes of death in Huntington's disease as reported on death certificates. *Genet Epidemiology* 1986;3:417–423.
24. Farrer LA. Suicide and attempted suicide in Huntington's disease: implications for preclinical testing of persons at risk. *Am J Med Genet* 1986;24:305–311.
25. Di Maio L Squiteri F, Napolitano G, et al. Suicide risk in Huntington's disease. *J Med Genet* 1993;30:293–295.
26. Lipe H, Schultz A, Bird TD. Risk factors for suicide in Huntington's disease: a retrospective case controlled study. *Am J Med Genet* 1993;48:231–233.

27. Bruyn GW. Huntington's chorea: historical, clinical and laboratory synopsis. In: Vinken PJ, Bruyn GW, eds., *Handbook of Clinical Neurology*. Amsterdam: North-Holland Publishing, 1968:268–378.

28. Davies SW, Turmaine M, Cozens BA, et al. Formation of neuronal intranuclear inclusions underlies the neurological dysfunction in mice transgenic for the HD mutation. *Cell* 1997;90:537–548.

29. Maat-Schieman MLC, Dorsman JC, Smoor MA, et al. Distribution of inclusions in neuronal nuclei and dystrophic neurites in Huntington's disease brain. *J Neuropathol Exp Neurol* 1999;58:129–137.

30. Wellington CL, Hayden MR. Caspases and neurodegeneration: on the cutting edge of new therapeutic approaches. *Clin Genet* 2000;57:1–10.

31. Gusella JF, Wexler NS, Conneally PM, et al. A polymorphic DNA marker genetically linked to Huntington's disease. *Nature* 1983;306:234–238.

32. Ambrose CM, Duyao MP, Barnes G, et al. Structure and expression of the Huntington disease gene: evidence against simple inactivation due to an expanded CAG repeat. *Somat Cell Mol Genet* 1994;20:17–38.

33. Kremer B, Goldberg YP, Andrew SE, et al. A worldwide study of the Huntington's disease mutation: the sensitivity and specificity of measuring CAG repeats. *N Engl J Med* 1994;330:1401–1406.

34. Rubinsztein DC, Leggo J, Coles R, et al. Phenotypic characterization of individuals with 30-40 CAG repeats in the Huntington disease gene reveals Huntington disease cases with 36 repeats and apparently normal elderly individuals with 36-39 repeats. *Am J Hum Genet* 1996;59:16–22.

35. Nance MA, Mathias-Hagen V, Breningstall G, et al. Analysis of a very large trinucleotide repeat in a patient with juvenile Huntington's disease. *Neurology* 1999;52:392–394.

36. Rubinsztein DC, Leggo J, Barton DE, et al. Site of (CCG) polymorphism in the HD gene. *Nat Genet* 1993;5:214–215.

37. McMurray CT. Mechanisms of DNA expansion. *Chromosoma* 1995;104:2–13.

38. Kovtun IV, McMurray CT. Trinucleotide expansion in haploid germ cells by gap repair. *Nat Genet* 2001;27:407–411.

39. Andrew SE, Goldberg YP, Hayden MR. Rethinking genotype and phenotype correlations in polyglutamine expansion disorders. *Hum Mol Genet* 1997;6:2005–2010.

40. De Rooij KE, de Koning Gans PAM, et al. Borderline repeat expansions in Huntington's disease. *Lancet* 1993;342:1491–1492.

41. Kremer B, Almqvist E, Theilmann J, et al. Sex-dependent mechanisms for expansions and contractions of the CAG repeat on affected Huntington disease chromosomes. *Am J Hum Genet* 1995;57:343–350.

42. Maat-Kievit A, Losekoot M, Zwinderman K, et al. Predictability of age at onset in Huntington disease in the Dutch population. *Medicine* 2002;81:251–259.

43. MacDonald ME, Barnes G, Srinidhi J, et al. Gametic but not somatic instability of CAG repeat length in Huntington's disease. *J Med Genet* 1993;30:982–986.

44. Andrew SE, Goldberg YP, Kremer B, et al. The relationship between trinucleotide (CAG) repeat length and clinical features of Huntington's disease. *Nat Genet* 1993;4:398–403.

45. Brinkman RR, Mezei MM, Theilmann J, et al. The likelihood of being affected with Huntington disease by a particular age, for a specific CAG repeat. *Am J Hum Genet* 1997;60:1202–1210.

46. Myers RH, Madden JJ, Teague JL, et al. Factors related to onset age of Huntington disease. *Am J Hum Genet* 1982;34:481–488.

47. Telenius H, Kremer HP, Theilmann J, et al. Molecular analysis of late onset Huntington's disease. *J Med Genet* 1993;30:991–995.

48. Kieburtz K, MacDonald M, Shih C, et al. Trinucleotide repeat length and progression of illness in Huntington's disease. *J Med Genet* 1994;31:872–874.

49. Claes S, Van Zand K, Legius E, et al. Correlations between triplet repeat expansion and clinical features in Huntington's disease. *Arch Neurol* 1995;52:749–753.

50. Gezondheidsraad. Commissie DNA diagnostiek. DNA diagnostiek. Rijswijk. Gezondheidsraad 1998. Publicatie nummer 1998/11.

51. Shaw MW. Testing for the Huntington gene: a right to know, a right not to know, or a duty to know. *Am J Med Genet* 1987;26:243–246.

52. Marshall FJ, Huntington Study Group. Interlaboratory variability of (CAG) in determinations in Huntington's disease. *Neurology* 1996;46:258.

53. Losekoot M, Bakker B, Laccone F, et al. A European pilot quality assessment scheme for molecular diagnosis of Huntington's disease. *Eur J Hum Genet* 1999;7:217–222.

54. Benitez J, Robledo M, Ramos C, et al. Somatic stability in chorion villi samples and other Huntington fetal tissues. *Hum Genet* 1995;96:229–232.

55. Gonzales-Gonzales MC, Trujillo MJ, Rodriguez de Alba M, et al. Huntington disease-unaffected fetus diagnosed from maternal plasma using QF-PCR. *Prenat Diagn* 2003;23:232–234.

56. Harper PS, Newcombe RG. Age at onset and life table risks in genetic counselling for Huntington's disease. *J Med Genet* 1992;4:239–242.

57. International Huntington Association and World Federation of Neurology Research Group on Huntington's Chorea. Guidelines for the molecular genetics predictive test in Huntington's disease. *J Med Genet* 1994;31:555–559.

58. Teltscher B, Polgar S. Objective knowledge about Huntington's disease and attitudes towards predictive testing of persons-at risk. *J Med Genet* 1981;18:31–39.

59. Schoenfeld M, Myers RH, Berkman B, et al. Potential impact of a predictive test on the gene frequency of Huntington's disease. *Am J Med Genet* 1984;18:423–429.

60. Evers-Kieboom G, Cassiman JJ, van de Berghe H. Attitudes towards predictive testing in Huntington's disease: a recent survey in Belgium. *J Med Genet* 1987;24:275–279.

61. Evers-Kieboom G, Swerts A, Cassiman JJ, et al. The motivation of at-risk individuals and their partners in deciding for or against predictive testing for Huntington's disease. *Clin Genet* 1989;35:29–40.

62. Kessler S, Field T, Worth L, et al. Attitudes of persons at risk for Huntington's disease toward predictive testing. *Am J Med Genet* 1987;26:259–270.

63. Mastromauro C, Myers RH, Berkman B. Attitudes toward presymptomatic testing in Huntington's disease. *Am J Med Genet* 1987;26:271–282.

64. Meissen GJ, Berchek RL. Intended use of predictive testing by those at risk for Huntington's disease. *Am J Med Genet* 1987;26:283–293.

65. Markel DS, Young AB, Penney JN. At-risk persons' attitudes toward presymptomatic and prenatal testing of Huntington's disease in Michigan. *Am J Med Genet* 1987;26:295–305

66. Bloch M, Fahy M, Fox S, et al. Predictive testing for Huntington's disease II: Demographic characteristics, life style patterns, attitudes and psychosocial assessment of the first fifty-one test candidates. *Am J Med Genet* 1989;32:217–224.

67. Craufurd D, Kerzin-Storror L, Dodge A, et al. Uptake of presymptomatic predictive testing for Huntington's disease. *Lancet* 1989:603–605.

68. Tyler A, Ball D, Craufurd D, the United Kingdom Huntington's Disease Prediction Consortium. Presymptomatic testing for Huntington's disease in the United Kingdom. *BMJ* 1992;304:1593–1596.

69. Maat-Kievit A, Vegter-vd Vlis M, Zoeteweij M, et al. The paradox of a better test for Huntington disease. *J Neurol Neurosurg Psychiat* 2000;69:579–583.

70. Morris MJ, Tyler A, Lazarou L, et al. Problems in genetic prediction for Huntington's disease. *Lancet* 1989;ii:601–603.

71. Meissen GJ, Mastromauro CA, Koroshetz WJ, et al. Predictive testing for Huntington's disease with the use of a linked DNA marker. *N Engl J Med* 1988;31:535–542.

72. Tibben A. What is knowledge but grieving? Thesis, Rotterdam, 1993.

73. Quaid KA, Morris M. Reluctance to undergo predictive testing by those at risk for Huntington's disease. *Am J Med Genet* 1993;45:41–45.

74. Codori AM, Hanson R, Brandt J. Self-selection in predictive testing for Huntington's disease. *Am J Med Genet* 1994a;54:167–173.

75. Codori AM, Brandt J. Psychological costs and benefits of predictive testing for Huntington's disease. *Am J Med Genet* 1994b;54:174–184.

76. Van der Steenstraten IM, Tibben A, Roos RA, et al. Predictive testing for Huntington's disease: non-participants compared with participants in the Dutch program. *Am J Hum Genet* 1994;55:618–625.

77. Bundey S. Few psychological consequences of presymptomatic testing for Huntington disease. *Lancet* 1997;349:4.

78. Bloch M, Adam S, Wiggins S, et al. Predictive testing for Huntington disease in Canada. The experience of those receiving an increased risk. *Am J Med Genet* 1992;42:499.

79. Dudok de Wit AC, Tibben A, Duivenvoorden HJ, et al., and the other members of the Rotterdam/Leiden Genetics Workgroup. Predicting adaptation to presymptomatic DNA testing for late onset disorders: who will experience distress? *J Med Genet* 1998;35:745–754.

80. Almqvist E, Bloch M, Brinkman R, et al. A world-wide assessment of suicide, suicide attempts or psychiatric hospitalisation after predictive testing for Huntington disease. *Am J Hum Genet* 1999;64:51293–1304.

81. Timman R, Maat-Kievit A, Roos R, et al. Adverse effects of predictive testing for Huntington disease underestimated: long-term effects 7-10 years after the test. *Health Psychol* 2004;23:189–197.

82. Bloch M, Hayden MR. Opinion: predictive testing for Huntington disease in childhood: challenges and implications. *Am J Hum Genet* 1990;46:1–4.

83. Harper PS, Clarke A. Should we test children for "adult" genetic children? *Lancet* 1990;335:1205–1206.

84. Braude PR, De Wert GM, Evers-Kieboom G, et al. Non-disclosure preimplantation genetic diagnosis for Huntington's disease: practical and ethical dilemmas. *Prenat Diagn* 1998;18:1422–1426.

85. Simpson SA, Zoeteweij MW, Nys K, et al. Prenatal testing for Huntington's disease: a European collaborative study. *Eur J Hum Genet* 2002;10:689–693.

86. Frets PG, Duivenvoorden HJ, Verhage F, et al. Factors influencing the reproductive decisions after genetic counselling. *Am J Med Genet* 1990;35:496–502.

87. Zoeteweij M, Geerinck-Vercammen CR, Maat-Kievit JA, et al. Prenatal testing for Huntington's disease: first results of a psychological follow-up study in the Netherlands. *Genet Couns* 1997;8:2147–148.

88. Harper PS, Sarfarazi M. Genetic prediction and family structure in Huntington's chorea. *BMJ* 1985;290:1929–1931.

89. Hayden MR, Kastelein JJP, Wilson RD, et al. First trimester prenatal diagnosis for Huntington's disease with DNA probes. *Lancet* 1987:1284–1285.

90. Quarrell OWJ, Tyler A, Upadhyaya M, et al. Exclusion testing for Huntington's disease in pregnancy with a closely linked DNA marker. *Lancet* 1987:1281–1283.

91. Millan FA, Curtis A, Mennie M, et al. Prenatal exclusion testing for Huntington's disease: problem of too much information. *J Med Genet* 1989;26:83–85.

92. Maat-Kievit JA, Vegter van der Vlis M, Zoeteweij M, et al. Experience in prenatal testing for Huntington's disease in The Netherlands: procedures, results and guidelines. *Prenat Diagn* 1999;19:450–457.

93. Evers-Kieboom G, Nys K, Harper P, et al. Predictive DNA-testing for Huntington's disease and reproductive decision making: a European Collaborative study. *Eur J Hum Genet* 2002;10:167–176.

94. Schulman JD, Black SH, Handyside A, et al. Preimplantation genetic testing for Huntington disease and certain other dominantly inherited disorders. *Clin Genet* 1996;49:57–58.

95. Sermon K, Goossens V, Seneca SM, et al. Preimplantation diagnosis for Huntington's disease (HD): Clinical application and analysis of the HD expansion in affected embryos. *Pren Diagn* 1998;18:1427–1436.

96. Sermon K, De Rijcke M, Lissens W, et al. Preimplantation genetic diagnosis for Huntington's disease with exclusion testing. *Eur J Hum Genet* 2002;10:591–598.

97. Adam S, Wiggins S, Whyte P, et al. Five year study of prenatal testing for Huntington disease: demand, attitudes and psychological assessment. *J Med Genet* 1993;30:549–556.

98. Maat-Kievit JA. Predictive testing for Huntington disease. Doctorate Thesis, Leiden June, 2001.

99. Tyler A, Quarrell OWJ, Lazarou LP, et al. Exclusion testing in pregnancy for Huntington's disease. *J Med Genet* 1990;27:488–495.

100. Tibben A, Frets PG, vd Kamp JJP, et al. Presymptomatic DNA testing for HD: pretest attitudes and expectations of applicants and their partners in the Dutch program. *Am J Med Genet* 1993a;48:10–61.

101. Tibben A, Duivenvoorden HJ, Niermeijer MF, et al. Presymptomatic DNA testing for Huntington disease: identifying the need for psychological intervention. *Am J Med Genet* 1993b;48:137–144.

102. Post SG. Huntington's disease: prenatal screening for late onset disease. *J Med Ethics* 1992;18:757–758.

103. Greenberg J. Huntington disease: prenatal screening for late onset disease. *J Med Ethics* 1993;19:121.

104. Benjamin CM, Adam S, Wiggins S, et al. Proceed with care: direct testing for Huntington Disease. *Am J Hum Genet* 1994;55:606–617.

105. Maat-Kievit A, Losekoot M, vd Boer-vd Berg H, et al. New problems in testing for Huntington disease: the issue of intermediate and reduced penetrance alleles. *J Med Genet* 2001;38:E12.

106. Leeflang EP, Zhang L, Tavare S, et al. Single sperm analysis of the trinucleotide repeats in the Huntington's disease gene: quantification of the mutation frequency spectrum. *Hum Mol Genet* 1995;4:1519–1526.

107. Chong SS, Almqvist E, Telenius H, et al. Contribution of DNA sequence and CAG size to mutation frequencies of intermediate alleles for Huntington disease: evidence from single sperm analyses. *Hum Molec Genet* 1997;6:301–309.

108. Legius E, Cuppens H, Dierick H, et al. Limited expansion of the (CAG)n repeat of the Huntington gene: a premutation? *Eur J Hum Genet* 1994;2:44–50.

109. McNeil SM, Novolletto A, Srinidhi J, et al. Reduced penetrance of the Huntington's disease mutation. *Hum Mol Genet* 1997;6:775–779.

110. Duyao M, Ambrose C, Myers R, et al. Trinucleotide repeat length: instability and age of onset in Huntington's disease. *Nat Genet* 1993;4:387–392.

111. Telenius H, Almqvist E, Kremer B, et al. Somatic mosaicism in sperm is associated with intergenerational (CAG)n changes in Huntington disease. *Hum Mol Genet* 1995;4:189–195.

112. Kelly TE, Allinson P, McGlennan RC, et al. Expansion of a 27 CAG repeat allele into a symptomatic Huntington disease-producing allele. *Am J Med Genet* 1999;87:91–92.

113. McGlennan RC, Allinson PS, Matthias-Hagen VL, et al. Evidence of an unstable paternal 27 CAG repeat allele in the huntingtin gene giving rise to clinically overt Huntington disease in a patient with the genotype17/38. *Am J Hum Genet* 1995;[Suppl 57]:A246.

114. Myers RH, MacDonald ME, Koroshetz WJ, et al. De novo expansion of a (CAG) in repeat in sporadic Huntington's disease. *Nat Genet* 1993;5:168–173.

115. Zuhlke C, Riess O, Bockel B, et al. Mitotic stability and meiotic variability of the (CAG) in repeat in the Huntington disease gene. *Hum Mol Genet* 1993;2:2063–2067.

116. Holmes SE, O 'Hearn E, Rosenblatt A, et al. A repeat expansion in the gene encoding junctophilin-3 is associated with Huntington disease-like 2. *Nat Genet* 2001;29:377–378.

117. Moore RC, Xiang F, Monaghan J, et al. Huntington disease phenocopy is a familial prion disease. *Am J Hum Genet* 2001;69:1385–1388.

118. Kremer B. Clinical neurology of Huntington's disease. In: Bates G, Harper PS, Jones L, eds., *Huntington's Disease* 3rd ed. Oxford Medical Publications, 2002

Routine Ultrasound for Dating

Heiner C. Bucher

Johannes G. Schmidt

William L. Martin

Khalid S. Khan

■ What Is the Problem that Requires Screening?

Poor perinatal outcome secondary to either postterm pregnancy, unrecognized multiple gestation, fetal anomalies, or growth restriction.

Ultrasound is used during pregnancy for diagnosis and screening. We focus on the effectiveness of ultrasound before 24 weeks' gestation for the prevention and management of postterm pregnancies and its relation to maternal and neonatal outcome. However, we recognize that the use of ultrasound is not easily separable into ultrasound for dating versus diagnosis of multiple gestation, malformations, or growth restriction. Ultrasound for the diagnosis of fetal malformations is covered in Chapter 24; that for growth restriction is in Chapters 31 and 32. The benefits of diagnosis are closely linked to the effectiveness and availability of treatment. If routine ultrasound improves the accuracy of the diagnosis of postterm pregnancy, multiple gestation, congenital anomalies, and fetal growth restriction, but does not affect pregnancy outcome, the problem may reside in the lack of an appropriate treatment for these conditions rather than the ultrasound per se.

What is the incidence/prevalence of the target condition?

A postterm pregnancy is one at 42 completed weeks (294 days) of gestation or more.[12] The prevalence of postterm pregnancy varies widely from 4% to 14%[3] due in part to differences among the populations examined and in part to differences in the measurements used to date the pregnancy. In a retrospective analysis of more than 1,700,000 notified births from the United Kingdom, the overall prevalence of postterm pregnancies was 6.2%.[4] Labor-induction policies at or around term (40–41 weeks of gestation) also affect the rate. For example, the prevalence of postterm pregnancy in Great Britain fell from 11.5% in 1958 to 4.4% in 1970, whereas the prevalence of labor induction rose from 13% to 26% in the same time period.[5]

Many population-based studies have relied on the first day of the last menstrual period to date the pregnancy. Such dates are often unreliable. In a study representative of all births in Sweden, the overall prevalence of postterm pregnancy was 12.2%.[3] In pregnancies with known dates, the postterm pregnancy rate was 10.2%, whereas it was 22.3% for pregnancies with an uncertain estimated date of confinement. There is only one series examining the rate of postterm pregnancy in women whose dates were based on basal body temperatures: the overall rate was 1% and the vast majority of women delivered before 294 days' gestation.

What are the sequelae of the condition that are of interest in clinical medicine?

Postterm pregnancies are associated with an increased risk of perinatal mortality and morbidity such as birth trauma and meconium aspiration syndrome. Due to low maternal morbidity and mortality after operative or vaginal delivery, obstetric decisions are increasingly affected by perinatal morbidity and mortality. As such, there has been growing adoption of a policy of labor induction before the onset of the postterm period.

Induction of labor. The frequency of labor induction in postterm pregnancies varies greatly according to local obstetric policy. For example, a population-based Norwegian study reported that 29.2% of postterm pregnancies versus 9.0% of term pregnancies were induced.[3] Furthermore, an analysis based on the comparison of postterm deliveries to those before 42 weeks' gestation may fail to recognize the progressively increasing rate of obstetric complications from 37 to 42 weeks' gestation.[6]

Maternal complications. Maternal complications during pregnancy are more common in postterm compared with those of term pregnancies.[3] In one study from Great Britain, labor at 41 weeks' gestation in primigravida was associated with a relative risk (RR) of 1.9 (95% confidence interval (CI), 1.6–2.2) for forceps delivery and a RR of 2.5 (95% CI, 1.8–3.3) for cesarean delivery.[6] The effect of gestational age on the rate of operative delivery was independent of birth weight. However, in another study, a policy of induction versus observation of pregnancy at 41 weeks' gestation or beyond modestly reduced the cesarean delivery rate (20.1% versus 22.0%; odds ratio [OR], 0.88; 95% CI, 0.78–0.99).[7]

Perinatal mortality. Several cohort studies reveal that gestation-specific fetal death and perinatal mortality rates reach a nadir at 40 weeks' gestation and then steadily increase thereafter.[4,8,9] For example, in one Swedish cohort study of more than 180,000 deliveries, the fetal death rates per 1,000 births at 41, 42, and 43 or more weeks gestation were 1.63, 2.02, and 3.46, respectively.[9] The corresponding OR (95% CI) for fetal death for weeks 41, 42, and 43 or more when compared with week 40 were 1.48 (1.13–1.95), 1.77 (1.22–2.56), and 2.90 (1.27–6.61), respectively. Gestation-specific fetal death rates expressed per total births, however, may incorrectly estimate the risk of fetal death. When using the proportion of ongoing pregnancies as the denominator, the risk of fetal death between 37 and 43 weeks' gestation increases sixfold.[4]

Large population-based studies indicate that fetal complications and perinatal mortality in postterm pregnancy are largely explained by fetuses that are small for gestational age.[8] The increased risk of death among small-for–gestational-age fetuses is impacted by the rate of lethal congenital malformations.[10] Approximately 25% of perinatal deaths in postterm pregnancies are due to malformations.[11] In one study, a policy at 41 weeks' gestation or beyond of induction versus watchful observation showed a trend toward reducing the perinatal mortality rate (0.09% versus 0.33%; OR, 0.41; 95% CI, 0.14–1.18).[7] Inaccurate control of the contribution of fetal malformation to the perinatal mortality rate in postterm pregnancies may lead to an overestimation of the effect of postterm delivery on neonatal outcome.

Perinatal morbidity. Higher rates of fetal distress, shoulder dystocia, and meconium aspiration occur in postterm-delivered infants in comparison with those delivered before 42 weeks' gestation.[8,10]

■ The Tests

Fetal sonographic biometry at less than 24 weeks' gestation.

What is the purpose of the tests?

Early-pregnancy ultrasonography provides a better estimate of the occurrence of postterm pregnancy by accurately dating the gestation compared with dating based on last menstrual period. However, routine ultrasound screening is used for accurate dating together with identification of multiple gestation, malformations, and growth restriction. What is unclear is whether routine ultrasound as practiced leads to a decrease in the overall perinatal morbidity and mortality. Accurate gestational age assessment also facilitates the cost-effective application of serological screening for markers of Down syndrome and/or neural tube defects (see Chapters 21–23), as the interpretation of these markers requires accurate dating.

What is the nature of the tests?

The gold standard for the assessment of gestational age is a documented time of ovulation/conception.[12] Compared with these standards, estimates derived using early ultrasound have proven to be within 9% of the known duration of gestation. Thus, the dating of pregnancy by ultrasound before 24 weeks' gestation is reasonably accurate. Prediction of the delivery date is a different matter. From 75% to 85% of pregnant women deliver within 2 weeks of their clinical estimated date of confinement.[13,14]

In a study of more than 4,000 pregnancies from a mixed socioeconomic population, the accuracy of the clinically predicted date of delivery in women with a known last menstrual period did not differ from that predicted by ultrasound examination up the 20th week of gestation.[15] According to menstrual history 84.7% and according to ultrasound 84.6% of women delivered within 2 weeks of their estimated date of delivery. However, among women with a suspect menstrual history, 69.7% of those clinically assessed and 81.2% of those with a sonographically determined due date delivered within 2 weeks' gestation. Thus, when the dates are in doubt, ultrasonography clearly improves the accuracy of gestational age dating.

Several sonographically derived fetal parameters are used to date the pregnancy. These include fetal crown–rump length, biparietal diameter, head circumference, and long bone length. The variability in the mean of all these estimates for dating is smaller before 24 weeks' gestation. Thus, a scan performed before 24 weeks' gestation is more accurate for the determination of gestational age than one performed subsequently.

It is unclear whether any single parameter is most accurate. Fetal crown–rump length measurements in the first trimester are reported as being accurate ± 5 days (2 SDs) in 95%.[16] In the second trimester, biparietal diameter or a combination of several sonographic parameters are the most accurate sonographic measure and predicts dates within a margin of ±7 to 11 days (2 SDs).[17]

What are the implications of testing?

What does an abnormal test result mean? A significant difference (generally defined as ≥ 2 SD, which corresponds to approximately 8–14 days) between a gestational age based on the last menstrual period and that based on the sonographic biometric parameters indicates that the due date should be changed to reflect the ultrasound.

An accurate ultrasound estimate of gestational age reduces the occurrence of labor induction for postterm pregnancy. The important question is whether routine ultrasound for dating improves maternal and perinatal outcome or whether ultrasound for dating should be reserved for pregnant women with suspect menstrual history or another indication. Only randomized controlled trials comparing routine with select ultrasound while incorporating a standard clinical approach to the management of the complication are capable of answering this question. Unfortunately, no studies have both randomized the use of ultrasound and have sufficiently standardized clinical management.

The impact of routine ultrasound on the induction rate and the overall pregnancy outcome was assessed in a meta-analysis by the Cochrane Collaboration of randomized controlled trials comparing routine with selective ultrasound.[18] That meta-analysis, in contrast with a previous one,[19] includes the RADIUS trial, a large randomized controlled trial of low-risk women.[20] The summary OR, based on six trials for induction of "postterm" pregnancy in groups with routine compared with groups with selective ultrasound, was 0.61 (95% CI, 0.52, 0.72), but there was heterogeneity across the trials for this finding. Perinatal mortality was not significantly lower in the routine ultrasound group

(OR, 0.86; 95% CI, 0.67, 1.12), although the OR for early pregnancy termination due to malformation was higher (OR, 3.19; 95% CI, 1.51, 6.60). Routine ultrasound was not associated with a reduction in the perinatal morbidity as crudely measured by 1- and 5-minute Apgar scores less than 7 (OR, 1.11; 95% CI 0.95–1.29 and 0.94; 95% CI, 0.69–1.29, respectively).

In the randomized controlled trial of routine versus selected ultrasound of low-risk pregnancies, the proportion of induced labor in the screened group was 25.1% compared with 24.7% in the control group.[21] According to the estimated gestational age at delivery, in the subgroup of women delivering at more than 42 weeks, 3.2% were in the screened group and 4.6% in the control group (difference –0.52%, 95% CI 0.95%–0.09%). However, it is noted that almost 45% of low-risk pregnancies randomized to the selected ultrasound group were believed by their caregiver to have an indication for ultrasound, an act that would likely dilute any differences between the groups.

Although this study included only women with a known menstrual history, there was a small but statistically significant difference in favor of the screened subjects in the subgroup of women who delivered after 42 weeks' gestation. However, there was no difference in neonatal outcome or any maternal complications such as induced labor and cesarean delivery. The rate of adverse perinatal outcome, defined as fetal or neonatal death up to 28 days of age or severe neonatal morbidity according to a 19-item list, was 5% in the screened group and 4.9% in the control group (RR, 1.0; 95% CI, 0.9, 1.2). There were no differences in perinatal outcome apparent in the subgroup of women with postterm pregnancies. The most likely explanation for this finding was the limited sensitivity of routine sonography for the detection of fetal malformation in this trial (see next section) coupled with the low rate of pregnancy termination after the diagnosis of a congenital malformation.

What does a normal test result mean?

The normal test result may take one of several forms depending on the underlying clinical circumstances. Typically, it means that the fetal biometric measurements are consistent with the woman's recalled last menstrual period or likely date of conception. In the absence of historical dating criteria, it can mean that the estimated date of confinement (EDC) will be based on this ultrasound result since the placental and fetal Doppler measured blood flows are normal and the fetal growth symmetrical. Lastly, a normal scan result may be one where the fetus has shown normal interval growth since a prior scan at least 3 weeks earlier.

What is the cost of testing?

Routine ultrasound screening in a low-risk population as examined in the trial by Ewigman et al.[20] added on average 1.6 scans per pregnancy. Screening more than 4 million pregnant women a year in the United States[22,23] at $200 per scan would increase medical costs of the pregnancy by $1.28 billion (1993). Based on the eligibility of 72% in this study, total costs for routine sonographic screening would still reach $921 million without any demonstrable benefit in perinatal and maternal outcome. However, estimates of the additional costs of routine ultrasound may vary considerably according to the number of selective scans effectuated in the control group. For example, in the study by Ewigman et al.,[18] 44.8% of the control group had at least one ultrasound, whereas in other trials the range of selective ultrasound in the control groups was between 10.2% and 77.0%. Thus, the incremental increase in health costs for routine ultrasound screening in the second trimester is likely much lower than previously estimated. A cost-effectiveness analysis in the UK National Health Service concluded that routine scanning in the second trimester may be relatively cost-effective considering the concomitant detection of anomalies.[24,25]

■ Conclusions and Recommendations

Opinion among both women and health care practitioners regarding the routine use of ultrasound has solidified in many, particularly resource-rich, countries. However, based on the available studies, routine one-stage ultrasound screening at up to 24 weeks' gestation does not improve perinatal outcome assessed by the perinatal mortality rate,[18] the live birth rate,[19] or a composite index of adverse perinatal outcomes.[20] But are these the appropriate endpoints? Is it logical to expect a tool, ultrasound, rather than the response to the tool to change outcome? Do women value being tested regardless of outcomes? A definitive answer regarding the advisability of routine second-trimester ultrasound screening is not possible based on available evidence alone. Although we consider the potential application of routine ultrasound to reduce the occurrence of postterm pregnancy, we also recognize the benefits of diagnosis are closely linked to the effectiveness and availability of treatment. This should encourage researchers to develop means to assess effectiveness of various management strategies of these conditions (e.g., the recent trial comparing immediate versus delayed delivery in growth-restricted infants).[26]

Routine ultrasound for dating does improve the identification of "true" postterm pregnancies. But, does improved diagnosis reduce maternal morbidity through avoidable intervention? A meta-analysis of the Cochrane Collaboration concludes that routine induction of labor in postterm pregnancies reduces perinatal mortality (OR, 0.20; 95% CI, 0.06–0.70).[27] The validity of this meta-analysis may be questioned for several reasons. The confidence intervals for the summary estimate are quite wide, six of the 13 included trials did not report perinatal mortality data, underlining the low power to obtain a reliable summary estimate from this study; several studies were included with quasi-randomization or improper randomization procedures; and a variety of different methods for labor induction were used. It is a widely accepted practice to induce labor after term has been reached, although the best available evidence indicates that routine induction of labor with vaginal prostaglandin E_2 increases the rate of delivery within 24 hours but does not alter the cesarean delivery rate compared with that of placebo or expectant management.[28] The studies of routine ultrasound reported cannot be used to address this issue because routine induction of labor was not the standard of care in postterm pregnancies and the sample size was too small to identify a decrease in rare events.

Another potential advantage of routine dating of pregnancy with ultrasound is the reduction of unnecessary administration of tocolysis (in cases of incorrectly diagnosed preterm labor). The RADIUS study found that routine scanning decreased the rate of tocolytic administration from 4.2% to 3.4%. Avoiding unnecessary intervention has clear benefits to patients and to the health care system.

Routine early-pregnancy (less than 24 weeks' gestation) ultrasound can be justified if it meets the following criteria : (1) It improves the health outcome about which patients care (i.e., death, disability, disfigurement, pain, anxiety); (2) the benefits outweigh the risks; and (3) the health effects outweigh the cost.[29] Routine ultrasound meets some of these criteria.[24] First, routine obstetric ultrasound can reduce perinatal mortality if congenital anomalies are appropriately identified and a modest number of patients elect pregnancy termination.[30] Second, the risks associated with the use of diagnostic ultrasound during pregnancy appear to be exceedingly low and limited to the potential risk of bio-effects and false-positive diagnoses. The false-positive rate of diagnostic ultrasound is also low (less than 2%) in experienced hands.

An accurate date of confinement is of benefit to women even with clear menstrual history if there are other reasons to be concerned about the precise date of confinement. A woman's choice of whether to have an ultrasound examination should be based on the best available information as to possible benefits and hazards. This information should include informing the woman that the effectiveness of routine ultrasound scanning is limited to the screening for malformations and its use for this purpose has implications including the risk of false-positive diagnosis and ethical issues surrounding termination of pregnancy. No other clear benefits have been demonstrated.

■ Summary

1 ■ What Is the Problem that Requires Screening?

Poor perinatal outcome secondary to either post maturity, unrecognized multiple gestation, fetal anomalies, or growth restriction. The focus of this chapter is on postterm pregnancy.

a. What is the incidence/prevalence of the target condition?

The prevalence of postterm pregnancy varies from 4% to 14%, possibly due in part to differences among the examined populations and in part to differences in the measurements used.

Continued

■ **Summary—cont'd**

b. *What are the sequelae of the condition that are of interest in clinical medicine?*
Postterm pregnancies are associated with adverse outcomes such as a higher rate of induced labor and maternal complications and increased perinatal mortality and morbidity. However, the increased perinatal mortality and morbidity rates are not necessarily explained by 'postterm' delivery per se.

2 ■ **The Tests**

a. *What is the purpose of the tests?*
To reduce the occurrence of postterm pregnancy by accurately dating the gestation. However, routine ultrasound screening is not separable into ultrasound for accurate dating to reduce the occurrence of postterm pregnancies from ultrasound to diagnose multiple gestation, malformations, and growth restriction.

b. *What is the nature of the tests?*
Fetal sonographic biometry before 24 weeks' gestation.

c. *What are the implications of testing?*
1. What does an abnormal test result mean?
A significant difference (≥ 2 SD/8 – 14 days) between the age assigned on the basis of the last menstrual period and that based on the sonographic biometric parameters indicates that the estimated date of confinement should be changed to reflect that of the ultrasound.
2. What does a normal test result mean?
Typically, one where the fetal biometric measurements are consistent with the woman's recalled last menstrual period or likely date of conception.

d. *What is the cost of testing?*
Routine scanning at less than 24 weeks' gestation may be relatively cost-effective when the total information gained is considered.

3 ■ Conclusions and Recommendations

Based on the available studies, ultrasound before 24 weeks' gestation does not improve perinatal outcome assessed by the perinatal mortality or live birth rate or by a composite index of adverse perinatal outcomes. Although, a definitive answer regarding the cost-effectiveness of routine second-trimester ultrasound screening is not possible based on published literature, in many countries this is already entrenched into practice largely for detection of fetal abnormalities and maternal reassurance. Thus the information gained about dating can thus be usefully employed to aid in monitoring fetal growth and assessing the need for induction for postterm.

References

1. World Health Organization. *Manual of the International Statistical Classification of Diseases, Injuries, and Causes of Death,* 9th ed. Geneva: WHO, 1977.
2. FIGO International Federation of Gynecology and Obstetrics. Report of the FIGO subcommittee on perinatal epidemiology and health statistics following a workshop in Cairo, November 11-18, 1984, on the methodology of measurement and recording of infant growth in the perinatal period. London: FIGO, 1986:54.
3. Bakketeig L, Bergsjø P. Post-term pregnancy: magnitude of the problem. In: Chalmers I, Enkin M, Keirse MJNC, eds. *Effective Care in Pregnancy and Childbirth.* Oxford: Oxford University Press, 1989:765–774.
4. Hilder L, Costeloe K, Thilaganathan B. Prolonged pregnancy: evaluating gestation-specific risk of fetal and infant mortality. Br J Obstet Gynecol 1998;105:169–173.
5. Chamberlain G, Philipp E, Howlett B, et al. *British Births, Vol. 2: Obstetric Care.* London: Heinemann Medical Books. 1978:292.
6. Saunders N, Paterson C. Effect of gestational age on obstetric performance: when is "term" over? *Lancet* 1991;338:1190–1192.
7. Sanchez-Ramos L, Olivier F, Delke I, et al. Labor induction versus expectant management for postterm pregnancies: a systematic review with meta-analysis. *Obstet Gynecol* 2003;101:1312–1318.
8. Campbell MK, Ostbye T, Irgens LM. Post-term birth: risk factors and outcomes in a 10-year cohort of Norwegian births. *Obstet Gynecol* 1997;89:543–548.
9. Divon MY, Haglund B, Nisell H et al. Fetal and neonatal mortality in the postterm pregnancy: the impact of gestational age and fetal growth restriction. *Am J Obstet Gynecol* 1988;178:726–731.
10. Calusson B, Cnattingius S Axelsson O. Outcomes of post-term births: The role of fetal growth restriction and malformations. *Obstet Gynecol* 1999;94:758–762.
11. Naeye R. Causes of perinatal mortality excess in prolonged gestations. *Am J Epidemiol* 1978;108:429–433.
12. Mac Gregor SN, Tamura RK, Sabbagha RE, et al. Underestimation of gestational age by conventional crown-rump length dating curves. *Obstet Gynecol* 1987;70:344–348.
13. Grennert L, Persson PH, Gennser G. Benefits of ultrasonic screening of a pregnant population. *Acta Obstet Gynecol Scand* 1978;78[Suppl]:5–14.
14. Kloosterman GJ. Epidemiology of postmaturity. In: Keirse MJNC, Anderson ABM, Bennebroek Gravenhorst J, eds., *Human Parturion.* The Hague: Leiden University Press, 1979:247–261.
15. Campell S, Warsof SL, Little D, et al. Routine ultrasound screening for the prediction of gestational age. *Obstet Gynecol* 1985; 65: 613–629.

16. Robinson HP, Fleming JEE. A critical evaluation of "crown-rump length" measurements. *Br J Obstet Gynaecol* 1975; 82:702–710.

17. Sabbagha RE. Gestational age. In: Sabbagha RE, ed., *Diagnostic Ultrasound Applied to Obstetrics and Gynecology*. Philadelphia: J.B. Lippincott, 1987:91–111.

18. Neilson JP. Ultrasound for fetal assessment in early pregnancy [Cochrane Review]. In: *The Cochrane Library, Issue 3*. Chichester, UK: John Wiley & Sons, 2004.

19. Bucher HC, Schmidt JG. Does routine ultrasound scanning improve outcome in pregnancy? A meta-analysis of various outcome measures. *BMJ* 1993;307:13–17.

20. Ewigman BG, Crane JP, Frigoletto FD et al. Effect of prenatal ultrasound screening on perinatal outcome. *N Engl J Med* 1993;329:821–828.

21. LeFevre ML, Bain RP, Ewigman BG, et al. A randomized trial if prenatal ultrasonographic screening: impact on maternal management and outcome. *Am J Obstet Gynecol* 1993;169:483–489.

22. National Center for Health Statistics. Vital statistics of the United States, 1988. Vol 1. Natality. Washington, DC: Government Printing Office, 1990. DHHS publication no. 90-1100.

23. National Center for Health Statistics. Vital statistics of the United States, 1988. Vol. 2 Mortality, Part A. Washington, DC: Government Printing Office, 1991. DHHS publication no. 91-1101.

24. Bricker L, Garcia J, Henderson J, et al. Ultrasound screening in pregnancy: a systematic review of the clinical effectiveness, cost-effectiveness and women's views. *Health Technol Assess* 2000;4:16:1–193.

25. Ritchie K, Boynton J, Bradbury I, et al. Routine ultrasound scanning before 24 weeks of pregnancy. Health Technology Assessment Report No. 5. Glasgow: NHS Quality Improvement Scotland, 2004.

26. Thornton JG, Hornbuckle J, Vail A, et al. Infant wellbeing at 2 years of age in the Growth Restriction Intervention Trial (GRIT): multicentred randomised controlled trial. *Lancet* 2004;364:513–520.

27. Crowley P. Elective induction of labour at 41+ weeks gestation. In: Chalmers I, ed., Oxford database of perinatal trials. Oxford: Oxford University Press (Version 1.2, disk issue 5; record 4144), 1991.

28. Kelly AJ, Kavanagh J, Thomas J. Vaginal prostaglandin (PGE2 and PGF2a) for induction of labour at term. In: *The Cochrane Library, Issue 3*. Chichester, UK: John Wiley & Sons, 2003.

29. Romero R. Routine obstetric ultrasound. *J Ultrasound Obstet Gynecol* 1993;3:303–307.

30. Saari-Kemppainen A, Karjalainen O, Ylostalo P, et al. Ultrasound screening and perinatal mortality: controlled trial of systematic one-stage screening in pregnancy. *Lancet* 1990; 336:387–391.

First Trimester Screening for Aneuploidy

Kevin Spencer

■ What Is the Problem that Requires Screening?

Major chromosomal aneuploidies that include the autosomal aneuploidies of trisomy 21 (Down syndrome), trisomy 13 (Patau syndrome), trisomy 18 (Edward syndrome), and to a lesser extent the sex aneuploids such as 45,X0 (Turner syndrome), 47,XXY (Klinefelter syndrome), and those with 47,XYY and triploidy (69,XXX or XXY).

What is the incidence/prevalence of the target condition?

The natural frequency of chromosomal abnormalities at birth approximates 6/1,000 births among women without any form of antenatal screening. The autosomal aneuploids are most frequent, with trisomy 21 the most common of the group having a historical birth prevalence of 1/800. The historical birth prevalences are summarized in Table 21–1.[2,3]

Although the birth rates of the major autosomal trisomies (13, 18, and 21) increase with advancing maternal age, this is not true for sex chromosome aneuploidies and triploidy. Thus, the general prevalence of age-related trisomies has increased over the past 20 years as a direct consequence of women postponing childbirth until later life, with the rate of trisomy 21 increasing from 1/740 to 1/500.[1]

Although the birth prevalence of the major chromosomal abnormalities approaches 6/1,000, the actual prevalence at any one time in pregnancy varies due to differing intrauterine lethality rates of the various conditions.[3] This means that there are a significantly greater number of affected fetuses in early pregnancy than at either mid gestation or at term.

There is also an increased risk of recurrence approximating 0.75% above the background maternal age risk in women who have delivered a fetus with an autosomal trisomy (but not in the case of the sex aneuploids or triploidy).[4]

Table 21-1	**Historical birth prevalence rates of common chromosome abnormalities**	

Aneuploidy		Prevalence
Autosomal		
	Trisomy 21	1/800
	Trisomy 18	1/6500
	Trisomy 13	1/12,500
Sex chromosomal		
	45,XO	1/2,500 females
	47,XXX	1/1,000 females
	47,XXY	1/500–1,000 males
	47,XYY	1/1,000 males
Other		
	Triploidy type 1	
	Triploidy type 2	

From Egan JF, Benn P, Borgida AF, et al. Efficacy of screening for fetal Down syndrome in the United States from 1974 to 1997. *Obstet Gynecol* 2000;96:979–985; and Hook EB. Prevalence, risk and recurrence. In: Brock DH, Rodeck CH, Ferguson-Smith MA, eds., *Prenatal Diagnosis and Screening*. Edinburgh: Churchill Livingstone, 1992:351–392.

What are the sequelae of the condition that are of interest in clinical medicine?

Trisomy 21. Langdon Down first described in his 1866 essay on "Observation of an ethnic classification of idiots" the phenotypic expression of the syndrome, which continues to bear his name.[5] Although in 1909 Suttleworth[6] described the association between the syndrome and increased maternal age, it was not until Lejune et al.[7] and Jacobs et al.[8] demonstrated in 1959 that the condition resulted from an extra copy of chromosome 21. This extra copy results either from nondisjunction or from a translocation. The syndrome requires either the whole or a segment of the long arm of chromosome 21, the distal portion of which is now known to determine the facial features, heart defects, mental IQ, and other clinical features. Most cases result from nondisjunction, and in 95% of these, the additional genetic material is of maternal origin.

The major clinical consequences of trisomy 21, apart from the learning disability with IQ scores ranging between 20 and 70, are the congenital heart defects that occur in 40% to 50% of individuals. Gastrointestinal complications occur in some 15% to 30%, with visual, ear, nose, and throat problems in 40% to 60% of children. The frequency of hypothyroidism is significantly increased, as is epilepsy. There is also a threefold increase in the incidence of leukemia. The average life expectancy has improved considerably over the past decade, approaching 50 years. With increased life expectancy, it was recognized that the many of the brains of adults with trisomy 21 adults have virtually all the neuropathological changes associated with Alzheimer dementia by age 40 years. Some studies report a prevalence of 8% at age 49 rising to 75% by age 60. Typical of many chromosomal anomalies, varied phenotypic expression is evident despite the same prime cause, and it is not possible to identify individuals who will develop a severe form from those who will be only mildly affected.

Trisomy 18. In 1960, Edwards et al.[9] first described this condition in which the median survival time was less than 1 week, 90% dying by 6 months, and less than 5% surviving to 1 year. Growth deficiency begins in utero and continues postnatally. Congenital heart disease and cardiopulmonary arrest are the most common causes of death. Survivors have profound physical and mental retardation.

Trisomy 13. Patau et al.[10] also described this condition in 1960, and like trisomy 18, the in utero characteristic feature is growth deficiency. The median survival time of infants is less than 1 week, with more than 80% of infants dying in the first month and only 3% surviving 6 months. Severe congenital heart and renal defects are the most common causes of death. Survivors are physically and mentally handicapped; blindness and deafness is common, and self-mutilating behavioral difficulties frequent.

Sex chromosomal aneuploidy. The sex chromosomal abnormalities are the most problematic to classify as a serious birth defects of the chromosomal aneuploidies.

The absent sex chromosome characteristic of Turner syndrome (45,X0) was first described in 1938. Features include short stature, gonadal dysgenesis, lymphedema, and congenital heart defects; no single feature is pathognomic. Infants born with Turner syndrome typically present clinically at puberty as only 10% have spontaneous puberty and fertility. Intellectual function is normal in most cases. Similar to the major autosomal trisomies, the in utero incidence of Turner syndrome is much higher than at birth. Again, the same genetic condition is expressed phenotypically in different ways. A significant proportion of early pregnancy losses in early pregnancy are 45,X0, whereas another group survive until around the 22 weeks and then spontaneously die. Such phenotypic variability makes antenatal screening and counseling difficult.

Klinefelter syndrome (47,XXY) is the most common sex chromosomal abnormality with a prevalence of 1/500 to 1,000 male births. Most individuals are identified during an investigation for delayed puberty, infertility, or gynecomastia. The abnormality is associated with relatively mild developmental delay in motor and language skills, coupled with behavioral difficulties. In some series, the IQ was 20 points below that of their siblings. An association with criminal behavior is suggested by an increased prevalence of Klinefelter in tall, mentally retarded criminals.

The 47,XXX karyotype is found in 1/1,000 females at birth. The vast majority of adult women with an extra X chromosome have normal puberty and reproductive capacity. The IQ is on average 10 points lower than that of siblings.

Triploidy. The triploid karyotype may be either 69,XXX or 69,XXY. It results from either an extra paternal set of chromosomes (diandric) or from an extra maternal set of chromosomes (digynic). Triploidy accounts for 15% of cytogenetically abnormal aborted fetuses. It is estimated to occur in 1% of conceptions, but high intra uterine lethality results in almost all being lost by the 25th week of gestation. Ninety-nine percent of affected fetuses do not survive to term, and the life expectancy for those that do is less than 1 year.

■ The Tests

What is the purpose of the tests?

The goal of antenatal screening programs is to provide specific information that allows couples to make informed reproductive decisions.[11] The goal is not to establish programs focused on eradicating disability. Antenatal screening programs identify a subgroup of women who are at sufficiently high risk of carrying a fetus affected by either trisomy 21 or one of the other major, chromosomal anomalies. This subgroup of women is then offered a diagnostic (invasive) test such as amniocentesis or chorionic villus sampling (CVS) followed by karyotyping of fetal tissue. Both of these invasive techniques entail a fetal loss rate 0.25% to 1% above the background rate for gestation, although rates vary greatly based on the experience of the operator.

What is the nature of the tests?

Biochemical and sonographic tests. The available tests may be either sonographic, biochemical, or a combination of both modalities for maximum yield. The probability of the fetus having trisomy 21, trisomy 13/18, or any of the other aneuploidies is calculated from the maternal age–specific risk (plus any adjustment for history), along with the results of an ultrasound examination during which the fluid at the back of the fetal neck (nuchal translucency [NT]) (Figure 21–1) is measured and the maternal serum concentration of two placental produced proteins (pregnancy-associated plasma protein-A [PAPP-A] and free beta-human chorionic gonadotropin [β-hCG]) ascertained. The blood test may be performed at the same time as the ultrasound examination as in a one-stop clinic for the assessment of risk (OSCAR) center[12–15] or sequentially with the blood sample obtained before or after the ultrasound examination. A combined risk assessment is given when all the results are available.

The concentrations of many biochemical markers vary with gestational age. These gestational fluctuations are removed by expressing the patient concentration as a ratio of the measured value to the median value for normal pregnancy at the same gestation to obtain a multiple of the median (MoM). Thus, a 1 MoM is normal, 2 MoM elevated, and 0.5 MoM reduced.

Only two currently recognized first-trimester maternal serum biochemical markers are of value screening for chromosomal anomalies. Free β-hCG is on

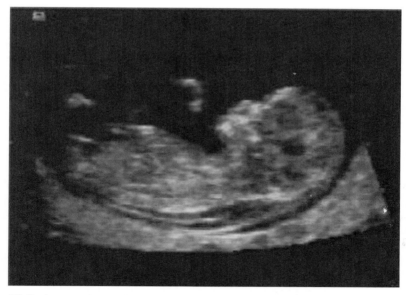

Figure 21-1   Increased nuchal translucency (NT) in a fetus with trisomy 21.

average 2 MoM[12] in pregnancies with a trisomy 21 fetus, whereas the levels are significantly reduced with trisomies 13 and 18 (0.5 and 0.3, respectively).[16–18] Unlike the second trimester, total hCG is a fairly poor discriminator for trisomy 21 in the first trimester.[19] PAPP-A is reduced to around 0.5 MoM in trisomy 21[12] and to 0.2 MoM in trisomies 13 and 18.[16–18] The distributions of the MoM values in normal and trisomy 21 pregnancies usually follow a Gaussian distribution when the MoM is log transformed. And although there is significant overlap of the two populations with all markers, it is possible to establish from the Gaussian distributions the likelihood of any one result coming from the population of results associated with fetal trisomy 21. An individual, patient-specific risk is calculated by multiplying the a priori risk (usually based on maternal age)[3] by the likelihood ratio. No single biochemical marker alone has sufficient clinical discrimination, and the most efficient screening program results by combining information from more than one marker. When the markers are independent, the likelihood ratio for each marker can simply be multiplied together to obtain the combined ratio. In clinical practice, the markers used correlate or provide similar information; thus, their likelihood ratios must be corrected by complex mathematical and statistical procedures.[20] The two biochemical markers together in the first trimester have detection rates no better than 65% at a 5% screen-positive rate,[12] making it slightly worse than second-trimester triple or quad biochemical screening.

The single most important sonographic marker of fetal aneuploidy in the first trimester is the fetal NT.[21] An echogenic area of fluid exists in all fetuses between the fetal skin and the soft tissue overlying the cervical spine

(Figure 21–1). Initial studies of high-risk populations identified an association between increased NT thickness and the presence of a fetal chromosomal anomaly.[22] Because the measurement is small (1–2.5 mm in normal pregnancies), it is necessary to use a standardized approach to measurement. The Fetal Medicine Foundation (FMF) approach to training, sonographer/obstetrician certification, and audit has become almost a universal standard in this area (www.fetalmedicine.com).[4] The NT measurement may be taken at the same time as the early pregnancy dating scan between 11 and 14 weeks' gestation. In most experienced hands, such examinations can be achieved in a 15-minute examination period. In studies that have used the FMF protocol, detection rates for trisomy 21 of are 70% to 75% with a 5% screen-positive rate.[23]

Recently, first-trimester screening with fetal NT and maternal serum biochemistry received approval from two national bodies. In the United Kingdom, the Nice Guidelines for Antenatal Care[24] and the Antenatal Screening Working Standards of the National Down's Syndrome Screening Programme[25] proposed that all women presenting for maternity care before 14 weeks' gestation be offered a combination of fetal NT and maternal serum biochemical measurement by 2007. In the United States, a recent American College of Obstetrics and Gynecology (ACOG) Committee Opinion on first-trimester screening for fetal aneuoploidy[26] endorsed the use of first-trimester screening in centers where appropriate ultrasound training and quality monitoring programs are in place and where appropriate early diagnosis is available.

What are the implications of testing?

Women who have a risk above a certain cutoff (usually 1/250–300) or whose risk is dramatically higher than their background age risk can consider the possibility of having an invasive diagnostic procedure such as amniocentesis or CVS followed by karyotyping of the fetal tissue. Karyotyping, whether by conventional G banding or molecular techniques such as fluorescent in-situ hybridization (FISH) or quantitative polymerase chain reaction (Q-PCR) (see Chapter 25), has a diagnostic accuracy of 99.9% or more.[27]

What does an abnormal test result mean? The screening test is not diagnostic, and the only way to be certain is to follow the screen result with a diagnostic test. Women who learn their fetus has a major chromosomal abnormality may opt for pregnancy termination.

In general population terms, a 1/300 trisomy 21 risk cutoff will label approximately 5% of pregnancies as at increased risk (sometimes referred to as screen positive) and the detection rate for trisomy 21 will be 90%.[12,13,28] In simple terms, nine of ten cases will be identified by screening. One factor often overlooked in screening programs is the fact that detection rates and (and thus screen-positive rates) vary considerably with maternal age. The detection rate falls in younger women, as does the screen-positive rate. Screening programs that quote only global detection and screen-positive rates may mislead the individual woman or couple. These issues need to be considered when counseling

Table 21-2	**Detection rate and false-positive rates for trisomy 21 in the first-trimester combined program**	
Maternal age, y	**Detection rate, %**	**False-positive rate, %**
20	78.8	2.3
25	80.6	2.9
30	83.8	4.0
35	89.7	8.7
38	93.9	15.9
40	96.1	24.4
44	98.8	47.1

women on the test and its results.[29] One study used modeling to calculate expected detection rates and screen-positive rates at various maternal ages in the first trimester using combined ultrasound and biochemical approaches.[30] Table 21–2 summarizes this data.

Combined risks for trisomies 13 and 18 are usually calculated because it is not possible to differentiate between these two situations on the basis of the raised NT or the reduced PAPP-A and free β-hCG.[16–18] Some cases of trisomy 13/18 will also have an increased risk of trisomy 21 by virtue of the raised NT, and others will have a normal trisomy 21 risk but an abnormal (> 1/150) trisomy 13/18 risk. Screening will identify 95% of trisomy 13/18 cases for an additional 0.3% false-positive rate.

Also among those women with an increased trisomy 21 risk will be some pregnancies affected by other chromosomal anomalies.[31,32] Table 21–3 summarizes the pattern of biochemical markers seen with the various aneuploidies. For all women who have a risk of greater than 1/300, the likelihood of having a fetus affected by trisomy 21 is 1/25, and the likelikhood of having a fetus affected by any chromosomal aneuploidy is 1/10. Thus nine in ten women will have a chromosomally normal fetus, and one in ten will have a fetus with a chromosomal abnormality. The overall positive predictive value of the trisomy 21 risk-screening test is around 5%.

Table 21-3	**Marker patterns in the first trimester with different chromosomal anomalies**		
Anomaly	**NT**	**Free β-hCG**	**PAPP-A**
Trisomy 21	↑ 2.5	↑ 2.0	↓ 0.5
Trisomy 18	↑ 3.5	↓ 0.3	↓ 0.2
Trisomy 13	↑ 2.5	↓ 0.5	↓ 0.3
Turner syndrome	↑ 7.0	↔	↓ 0.5
Triploidy I	↑ 2.5	↑ 8.0	↓ 0.8
Triploidy II	↔	↓ 0.2	↓ 0.1

β-hCG, beta human chorionic gonadotropin; NT, nuchal translucency; PAPP-A, pregnancy-associated plasma protein-A.

Screening by OSCAR clinics has been in operation at two centers in the United Kingdom since 1998.[13,15,28] The results of the first 3 years of screening women of all maternal ages at these centers is published, with detection rates of 92% for trisomy 21 and 96% for all aneuploids, with a screen-positive rate below 5%.[13,28] Patient acceptance of screening was high (97%) indicating that early one-stop screening is acceptable to women. Even the screening of twin pregnancies with such a procedure seems clinically effective identifying three of four twin pregnancies discordant for trisomy 21.[33,34] For the 8% women who present too early for NT (i.e., ultrasound examination shows them to be prior to 11 weeks 0 days [crown–rump length, 45 mm]), it is a simple task to reschedule a new visit at the appropriate gestation. For the 5% those presenting too late for NT (i.e., beyond 13 weeks 6 days, crown–rump length, 84 mm), second-trimester biochemical screening can be performed.

In instance where the karyotype is normal, but the risk driven by an increased NT, there is an increased probability the fetus has a major heart defect. In one study of 1,319 chromosomally normal fetuses with an increased NT, the prevalence of major cardiac defects was 4.5% and correlated directly to the size of the NT.[35] Thus, the rate was 3.1% where the NT ranged from 3.5 to 4.4 mm, but rose to 30.3% when the NT was equal to or above 6.5 mm. In another study, the prevalence was 0.31% in fetuses with an NT below 2.5 mm but 5% in those with an NT greater than 3.4 mm.[36]

In an analysis of outcomes in the same group of 1,319 chromosomally normal fetuses,[37] the overall probability of a livebirth with no defects when the NT was above 3.4 mm fell from 85.9% in fetuses with an NT between 2.5 and 3.4 mm to 31.2% in fetuses with an NT greater than 6.4 mm. Thus, an increased NT is a sign of poor pregnancy outcome. Souka et al.[37] proposed a cascade method of investigating such pregnancies over the ensuing next 10 weeks.

In instances where the karyotype is normal and the increased risk driven by the biochemical parameters, a potential adverse outcome may also be suspected, although the pattern is one more of lowered levels of PAPP-A and, to a lesser extent, free β-hCG, and is associated with miscarriage, preeclampsia, growth restriction, or low birth weight.[38–42] However, the sensitivity is quite poor—being equivalent to second-trimester biochemical screening.[43]

What does a normal test result mean? If the initial risk is lower than the usual cutoff of 1/300, approximately 95% of women will be classified as 'low risk'. They are accurately reassured their pregnancy is not affected by one of the major aneuploidies. The negative predictive value of the trisomy 21 screening test is 99.98%, though unfortunately 1/10 trisomy 21 fetus will be classified into the low-risk group. However, this is much better than can be achieved using second-trimester biochemical screening, screening by maternal age alone, or relying on nonspecific ultrasound signs in the second trimester.[44]

What is the cost of testing?

Costs in a private health care system in which women self-select themselves for screening are often based on the economics of what the market will stand rather than the actual cost of delivering the service; in other systems, it may be based on what reimbursement costs have been agreed or are allowed. In state-funded health care systems, universal screening programs may be developed where the cost of the program is viewed from a societal perspective, balancing the costs of detection against the costs of lifetime care for an individual with the disease. Other costs, which are difficult to factor into such economic appraisals, are the human and individual costs. Indeed some have argued that a cost-effectiveness analysis is not yet an appropriate tool to justify antenatal screening.[45] Authors of a systematic review of the economic evaluations of antenatal screening (ten studies of trisomy 21 screening, predominantly second-trimester biochemical screening) reported that there are clear economic arguments for trisomy 21 screening.[46] However, the same review highlighted the poor methodologic quality of most evaluations that seem only to consider basic cost and not institutional overheads; some included only the incremental costs of moving from a two-marker to a three-marker program.

First-trimester screening costs were evaluated in five other studies but, again, they compared only the incremental costs moving from one strategy to another.[47-51] Most agreed that first-trimester combined screening was more cost-effective than screening by maternal age alone or screening by second-trimester biochemistry. In our own point of care program, we estimated that the cost of provision of a simultaneous NT and biochemical testing program for a population of 4,500 women screened actually has an institutional saving of £3,000 and an individuals saving of £7,000 compared with the cost of providing such a service in a sequential way.[15] In the United Kingdom, typical private patient charges for such combined first-trimester screening approximate £100 to £150 per patient, with any invasive testing charges on top. In a crude costing analysis that did not include any institutional overhead or any costs associated with counseling or midwifery, Wald et al.[52] suggested a unit cost of £15 for the combined test. We believe this cost is unrealistic, and our estimates place the cost much closer to £35 per test (see related discussions in Chapters 21–23).

One of the difficulties in comparing costs and economic evaluations from different countries is the question of how transportable they are to different health care systems and different economies. In various cost-effectiveness analyses, the appropriate excess lifetime support costs of a person with trisomy 21 remains unclear. In the United Kingdom, one frequently quoted figure is that derived by Shackley et al.[53] who calculated a figure of £79,500 at 1990 prices, whereas Gill et al.[54] calculated that it was £156,660 at 1983 prices. A commonly used excess lifetime support cost in the United States is the one derived by Waitzman et al.[55] at $451,000 for 1989 prices and when adjusted for inflation in various cost analysis studies[56-58] reaches a figure of $677,692 (£387,252) at 2002 prices.[59] If one adjusts the UK figure of Gill et al.[54] by the retail price index 1983 to 2002, this would equate to £284,024, a figure that is still 25% lower than the US figure, but more realistic than the Shackley et al.[53] figure.

Another difficulty comparing costs and economic evaluations from different countries is the relative cost of health care provision. For example, Gilbert et al.[48] estimated ultrasound NT costs at £4.44 per woman and this figure has been used by others.[52] However, this cost did not include equipment costs, space, or institutional overheads. A more realistic cost for first-trimester ultrasound is that calculated by Henderson et al.[60] at £14.31. As has been pointed out[59] such costs are far below the cost of an ultrasound examination in the United States where the estimated cost for combined NT and biochemical screening in one study has been estimated at $130 (£75) rather then the $26 (£15) estimated by Wald et al.[52] or Gilbert et al.[48] or our in-house estimates of $61 (£35).

Clearly much depends on the cost input and the overall program costs and the excess lifetime support cost that is being balanced against. If we take the UK figures of Gill et al.[54] for excess lifetime support cost, adjusted to 2002 as £284,024 and if we adjust the program costs of Gilbert et al.[48] using a more realistic cost for ultrasound and biochemistry, the overall program costs for screening a population of 10,000 women would be £436,800. With a birth prevalence of 1:500, 20 cases with trisomy 21 would be live born if no screening took place. The societal costs therefore would be 20 × £284,024 or £5.6 million ($9.9 million). Assuming an 80% uptake of screening, four live-born cases with trisomy 21 would occur in the 2,000 women not screened. In the remaining 8,000, assuming an 85% detection rate, 2.4 cases would be missed and reach term. Of the remaining 13.6 cases, assuming uptake of CVS or amniocentesis was 80%, 10.88 births could be potentially avoided. If 90% of those with diagnosed trisomy 21 accepted termination, the birth of 9.88 of the 20 cases could be avoided. Thus the cost per case avoided is £436,800/9.88 or £44,210 compared with the excess lifetime cost of £284,024. Even if the uptake of screening fell to only 50%, the uptake of CVS was only 50%, and the uptake of termination was 50%, the birth of 2.15 cases would be averted at a cost per cases of £203,162 which would still be lower than the excess lifetime cost per individual.

In reality, cost-effectiveness arguments are fraught with error and assumptions that may not be valid. Antenatal screening, however, should not be about cost avoidance or the eradication of individuals with disability. Antenatal screening is concerned with providing couples with information by which they can make reproductive decisions that are appropriate from them.[61]

■ Conclusions and Recommendations

The past decade has witnessed considerable focus on moving antenatal screening earlier into the first trimester. When women's views are elicited, there is a clear preference for screening at the earliest possible time in pregnancy.[50-53] Earlier screening should provide women with earlier reassurance and, if termination of pregnancy is decided for an abnormality, it can be completed before fetal movements are evident when the procedure related risks are lowest.[49] In addition to detecting 90% of fetuses with trisomy 21, first-trimester screening identifies over 90% of other chromosomal aneuploidies, with a screen-positive rate of around 4% to 5%. The fact that some trisomy 21 and other chromosomally abnormal pregnancies detected in the first trimester will be spontaneously lost before term is not a strong argument against early screening. For these women, the findings may provide important information with regard to future reproductive decisions and the potential to prevent a late loss of unknown cause. Nor is an ethical objection to pregnancy termination a strong argument against screening as fore knowledge of a fetal abnormality provides the patient an opportunity to learn about a complex problem in detail, and may alter the type and location of pregnancy care.

Although improvements in screening performance have previously been measured by increased detection rates, little attention or research has focused on service delivery and counseling or how it may affect maternal and family anxiety and stress at a time when they should be celebrating. Screening necessarily generates anxiety because it identifies individuals with a high risk of having a child with a serious disorder. An "increased risk" result makes awareness of the risk both real and personal at a particularly poignant time because of the strong emotions associated with pregnancy. The screening service should be conducted so that the general environment of screening, the information offered, and the personal support are tailored to show the anxiety generated by screening is temporary and minimal, thus helping couples to make the decisions they feel are appropriate for them.

Clearly, screening should not be confined to simply performing tests and reporting risks. Couples need appropriate knowledge of the screening test, together with its limitations, so they can make a truly informed decision on screening. They need to consider their possible action if a screening result suggests that a diagnostic procedure is indicated and if an anomaly is diagnosed. It is important for them to understand that "increased risk" (or "screen positive") does not necessarily mean the pregnancy is affected. Equally, they should understand that "not at increased risk" (or "screen negative") does not provide complete reassurance there is no risk. For those couples who desire to know what the future holds, first-trimester combined screening in centers with the relevant experience in measuring NT as defined by the FMF and suitably qualified laboratory programs offers the best opportunity of either reassurance or the knowledge that the pregnancy is affected by a chromosomal abnormality.

■ **Summary**

1 ■ **What Is the Problem that Requires Screening?**

Fetal aneuploidy.

a. *What is the incidence/prevalence of the target condition?*

The birth prevalence of the major chromosomal abnormalities approaches 6/1,000.

b. *What are the sequelae of the condition that are of interest in clinical medicine?*

The major clinical consequences of trisomy 21 include mental retardation with IQ scores ranging between 20 and 70, congenital heart defects in 50%, gastrointestinal complications in 30%, and visual, ear, nose, and throat problems in 40% to 60%. The frequency of hypothyroidism is significantly increased, as is epilepsy. There is also a threefold increase in the incidence of leukemia. The average life expectancy has improved considerably over the past decade, approaching 50 years. Trisomies 13 and 18 along with triploidy are essentially lethal. Sex chromosome abnormalities have a variable phenotype.

2 ■ **The Tests**

a. *What is the purpose of the tests?*

To identify pregnancies at sufficiently high risk for a fetus with a major chromosome abnormality.

b. *What is the nature of the tests?*

First-trimester ultrasound and maternal biochemistry.

c. *What are the implications of testing?*

1. What does an abnormal test result mean?

An abnormal test means further diagnostic testing should be offered. More than 90% of fetuses with a major chromosome abnormality are included within the approximately 5% of the population labeled screen-positive. Screen-positive women have a likelihood of carrying a child with a major chromosome abnormality that exceeds the risk of a pregnancy loss from invasive testing. Pregnancy termination should be an option for women whose fetus has a major chromosome abnormality.

2. What does a normal test result mean?

If the initial risk is lower than the usual cutoff of 1/300, then approximately 95% of women will be classified as 'low risk' for major aneuploidies. The negative predictive value of the trisomy 21 screening test is 99.98%.

d. *What is the cost of testing?*

The costs per case averted in the United Kingdom is in the order of £44,210 compared with the excess lifetime support costs of a person with trisomy 21 syndrome of £284,024. The individual cost per screen at UK National Health Service prices and conditions is approximately £45.

3 ■ Conclusions and Recommendations

First-trimester screening for fetal aneuploidy provides for efficient screening of the population that is cost-effective in terms of societal expenditures.

References

1. Egan JF, Benn P, Borgida AF, et al. Efficacy of screening for fetal Down syndrome in the United States from 1974 to 1997. *Obstet Gynecol* 2000;96:979–985.
2. Hook EB. Prevalence, risk and recurrence. In: Brock DH, Rodeck CH, Ferguson-Smith MA, eds., *Prenatal Diagnosis and Screening*. Edinburgh: Churchill Livingstone, 1992:351–392.
3. Snijders RJM, Sebire NJ, Nicolaides KH. Maternal age and gestational age specific risks for chromosomal defects. *Fetal Diag Ther* 1995;10:356–357.
4. Nicolaides KH, Sebire NJ, Snijders RJM. *The 11-14 Weeks Scan: the Diagnosis of Fetal Abnormalities*. London: Parthenon Publishing, 1999.
5. Down, J.L. Observations on an ethnic classification of idiots. *Lond Hosp Rep* 1866:3;259–262
6. Shuttleworth GE. Mongoloid imbecility. *Br Med J* 1909:2;661–665.
7. Lejeune J, Gautier M, Turpin R. Etudes des chromosomes somatiques de neuf enfants mongoliens. *C R Acad Sci* 1959:248;1721.
8. Jacobs PA, Baikie AG, Court Brown WM, et al. The somatic chromosomes in mongolism. *Lancet* 1959:1;710.
9. Edwards JH, Harnden DG, Cameron AH, et al. A new trisomic syndrome. *Lancet* 1960:1;787–790.
10. Patau K, Smith DW, Therman E, et al. Multiple congenital anomaly caused by an extra autosome. *Lancet* 1960:1;790–793.

11. Royal College of Obstetricians and Gynaecologists. Recommendations arising from the 32nd Study Group: screening for down syndrome in the first trimester. In: Grudzinskas JG, Ward RHT, eds., *Screening for Down Syndrome in the First Trimester.* London: RCOG Press, 1997:353–356.

12. Spencer K, Souter V, Tul N, et al. A screening program for trisomy 21 at 10-14 weeks using fetal nuchal translucency, maternal serum free β-human chorionic gonadotropin and pregnancy-associated plasma protein-A. *Ultrasound Obstet Gynecol* 1999;13:231–237.

13. Spencer K. Point of care screening for chromosomal anomalies in the first trimester. *Clin Chem* 2002;48:403–404.

14. Spencer K, Spencer CE, Power M, et al. Screening for chromosomal abnormalities in the first trimester using ultrasound and maternal serum biochemistry in a one stop clinic: a review of three years prospective experience. *Br J Obstet Gynaecol* 2003;110:281–286.

15. Spencer K. Screening at the point of care: Down syndrome—a case study. In: Price CP, St John A, Hicks JM, eds., *Point of Care Testing.* Washington: AACC Press, 2004:333–339.

16. Tul N, Spencer K, Noble P, et al. Screening for trisomy 18 by fetal nuchal translucency, maternal serum free β-hCG and PAPP-A at 10-14 weeks of gestation. *Prenat Diagn* 1999;19:1035–1042.

17. Spencer K, Ong C, Skentou H, et al. Screening for trisomy 13 by fetal nuchal translucency thickness and maternal serum free β-hCG and PAPP-A at 10-14 weeks. *Prenat Diagn* 2000;20:411–416.

18. Spencer K, Nicolaides KH. A first trimester trisomy 13/trisomy 18 risk algorithm combining fetal nuchal translucency thickness, maternal serum free β-hCG and PAPP-A. *Prenat Diagn* 2002;22:877–879.

19. Spencer K, Berry E, Crossley JA, et al. Is maternal serum total hCG a marker of trisomy 21 in the first trimester of pregnancy. *Prenat Diagn* 2000;20:311–317.

20. Reynolds T, Penney M. The mathematical basis of multivariate risk analysis: with special reference to screening for Down syndrome associated pregnancy. *Ann Clin Biochem* 1990;27: 452–458.

21. Snijders RJM, Noble P, Sebire N, et al. UK multicentre project on assessment of risk of trisomy 21 by maternal age and fetal nuchal-translucency thickness at 10-14 weeks of gestation. *Lancet* 1999;18:519–521.

22. Pandya PP, Snijders RJM, Johnson SP, et al. Screening for fetal trisomies by maternal age and fetal nuchal translucency thickness at 10-14 weeks of gestation. *Br J Obstet Gynaecol* 1995;102:957–962.

23. Nicolaides KH. Screening for chromosomal defects. *Ultrasound Obstet Gynecol* 2003;21:313–321.

24. National Institute for Clinical Excellence. Antenatal care: routine care for the healthy pregnant woman. Clinical Guidance No. 6, 2003.

25. National Down's Syndrome Screening Programme for England. *Antenatal Screening—Working Standards,* 2004.

26. ACOG Committee Opinion No. 296. First trimester screening for fetal aneuploidy. *Obstet Gynecol* 2004;104:215 –217.

27. Hulten MA, Dhanjal S, Pertl B. Rapid and simple antenatal diagnosis of common chromosome disorders: advantages and disadvantages of the molecular methods of FISH and QF-PCR. *Reproduction* 2003;126:279–297.

28. Bindra R, Heath V, Liao A, et al. One stop clinic for assessment of risk for trisomy 21 at 11-14 weeks: a prospective study of 15,030 pregnancies. *Ultrasound Obstet Gynecol* 2002;20:219–225.

29. Reynolds TM, Nix AB, Dunstan FD, et al. Age-specific detection and false positive rates: an aid to counseling in Down's Syndrome risk screening. *Obstet Gynecol* 1993;81:447–450.

30. Spencer K. Age related detection and false positive rates when screening for Down's Syndrome in the first trimester using fetal nuchal translucency and maternal serum free a-hCG and PAPP-A. *Br J Obstet Gynaecol* 2001;108:1043–1046.

31. Spencer K, Tul N, Nicolaides KH. Maternal serum free β-hCG and PAPP-A in fetal sex chromosome defects in the first trimester. *Prenat Diagn* 2000;20:390–394.

32. Spencer K, Liao AWJ, Skentou H, et al. Screening for triploidy by fetal nuchal translucency and maternal serum free β-hCG and PAPP-A at 10-14 weeks of gestation. *Prenat Diagn* 2000;20:852–853.

33. Spencer K, Nicolaides KH. Screening for trisomy 21 in twins using first trimester ultrasound and maternal serum biochemistry in a one stop clinic: a review of three years experience. *Br J Obstet Gynaecol* 2003;110:276–280.

34. Spencer K. Non-invasive screening tests. In: Blickstein I, Keith L, eds., *Multiple Pregnancy: Epidemiology, Gestation and Perinatal Outcome.* London: Parthenon, 2004.

35. Ghi T, Huggon IC, Zosmer N, et al. Incidence of major structural cardiac defects associated with increased nuchal translucency but normal karyotype. *Ultrasound Obstet Gynecol* 2001;18:610–614.

36. Mavrides E, Cobian-Sanchez F, Tekay A, et al. Limitations of using first trimester nuchal translucency measurement in routine screening for major congenital heart defects. *Ultrasound Obstet Gynecol* 2001;17:106–110.

37. Souka AP, Krampl E, Bakalis S, et al. Outcome of pregnancy in chromosomally normal fetuses with increased nuchal translucency in the first trimester. *Ultrasound Obstet Gynecol* 2001;18:9–17.

38. Ong CYT, Liao AW, Spencer K, et al. First trimester maternal serum a-human chorionic gonadotrophin and pregnancy associated plasma protein A as predictors of pregnancy complications. *Br J Obstet Gynaecol* 2000;107:1265–1270.

39. Smith GCS, Stenhouse EJ, Crossley JA, et al. Early pregnancy levels of pregnancy associated plasma protein A and the risk of intrauterine growth restriction, premature birth, preeclampsia, and stillbirth. *J Clin Endocrinol Metab* 2002;87:1762–1767.

40. Smith GCS, Stenhouse EJ, Crossley JA, et al. Early pregnancy origins of low birth weight. *Nature* 2002;417:916.

41. Yaron Y, Heifetz S, Ochshorn Y, et al. Decreased first trimester PAPP-A is a predictor of adverse outcome. *Prenat Diagn* 2002;22:778–782.

42. Tul N, Pusenjak S, Osredkar J, et al. Predicting complications of pregnancy with first trimester maternal serum free β-hCG, PAPP-A and inhibin-A. *Prenat Diagn* 2003;23:990–996.

43. Spencer K. Second trimester antenatal screening for Down syndrome and the relationship of maternal serum biochemical markers to pregnancy complication with adverse outcome. *Prenat Diagn* 2000;20:652–656.

44. Wald NJ, Kennard A, Hackshaw A, et al. Antenatal screening for Down's syndrome. *Health Technol Assessment* 1998;2:11–112.

45. Ganiats TG. Justifying prenatal screening and genetic amniocentesis programs by cost-effectiveness analyses: a re-evaluation. *Med Decis Making* 1996;16:45–50.

46. Petrou S, Henderson J, Roberts T, et al. Recent economic evaluations of antenatal screening: a systematic review and critique. *J Med Screen* 2000;7:59–73.

47. Vintzileos AM, Ananth CV, Smulian JC, et al. Cost-benefit analysis of prenatal diagnosis for Down syndrome using the British or the American approach. *Obstet Gynecol* 2000;95:577–583.

48. Gilbert RE, Augood C, Gupta R, et al. Screening for Down's syndrome: effects, safety, and cost effectiveness of first and second trimester strategies. *BMJ* 2001;323:423–425.

49. Caughey AB, Kuppermann M, Norton ME, et al. Nuchal translucency and first trimester biochemical markers for down syndrome screening: a cost-effectiveness analysis. *Am J Obstet Gynecol* 2002;187:1239–1245.

50. Christiansen M, Olesen Larsen S. An increase in cost effectiveness of first trimester maternal screening programmes for fetal chromosome anomalies is obtained by contingent testing. *Prenat Diagn* 2002;22:482–486.

51. Cusick W, Buchanan P, Hallahan TW, Krantz DA, Larsen JW, Macri JN. Combined first trimester versus second trimester serum screening for Down syndrome: a cost analysis. *Am J Obstet Gynecol* 2003;188:745–751.

52. Wald NJ, Rodeck C, Hackshaw AK, et al. First and second trimester antenatal screening for Down's syndrome: the results of the Serum, Urine and Ultrasound Screening Study (SURUSS). *Health Technol Assess* 2003;7:11.

53. Shackley P, McGuire A, Boyd PA, et al. An economic appraisal of alternative pre-natal screening programmes fro Down's syndrome. *J Public Health Med* 1993;15:175–184.

54. Gill M, Murday V, Slack J. An economic appraisal of screening for Down's Syndrome in pregnancy using maternal age and serum alpha fetoprotein concentration. *Soc Sci Med* 1987; 24:725–731.
55. Waitzman NJ, Romano PS, Scheffler RM. Estimates of the costs of birth defects. *Inquiry* 1994;33:188–205.
56. Waitzman N, Romano P, Scheffler R, et al. Economic costs of birth defects and cerebral palsy—United States, 1992. *MMWR Recomm Rep* 1995;44:694–699.
57. Beazoglou T, Heffley D, Kyriopoulos J, et al. Economic evaluation of prenatal screening for Down syndrome in the USA. *Prenat Diagn* 1998;18:1241–1252.
58. Cunningham GC, Tompkinson DG. Cost and effectiveness of the California triple maker prenatal screening program. *Genet Med* 1999;1:199–206.
59. Biggio JR, Morris C, Owen J, et al. An outcome analysis of five prenatal screening strategies for trisomy 21 in women younger than 35 years. *Am J Obstet Gynecol* 2004;190:721–729.
60. Henderson J, Bricker L, Roberts T, et al. British National Health Service's and women's costs of antenatal ultrasound screening and follow-up tests. *Ultrasound Obstet Gynaecol* 2002;20:154–162.
61. RCOG. Recommendations arising from the 32nd Study Group: screening for Down syndrome in the first trimester. In: Grudzinskas JG, Ward RHT, eds., *Screening for Down syndrome in the first trimester.* London: RCOG Press, 1997:353–356.
62. Lawson HW, Frye A, Atrash HK, et al. Abortion mortality, United States, 1972–1987. *Am J Obstet Gynecol* 1994;171:1365–1372.
63. Kornman LH, Wortelboer MJM, Beekhuis JR, et al. Women's opinions and the implications of first-versus second trimester screening for fetal Down's syndrome. *Prenat Diagn* 1997;17:1011–1018.
64. Mulvey S, Wallace EM. Women's knowledge of and attitudes to first and second trimester screening for Down's syndrome. *Br J Obstet Gynaecol* 2000;107:1302–1305.
65. Monni G, Ibba RM, Zoppi MA. Antenatal screening for Down's syndrome. *Lancet* 1998;352: 1631–1632.
66. Spencer K, Aitken D. Factors affecting women's preference for type of prenatal screening test for chromosomal anomalies. *Ultrasound Obstet Gynecol* 2004;24:735–739.

Second Trimester Screening for Aneuploidy (Ultrasound and Biochemistry)

Lami Yeo

Anthony M. Vintzileos

■ What Is the Problem that Requires Screening?

Fetal Trisomy 21 (Down Syndrome) and Trisomy 18 (Edwards Syndrome).

Both trisomy 21 and trisomy 18 occur when the fetal cells contain three (vs. two) copies of chromosomes number 21 or 18, respectively. Autosomal trisomies are primarily the result of meiotic nondisjunction, the prevalence of which increases with maternal age. Occasionally, they can result from an unbalanced translocation. Balanced translocations occur when chromatin material is exchanged between chromosomes, but the exchanged material is intact. Although those individuals carrying the balanced translocation are phenotypically normal, they produce unbalanced rearrangements in offspring (with transmission of extra chromatin material from chromosome 21 or 18), leading to trisomy 21 or trisomy 18.

What is the incidence/prevalence of the target condition?

Trisomy 21 is the most common autosomal trisomy among liveborn infants. In the United States, it occurs in approximately 1/504 pregnancies during the second trimester[1] and in 1/800 live births. Trisomy 18 is the second most common autosomal trisomy and occurs in 1/3,000–6,000 births; however, the actual prevalence will vary according to gestational age because fetal demise or stillbirth is common. It is estimated that 50% to 90% of fetuses with trisomy 18 alive at 16 weeks will not be born alive.[2] For both disorders, the prevalence increases with maternal age. For instance, the age-related risk for trisomy 21 at second-trimester amniocentesis is 1:1,176, 1:274, and 1:23 for the 20, 35, and 44-year-old woman, respectively.[3] It follows then, that the prevalence will also depend on the mean age of all pregnant women in a particular population. Over the last three decades, there has been a fundamental shift in birth trends, with more births occurring to women 35 years or older.[1] Therefore, the prevalence of fetal trisomy 21 (during the second trimester) has increased from 1/740 in 1974 to 1/504 in 1997. Like trisomy 18, the prevalence of trisomy 21 in the second trimester is higher than at term because about 23% of trisomy 21 fetuses are lost spontaneously between the second trimester and term.[4]

It should be noted that all pregnancies theoretically are at risk of fetal aneuploidy, not just women of advanced maternal age. Other factors that increase one's risk include a history of fetal aneuploidy, abnormal biochemical screening results, fetal anomalies detected sonographically, and a known balanced, structural rearrangements in one of the parents.

What are the sequelae of the condition that are of interest in clinical medicine?

Trisomy 21 is the single most common genetic cause of mental retardation and is associated with long-term survival. Although people affected with trisomy 21 have characteristic craniofacial features, significant medical problems can also occur. They include hypothyroidism, respiratory infections, seizures, eye disorders (such as myopia and cataracts), Alzheimer disease (premature onset), leukemia, hearing loss, and atlantoaxial instability. Cardiac defects are present in 40% to 50%, and gastrointestinal abnormalities such as duodenal atresia/stenosis or tracheoesophageal fistula are seen in 15% to 30%.

Trisomy 18 fetuses, on the other hand, have a uniformly poor prognosis, being associated with profound neurologic damage and mental deficiency in newborns. Diverse and multiple anatomic abnormalities can occur in almost every organ system. Cardiac malformations occur in about 90% of cases. If liveborn, 50% survive 1 month, fewer than 5% survive a year, and only a few survive to 10 years.

Virtually all trisomy 13 fetuses have malformations. For additional information, see Chapter 14.

There is no corrective treatment. Due to the described sequelae, pregnancy termination should be an option.

■ The Tests

Second-trimester maternal biochemistry and genetic sonography.

What is the purpose of the tests?

To identify those women in the second trimester at high risk of having a fetus with trisomy 21 and trisomy 18, and would thus warrant offering further antenatal testing (genetic sonography or genetic amniocentesis).

What is the nature of the tests?

Both invasive and noninvasive tests have been used. The first method of screening for fetal trisomy 21 began in the early 1970s and was based on maternal age. All women age 35 years or older were offered invasive testing. The age threshold was selected for two reasons: first, only 5% of the pregnant population were older than 35 years in the 1970s (screen-positive rate 5%); and second, it was at age 35 when the risk for midtrimester fetal trisomy 21 was thought to approximate the risk of a pregnancy loss due to amniocentesis (1/200). Presently, screening tests in the second trimester are noninvasive.

Maternal biochemical screening (triple or quadruple). A new method of screening was first developed in the 1980s that incorporated both maternal age and the measurement of one or more maternal biochemical serum markers (e.g., beta human chorionic gonadotropin [β-hCG], α-fetoprotein [AFP], unconjugated estriol) in the second trimester. Recently, there new analytes have been added (dimeric inhibin A) (the so-called quadruple screen).

Maternal age as a screening method currently identifies at best 47% of trisomy 21 cases, with a screen-positive rate that has been increasing in recent years (13% to 14%).[1] Based on maternal age alone, roughly 140 amniocenteses must be performed to detect one trisomy 21 fetus,[5] implying that one normal fetus may be lost for every two trisomy 21 fetuses identified.

Maternal biochemical serum screening for fetal trisomy 21 in low-risk (younger than 35 years old) stemmed from the observation in the mid-1980s that the mean level of maternal serum AFP in trisomy 21 pregnancies was 0.7 multiple of the median (MoM).[6] Later, it was realized that the maternal serum hCG levels were higher (2.04 MoM) and the unconjugated estriol levels lower (0.79 MoM) in trisomy 21 pregnancies.[7] By using the relative risks derived from maternal serum levels of these three analytes, the maternal age–related risk can be adjusted and a triple screen risk for fetal trisomy 21 then calculated for each individual patient.

In the low-risk population, the triple screen identifies approximately 60% of all trisomy 21 pregnancies as being at increased with a 5% screen-positive rate. However, this approach used in isolation still requires approximately 60 to 70 amniocenteses to detect one fetus with trisomy 21.[5] As a result, one normal fetus may be lost as a complication from amniocentesis for every three to four trisomy 21 fetuses detected. Accordingly, the process of routinely offering amniocentesis to all women has been challenged by some. In women older than 35 years, the triple screen will detect 75% or more of all trisomy 21 cases, plus some other types of aneuploidy.[8] Because the maternal age–related risk of trisomy 21 is the basis of the serum screening protocol, both the trisomy 21 detection rate and the screen-positive rate increase with maternal age. Depending on the laboratory used, varying screen-positive cutoffs may be used. The most commonly used cutoff is equivalent to the risk of a 35-year-old woman having a trisomy 21 fetus (1/250–300) in the second trimester. Recently, the most promising new analyte that has emerged, dimeric inhibin A, and was combined with the three traditional analytes. The resulting quadruple screen detects 67% to 76% of fetal trisomy 21 in low-risk women, with a screen-positive rate of 5% or less.[9]

Serum screening is most accurate (and sensitive) when performed between 16 and 18 weeks' gestation, although it can be done anytime between 15 and 20 weeks' gestation. Accurate dating of the pregnancy is essential as errant dates will affect the calculated triple/quadruple screen risk and generate both false-positive and false-negative results. The triple screen will also detect about 60% to 75% of fetuses with trisomy 18 when a separate analysis is performed that seeks low levels of all 3 analytes with or without consideration of maternal age.[10]

Genetic sonography. Genetic sonography is a targeted sonographic examination in the second trimester for fetal aneuploidy (most specifically for trisomy 21) that searches for the presence of fetal structural anomalies, abnormal fetal biometry and other sonographically detectable markers of aneuploidy.[11] There has been a wealth of information published regarding the specific use of genetic sonography for detecting fetal trisomy 21 antenatally. Many women will use the information derived from this sonogram to obtain a new adjusted trisomy 21 risk to help guide their decision about amniocentesis, instead of choosing invasive testing automatically as a first option. In essence, it optimizes the selection of candidates for invasive testing in order to diminish procedure-related losses of normal fetuses, without significantly decreasing detection rates. The authors believe it should be offered only to high-risk women (advanced maternal age, abnormal serum screening, or both).

Because only 25% of second-trimester fetuses with trisomy 21 have sonographically detectable major anomalies,[5] the search must involve other markers to increase sensitivity. This practice assumes that the risk derived from biochemical markers is independent of the risk derived from sonographic markers. This assumption remains to be tested.

A number of second-trimester sonographic markers for aneuploidy have been identified including short long bones, pyelectasis, increased nuchal fold thickness, choroid plexus cysts, short ear length, hyperechoic bowel, echogenic intracardiac focus, sandal gap, hypoplastic mid-phalanx of fifth digit, clinodactyly, and more recently, absent nasal bone. Each by itself, however, has a low to moderate sensitivity for trisomy 21. In addition, many of these antenatal sonographic findings may not necessarily increase the aneuploidy risk when seen in isolation in low-risk women and in fact are commonly seen in the euploid fetus. However, when seen with multiple other sonographic anomalies or markers, or in high-risk women, the risk of aneuploidy increases.

Thickening of the nuchal fold in second trimester appears to be the single most sensitive and specific marker for fetal trisomy 21 (sensitivity 40% and false-positive rate of 0.1%),[12] although absent nasal bone has also recently been shown to have a 41% sensitivity and 100% specificity for fetal trisomy 21.[13] Short femur length (measured to expected length < 0.91) may occur in 24% of trisomy 21 fetuses,[14] whereas a short humerus (measured to expected length < 0.90) identifies 50% of trisomy 21 fetuses, with a false-positive rate of 6.25%.[15] Unfortunately, there tends to be a large overlap in bone measurements between normal and affected fetuses. Isolated echogenic bowel has a reported sensitivity of 7% to 12.5%, whereas an isolated echogenic intracardiac focus has a sensitivity of 18%.[15] The sensitivity of pyelectasis (anteroposterior diameter renal pelvis more than 4 mm in second trimester) for trisomy 21 is 25%.[15] We recently examined the sensitivity for fetal trisomy 21 by sonographic ear length.[16] Of 51 trisomy 21 fetuses, 41% had an ear length below the tenth percentile. Although an association between choroid plexus cysts and trisomy 18 is established, there is no association with fetal trisomy 21 when isolated.

In 1996, we described the use of second-trimester genetic sonography to guide the clinical management of women at high-risk of fetal trisomy 21.[17] Subsequently, we analyzed our data in 1999 and counseled women that in the presence of a normal genetic sonogram, the likelihood of fetal trisomy 21 was reduced by at least 80% from the a priori risk (triple screen, or if unavailable, maternal age).[18] In our unit, we target many specific aneuploidy markers when performing genetic sonography (Table 22–1). In conjunction with maternal age or biochemical serum screening, we use the results of genetic sonography to adjust the risk of fetal trisomy 21 for each high-risk patient, based on our accuracy. An adjusted risk is considered abnormal if it is greater than 1:270. The risk of fetal trisomy 21 rises with the number of markers present. The a-priori risk is based on first, serum screening or on maternal age if serum screening was not performed. For example, assuming independence, if the a-priori risk of fetal trisomy 21 is 1:274 and the genetic scan is normal, the new adjusted risk of fetal trisomy 21 will be 1:274 times 0.20 (1:1370) (at least 80% reduction) and this new risk is discussed with the patient. However, women are always counseled that genetic sonography can never reduce their risk of having a trisomy 21 fetus down to 0%. We follow the practice guidelines shown in Figure 22–1.

Table 22-1	**Genetic sonography aneuploidy markers (Robert Wood Johnson Medical School)**
Aneuploidy markers	
Structural anomalies including cardiac (four chamber and outflow tracts)	
Short femur (observed/expected <10%)	
Short humerus (observed/expected <10%)	
Pyelectasis (anteroposterior diameter of renal pelvis ≥4 mm)	
Nuchal fold thickening (≥6 mm)	
Echogenic bowel (similar echogenicity to iliac bones)	
Choroid plexus cysts (>10 mm)	
Hypoplastic middle phalanx of the fifth digit	
Wide space between first and second toes (sandal gap)	
Two vessel umbilical cord	
Echogenic intracardiac focus, short tibia, short fibula, short ear (since October 1997)	
Absent nasal bone (since 2003)	

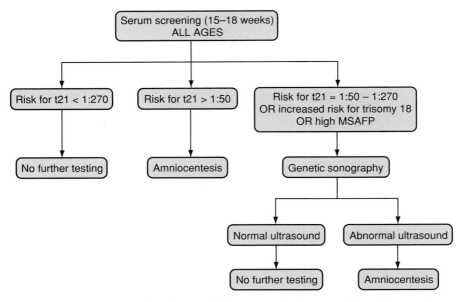

Figure 22-1 Proposed cost-effective use of ultrasonography for prenatal genetic screening trisomy 21. *MSAFP*, maternal serum α–fetoprotein.

Although intuitively it might seem that detecting certain markers (such as cardiac defects, thickened nuchal fold) in isolation are very "strong" and would increase the risk of trisomy 21, in our experience we have most frequently found these markers in combination with other markers. Currently, we accept either a triple or quadruple screen risk for the a priori risk because most of our data were generated from high-risk women who have had these serum tests performed. Recent data indicate that combining second-trimester genetic sonography with traditional serum markers may significantly improve the diagnostic accuracy of trisomy 21 fetuses.[19]

By combining multiple aneuploidy markers, the sensitivity for trisomy 21 may be increased to more than 80%, with false-positive rates of 10% to 15% (by defining as abnormal any sonographic exam with at least one abnormal marker present). Many published studies have examined the efficacy of genetic sonography to detect trisomy 21 in high-risk populations. The overall sensitivity is 77% (50%–93%) and the false-positive rate is 13% (7%–17%) when defining the sonogram as abnormal with at least one abnormal marker.[11] In 1998, a large collaborative study from 11 centers (including our own) examined the sensitivity of sonography in detecting fetal trisomy 21.[20] The study concluded that 85% of trisomy 21 fetuses had at least one abnormal finding on ultrasound. In 2003, an eight-center study (including our own) evaluated the utility of second-trimester genetic sonography among high-risk pregnancies, including 176 trisomy 21 fetuses.[21] The sensitivity for trisomy 21 was 72%, with a range of 64% to 80% at the various sites. Importantly, about half (47%) of trisomy 21 fetuses had a thickened nuchal fold of 5 mm or more, making this marker the one with the highest sensitivity. Many researchers have concluded that the risk adjustment for trisomy 21 is institution-specific and that the data from one may not apply to other centers. In addition, some believe that the use of genetic sonography should be limited only to specialized centers.[8]

Although genetic sonography has been recommended to screen the general population, we believe it should be applied only to high-risk women. First, applying genetic sonography to low-risk women may be precarious due to the low positive predictive value in this population. In low-risk women, the a-priori risk of fetal trisomy 21 may be so decreased that finding only one aneuploidy marker does not usually raise the risk enough to justify invasive testing. Accordingly, it is expected that the positive predictive value (and perhaps even the sensitivity) of genetic sonography for fetal trisomy 21 may be decreased in the low-risk patient. Second, significant expertise is required to rule out fetal abnormalities (especially subtle cardiac defects) and this is not widely available. Third, the accuracy of aneuploidy markers in the second trimester has been studied mainly in high-risk populations, and extrapolating this to the low-risk patient is inappropriate. In low-risk women, isolated markers (with the exception of thickened nuchal fold or organ structural abnormalities) should not be used as an indication for invasive testing. It is essential to remember that because the sensitivity of an isolated marker (with the possible exception of thickened nuchal fold) is so low, clinicians should not recommend amniocentesis in low-risk women.[22] The incidental findings of an organ/structural abnormality (with a few exceptions, such as gastroschisis) or two or more aneuploidy markers in a low-risk patient should trigger counseling and amniocentesis after informed consent. The patient should be informed that if one extrapolates the genetic ultrasound accuracy from high-risk to low-risk women, then the risk of trisomy 21 is most likely high enough to justify offering genetic amniocentesis. In such women, we have found that the risk for trisomy 21 is higher than the risk of amniocentesis-related fetal loss, regardless of maternal age or serum screening results (unless the a priori risk is less than 1:10,000).

As for fetal trisomy 18, the published results of antenatal sonography have been variable, but with high sensitivity (64%–100%) particularly when part of a complete, anatomic survey.[23] We have found that by performing a thorough survey, all trisomy 18 fetuses had four or more sonographic abnormalities; in fact, one patient had 19 individual fetal abnormalities. Almost every organ system can be affected, and intrauterine growth restriction is common. The most sensitive markers for trisomy 18 were short ear length (96%), bilateral clenched or closed hands or overlapping digits (95%), and central nervous system anomalies (87%). In addition, 92% of the trisomy 18 fetuses had at least two of four minor sonographic abnormalities (upper extremities/hands, lower extremities/feet, face, ear). Other investigators have also reported abnormal hands to be the most common fetal sonographic abnormality in trisomy 18.[24]

Choroid plexus cysts (CPCs) are common in normal fetuses (0.3%–3.6%). However, they are also associated with trisomy 18. Thus, amniocentesis has been considered and offered in the past even if they are isolated. In our study, although half of the trisomy 18 fetuses had CPC, they were never isolated and were always associated with multiple other sonographic abnormalities.[23] In another study of 98 fetuses with isolated CPC, none had aneuploidy, while 100% of the 13 fetuses with CPC and major anatomic abnormalities had trisomy 18.[25] However, it is imperative to ensure that the cysts are truly isolated by performing a detailed fetal survey. In our experience, the risk of aneuploidy is very low and does not justify invasive testing if no other abnormalities are found (especially when ear length is normal and hands are open). Others agree that the detection of isolated CPCs should not alter obstetric management after a high-quality ultrasound, assuming the patient is otherwise considered at low risk for fetal aneuploidy.[26] Therefore, much like genetic sonography in screening for fetal trisomy 21, normal findings from a complete sonographic survey in experienced hands should "decrease" a patient's risk of trisomy 18 (regardless of the presence/absence of CPC or abnormal serum screening results) to an extremely low level sufficient to avoid amniocentesis after appropriate patient counseling.[23]

What are the implications of testing?

What does an abnormal test result mean? Provided that the dating used for the serum screening calculation is correct, the woman is at increased risk of carrying a fetus with trisomy 21 or trisomy 18. Genetic counseling with genetic sonography should be offered. If the ultrasound adjusted risk of fetal trisomy 21 from genetic sonography is abnormal (>1/250–1/300), or a fetal anatomy survey has structural abnormalities, the patient is counseled that there is an increased risk of fetal aneuploidy, such as trisomy 21 or trisomy 18 and invasive testing offered. This may be either amniocentesis or cordocentesis depending upon the urgency of the diagnosis.

Over a 10-year period, we have evaluated 5,299 fetuses with genetic sonography in our unit. The overall sensitivity for trisomy 21 and trisomy 18 with an abnormal genetic sonogram (presence of one or more abnormal sonographic markers) was 87% and 100%, respectively. The specificity and positive and negative predictive values of genetic sonography to detect fetal trisomy 21 was 91%, 11%, and 99.8%, respectively. Although the overwhelming majority (85%) had normal sonograms with no abnormal markers seen, 12% had one abnormal marker present, and 3% had two or more abnormal markers present. About two thirds of trisomy 21 fetuses had two or more abnormal sonographic markers seen. We have found that the amniocentesis rate increases in direct proportion to the number of abnormal sonographic markers identified, with almost 100% of women choosing invasive testing when four or more markers are seen.

What does a normal test result mean? Women who have a low trisomy 21 risk below the cutoff (typically 1:270) whether based on serum screening alone or the new adjusted risk for trisomy 21 based on genetic sonography are not offered further testing. However, it is absolutely vital that both the physician and patient clearly understand that these are only screening tests (not diagnostic), and that a negative screening test does not imply the fetus is unaffected with trisomy 21, but only unlikely to be. Triple screen testing has a sensitivity of 60% for fetal trisomy 21; this implies that 40% of women with a trisomy 21 fetus will have "negative" results. The only definitive way to know that a fetus is, or is not affected with aneuploidy is to undergo karyotype testing. Only 3% have chosen amniocentesis in our unit over a 10-year period when their genetic ultrasound is normal. A total of 4,951 women have avoided amniocentesis; if the fetal loss rate directly related to amniocentesis is estimated to be between 1/100 and 1/300, then this amounts to between 17 and 50 fetal lives saved.

What is the cost of testing?

The total cost of second-trimester serum screening is approximately $80.[27] Although universal amniocentesis ideally will detect all trisomy 21 fetuses, this process will not be acceptable to all women and is not what occurs in daily practice. We recently analyzed the costs for universal amniocentesis and genetic sonography in high-risk women, and found that genetic sonography was cost-effective if the sensitivity for detecting trisomy 21 was 75% and higher.[28] Based on data derived from a nationwide medical cost-profiling company, genetic sonography costs about $300, whereas an amniocentesis package (genetic counseling, sonographic guidance during procedure, amniocentesis, karyotype, and AFP testing of the amniotic fluid) costs $1,200. We also found that genetic sonography had the following benefits (when compared with universal amniocentesis): Total cost to identify a fetus with trisomy 21 was $51,000 (compared with $120,000), a savings of $38 million (9%) and a decrease in the loss of normal fetuses of 87% (1,116 fetuses) as the result of avoiding amniocentesis.[28]

In a recent cost analysis of trisomy 21 screening in women with advanced maternal age, the authors found that screening by age alone would result in the 100% detection of trisomy 21 cases in this cohort, but would require over 530,000 amniocenteses and result in 2,653 procedure-related losses.[29] On the other hand, combining age with serum screen and genetic sonography would detect 97.6% of trisomy 21 cases in the advanced age cohort, but would require only 119,791 amniocenteses and result in 599 procedure-related losses. The projected cost per trisomy 21 case detected (using age screening) was $219,109 versus $155,992 (using serum screening and genetic sonography). Therefore, the combination of advanced maternal age, serum screen, and genetic sonography would result in the fewest procedure-related losses, and lowest cost per trisomy 21 case detected.

Others have also found genetic sonography to be cost-effective in women younger than 35 years old who are at moderate risk of trisomy 21 (1:191 to 1:1,000) based on triple screen results, as well as in advanced maternal age women, who declined amniocentesis after second-trimester genetic counseling.[30] Offering genetic ultrasounds to these women is associated with cost-savings for most acceptable genetic sonography accuracies.

Recently, we performed an economic evaluation of various antenatal diagnostic strategies for women at increased risk of fetal trisomy 18 (either fetal CPCs discovered on ultrasound or an abnormal triple screen).[31] Universal amniocentesis of all at-risk women was compared with universal targeted genetic sonography of all at-risk women (with amniocentesis reserved only for those with abnormal sonography results). The first strategy generated an annual cost of $12 million and 40 fetal losses as a result of amniocenteses; however, the second strategy of targeted genetic sonography generated costs of only $5 million and eight fetal losses, respectively. Therefore, routine second-trimester amniocentesis in those women at increased risk of fetal trisomy 18 was not justified from the cost-benefit point of view.

Figure 22–2 illustrates a proposed cost-effective use of ultrasonography for prenatal genetic screening.

■ Conclusions and Recommendations

Fetal Down syndrome and trisomy 18 have significant implications for the pregnant woman, her family, and society at large. As a result, there is a need to identify these aneuploidies antenatally. Although invasive forms of testing provide almost 100% diagnostic accuracy for aneuploidy, there may be considerable, inherent risks to the procedures such as pregnancy loss. Accordingly, many women choose screening tests in the second trimester, and then based on the results, determine whether further invasive, diagnostic testing is necessary. In the second trimester, currently accepted methods of screening for aneuploidy involve the performance of ultrasonography and/or biochemical testing, as they clearly provide higher sensitivities than maternal age alone. In point, maternal age should be used for screening only as a last resort. For serum screening to be effective, pregnancy dating must be accurate and awareness of sonographic markers and abnormalities for the detection of these syndromes is essential. A complete, targeted, and thorough exam should be offered and performed in all women to increase sensitivity. Genetic sonography, in conjunction with maternal age or serum screening, adjusts the risk of fetal trisomy 21 for each individual patient, and presently should be offered to high-risk women only. Performing a detailed and complete prenatal ultrasound has high sensitivity for detecting fetal trisomy 18. In addition, the detection of isolated CPCs after a high-quality

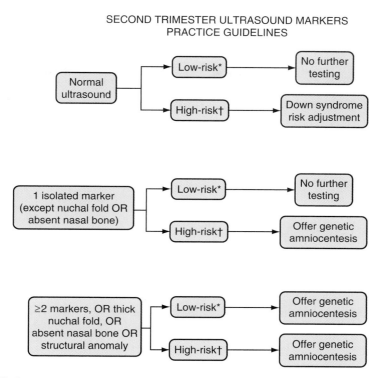

Figure 22–2 Algorithm for clinical management based on results of second-trimester ultrasound (presence or absence of ultrasound markers). *Maternal age, less than 35 years and/or serum screen less than 1:274; †Maternal age older than 35 and/or serum screen ≥ 1:274.

ultrasound should not alter obstetric management assuming the patient is otherwise considered at low risk of fetal aneuploidy. Both physician and patient must understand that negative screening tests do not imply the fetus is unaffected with trisomy 21 or trisomy 18, as there can be false-negative results.

Genetic sonography is cost-effective compared to maternal age screening if the sensitivity for detecting trisomy 21 is more than 75% in women younger than 35 years who are at moderate risk for trisomy 21 (based on triple screen results) and in advanced maternal age women who decline amniocentesis after second-trimester genetic counseling. In addition, routine second-trimester amniocentesis in those women at increased risk of fetal trisomy 18 (CPCs discovered on ultrasound or an abnormal triple screen) is not justified from the cost-benefit point of view.

■ **Summary**

1 ■ What Is the Problem that Requires Screening?

Fetal trisomy 21 (Down syndrome) and trisomy 18 (Edwards syndrome).

a. What is the incidence/prevalence of the target condition?

Trisomy 21 occurs in 1/504 pregnancies during the second trimester and in 1/800 livebirths in the United States. Trisomy 18 occurs in 1/3,000–6,000 births. The prevalence for both disorders increases with maternal age.

b. What are the sequelae of the condition that are of interest in clinical medicine?

Trisomy 21 is associated with mental retardation and significant medical problems. Trisomy 18 fetuses have a uniformly poor prognosis with multiple abnormalities in organ systems.

2 ■ The Tests

Age, maternal biochemical screening, genetic sonography.

a. What is the purpose of the tests?

To identify pregnancies at high-risk of fetal trisomy 21 or trisomy 18.

b. What is the nature of the tests?

Biochemical screening involves either three or four analytes, which gives a risk of fetal trisomy 21 and trisomy 18. Second-trimester genetic sonography for fetal aneuploidy (most specifically trisomy 21) searches for markers/abnormalities and gives an adjusted risk of trisomy 21. It is only offered and performed in high-risk women. A complete targeted sonographic survey can identify abnormalities in virtually all cases of fetal trisomy 18.

c. What are the implications of testing?

1. What does an abnormal test result mean?

The patient is at increased risk of carrying a fetus with trisomy 21 or trisomy 18, and genetic counseling with genetic sonography or direct fetal karyotyping should be offered.

2. What does a normal test result mean?

Those who have a low trisomy 21 or trisomy 18 risks, that is below the cutoff, are offered no further testing. However, both the patient and clinician must understand these are only screening tests (not diagnostic), and a negative screening test does not imply the fetus is unaffected with aneuploidy.

d. What is the cost of testing?

The costs for serum screening, genetic sonography, and amniocentesis package are $80, $300, and $1,200, respectively. Genetic sonography can be cost-effective if certain criteria are met, and it has certain benefits when compared with universal amniocentesis. Routine amniocentesis in women at increased risk of fetal trisomy 18 is not justified from a cost-benefit point of view.

3 ■ Conclusions and Recommendations

Prenatal screening tests for aneuploidy can involve biochemical testing and/or ultrasonography. To be effective, certain criteria should be met. Genetic sonography adjusts the risk of fetal trisomy 21 for each individual patient and should be offered to high-risk women only. Performing a detailed and complete prenatal scan has high sensitivity for detecting fetal trisomy 18. Negative screening tests, however, do not imply the fetus is unaffected with aneuploidy. Genetic sonography can be cost-effective if certain criteria are met, and it has certain benefits when compared with universal amniocentesis. Routine amniocentesis in women at increased risk of fetal trisomy 18 is not justified from a cost-benefit point of view.

References

1. Egan JF, Benn P, Borgida AF, et al. Efficacy of screening for fetal Down syndrome in the United States from 1974 to 1997. *Obstet Gynecol* 2000;96:979–985.
2. Hook EB, Woodbury DF, Albright SG. Rates of trisomy 18 in livebirths, stillbirths, and at amniocentesis. *Birth Defects* 1979;XV:81–93.

3. Snijders RJ, Sundberg K, Holzgreve W, et al. Maternal age- and gestation-specific risk for trisomy 21. *Ultrasound Obstet Gynecol* 1999;13:167–170.
4. Cuckle HS, Wald NJ. Screening for Down's syndrome. In: Lilford RJ, ed., *Prenatal Diagnosis and Prognosis*. London: Butterworth, 1990:67–92.
5. Vintzileos AM, Egan JF. Adjusting the risk for trisomy 21 on the basis of second trimester ultrasonography. *Am J Obstet Gynecol* 1995;172:837-844.
6. Cuckle HS, Wald NJ, Lindenbaum RH. Maternal serum alpha-fetoprotein measurement: a screening test for Down syndrome. *Lancet* 1984;1:926–929.
7. Haddow JE, Palomaki GE, Knight GJ, et al. Prenatal screening for Down's syndrome with use of maternal serum markers. *N Engl J Med* 1992;327:588–593.
8. American College of Obstetricians and Gynecologists. Prenatal diagnosis of fetal chromosomal abnormalities: 2003 Compendium of Selected Publications, 2003:547–557.
9. Wald NJ, Densem JW, George L, et al. Prenatal screening for Down's syndrome using inhibin-A as a serum marker. *Prenat Diagn* 1996;16:143–153.
10. Palomaki GE, Haddow JE, Knight GJ, et al. Risk-based prenatal screening for trisomy 18 using alpha-fetoprotein, unconjugated oestriol and human chorionic gonadotropin. *Prenat Diagn* 1995;15:713–723.
11. Yeo L, Vintzileos AM. The use of genetic sonography to reduce the need for amniocentesis in women at high-risk for Down syndrome. *Semin Perinatol* 2003;27:152–159.
12. Benacerraf BR, Barss BA, Laboda LA. A sonographic sign for the detection in the second trimester of the fetus with Down's syndrome. *Am J Obstet Gynecol* 1985;151:1078–1079.
13. Vintzileos A, Walters C, Yeo L. Absent nasal bone in the prenatal detection of fetuses with trisomy 21 in a high-risk population. *Obstet Gynecol* 2003;101:905–908.
14. Nyberg DA, Resta RG, Hickok DE, et al. Femur length shortening in the detection of Down syndrome: is prenatal screening feasible? *Am J Obstet Gynecol* 1990;162:1247–1252.
15. Bromley B, Benacerraf BR. The genetic sonogram scoring index. *Semin Perinatol* 2003;27:124–129.
16. Yeo L, Guzman ER, Ananth CV, et al. Prenatal detection of fetal aneuploidy by sonographic ear length. *J Ultrasound Med* 2003;22:565–576.
17. Vintzileos AM, Campbell WA, Rodis JF, et al. The use of second-trimester genetic sonogram in guiding clinical management of women at increased risk for fetal trisomy 21. *Obstet Gynecol* 1996;87:948–952.
18. Vintzileos AM, Guzman ER, Smulian JC, et al. Indication-specific accuracy of second-trimester genetic ultrasonography for the detection of trisomy 21. *Am J Obstet Gynecol* 1999;181:1045–1048.
19. Bahado-Singh R, Cheng CC, Matta P, et al. Combined serum and ultrasound screening for detection of fetal aneuploidy. *Semin Perinatol* 2003;27:145–151.
20. Persutte WH, Hobbins JC, Nyberg DA, et al. Trisomy 21 multicenter collaborative project [abstr]. *Am J Obstet Gynecol* 1998;178:S22.
21. Hobbins JC, Lezotte DC, Persutte WH, et al. An eight center study to evaluate the utility of midterm genetic ultrasounds among high-risk pregnancies. *J Ultrasound Med* 2002;22:33–38.
22. Hobbins JC, Bahado-Singh RO, Lezotte DC. The genetic sonogram in screening for Down syndrome; response to the JAMA study. *J Ultrasound Med* 2001;20:269–272.
23. Yeo L, Guzman ER, Day-Salvatore D, et al. Prenatal detection of fetal trisomy 18 through abnormal sonographic features. *J Ultrasound Med* 2003;22:581–590.
24. Benacerraf BR, Miller WA, Frigoletto FD. Sonographic detection of fetuses with trisomies 13 and 18: accuracy and limitations. *Am J Obstet Gynecol* 1988;158:404–409.
25. Yeo L, Guzman ER, Vintzileos AM, et al. Isolated vs. non-isolated choroid plexus cysts: their relationship to aneuploidy and other congenital anomalies [abstr]. *Am J Obstet Gynecol* 1999;180:S58.
26. Nyberg DA, Souter VL. Chromosomal abnormalities. In: Nyberg DA, McGahan JP, Pretorius DH, Pilu G, eds., *Diagnostic Imaging of Fetal Anomalies*. Philadelphia: Lippincott Williams and Wilkins, 2003:881.
27. Cusick W, Vintzileos AM. Fetal Down syndrome screening: a cost effectiveness analysis of alternative screening programs. *J Matern Fetal Med* 1990;8:243–248.

28. Vintzileos AM, Ananth CV, Fisher AJ, et al. An economic evaluation of second-trimester genetic ultrasonography for prenatal detection of Down syndrome. *Am J Obstet Gynecol* 1998;179:1214–1219.
29. Hartnett J, Borgida AF, Benn PA, et al. Cost analysis of Down syndrome screening in advanced maternal age. *J Matern Fetal Neonatal Med* 2003;13:80–84.
30. Devore GR. Is genetic ultrasound cost-effective? *Semin Perinatol* 2003;27:173–182.
31. Vintzileos AM, Ananth CV, Fisher AJ, et al. An economic evaluation of prenatal strategies for detection of trisomy 18. *Am J Obstet Gynecol* 1998;179:1220–1224.

23

Biochemical Screening for Fetal Abnormalities

George J. Knight

Glenn E. Palomaki

James E. Haddow

■ What Is the Problem that Requires Screening?

Fetal neural tube defects, abdominal wall defects.

Neural tube defects are central nervous system malformations resulting from failure of the neural tube to close anywhere along the neural axis between the third and fourth weeks of gestation. Anencephaly occurs when closure is incomplete at the cephalic end of the neural tube. Spina bifida occurs when closure is incomplete more caudally. These two malformations together account for nearly all neural tube defects and occur in approximately equal proportions. Encephalocele, a much less common lesion, is created when neural tube closure fails to occur in the posterior region of the skull.

A neural tube defect is characterized as being closed when it is covered by skin or a thick membrane. An open neural tube defect is either uncovered or covered by only a thin, permeable membrane. Virtually all cases of anencephaly, and approximately 80% of spina bifida cases are open. Encephaloceles are nearly always closed. The pathophysiologic basis of the screening test is leakage of AFP from an open lesion into the amniotic fluid and then into the maternal circulation. The α-fetoprotein (AFP) screening test, therefore, cannot detect closed lesions.

There are two main types of abdominal wall defects. Gastroschisis is a paraumbilical defect usually on the right side of the anterior abdominal wall lateral to the umbilical vessels. Left-sided defects are rare. Omphalocele is an extraembryonic hernia due to the arrest of ventral medial migration of the dermatomyotomes. It is associated with other malformations more than 60% of the time.

What is the incidence/prevalence of the target condition?

In the 1970s the birth prevalence of neural tube defects approximated 2/1,000 in the northeastern United States and 1/1,000 in California.[1] The rate of occurrence of these malformations fell in the United States during the 1970s, prior to widespread introduction of antenatal screening and diagnosis.[2] The discovery that folic acid supplements can reduce neural tube defects further confounds estimates of the current rate of neural tube defects.[3] The March of Dimes and other organizations actively promote preconceptional folic acid supplements, and the US Food and Drug Administration has authorized fortification of cereal grains. It is estimated these activities have reduced the prevalence of neural tube defects by 20% in the United States,[4] and further estimated that 75% of these defects could be eliminated if the folic acid intake were optimal.[5] The prevalence of neural tube defects in the absence of antenatal screening and pregnancy termination is therefore poorly defined. As a direct result, the use of patient risk demographics to identify women at high risk of fetal neural tube defects, as is the norm for trisomy 21 screening, is questionable.

Neural tube defects generally follow a multifactorial inheritance pattern. Both genetic and environmental factors have an etiologic role, and the risk of recurrence in future pregnancies rises with each affected pregnancy. Rates are higher in the East than in the West, and black women have two- to threefold lower rates than white women.[6] A woman who has delivered one child with a neural tube defect is ten times more likely than a woman in the general population to have a second affected pregnancy. If that same woman delivers a second affected child, her risk with each subsequent pregnancy rises to 20 times that of a woman in the general population.[7]

The annual prevalence of gastroschisis approximates 1/2,500–3,000 live births with an equal sex ratio. There appears to be an increasing annual prevalence of gastroschisis not entirely explained by increased recognition of the problem. Population-based studies suggest an association with nonsteroidal anti-inflammatory drug use in the first trimester. Omphalocele has an annual prevalence of 1/2,500 to 1/5,000 pregnancies.

What are the sequelae of the condition that are of interest in clinical medicine?

Anencephaly is incompatible with life. Vital functions may continue for hours or days after birth, but viability beyond that time is rare. Nearly all cases of anencephaly are now detected during the second trimester via either ultrasound or biochemical screening. Pregnancy termination is usually chosen.

Spina bifida is variable in severity, but, as a rule, open defects have a worse prognosis than closed ones. With aggressive medical and surgical management, approximately 70% of individuals survive the first 5 years of life. One study reported that at the end of 5 years, survivors had spent an average of more than 6 months in hospital and undergone six major surgical procedures.[8] The most common problems are hydrocephaly (associated with Arnold-Chiari malformation), paralysis of the lower limbs (the level of paralysis is defined by the location of the lesion), and problems with bowel and bladder function. Open spina bifida is now regularly detected antenatally during the second trimester. Some choose pregnancy termination; others choose to continue the pregnancy and prepare for managing the medical and surgical problems after birth of the affected baby.

An alternative for selected women with an affected fetus may be *in utero* repair of open spina bifida or myelomeningocele.[9] The US National Institute of Child Health and Human Development is conducting a study (Management of Myelomeningocele Study) to determine whether in utero surgical correction of spina bifida is safer and more effective than traditional surgery performed a few days after birth. Information on the status and findings of this study is available at www.spinabifidamoms.com. Preliminary reports suggest a decrease in the need for ventriculoperitoneal shunting without improvement in motor function.

■ The Tests

The measurement of α-fetoprotein in the maternal serum.

What is the purpose of the tests?

To identify women at increased risk of having a fetus with an open neural tube defect.

What is the nature of the tests?

The concentration of AFP is measured in a maternal blood sample drawn between 15 weeks and 20 weeks of gestation. The optimum screening window for detecting open spina bifida is 16 to 18 weeks' gestation. Prior to 15 weeks, the detection rate is reduced.[10,11] If screening is performed at 21 weeks' gestation or later, diagnostic options are limited and termination after diagnosis may no longer be available.

The woman's AFP value is expressed as a multiple of the laboratory's median AFP values (MoM) at her gestational age. Among other benefits, the conversion of test results to MoM takes into account the 15% per week increase in average AFP values at this time in pregnancy. The MoM is adjusted by the laboratory for the variables that affect AFP levels (see next page).

Women with MoM values above a specified cutoff level are considered screen positive and are referred for counseling and diagnostic procedures. Most screening programs use a cutoff of 2.0 or 2.5 MoM, with the latter being more common. Selecting a MoM cutoff is a compromise between maximizing the detection of neural tube defects and minimizing the number of women requiring follow-up diagnostic procedures. At a 2.5-MoM cutoff, approximately 70% of open spina bifida and 90% of anencephalic pregnancies can be detected, with 2% of women having a screen-positive test. At a lower cutoff of 2.0 MoM, the detection rate is increased to 85% and 95%, respectively, but the proportion of women with a screen-positive test increases to approximately 4%.

The laboratory will request certain demographic and clinical information on the laboratory requisition slip that is needed to interpret the AFP test result. This data include the following:

Gestational age: The single most important factor affecting the interpretation of AFP values is the estimation of gestational age. An estimation of gestational age by physical examination is the least reliable dating method and will decrease screening performance. Use of the first day of the last menstrual period (LMP) is acceptable but not optimal for the purpose of antenatal screening. Ultrasound dating by measurement of fetal crown rump length in the first trimester or by biparietal diameter in the second trimester is preferred over LMP dating because it increases the detection rate for open neural tube defects and reduces the screen-positive rate. Optimal screening performance is achieved when the pregnancy is dated using *only* the biparietal diameter measurement. This measurement is smaller than expected in fetuses with open spina bifida (leading to an underestimation of the gestational age), resulting in an artifactual increase in the calculated AFP MoM value, thereby increasing the detection rate.[12]

Maternal weight: On average, heavier women have lower and lighter women higher AFP values. This effect is attributed to the larger blood volume of heavier women, which dilutes the AFP entering the maternal serum, whereas the smaller blood volume of lighter weight women concentrates the AFP. Routine adjustment of the AFP MoM value for maternal weight will increase the detection rate for open neural tube defects and lower the proportion of women with a screen-positive test result.[13] Recent studies also show that heavier weight women have a two- to threefold increased risk of open spina bifida.[14,15] This strengthens the justification for taking maternal weight into account when screening for this disorder. Adjusting maternal serum AFP levels for maternal weight is considered standard laboratory practice.[16]

Maternal race: The AFP levels of black women are on average 10% to 15% higher than those of white women.[17] This difference is taken into account either by adjusting individual MoM values from black women (when medians from the white population are used) or by using race-specific median values. In addition, the birth prevalence of open neural tube defects in black women is approximately one third to one half that of white women.[1] The difference in birth prevalence may be taken into account by raising the screening cutoff for black women (e.g., from 2.5 to 3.0 MoM).

Maternal insulin-dependent diabetes: The AFP levels of women with insulin-dependent diabetes before pregnancy are on average 20% lower than those of nondiabetic women.[18] These differences are taken into account by adjusting the individual MoM values upward. In addition, the birth prevalence of open neural tube defects is three to five times higher than in a comparable nondiabetic population.[19] This higher prevalence may be taken into account by lowering the screening cutoff level (e.g., from 2.5 to 2.0 MoM).

Multiple fetal pregnancy: Levels of AFP are higher in multiple fetal pregnancy, approximately in proportion to the number of fetuses. For example, levels in twin pregnancies are double those in singleton pregnancies. This difference can be taken into account by raising the screening cutoff (e.g., from 2.5 to 4.0 MoM). However, the screening performance will remain inferior to that achievable with singleton pregnancies—58% detection of open spina bifida with an 8% false-positive rate.[20] In addition, the prevalence of neural tube defects is twice as high as in singleton pregnancies.[21] The AFP screening performance in triplet and quadruplet pregnancies is poorly defined, and measurements from such pregnancies are usually not interpreted.

Family history of neural tube defects: A woman with a close family member affected by a neural tube defect is at a five- to tenfold increased risk of having an affected fetus.[7] Many physicians consider these risks sufficiently high to bypass maternal serum screening and instead recommend direct diagnostic testing with ultrasound. If AFP screening measurements are performed in such women, it is important to take the increased risk into account by either adjusting the value to reflect the higher individual risk or by lowering the MoM cutoff level (or both).

What are the implications of testing?

What does an abnormal test result mean? An elevated AFP MoM value (screen positive) may indicate the presence of an open neural tube defect and indicates the need for additional investigations. One option is to request a second serum sample and, if the second sample tests negative, recommend no further action. Repeated testing has the effect of reducing the number of women offered an additional ultrasound examination in a referral laboratory with little loss of detection. In practice, many screening programs have a two-tiered protocol based on the degree of the AFP elevation. For example, if a cutoff of 2.0 MoM is being used, a repeated sample may be recommended only if the value is between 2.0 and 3.0 MoM. This policy acknowledges that a serum with a value above 3.0 MoM is unlikely to drop back into the normal range upon repeated testing. If the original sample is above 3.0 MoM, and the pregnancy is dated by LMP, the next step is to confirm gestational age. When the gestational age estimate by ultrasound is more advanced than that obtained using the last menstrual period (generally defined as being at least 8–14 days), the AFP result is reinterpreted by the laboratory. The routine ultrasound examination will also identify anencephalic pregnancies, along with other conditions associated with elevated AFP levels, such as multiple pregnancy or fetal death.

Historically, when no explanation was found for the elevated AFP (approximately 1% of all pregnancies tested) after a low-level ultrasound examination for dates, viability, and fetal number, the screen-positive women were counseled and offered amniocentesis where the amniotic fluid AFP and acetylcholinesterase were measured. An elevated amniotic fluid AFP level and a positive acetylcholinesterase test are found in more than 98% of open spina bifida cases with a false-positive rate of less than 0.3%.[22] It was also common practice to perform chromosomal analysis of these fluids. The cost-effectiveness of this practice when associated with a normal high-resolution ultrasound examination is dubious, especially because the yield of serious chromosomal defects is low in such samples;[23-25] however, given that the expense of amniocentesis and risk of fetal loss has already been incurred, karyotyping seems prudent.

Currently, it is now common for women with an elevated maternal serum AFP to be referred to a high-risk perinatal center for high-resolution ultrasound examination in place of amniocentesis.[26] Anencephaly is readily diagnosed, and the ultrasound diagnosis of open spina bifida is significantly enhanced by visualization of two cranial "fruit" signs associated with this condition. The first sign results because the frontal region of the fetal skull is pinched, giving the skull an overall "lemon" shape rather than the normal egg shape (found in 86% of affected and 0.23% of unaffected pregnancies).[27] The second is the "banana" sign, in which the two cerebellar hemispheres adopt a bow shape because the transverse diameter of the cerebellum is reduced or not seen (found in 93% of affected and 0.05% of unaffected pregnancies).[27] The presence of one or both of these signs alerts the sonographer to carefully examine the spine to identify the spinal defect. This policy of replacing ultrasound examination for amniocentesis has been questioned because the detection rate will be operator dependent.[28] That said, many fetal medicine ultrasound laboratories are confident with the sonographic diagnosis as long as the quality of the examination is good. The optimal policy for any given geographic area and institution requires common sense. When available, high-resolution ultrasound examination by an individual experienced in the diagnosis of fetal malformation can replace the need for most amniocenteses. If such expertise is unavailable, it is prudent for the practitioner to rely on amniocentesis.

In addition to its association with open neural tube defects, an elevated maternal serum AFP level is frequently found in cases of open ventral wall defects (omphalocele and gastroschisis).[29] The maternal serum AFP level tends to be much higher with gastroschisis because, unlike omphaloceles, a gastroschisis is not covered by peritoneum. AFP screening, as described above, will detect virtually all cases of gastroschisis and about 70% of cases of omphalocele.

Informed counseling is essential to a successful screening program. The woman should understand that this is a screening test. Clinicians should also be aware that an elevated serum AFP where structural malformation has been ruled out is associated with a variety of adverse pregnancy outcomes, including intrauterine death, preterm delivery, fetal growth restriction, and low birthweight.[30,31] Although physicians may choose to increase antenatal surveillance in such cases, no intervention has been shown systematically to be effective in improving pregnancy outcome.[32,33]

Antenatal diagnosis of an open neural tube defect will lead to a change in the management of the pregnancy. Some women, after appropriate and nondirective genetic counseling, may choose pregnancy termination. Others choose to continue the pregnancy, but the location of delivery is altered to provide optimal neonatal care.

In contrast to the situation with elevated AFP values, women with low AFP values are not at increased risk of adverse outcomes once in utero fetal death or missed abortion has been ruled out.[34] In a study of over 800,000 pregnancies, AFP values below 3 µg/L occurred only in 1 in 56,000 pregnancies, after technical errors and sample mix-up had been ruled out.[35] Existing fetal death was the most common explanation for the low value, particularly when associated with low or nondetectable human chorionic gonadotropin (hCG). However, low AFP levels in viable pregnancies are associated with increased risk of trisomy 21,[36] and trisomy 18[37] (see Chapters 21, 22). AFP is one of the makers used in the triple test (AFP, unconjugated estriol, and human chorionic gonadotrophin) or quad test (triple test plus dimeric inhibin A) to screen for these trisomies. The laboratory will automatically take the AFP result into account when calculating risk of these conditions.

What does a normal test result mean? A normal test means it is unlikely the fetus has either an open spine defect or an abdominal wall defect. It is essential, therefore, that both the clinician and the woman understand that a negative screening test reduces, but does not eliminate the risk of having a fetus with a neural tube defect. Approximately 20% to 30% of cases of fetal open spina bifida are associated with maternal serum AFP levels below the screening cutoff. In addition, skin-covered cases of spina bifida are not detectable by AFP screening (closed spina bifida).

What is the cost of testing?

The same serum specimen is used for both neural tube defect and Down syndrome screening. Therefore, the fixed charges for drawing, transporting, logging in the specimen, and interpreting and reporting test results are shared costs. Consequently, the incremental cost for adding one, two, or more analytes is less than the charge than if each analyte were treated as a separate specimen. It can also be difficult in some healthcare systems such as the United States to provide a definitive cost for the testing because list prices are often discounted, capped, or the cost of the testing is bundled in with other test costs. Another issue affecting test cost is the support services that the laboratory provides to the physician. The American College of Obstetricians and Gynecologists recommends offering AFP testing for neural tube defects only as part of an antenatal screening program.[38] The responsibilities of any screening program include rapid communication of positive test results, availability of expert advice, and access to diagnostic follow-up testing. It is of particular importance that the laboratory is able to promptly reinterpret the AFP test when new information is provided by the physician (e.g., ultrasound revision of gestational age). When full program services are included, the total charge for AFP as used for both neural tube and trisomy 21 screening is in the range of $40 to $100. Costs are reported to be considerably less outside the United States. One study estimated the cost of the triple test (which would include AFP) at £11 ($18) and £13 ($21) for the quad test.[39] The cost estimates were based on consumables and staff time. These costs would appear to be unrealistically low, even in a government-funded health care system. A more reasonable estimate would need to include the cost of equipment and maintenance, sample collection and transport, log in and reporting, and facility overhead.

California has estimated the cost-effectiveness of their triple-marker program for the detection of neural tube defects (and other open defects) and trisomy 21 for the period of 1995 to 1997. California is in a unique position to make this calculation, because the entire program is administered and controlled by the state. During this time, the total cost to run the program was about $69 million, or $34.5 million for the neural tube defect component if the costs are apportioned equally. The estimated avoided costs (medical care, developmental services, and special education) for 109 spina bifida, 224 anencephaly, 20 gastroschisis, and 14 omphalocele cases identified by the screening program was $44 million in 1996 dollars. This yields a cost-benefit ratio of $1.27 for every $1.00 spent on the screening program for open fetal defect screening. This calculation may overstate the benefit for neural tube defect screening, because the costs are split evenly between neural tube defects and trisomy 21 screening. A further consideration is that the excess costs in 1988 for raising a child with trisomy 21 were greater than for spina bifida—$410,000 ($642,000 in 2003 dollars) and $285,000 ($404,000 in 2003 dollars), respectively. Societal cost-effectiveness evaluations assume a percentage of women choose pregnancy termination after being informed and appropriately counseled by trained personnel.

■ Conclusions and Recommendations

Spina bifida is variable in severity, but clearly has a long-term impact on the affected individual, family members, and society. More than 95% of neural tube defect cases occur to pregnant women with no history of these abnormalities. Thus, an obstetric or family history is not a useful screening tool. Screening using AFP levels is sensitive and specific when part of an organized screening program. Available data suggest that if at least 25% of women opt for pregnancy termination, there is a net cost benefit to society. Consequently, nearly all pregnant women seen for prenatal care prior to 20 weeks' gestation should be offered AFP evaluation. Women with a history of neural tube defects, with a suspicious ultrasonographic finding, or with insulin-dependent diabetes mellitus prior to pregnancy, should be considered candidates for a targeted ultrasound performed within a skilled unit.

■ **Summary**

1 ■ What Is the Problem that Requires Screening?

Fetal neural tube defects, abdominal wall defects.

a. What is the incidence/prevalence of the target condition?

The birth prevalence of neural tube defects varies according to such conditions as geographic location, racial origin, and time. Folic acid supplementation has reduced birth prevalence, but prevalence is still reported as 1–2/1,000.

b. What are the sequelae of the condition that are of interest in clinical medicine?

Anencephaly is not compatible with life. Spina bifida is variable in severity, but, as a rule, open defects have a worse prognosis than closed: 30% die within the first 5 years despite medical care. Gastroschisis is usually isolated, while the association of omphalocele with other malformations is high.

2 ■ The Tests

a. What is the purpose of the tests?

To identify pregnancies at high risk of a fetus with open neural tube defect.

b. What is the nature of the tests?

Measurement of the maternal serum AFP level between 15 and 20 weeks' gestation.

c. What are the implications of testing?

1. What does an abnormal test result mean?

An elevated AFP level may indicate the presence of an open neural tube defect and suggests the need for additional investigations. Approximately 80% of neural tube defects are associated with an elevated AFP. In the screen-positive pregnancies where no explanation can be found (1%–2% of pregnancies tested), the women are counseled and offered high-resolution ultrasound examination by trained personnel and/or amniocentesis. AFP screening will detect

■ **Summary**

virtually all cases of gastroschisis and about 70% of cases of omphalocele.

2. What does a normal test result mean?

A negative screening test result considerably reduces but does not eliminate the risk of having a fetus with a neural tube defect or abdominal wall defect.

d. What is the cost of testing?
AFP is almost always ordered as part the triple or quad test in the second trimester of pregnancy. Costs in the United States for these tests range from $40 to $100.

3 ■ **Conclusions and Recommendations**

Spina bifida has a long-term impact on the affected individual, family members, and society. More than 95% of neural tube defect cases occur to pregnant women with no prior history of these abnormalities. Screening using AFP is sensitive and specific when part of an organized screening program.

References

1. Greenburg F, James LM, Oakley GP. Estimates of birth prevalence rates of spina bifida in the United States from computer-generated maps. *Am J Obstet Gynecol* 1983;145:570–573.
2. Metropolitan Atlanta Congenital Defects Program, Birth Defects Monitoring Program: *Congenital Malformations Surveillance*. Atlanta: U.S. Department of Health & Human Services, 1993.
3. MRC Vitamin Study Research Group. Prevention of neural tube defects: results of the Medical Research Council Vitamin Study. *Lancet* 1991;338:131–137.
4. Centers for Disease Control and Prevention (CDC). Spina bifida and anencephaly before and after folic acid mandate—United States, 1995–1996 and 1999–2000. *MMWR Morb Mortal Wkly Rep* 2004;53:362–365.
5. Wald NJ. Folic acid and the prevention of neural-tube defects. *N Eng J Med* 2004;350:101–103.
6. Johnson AM. Racial differences in maternal serum screening. In: Mizejewski JG, Porter IH, eds., *Alpha-fetoprotein and Congenital Disorders*. New York: Academic Press, 1985:183–196.
7. Little J. Risks in siblings and other relatives. In: Elwood JM, Little J, Elwood JH, eds., *Epidemiology and Control of Neural Tube Defects*. Oxford: Oxford University Press, 1992:604–676.
8. Althouse R, Wald N. Survival and handicap of infants with spina bifida. *Arch Dis Child* 1980;55:845–850.
9. Walsh DS, Adzick NS. Foetal surgery for spina bifida. *Semin Neonatol* 2003;8:197–205.

10. Wald NJ, Cuckle H, Brock JH, et al. Maternal serum-alpha-fetoprotein measurement in antenatal screening for anencephaly and spina bifida in early pregnancy: report of U.K. collaborative study on alpha-fetoprotein in relation to neural-tube defects. *Lancet* 1997;i:1323–1332.

11. Sebire NJ, Spencer K, Noble PL, et al. Maternal serum alpha-fetoprotein in fetal neural tube and abdominal wall defects at 10 to 14 weeks of gestation. *Br J Obstet Gynaecol* 1997;104:849–851.

12. Wald NJ, Cuckle HS, Boreham J. Alpha-fetoprotein screening for open spina bifida: Effect of routine biparietal measurement to estimate gestational age. *Rev Epidemiol Sante Publique* 1984;32:62–69.

13. Johnson AM, Palomaki GE, Haddow JE. Maternal serum a-fetoprotein levels in pregnancies among black and white women with fetal open spina bifida: a United States collaborative study. *Am J Obstet Gynecol* 1990;162:328–331.

14. Waller DK, Mills JL, Simpson JL, et al. Are obese women at higher risk for producing malformed offspring? *Am J Obstet Gynecol* 1994;170:541–548.

15. Haddow JE, Palomaki GE. Haddow JE, et al. Is maternal obesity a risk factor for open neural tube defects? *Am J Obstet Gynecol* 1995;172:245–247.

16. Neveux LM, Palomaki GE, Larrivee DA, et al. Refinements in managing weight adjustment for interpreting prenatal screening results. *Prenat Diagn* 1996;16:1115–1119.

17. Baumgarten A. Racial difference and biological significance of maternal serum alpha-fetoprotein. *Lancet* 1986;ii:573.

18. Greene MF, Haddow JE, Palomaki GE, et al. Maternal serum alpha-fetoprotein levels in diabetic pregnancies. *Lancet* 1988;ii:345–346.

19. Adams MJ, Windham GC, James LM. Clinical interpretation of maternal serum alpha-fetoprotein concentrations. *Am J Obstet Gynecol* 1984;148:241–254.

20. Cuckle H, Wald NJ, Stevenson JD, et al. Maternal serum alpha-fetoprotein screening for open neural tube defects in twin pregnancies. *Prenat Diagn* 1990;10:71–77.

21. Wald NJ, Cuckle HS. Recent advances in screening for neural tube defects and Down's syndrome. *Baillieres Clin Obstet Gynaecol* 1987;1:649–676.

22. Wald N, Cuckle H, Nanchahal K. Amniotic fluid acetylcholinesterase measurement in the prenatal diagnosis of open neural tube defects. Second report of the Collaborative Acetylcholinesterase Study. *Prenat Diagn* 1989;8:813–829.

23. Feuchtbaum LB, Cunningham G, Waller DK, et al. Fetal karyotyping for chromosome abnormalities after an unexplained elevated maternal serum alpha-fetoprotein screening. *Obstet Gynecol* 1995;86:248–254.

24. Thiagarajah S, Stroud CB, Vavelidis F, et al. Elevated maternal serum alpha-fetoprotein levels: what is the risk of fetal aneuploidy? *Am J Obstet Gynecol* 1995;173:388–391.

25. Hiett AK, Callaghan CM, Brown HL, et al. The association of aneuploidy and unexplained elevated maternal serum alpha-fetoprotein. *J Perinatol* 1998;18:343–346.

26. Nadel AS, Green JK, Holmes LB, et al. Absence of need for amniocentesis in patients with elevated levels of maternal serum alpha-fetoprotein and normal ultrasonographic examinations. *N Engl J Med* 1990;324:769–772.

27. Wald N, Kennard A, Donnenfeld A, et al. Ultrasound scanning for congenial abnormalities. In: Wald N, Leck I, eds. *Antenatal and Neonatal Screening.* Oxford: Oxford University Press, 2000:441–469.

28. Wald NJ, Cuckle HS, Haddow JE, et al. Sensitivity of ultrasound in detecting spina bifida. *N Engl J Med* 1991;324:769–770.

29. Palomaki GE, Hill LE, Knight GJ, et al. Second trimester maternal serum, alpha feto-protein levels in pregnancies associated with gastroschisis and omphalocele. *Obstet Gynecol* 1988;71:906–909.

30. Haddow JE, Knight GJ, Kloza EM, et al. Alpha feto-protein, vaginal bleeding, and pregnancy risk. *Br J Obstet* 1986;93:589–595.

31. Katz VL, Chescheir NC, Cefalo RC. Unexplained elevations of maternal serum alpha-fetoprotein. *Obstet Gynecol Surv* 1990;45:719–726.

32. Goldenberg RL, Cliver SP, Bronstein J, et al. Bed rest in pregnancy. *Obstet Gynecol* 1994;84:131–136.

33. Huerta-Enochian G, Katz V, Erfurth S. The association of abnormal α-fetoprotein and adverse pregnancy outcome: does increased fetal surveillance affect pregnancy outcome? *Am J Obstet Gynecol* 2001;184:1549–1555.
34. Haddow JE, Hill LE, Palomaki GE, et al. Very low versus undetectable maternal serum alpha-fetoprotein values and fetal death. *Prenat Diagn* 1987;7:401–406.
35. Muller F, Dreux S, Sault C, et al. Very low alpha-fetoprotein in Down syndrome maternal serum screening. *Prenat Diagn* 2003;23:584–287.
36. Merkatz IR, Nitowsky HM, Macri JN, et al. An association between low maternal serum alpha-fetoprotein and fetal chromosomal abnormalities. *Am J Obstet Gynecol* 1984;148:866–894.
37. Canick JA, Palomaki GE, Osathanondh R. Prenatal screening for trisomy 18 in the second trimester. *Prenat Diagn* 1990;10:546–548.
38. ACOG. *Prenatal Detection of Neural Tube Defects: Technical Bulletin 99.* Washington, DC: American College of Obstetricians and Gynecologists, 1986.
39. Gilbert RE, Augood C, Gupta R, et al. Screening for Down's syndrome: effects, safety, and cost effectiveness of first and second trimester strategies. *BMJ* 2001;323:423–425.

Routine Ultrasonography for the Detection of Fetal Structural Anomalies

Juriy W. Wladimiroff

■ What Is the Problem that Requires Screening?

Fetal structural anomalies.

What is the incidence/prevalence of the target condition?

About 2% to 3% of newborns have detectable congenital structural anomalies, 20% to 30% of which result in perinatal death.[1] Congenital anomalies contribute to 15% of all perinatal deaths, and a further 10% to 15% of deaths in the United Kingdom during the first year of life.

What are the sequelae of the condition that are of interest in clinical medicine?

Perinatal mortality is now in the range of 7–8/1,000 births in industrialized countries. The improvement reflects predominantly enhanced intrapartum and neonatal care. Intrauterine growth restriction (IUGR), preterm delivery, and congenital disease are still major determinants of perinatal mortality and morbidity. Thus, the prevention and early detection of congenital anomalies has become an important part of antenatal care.

Major fetal structural anomalies are associated with preterm delivery, perinatal mortality and morbidity, unwarranted obstetric surgery, and prolonged postnatal hospitalization, all of which exact emotional, social, and financial hardship upon the involved families and society. The antenatal detection of major fetal malformations allows the woman a range of options varying from pregnancy termination to possible intrauterine treatment and adjustment of obstetric management. The latter concerns the immediate availability of specialized neonatal care for the structurally abnormal infant. The potential advantage of antenatal diagnosis of major but nonlethal fetal malformations is modification of the timing, mode, and geographic location of the delivery.

Forewarned, the parents can avoid the delivery of a child in a hospital ill prepared to care for the problem.

■ The Tests

Detailed ultrasound examination of the fetus.

What is the purpose of the tests?

To identify major fetal structural anomalies before 24 weeks' gestation.

What is the nature of the tests?

Fetal anomaly scanning entails a detailed examination of fetal morphology and physiologic function. The reported accuracy of ultrasound for the detection of fetal anomalies depends on the case definition in terms of the nature and the seriousness of the malformation, the skill and experience of the ultrasonographer, the quality of the ultrasound equipment, the gestational age at which the scan is performed, and availability of verification of anomalies. Accuracy estimates are further compromised by inadequate ascertainment of newborns with structural anomalies not readily apparent at birth.[2]

There are two approaches. Screening may be universal or targeted at women with an increased risk of having a fetus with a structural malformation.

Universal screening. The vast majority of malformed fetuses occur in pregnancies not known to have clinical risk factors. These examinations include documentation of fetal viability, gestational age, number, placental location, and a survey of major fetal structural anomalies. The effectiveness of screening low-risk populations by such means of ultrasound has been challenged demonstrating that an appropriately trained sonographer is of paramount importance.[3]

Targeted screening. Targeted screening refers to the examination of women at increased risk of having children with structural anomalies. Two distinct risk situations can be distinguished for indication-based ultrasound examinations:

Risk factors known prior to pregnancy: Screening is targeted at women at increased risk of fetal structural anomalies because of one or more specific risk factors known *before* the current pregnancy, such as a previously affected infant, a parent with a structural anomaly, maternal type 1 diabetes mellitus, or maternal use of antiepileptic drugs or certain psychopharmacokinetic drugs (including lithium) associated with an increased risk of fetal cardiac anomalies. There is still agreement that the 18- to 22-week scan is the ideal time for a cardiac investigation because 24 weeks' gestation is the legal upper limit for pregnancy termination in many countries. The overall prevalence of major fetal structural anomalies in this increased-risk group is 3% to 5%.[4,5] Parents in this group often opt for pregnancy termination if the fetus is structurally abnormal. Lie et al.[6] observed in 1994 that among women whose first infant had a birth defect, the risk of the same defect in the second infant was 7.6 times higher than expected (95% confidence interval [CI], 6.5–8.8), whereas the risk of a different defect was 1.5 times higher (95% CI, 1.3–-1.7) than expected.

Risk factors found during pregnancy: Diagnostic investigations for suspected fetal pathology are also based on abnormal obstetric findings that manifest during the present pregnancy. In early pregnancy, it is fetal nuchal translucency, which is not only associated with chromosomal abnormality, notably trisomy 21, but also with a wide range of single and multiple fetal anomalies. Particularly, the prevalence of major cardiac defects is substantially higher.[7] Abnormal findings in late pregnancy include hydramnios, oligohydramnios, severe fetal growth restriction, and fetal cardiac dysrhythmias. These findings are strongly associated with fetal structural anomalies.

The prevalence of fetal structural anomalies in this category approximated 35% to 40% in the late 1980s,[4] but has now increased to 55% to 60% due to more efficient referrals from primary and secondary obstetric care centers.[5] More than one organ system is involved in some 20% of cases, and is often based on the presence of a particular syndrome or chromosome abnormality.[5]

What are the implications of testing?

What does an abnormal test result mean? An abnormal scan, when performed by a qualified sonographer/sonologist, means the fetus is highly likely to have an anomaly. Where indicated, swift information on the fetal chromosome pattern is essential for optimal counseling and obstetric management. For example, preterm labor is neither inhibited nor is intrauterine hypoxemia treated by cesarean delivery if trisomy 13 or trisomy 18 is diagnosed. Aneuploidy can be rapidly detected using fluorescence in situ hybridization (FISH) with DNA probes specific for chromosomes 13, 18, 21, X, and Y.[8] In the case of a fetal anomaly compatible with life (for example, intestinal atresia, unilateral hydronephrosis), the mode (vaginal or caesarean delivery), timing (preterm or term), and location (academic or nonacademic center) of the delivery are discussed with the neonatologist and the organ specialist (pediatric surgeon or cardiologist, for example). In case of major pregnancy malformation, pregnancy termination may be an option.

Verification of the diagnosis is feasible in case of pregnancy termination for a major fetal anomaly followed by a proper postmortem examination. Some mild lesions, such as those involving the heart or urinary tract, may remain asymptomatic during intrauterine life and even after birth. Furthermore, certain anomalies such as renal pyelectasis or small cardiac ventricular defects may be transient.[9]

The overall sensitivity as reported in 1993 of ultrasound for the detection of congenital anomalies was 53% and the specificity 99%.[10–15] Sensitivity and specificity varied by organ system, with the lowest percentages for fetal facial structures and the cardiovascular system. The inclusion of minor anomalies with a high prevalence that are easily detected by antenatal ultrasound distorts the overall sensitivity of the examination. For instance, 63% of the anomalies detected in a group of more than 8,500 unselected women at 19 weeks' gestation were of renal origin and of a minor nature that are easily detected antenatally. In contrast, a high proportion of benign cardiac anomalies are not diagnosed antenatally,[16] especially when based on the presence or absence of a normal four-chamber view (16.7% for major, 4.5% for both major and minor). It is now clear that the routine cardiac scan in an unselected population of women should also include the visualization of the arterioventricular connections.[17] Because the antenatal diagnostic rate of cardiac anomalies appears essentially confined to major anomalies, antenatally diagnosed fetal congenital heart disease is associated with a poorer outcome than that diagnosed after birth.[18]

The relatively low diagnostic rate of congenital heart disease in unselected women was also highlighted by a study of 20 centers in 12 European countries (Euroscan study) reporting an overall detection rate of 25% (Table 24–1).[17,19] The rate was lowest (8%) in countries with no screening and in Eastern Europe, and highest (19%–48%) in Western Europe (Table 24–1). The overall detection rate was only 16% in cases of isolated congenital heart disease. Malformations

Table 24-1   **Data from the Euroscan study**

Type of anomaly	Detection rate	Authors
Neural tube defects	62%–97%	Boyd et al., 2000[a]
Congenital heart disease	11%–48%	Garne et al., 2001; Stoll et al., 2001[b]
Limb reduction deficiencies	0%–64%	Stoll et al., 2000[c]
Cleft lip with or without cleft palate	0%–75%	Clementi et al., 2000[d]
Omphalocele	0%–100%	Barisic et al., 2001[e]
Gastroschisis	18%–100%	Barisic et al., 2001[e]
Gastrointestinal anomalies	38%–72%	Barisic et al., 2001[e]
Diaphragmatic hernia	29%–100%	Garne et al., 2002[f]

[a]Boyd PA, Wellesley DG, De Walle HEK, et al. Evaluation of the prenatal diagnosis of neural tube defects by fetal ultrasonographic examination in different centres across Europe. *J Med Screening* 2000;7:169–174.

[b]Stoll C, Garne E, Clementi M; EUROSCAN Study Group. Evaluation of prenatal diagnosis of associated congenital heart diseases by fetal ultrasonographic examination in Europe. *Prenat Diagn* 2001;21:243–52.

[c]Stoll C, Wiesel A, Queisser-Luft A, et al. Evaluation of the prenatal diagnosis of limb reduction deficiencies. EUROSCAN Study Group. *Prenat Diagn* 2000;20:811–818.

[d]Clementi M, Tenconi R, Bianchi F, Stoll C. Evaluation of prenatal diagnosis of cleft lip with or without cleft palate and cleft palate by ultrasound: experience from 20 European registries. EUROSCAN study group. *Prenat Diagn* 2000;20:870–875.

[e]Barisic I, Clementi M, Hausler M, Gjergja R, Kern J, Stoll C; Euroscan Study Group. Evaluation of prenatal ultrasound diagnosis of fetal abdominal wall defects by 19 European registries. *Ultrasound Obstet Gynecol* 2001;18:309–16.

[f]Garne E, Haeusler M, Barisic I, et al. Congenital diaphragmatic hernia: evaluation of prenatal diagnosis in 20 European regions. *Ultrasound Obstet Gynecol* 2002;19:329–333.

[g]Garne E, Stoll C, Clementi M; Euroscan Group. Evaluation of prenatal diagnosis of congenital heart diseases by ultrasound: experience from 20 European registries. *Ultrasound Obstet Gynecol* 2001;17:386–91.

affecting ventricular size were detected in 50% of cases. The authors concluded that there is no difference in detection or in gestational age at detection between countries employing one scan in the second trimester and those conducting two anomaly scans. However, the detection rate was lower in countries were there was no routine ultrasound scanning policy. Notably, a high maternal body mass was associated with a lower anomaly detection rate. In experienced hands, a sensitivity of 74% for cardiac lesions overall can be achieved. Color-coded Doppler ultrasonography, which permits visualization of blood flow direction, improves the detection of these small defects.[20,21]

What does a normal test result mean? Normal findings are generally reassuring given the high specificity achieved by ultrasound examinations by trained sonographers and the relatively low prevalence of major fetal structural anomalies.[22]

What is the cost of testing?

Any economic evaluation of the potential benefit from screening pregnancies with ultrasound is complex for at least two reasons: (a) it involves many tangible costs of antenatal care that typically pertain to local remuneration structures; (b) the accuracy of anomaly screening can vary widely between centers. The limited information available on antenatal ultrasound screening is often contradictory. The Helsinki ultrasound randomized trial[23] supported the implementation of a one-stage ultrasound screening program based on a beneficial cost-effectiveness ratio. However, subsequent proposals based on economic analysis will likely fall short of implementation because official bodies may fail to fund health interventions based on such screening programs to avoid the abortion/anti-abortion debate. In the late 1990s, Roberts et al.[24] compared the cost-effectiveness of different programs of routine antenatal ultrasound screening to detect four key fetal anomalies: serious congenital heart disease, spina bifida, trisomy 21, and lethal anomalies. The cheapest but not the most effective screening program consisted of a single scan. They concluded that the overall allocation of resources for routine ultrasound screening in the United Kingdom was not economically efficient, but that certain scenarios for ultrasound screening are potentially within the range of cost-effectiveness reached by other, possibly competing, screening programs.

■ Conclusions and Recommendations

The impact of routine ultrasonography on perinatal morbidity or mortality is determined by a range of complex issues involving both financial and societal costs, the skill of the ultrasonographers involved in the screening program, and the societal view of severely malformed fetuses.[25]

The early detection of fetal structural anomalies reduces perinatal mortality and morbidity by one of two mechanisms. First, it can reduce mortality by converting neonatal or perinatal deaths to elective terminations of pregnancy. Second, it may reduce morbidity by optimizing the circumstances surrounding the delivery of a fetus with a major but not necessarily lethal anomaly. Several studies have tried to determine the impact of routine ultrasonography on fetal outcome. In the Helsinki trial, 9,010 pregnant women were randomized either to routine ultrasound investigation between 16 and 20 weeks' gestation (the screening group) or to selective ultrasonography (i.e., indication based [the control group]). Perinatal mortality was significantly lower in the screening group (4.6/1,000) compared with the control group (9/1,000). This near 50% reduction in perinatal mortality was due mostly to pregnancy terminations for reasons of fetal structural anomalies, which emphasizes the importance of anomaly scanning before 22 weeks' gestation. Furthermore, it demonstrates the potential impact of the women's attitudes to pregnancy termination on the efficacy of routine ultrasound examination, in terms of perinatal mortality. Less clear is the benefit of early detection of nonlethal fetal structural anomalies and the impact of adjustment of obstetric management on perinatal mortality. Additional study is needed.

It should be emphasized again that scanning expertise strongly determines the detection rate of malformed fetuses. Adequate training is a prerequisite for the level of scanning required to achieve a high detection rate. Ultrasound investigation for fetal structural anomalies should be performed by a specifically staffed and trained unit when the fetus is between 18 and 22 weeks of gestation. The impact on perinatal outcome is determined mainly by the percentage of women who decide to terminate their pregnancy if a major fetal structural anomaly is diagnosed.

■ Summary

1 ■ What Is the Problem that Requires Screening?

Fetal structural anomalies.

a. *What is the incidence/prevalence of the target condition?*
About 2% to 3% of the newborns have detectable major structural pathology, 20% to 30% of which result in perinatal death.

b. *What are the sequelae of the condition that are of interest in clinical medicine?*
Death or life-long suffering for the affected individual.

Continued

2 ■ The Tests

Ultrasound for the detection of fetal malformations by trained personnel.

a. What is the purpose of the tests?

To diagnose major structural fetal anomalies.

b. What is the nature of the tests?

Screening may be either targeted or universal. The accuracy of ultrasound examinations for the detection of fetal structural anomalies is determined by the sonographer's level of experience, the equipment used, and the woman's physical characteristics. The reported accuracy varies markedly depending on the organ/structure.

c. What are the implications of testing?

1. What does an abnormal test result mean?

   The fetus is highly likely to have a structural malformation.

2. What does a normal test result mean?

   Normal findings are generally reassuring and indicate the fetus is unlikely to have a major structural malformation.

d. What is the cost of testing?

A study in the United Kingdom demonstrated that certain scenarios for ultrasound screening are potentially within the range of cost-effectiveness. A reduction in costs in cases amenable to biventricular repair and in transposition of the great arteries has been established following antenatal echocardiography.

3 ■ Conclusions and Recommendations

Routine ultrasound performed on the fetus by trained sonographers between 18 and 22 weeks' gestation has high specificity and good sensitivity. Cost benefits to society reflect mainly the rate of pregnancy termination for lethal or potentially lethal malformations. Such an analysis does not include potential benefits of enhanced dating and early diagnosis of multiple gestations.

References

1. Morrison I. Perinatal mortality: basic considerations. *Semin Perinatol* 1985;9:144–150.
2. De Vore G. Opinion: financial implications of routine screening ultrasound. *Ultrasound Obstet Gynecol* 1996;7:307–308.
3. Ewigman BG, Crane JP, Frigoletto FD, et al. A randomized trial of prenatal ultrasound screening in a low risk population: impact on perinatal outcome. *N Engl J Med* 1993;329:821–827.
4. Wladimiroff JW, Sachs ES, Reuss A, et al. Prenatal diagnosis of chromosome abnormalities in the presence of fetal structural defects. *Am J Med Genet* 1988;29:289–291.
5. Wladimiroff JW, Cohen-Overbeek TE, Ursem NT, et al. Twenty years of experience in advanced ultrasound scanning for fetal anomalies in Rotterdam. *Ned Tijdschr Geneeskd* 2003;147: 2106–2110.
6. Lie RT, Wilcox AJ, Skjaerven R. A population based study of the risk of recurrence of birth defects. *N Engl J Med* 1994;331:1–4.
7. Ghi T, Huggon IC, Zosmer N, et al. Incidence of major structural cardiac defects associated with increased nuchal translucency but normal karyotype. *Ultrasound Obstet Gynecol* 2001;18:610–614.
8. Weremowicz S, Sandstrom DJ, Morton CC, et al. Fluorescence in situ hybridization (FISH) for rapid detection of aneuploidy experience in 911 prenatal cases. *Prenat Diagn* 2001;21:262–269.
9. Tabor A, Zdravkovic M, Perslev A. Screening for congenital malformations by ultrasonography in the general population of pregnant women: factors affecting the efficacy. *Acta Obstet Gynecol Scand* 2003;82:1092–1098.
10. Rosendahl H, Kivenen S. Antenatal detection of congenital malformations by routine ultrasonography. *Obstet Gynecol* 1989;73:947–951.
11. Saari-Kemppainen A, Karjalainen O, Ylostalo P, et al. Ultrasound screening and perinatal mortality: controlled trial of systematic one-stage screening in pregnancy: the Helsinki Ultrasound Trial. *Lancet* 1990;i:387–391.
12. Levi S, Hyjazi Y, Schaaps JD, et al. Sensitivity and specificity of routine antenatal screening for congenital anomalies by ultrasound: the Belgian multicentric study. *Ultrasound Obstet Gynecol* 1991;1:102–110.
13. Chitty LS, Hung GH, Moore J, et al. Effectiveness of routine ultrasonography in detecting fetal structural anomalies in a low risk population. *BMJ* 1991;303:1165–1169.
14. Shirley IM, Bottomly F, Robinson VP. Routine radiographer screening for fetal abnormalities by ultrasound in a unselected population. *Br J Radiol* 1992;65:564–569.
15. Luck CA. Value of routine ultrasound scanning at 19 weeks: a four year study of 8,849 deliveries. *Br Med J* 1992;304;1474–1478.
16. Buskens E, Grobbee DE, Frohn-Mulder IME. Efficacy of routine fetal ultrasound screening for congenital heart disease in normal pregnancy. *Circulation* 1996;94:67–72.
17. Garne E, Stoll C, Clementi M. Evaluation of prenatal diagnosis of congenital heart disease by ultrasound: experience from 20 European Registries. *Ultrasound Obstet Gynecol* 2001;17:386–391.
18. Levi S, Zhang WH, Alexander S. Short-term outcome of isolated and associated congenital heart defects in relation to antenatal ultrasound screening. *Ultrasound Obstet Gynecol* 2003;21:532–538.
19. Clementi M, Stoll C.The Euroscan study [editorial]. *Ultrasound Obstet Gynecol* 2001;18:297–300.
20. Stewart PA, Wladimiroff JW. Fetal echocardiography and color Doppler flow imaging: the Rotterdam experience. *Ultrasound Obstet Gynecol*. 1993;3:3168–3175.
21. Chaoui R, Hoffmann J, Heling KS. Three-dimensional (3D) and 4D color Doppler fetal echocardiography using spatio-temporal image correlation (STIC). *Ultrasound Obstet Gynecol* 2004;23:535–545.
22. Levi S, Crouzet P, Schaaps JP, et al. Ultrasound screening for fetal malformations. *Lancet* 1989;I:678.
23. Leivo T, Tuominen R, Saari-Kemppainen A. Cost-effectiveness of one-stage ultrasound screening in pregnancy: a report from the Helsinki ultrasound trial. *Ultrasound Obstet Gynecol* 1996;7:309–314.

24. Roberts T, Mugford M, Piercy J. Choosing options for ultrasound screening in pregnancy and comparing cost-effectiveness: a decision analysis approach. *Br J Obstet Gynaecol* 1998;105:960–970.

25. Gomez KJ, Copel JA. Ultrasound for fetal structural anomalies. *Curr Opin Obstet Gynecol* 1993;5:204–210.

26. Boyd PA, Wellesley DG, De Walle HEK, et al. Evaluation of the prenatal diagnosis of neural tube defects by fetal ultrasonographic examination in different centres across Europe. *J Med Screening* 2000;7:169–174.

27. Stoll C, Wiesel A, Queisser-Luft A, et al. Evaluation of the prenatal diagnosis of limb reduction deficiencies. EUROSCAN Study Group. *Prenat Diagn* 2000;20:811–818.

28. Clementi M, Tenconi R, Bianchi F, Stoll C. Evaluation of prenatal diagnosis of cleft lip with or without cleft palate and cleft palate by ultrasound: experience from 20 European registries. EUROSCAN study group. *Prenat Diagn* 2000;20:870–875.

29. Garne E, Haeusler M, Barisic I, et al. Congenital diaphragmatic hernia: evaluation of prenatal diagnosis in 20 European regions. *Ultrasound Obstet Gynecol* 2002;19:329–333.

30. Garne E, Stoll C, Clementi M; Euroscan Group. Evaluation of prenatal diagnosis of congenital heart diseases by ultrasound: experience from 20 European registries. *Ultrasound Obstet Gynecol* 2001;17:386–91.

25

Molecular Tests for Antenatal Detection of Aneuploidy

Gill M. Grimshaw

■ What is the Problem that Requires Screening?

Fetal aneuploidy.

What is the incidence/prevalence of the target condition?

The birth prevalence of fetal aneuploidy is about 1%. See related material in Chapters 21 and 22.

What are the sequelae of the condition that are of interest in clinical medicine?

These are described in Chapters 21 and 22.

■ The Tests

What is the purpose of the tests?

The provision of a clinically useful, rapid fetal karyotype.

What is the nature of the tests?

Antenatal testing for fetal aneuploidy is a two-stage process. In the first stage, a risk assessment and noninvasive tests are conducted to assign a value to the likelihood of a fetal abnormality (see Chapters 21 and 22). If this risk is above a specific threshold, the obstetrician is likely to be presented with a distressed woman who demands a diagnostic test to either confirm an abnormality or reassure her that the fetus is normal.

Conventional karyotyping. Obstetricians traditionally offer pregnant women a test based on cultured fetal cells. These cells are obtained either from aspirated amniotic fluid or from a biopsy of the chorionic villae. Not all attempts to obtain fetal cells by amniocentesis or chorionic villus sampling (CVS) are successful; in now out-of-date studies, 2% of all attempts to obtain amniotic fluid are unsuccessful, and between 1.3% and 5% of CVS attempts fail.[1–3] Although these rates have declined, the risk remains. In addition, culture failure occurs in a small number of cases—the average UK failure rate in 1999 was 0.3%.[4] There is also a small possibility (0.2% of cultures) of misleading results due to overgrowth of maternal cells.[5] Successfully cultured cells are examined under a microscope for structural or numerical abnormality. This test, referred to as karyotyping, is a reliable and accurate test for the detection of aneuploidies. The detection rate for Down syndrome in successfully cultured samples is 99.7%.[6] The main disadvantage of karyotyping this way is that it is nonautomated and lengthy procedure that requires specialist scientific expertise; it is therefore slow and expensive. There are also large variations in the rate at which cells from individual specimens grow. This leads to a wide range of reporting times that are unpredictable for the individual. The mean time to diagnosis for fetal karyotyping in the United Kingdom is 13.4 days (range, 7.3–20.2 days).[7] As a result, obstetricians typically advise couples the wait for a result following amniocentesis may be up to 3 weeks. Yet, some laboratories now record an average time of 7 days to reporting the results with improved methods.[8,9]

There are several drawbacks to using karyotyping. First, fetal cells can only be obtained by an invasive procedure, and the act of obtaining them carries a risk of pregnancy loss (typically 0.5% to 1%[10]). Second, women who have come through a screening program for trisomy 21 may not be told or may not be aware that the test will identify other aneuploidies. Third, the test is slow and requires a high degree of scientific training to interpret and report results. Waiting for diagnostic test results can place a marked psychological burden on women and their partners. Last, some of the abnormalities that may be disclosed have unknown or little effect on the current infant.

Molecular tests. As molecular tests capable of replicating DNA have evolved, they hold the promise of more rapid results at less cost. In addition, it may be possible to use smaller samples or fewer fetal cells for the analysis because all are based on DNA amplification. It may also be possible to automate the analysis. Molecular methods therefore appear to offer the potential for rapid, inexpensive tests for antenatal diagnosis. Unlike karyotyping, molecular tests will not detect all aneuploidies. Instead, each chromosome to be tested requires a specific probe. Currently, molecular tests are designed only to detect numerical abnormalities of the more common chromosome disorders. The panel commonly used comprises trisomies 21, 18, and 13 and sex chromosome abnormalities.

Two main types of molecular methods are currently used for the antenatal diagnosis of chromosome abnormalities, although molecular technologies are evolving rapidly and new methods may prove equally suitable. The two methods used are fluorescence in situ hybridization (FISH) and quantitative polymerase chain reaction (Q-PCR). Other methods now available use small amounts of fetal cells and have the advantage of offering a choice of probes for specific DNA sequences (for example, multiplex ligation-dependent probe amplification [MLPA][11] and multiplex amplifiable probe hybridization [MAPH][12]). None of these methods require lengthy culture of fetal cells.

The application of FISH is common in some obstetric clinics. It involves the use of chromosome-specific probes that have fluorescent labels attached. The probes are applied to cellular preparations, and detection systems consisting of fluorescence microscopy or other similar image analysis systems are used to examine the cells. The scientific skills of a cytogeneticist are still required in many laboratories to examine the cellular preparations, although this method may be amenable to some form of automation.

The Q-PCR test is an alternative to FISH. It is based on a versatile and widely used amplification technique through which even the smallest amount of a DNA target can be amplified to provide quantities that are detectable and identifiable. Amplification uses DNA polymerase to catalyze the rapid synthesis of new strands of DNA from an original strand using a primer. Detection requires an expensive DNA analyzer.

Comparisons of FISH, Q-PCR and karyotyping when used for antenatal detection of chromosome abnormality are found in Tables 25–1 and 25–2. Not included in the prior discussion is the potential to test for the presence of a unique proteomic fingerprint to identify certain types of fetal aneuploidy.

Sensitivity and specificity. There are two ways of representing the implications of an abnormal result when molecular tests are used in place of karyotyping. First, "panel" sensitivity and specificity reflect the test's ability to detect any chromosomal abnormality from the panel. Second, molecular tests are designed to detect any detectable chromosomal abnormality. The performance measures calculated in this scenario are the "overall" sensitivity and specificity. The question is then "how many chromosomal abnormalities will be missed using molecular tests?" Since molecular methods detect only what they are designed to detect, numerous uncommon chromosome abnormalities may remain undetected unless other diagnostic procedures, for example an ultrasound examination, disclose an abnormality. Arguably, this is more satisfactory from an ethical view because the mother will be aware of and give consent to testing for specific chromosomal abnormalities. It is at the same time important that clinicians and parents acknowledge that some fetal chromosome abnormalities may remain undetected using molecular methods, a fact not all couples will find acceptable. Throughout this chapter, we will consider the traditional karyotype as the gold standard.

Panel sensitivity and specificity: During a study in the United Kingdom to evaluate molecular tests[13] 902 FISH and 3,318 Q-PCR tests were compared to karyotyping for the detection of numerical chromosomal abnormalities 21, 13, and 18 and sex chromosomal abnormalities In this series, no abnormalities were missed by FISH, although Q-PCR gave one false-positive result. Some

Table 25–1	**Comparing molecular methods, FISH and Q-PCR**	
	FISH	**Q-PCR**
Advantages	Analysis completed in 24–48 h	Analysis completed in 24–48 h
	Application in cytogenetic labs well developed; all large laboratories use FISH in routine practice, though not for prenatal interphase trisomy detection	Quantitative interpretation of profiles is less subjective than interpreting FISH results
	Protocols for simultaneous detection of aneuploidy for chromosomes 21, 13, 18, X, and Y well developed and tested	Less labor-intensive, both in terms of time and expertise, than FISH
		Q-PCR analysis already automated
Disadvantages	Interpretation of results more subjective than in quantitative Q-PCR	Application for aneuploidy diagnosis much less well developed than FISH, but DNA laboratories use Q-PCR in routine practice for other conditions
	More labor-intensive, both in terms of time and expertise, than Q-PCR	Protocols for simultaneous detection of aneuploidy for chromosomes 21, 13, 18, X, and Y (multiplexing) less well developed
	Consumables costs higher than Q-PCR	
	More difficult to automate than Q-PCR	Capital costs considerably higher than FISH
	Not able, without further development, to detect structural chromosomal abnormalities	Not able, without further development, to detect structural chromosomal abnormalities

FISH, fluorescence in situ hybridization; Q-PCR, quantitative polymerase chain reaction.

Table 25–2	**Comparing karyotyping with molecular tests**	
	Karyotyping	**Molecular tests**
Advantages	Can detect numerical AND structural chromosome abnormalities	Analysis completed in 24–48 h
	High-quality, well-developed test with national quality assurance systems in place	Molecular tests more readily automated
Disadvantages	Results can take up to 3 weeks	Not able, without further development, to detect structural chromosomal abnormalities
	More labor-intensive, both in terms of time and expertise, than Q-PCR	
	Reading cannot readily be automated	
	Detects abnormalities with little or unknown clinical significance	

Q-PCR, quantitative polymerase chain reaction.

samples were heavily contaminated by maternal blood and had to be excluded from testing because Q-PCR is sensitive to maternal contamination. Table 25–3 provides the calculated test parameters (panel sensitivity and specificity) from this series for both molecular techniques and shows the relative failure rates of the test based on the detection of the abnormalities it is designed to detect.

Overall sensitivity and specificity: Using a database of all karyotyping tests conducted during an 11-year period (1988–1999) that is maintained by the Regional Genetic Service in the West Midlands, United Kingdom,[6] it was possible to calculate the number and nature of cases that would have been missed should molecular testing be substituted for karyotyping. The subjects were sub grouped into (a) "low risk"—selection for amniocentesis based solely on the risk assessment for trisomy 21 during antenatal screening using risk factors such as maternal age and serum testing, and (b) "high risk"—where pregnancies were identified as having an additional risk, arising from reproductive history, in particular family history indicative of chromosome abnormalities (including either parent being a carrier of a structural chromosome abnormality) or abnormal ultrasound scan.

Tables 25–4 through 25–6 illustrate the prevalence of chromosomal abnormalities other than trisomies 21, 13, and 18 and numerical sex chromosome abnormalities that would have been undetected if molecular tests were substituted for karyotyping low-risk pregnancies. Most undetectable abnormalities from both high- and low-risk groups (236/378) were judged not to be clinically significant. Thirty-four percent (84 cases) of the 245 low-risk pregnancies identified as having an other chromosomal abnormality were judged to be clinically significant.[13] Thus, 2.7/1,000 women (0.27% or 84/30,861) tested for an enhanced risk would have had a child with an chromosomal abnormality undetected by the substitute molecular test. Fifty percent of these abnormalities consisted of mosaicism where the impact of the chromosome abnormality on clinical outcome is difficult to predict. It was calculated that 26/1,000 (58/2,193) high-risk pregnancies would be undetected if molecular tests were substituted

Table 25–3 **Panel sensitivity and specificity for molecular tests compared with karyotyping**

| Test | Failed to complete test,[a]% | Completed tests | |
		"Absolute" sensitivity	"Absolute" specificity
FISH	3.13[b]	1.00	1.00
Q-PCR	3.66[b]	0.9565	0.9997
Karyotyping	1.09	—	—

FISH, fluorescence in situ hybridization; Q-PCR, quantitative polymerase chain reaction.
[a]Including all tests where no result obtained.
[b]Samples with visible maternal cell contamination excluded.

Table 25–4   Chromosome abnormalities detected antenatally by a karyotyping service (11 years' data)

	Prevalence[a]		
	Low risk[b]	High risk[c]	Total
Total cases tested	30,861	2,193	33,054
Trisomy 21[d]	390 (1.3%)	74 (3.4%)	464 (1.4%)
Trisomies 13 and 18	63 (0.2%)	71 (3.2%)	134 (0.4%)
Sex chromosome abnormalities	65 (0.2%)	22 (1.0%)	87 (0.3%)
Other abnormalities	245 (0.8%)	133 (6.1%)	378 (1.1%)
Total abnormalities	763 (2.5%)	300 (13.7%)	1,063 (3.2%)

[a]Based on those tested, rates are therefore dependent on selection criteria for amniocentesis.
[b]Also included in this category were de novo abnormalities.
[c]Case selection based on familial history, previous pregnancy, or abnormal scan.
[d]If the molecular test for Down syndrome only is used, triploidy would appear to be Down syndrome and is therefore included in this column. If a test for trisomies 18, 13, and 21 was used, triploidy would be identified. Figures for numbers of triploidy are included as appropriate.

for karyotyping. This contrasts with the much lower figure for low-risk pregnancies and underlines the importance of karyotyping these women.

From Tables 25–4 and 25–5, the percentage of abnormalities that would have remained undetected per year can be calculated. Currently two molecular test configurations are available: one that tests for trisomy 21 only and one that tests for trisomy 21, 18, 13 and numerical sex chromosomal abnormalities. Table 25–6 shows the estimated number of cases that would remain undetected if karyotyping for low-risk pregnancies were replaced by either of these molecular test configurations. Using these data, the "overall" test performance is calculated (Table 25–7). Clearly, if molecular testing is used only for trisomy 21, then

Table 25–5   Estimated annual rates of various abnormalities detected for all those selected for amniocentesis based on data in Table 25–4A

	Cases
Average throughput per annum	3,005
Average total abnormalities detected	97 (100%)
Trisomy 21	42 (43.3%)
Trisomy 18	9 (9.3%)
Trisomy 13	4 (4.1%)
Numerical sex chromosome abnormalities	8 (8.2%)
Total "other" abnormalities	34 (35.1%)
Clinically significant "other" abnormalities	13 (13.4%)
Average total clinically significant abnormalities	75 (77.3%)

Columns are rounded to the nearest whole number; values in the totals column may reflect these rounding errors.

Table 25–6   Estimated clinically significant defects that would not have been detectable per annum if karyotyping were always performed for high-risk cases and molecular tests for lower risk cases

Testing regime	Clinically significant defects not detected per annum in West Midlands (%)[a]
Molecular test for Down only (trisomy 21)	21 (30.7)
Molecular test for trisomies 21,18, 13, and numerical sex chromosome abnormalities	6 (9.2)

[a]As percentage of total clinically significant cases detected.

many more common chromosomal abnormalities will be missed and the "overall" sensitivity relative to karyotyping unacceptably low.

What are the implications of testing?

What does an abnormal test result mean? The fetus has one of the chromosomal abnormalities from the panel (trisomy 21, 18, or 13 or sex chromosomal abnormalities). No further testing is needed and the woman should be given nondirective genetic counseling and offered pregnancy termination where indicated.

What does a normal test result mean? A normal test result eliminates out one or more of the chromosomal abnormalities from the panel. However, a normal test result does not exclude the presence of other chromosomal abnormalities. In women at increased risk of chromosomal abnormality—for instance because of abnormal ultrasound findings—further conventional karyotyping and counseling should be offered.

Table 25–7   Overall test performance if molecular tests are substituted appropriately for karyotyping

Molecular test regime compared with karyotyping	"Relative" sensitivity	"Relative" specificity
FISH test for Down syndrome only (trisomy 21)	0.6478	0.9999
Q-PCR test for Down syndrome only (trisomy 21)	0.6196	0.9996
FISH test for trisomies 21,18, and 13 and X,Y abnormalities	0.8605	0.9999
Q-PCR test for trisomies 21,18, and 13 and X,Y abnormalities	0.8234	0.9996

FISH, fluorescence in situ hybridization; Q-PCR, quantitative polymerase chain reaction.

What is the cost of testing?

The data presented in the previous section suggest that molecular tests cannot be a complete substitute for karyotyping unless the technology is developed improved. In theory, it is possible to develop FISH or Q-PCR that can detect many more abnormalities. However, the mean cost per test will rise as probes are added. The most efficient solution may be to conduct testing in a targeted fashion. Choices to be made include local assessment of the most appropriate method, Q-PCR or FISH; whether to test for trisomy 21 or some other combination of more common abnormalities; and in what combination karyotyping and molecular methods should be used.

As Q-PCR is suitable for high volumes of automated tests, it offers economies of scale not possible with FISH. Furthermore, Q-PCR requires a lower level of scientific input to produce and interpret results. Therefore, the actual cost of the Q-PCR test is much lower than FISH at higher volumes and in industrialized settings. However, many clinics have a relatively small sample volumes, which could be tested in laboratories where specimens from other specialties are also processed using FISH. In this instance, the cost per test is reduced because the more expensively trained staff is already employed within the laboratory for other purposes and the costs spread across multiple activities. The influence of throughput on the economies of molecular testing compared to traditional karyotyping is shown in Figure 25–1.

For the remainder of this section, only two configurations are considered. These configurations were those identified by obstetricians and specialist nurses

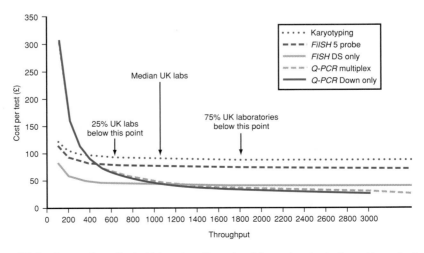

Figure 25-1 Comparing effect of laboratory throughput for molecular tests and karyotyping.

as the ones most likely to be requested by antenatal clinics.[13] The first configuration is to test for trisomy 21 only. The second is to test for five chromosomal abnormalities (trisomy 21, 13, 18 and numerical sex chromosomal abnormalities in a five-probe configuration). Clinicians were satisfied with this configuration provided traditional karyotyping was available for specific women.

First, the configurations are considered from the perspective of the testing options offered to women at high risk of having a fetus with a chromosomal abnormality. The two extremes would be the complete replacement of karyotyping with molecular testing or to not use molecular tests at all (i.e., the status quo).

The protocols summarized in Table 25–8 and Figure 25–2 are considered in turn with reference to the status quo, where the cost of karyotyping for all women at risk is currently around £2,200 ($3,170, 2001 data[7]) per case detected.

Option 1: Complete replacement of karyotyping by molecular testing. The overwhelming advantage of this option is all women tested get a rapid result. This reduces anxiety considerably for the couple. However, some clinically significant abnormalities will not be detected. The cost per case detected for a one-test–for-all option is illustrated in Table 25–9 for both configurations. Because so many cases would remain undetected, only the five-probe Q-PCR version reduces the cost per case detected.

Option 2: Offering all women molecular testing plus karyotyping. This option would replace karyotyping alone as the reference test, because it has the advantage of a rapid result for the most common abnormalities but also provides the potential reassurance of excluding rare abnormalities. However, the dilemma of how to inform couples about results that are not clinically significant remains as it currently does for karyotyping alone. This is a very expensive

Table 25–8   Possible protocols for antenatal testing for chromosome abnormalities

Testing regime option		Summary	
1		New gold standard, molecular test and karyotyping for all women	
2	A	Local or national decision:	Karyotyping only for all women
	B	"One for all" option	Molecular testing only for all women
3		Molecular testing for all women, some samples also karyotyped	
4		Karyotyping for all women, selected samples given additional molecular test	
5	A	"Either-or" option	Some samples karyotyped, some molecular testing, clinician's choice.
	B		Variant of 5A, based on parental choice

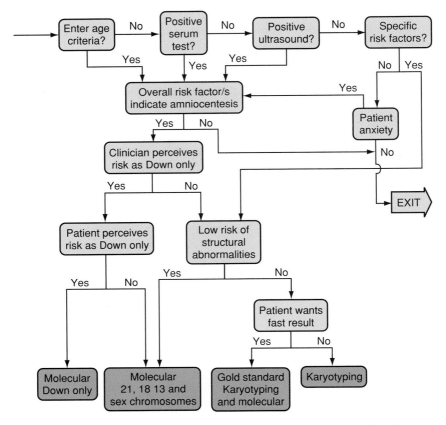

Figure 25–2 Flow chart for enabling clinician and patient choice for antenatal testing.

Table 25–9	**Percentage variation in cost per case detected for Options 1 and 2 compared with karyotyping for average U.K. laboratory throughput (1,000 cases per annum)**				
		Option 1: Molecular test only for all		**Option 2: Karyotyping and molecular tests for all.**	
Test configuration		**Difference in cost, %**	**Positive cases undetectable[b]**	**Difference in cost, %**	**Positive cases undetectable[b]**
Q-PCR[a]	Tri-21 only	+29	15	+49	0
	Five-probe	−19	4	53	0
FISH	Tri-21 only	+23	15	+47	0
	Five-probe	+28	4	84	0

FISH, fluorescence in situ hybridization; Tri-21, trisomy 21; Q-PCR, quantitative polymerase chain reaction.
[a]Q-PCR is very sensitive to throughput and percentage will fall below that for FISH at higher throughputs.
[b]These refer to clinically significant cases undetectable per 1,000 women tested.

option compared to the others (Table 25–9). The cost per quality-adjusted life-year is calculated to be between £23,000 and £26,000 ($33,000 to $37,500, 2001 data) for this option.[7]

Option 3: Molecular testing with karyotyping for high-risk cases. As most women coming forward for diagnostic tests have had an increased risk assessment for trisomy 21, it can be argued that a diagnostic test that rapidly and accurately tests for trisomy 21 only is the most ethical solution. However, in practice, the five-probe test for this majority and karyotyping plus molecular test for the higher risk cases (e.g., family history, previous pregnancy, or abnormal scan) offers a reasonable compromise between the status quo and Option 1. Table 25–10 illustrates the costs per case detected compared with karyotyping as well as the number of cases that would remain undetected.

Option 4: Karyotyping for all, with some women offered molecular tests. One possibility is to continue to offer karyotyping to all, but in addition offer a rapid result to those with the highest risk of abnormality. The cost per case detected can be seen in Table 25–10 for this option. It is clear that no cases would remain undetected. However, there is an issue of equity since 92% of those tested receive a reassuring result and waiting times for these couples are not reduced. This negates the advantage of the faster tests.

Option 5: Either-or option: clinician or parental choice for only one test. In many clinics, Option 5 is attractive, where either the parents or the clinicians

Table 25–10 **Percentage variation in cost per case detected for Options 3 and 4 compared with karyotyping for average U.K. laboratory throughput (1,000 cases per annum)**

Test configuration		Option 3: Molecular test for all plus karyotyping for high risk		Option 4: Karyotyping for all plus molecular for some	
		Difference in cost[c] per case detected, %	Positive cases undetectable[b]	Difference in cost[c] per case detected, %	Positive cases undetectable[b]
Q-PCR[a]	Tri-21 only	−9	9.1	+3	0
	5 probe	−23	2.5	+3	0
FISH	Tri-21 only	−13	9.1	+3	0
	5 probe	+17	2.5	+6	0

FISH, fluorescence in situ hybridization; Tri-21, trisomy 21; Q-PCR, quantitative polymerase chain reaction.
[a]Q-PCR is very sensitive to throughput and percentage will fall below that for FISH at higher throughputs.
[b]These refer to clinically significant cases undetectable per 1.000 women tested.
[c]Compared with karyotyping only for all women.

choose the most suitable test. Parents who have received an assessment for their risk of trisomy 21 may choose to have a rapid test. Table 25–9 demonstrates that for most laboratories it would be cost-effective to offer a test in this situation that was configured for trisomy 21, 18, and 13 and numerical sex chromosomal abnormalities. Laboratories may choose to offer FISH where there is a low volume of tests but the demand from other services for tests that require a high level of scientific input. In contrast, laboratories may offer Q-PCR where there is a high volume of similar tests. Laboratories with a throughput of around 1500 specimens can offer a Q-PCR five-probe test at the same cost as a trisomy 21–only FISH test.

Surveys of parents from two areas in the United Kingdom indicated that around 60% would opt for a rapid test result and that test anxiety quickly returns to the pretest levels. If 60% of parents or clinicians opt for molecular tests, the cost per clinically significant case detected is 21% lower than cost of karyotyping all (status quo) if multiplex Q-PCR is used, with the cost per case detected falling from £2,800 to around £2,300. As a result, the United Kingdom's direct testing costs would fall by 25%. However if choices were reversed (i.e., only 30% opt for molecular tests), then the costs would be similar to offering karyotyping to all.

■ Conclusions and Recommendations

With karyotyping, the specimen can be rapidly transported to the laboratory and there is time, while waiting for results, to allocate appointments for the provision of results and any counseling that may be required. Rapid tests place clinics under pressure as the source of delay in receiving results may switch from the laboratory to the clinic. Thus, if molecular tests are introduced, it may not be solely a question of replacing the technology, but also of examining the logistics and systems associated with the test.

The wide-scale introduction of molecular tests would undoubtedly be an opportunity for services to examine the various clinical protocols and options. Currently, demand is limited by the invasive nature of the test and subsequent rate of a pregnancy loss. Severe demands may be placed on laboratory services once a maternal blood sample can be used to obtain fetal cells. If regionally or nationally centralized services for antenatal testing are considered, then Q-PCR may offer economies of scale. One of the most cost-effective options for clinics is parental choice. Within this option, protocols for case selection of high-risk individuals must be developed as overall costs would otherwise rise above current UK testing costs if more than 20% of women are offered new gold standard (Option 1) FISH, or 50% of patients offered this regime use Q-PCR. There is the additional cost of training the professionals to appropriately counsel the couples as to their options and the potential for false-negative test results.

It should be recognized that one of the important potential disadvantages of molecular tests, if used to replace karyotyping within a screening program, is that some abnormalities will be undetected. The risk of a false-negative for a few women should be balanced against the advantages of molecular tests. Within a screening program, there may be serious medicolegal consequences arising from a lack of understanding that the program will miss nontargeted abnormalities.

■ Summary

1 ■ **What Is the Problem that Requires Screening?**

Fetal aneuploidy.

a. What is the incidence/prevalence of the target condition?
The birth prevalence of fetal aneuploidy is about 1%.

b. What are the sequelae of the condition that are of interest in clinical medicine?
These are described in Chapters 21 and 22.

2 ■ **The Tests**

a. What is the purpose of the tests?
Rapid karyotyping.

b. What is the nature of the tests?
Antenatal testing for fetal aneuploidy is a two-stage process. In the first stage, a risk assessment is performed and non-invasive tests conducted to assign a likelihood of a fetal abnormality being present. When that risk is increased, obstetricians traditionally offer pregnant women a test based on cultured fetal cells. Two new methods allow for the rapid antenatal diagnosis of a chromosome abnormality, fluorescence in situ hybridization (FISH) and quantitative polymerase chain reaction (Q-PCR). In this context, FISH and Q-PCR probes specific for trisomy 21, 18, and 13 and numerical sex chromosomal abnormalities (five-probe configuration) are commonly used.

Continued

■ **Summary—cont'd**

c. *What are the implications of testing?*

1. What does an abnormal test result mean?

   The fetus has one of the chromosomal abnormalities from the panel (trisomy 21, 18, 13 or sex chromosomal abnormalities). No further testing is needed and the woman should be given nondirective genetic counseling and offered pregnancy termination where indicated.

2. What does a normal test result mean?

   A normal test result rules out one or more of the chromosomal abnormalities from the panel. However, a normal test result does not exclude other chromosomal abnormalities. In women at increased risk of chromosomal abnormality—for instance those with abnormal ultrasound findings—conventional karyotyping and counseling should be offered.

d. *What is the cost of testing?*

Depending on the strategy selected, there may be savings of up to 23% or additional costs of 29%.

3 ■ Conclusions and Recommendations

Rapid karyotyping by molecular testing is a promising adjuvant option in testing for fetal aneuploidy. However, molecular testing cannot fully replace conventional karyotyping within a screening program for chromosomal abnormalities.

References

1. Wald NJ, Kennard A, Hackshaw A, et al. Antenatal screening for Down's syndrome [review]. *Health Technol Assess* 1998;2:i–iv.
2. MRC Working Party on Evaluation of Chorionic Villus sampling. MRC Working Party European Trial of Chorionic Villus sampling. *Lancet* 1991;337:1491–1499.
3. Lippman A, Tomkins D, Shime J, et al. Canadian multi-centre randomised trial of chorionic villus sampling and amniocentesis. *Prenat Diag* 1992;12:385–476.
4. Whiteman DAH, Klinger K. Efficiency of rapid in situ hybridization methods for prenatal diagnosis of chromosomal abnormalities causing birth defects. *Am J Hum Genet* 1991;49[Suppl A]:1279.
5. Connor JM, Ferguson-Smith MA. *Essential Medical Genetics*. Oxford: Blackwell, 1993.
6. Roberts E, Ely A, Hulten M, et al. The impact of FISH/PCR technology on routine prenatal diagnosis for chromosome abnormality. *Cytogenet Cell Genet* 1999;85:9–12.

7. Department of Health. *Report of Genetics Research Advisory Group.* London: Department of Health, 1995.

8. Howe D, Gornal R, Wellesley D, et al. Six year survey of screening for Down's syndrome by maternal age and mid-trimester ultrasound scan. *BMJ* 2000;320:606–610.

9. NEQAS. UK national external quality assessment scheme: report for clinical cytogenetics. *Clinical Cytogenet* 1999.

10. Tabor A, Madsen M, Obel E, et al. Randomised controlled trial of genetic amniocentesis in 4606 low-risk women. *Lancet* 1986;i:1287–1293.

11. Slater HR, Bruno DL, Ren H, et al. Rapid, high throughput prenatal detection of aneuploidy using novel quantitative method (MLPA). *J Med Genet* 2003;40:907–912.

12. Armour, JA, Sismani, C, Patsalis, PC, and Cross, G. Measurement of locus copy number by hybridisation with amplifiable probes. *Nucleic Acids Res* 2000;28:605–609.

13. Grimshaw GM, Szczepura A, Hultén M, et al. Evaluation of molecular tests for prenatal diagnosis of chromosome abnormalities. *Health Technol Assess* 2003;7:1–146.

26

Thrombophilia and Pregnancy Complications: Preeclampsia, (Late) Intrauterine Fetal Death, and Thrombosis

Christianne J. M. de Groot

Eric A. P. Steegers

■ What Is the Problem that Requires Screening?

Thrombophilia defines a group of disorders associated with an increased tendency for the development of thrombosis. It may be genetically determined, acquired, or both. Acquired causes include prolonged immobilization, surgery, trauma, previous thrombosis, antiphospholipid antibodies, use of certain hormonal contraceptives, mild to moderate hyperhomocysteinemia, pregnancy, preeclampsia, and the puerperium. Inheritable causes include common gene mutations (Factor V Leiden, prothrombin 20210A allele), rare gene mutations (antithrombin, protein C and S deficiencies), and very rare causes (dysfibrinogenemia) (Table 26–1). Acquired and genetic causes frequently interact, making it difficult to decide which patient to test for an inherited thrombophilia, what tests to perform, and when to order them.[1] In most patients with an inherited thrombophilia, thrombosis is the result of impaired neutralization of thrombin or a failure to control the generation of thrombin. Normal pregnancy is associated with major alterations of hemostasis, including increased concentrations of most clotting factors, decreased concentrations of some natural anticoagulants, and reduced fibrinolytic activity. As pregnancy progresses and into the puerperium, these changes result in a shift of the overall balance toward hypercoagulability. It is, therefore, not surprising that thrombophilias often first manifest clinically in pregnancy.

Successful pregnancy outcome is dependent on normal trophoblast invasion into the uterine vasculature with the development and maintenance of an adequate uteroplacental circulation. Inadequate invasion by the trophoblast and

Table 26–1	**Prevalence of heritable thrombophilias in the general population and the risk of venous thromboembolism**			
Heritable thrombo- philias		**Prevalence "general" population**	**Risk of venous thrombo- embolism (7, 24, 25)**	**Prevalence gestational venous thrombo- embolism (4)**
Common- mutations	Factor V Leiden	2%–15%	Three- to eightfold	30%–50%
	Prothrombin 20210A	2%–6%	Threefold	10%–20%
Rare mutations	Antithrombin deficiency	0.02%	25- to 50-fold	1%–5%
	Protein C deficiency	0.2%–0.4%	10- to 15-fold	1%–5%
	Protein S deficiency	Unknown	Twofold	2%–10%
Very rare causes	TAFI (> 1,220 U/L)		Twofold	
	High factor VIII (> 1,500 U/L)		Fivefold	
	Factor IX (> 1,280 U/L)		2.5-fold	
	Factor XI (> 1,200 U/L)		Twofold	
Complex/ mixed	Hyperhomo- cystinemia (MTHFR 677 TT)	11% (24)		10%–20%

TAFA, thrombin activatable fibrinolysis inhibitor; U/L, units per liter.

damage to the maternal vessels supplying the placenta can impair flow and generate prothrombotic changes in the vessel wall.[2] There is now evidence that abnormalities of the placental vasculature characterized by thrombosis, leading to inadequate uteroplacental circulation, are associated with several poor pregnancy outcomes including preeclampsia, fetal growth restriction, and intrauterine death. However, studies describing the association of thrombophilia with (poor) pregnancy outcome are inconsistent, which may reflect inadequate sample size, inconsistent case definition, potential selective bias, retrospective design, and false-positive test results. In this chapter, we address pregnancy complications potentially associated with thrombophilia including preeclampsia, late fetal death, and thrombosis.

What is the incidence/prevalence of the target condition?

The frequencies of the major inherited thrombophilias vary substantially within healthy populations and among patients with venous thrombosis. The prevalence is higher among healthy whites than Asians and blacks, and among patients with venous thrombosis (also in pregnancy) than in healthy subjects

(Table 26–1). Heritable thrombophilias are present in at least 15% of the Western populations and underlie approximately 50% of episodes of venous thromboembolism in pregnancy.[2] This prevalence is likely to increase as new disorders are discovered. The simultaneous occurrence of several thrombophilias is not rare.[3]

The first three inherited thrombophilias described as risk factors for venous thrombosis were all defects in the anticoagulant pathways: deficiencies in antithrombin, protein C, and protein S. Together, they are found in approximately 15% of families with inherited thrombophilia.[4] All are inherited as autosomal dominant disorders except for protein C deficiency, which is an autosomal recessive disorder. More recently, a genetic risk factor associated with resistance to activated protein C, the factor V Leiden mutation (R506Q)[5] and a genetic risk factor with increased prothrombin (prothrombin 20210A allele or Factor II G20210A mutation[6]) were described. These mutations of genes for procoagulant factors are more prevalent than defects in the anticoagulant pathways. Factor V Leiden accounts for most but not all cases of activated protein C (APC) resistance.[7] Factor V Leiden and prothrombin 20210A mutation together are found in up to 63% of the thrombophilia families.[4]

Hyperhomocystinemia is usually the result of an acquired cause (low intake of folate or vitamins B_6 or B_{12}), and only rarely is it related to the heterozygous cystathionine beta-synthase (CS) mutation and associated with venous and arterial thrombosis. A common variant in the gene for methylene tetrahydrofolate reductase (677 TT MTHFR) is associated with mildly elevated homocysteine levels.

Additional markers of thrombophilia are described implicating disorders of the fibrinolytic system including thrombin activatable fibrinolysis inhibitor (TAFI) and elevated coagulation factors such as factors VIII, IX, and XI. These mutations will not be discussed, because little is known about them in relation to pregnancy complications.

What are the sequelae of the condition that are of interest in clinical medicine?

Preeclampsia. Preeclampsia is defined as hypertension (diastolic blood pressure (≥90 mm Hg) new to pregnancy; manifested after 20 weeks' gestation; associated with proteinuria (>0.3 g per 24-hour period) that resolve after pregnancy. The reported prevalence of pregnancy-related hypertension ranges from 2% to 35% depending on the diagnostic criteria used and the population studied.[8] Severe preeclampsia is defined as hypertension of 160/110 mm Hg or higher or proteinuria above 5 g per 24-hour period or eclampsia or HELLP (hemolysis, elevated liver enzymes, low platelet count syndrome). The association of thrombophilia and preeclampsia is widely reported and supported by the results of a recently published meta-analysis of almost 3,000 women who developed preeclampsia during pregnancy.[9] Although the results of this meta-analysis concluded there was an association between factor V Leiden and preeclampsia (odds ratio [OR], 2.25; 95% confidence interval [CI], 1.50–3.38), the five largest studies in the analysis found no such association (OR, 1.21; 95% CI, 0.84–1.74). Moreover, studies published in 2001 and 2002 also failed to find an association, in stark contrast with earlier studies,[10] and there is a large and statistically significant heterogeneity among the results of different studies. It appears any relationship is modest.

Meta-analysis indicates that there is no association with the prothrombin 20210A allele and preeclampsia (1,400 women) and only weak association with MTHFR C677T homozygosity and *severe* preeclampsia (OR, 2.84; 95% CI, 1.95–4.14).[10]

Intrauterine fetal death. Intrauterine fetal death occurs in approximately 1% of early pregnancies (embryo or fetus < 20 weeks' gestation) and in 0.5% of pregnancies after 20 weeks.[11] In one recent review, a strong association was observed between second/third trimester fetal loss and the presence of factor V Leiden.[12] The OR rose with an increasing number of previous losses and those occurring later in pregnancy. The overall OR for the presence of factor V Leiden for combined second-/third-trimester fetal loss was 1.2 (95% CI, 0.6–2.5), whereas it was 2.8 (95% CI, 1.3–6.2) for third-trimester fetal loss only. The OR was 10.7 (95% CI, 4.0–28.5) for women who experienced two or more fetal losses. Sarig et al.[13] also reported a significant higher percentage of thrombophilia (one or more defects) in women with late pregnancy wastage (> 24 weeks' gestation). Likewise, Martinelli et al.[14] observed that both factor V Leiden and factor II mutations are associated with a tripling of the risk for a late fetal loss. In contrast, others find no association between factor V Leiden or factor II mutations and late fetal loss[15] defined as 27 weeks' gestation after excluding women with severe hypertensive disorders.[16] More convincingly, Völzke et al.[17] were unable to demonstrate in a population-based sample any association between factor V Leiden and late fetal loss (> 28 weeks' gestation). Women with protein C or S deficiency have an increased risk of fetal loss (after 28 weeks[18,19]). The risk of fetal loss is even greater for women with an antithrombin deficiency and in those with combined defects (OR 5.2 [95% CI, 1.5–18.1], and OR 14.3 [95% CI, 2.4–86], respectively).[18]

Unexplained fetal loss is not associated with a mutation in the *MTHFR* gene.[11,19]

Thrombosis. While thrombosis is the greatest, single cause of maternal death in many developed countries, most thromboembolic events during pregnancy are not fatal. However, these nonfatal events are responsible for long-term morbidity.[20] The incidence of thromboembolism in one retrospective study of 72,201 deliveries was 0.74/1,000 pregnancy years, which is about eight times that of nonpregnant women of the same age range.[21] The risk of venous thrombosis in the puerperium is further increased about 25 times (2.50/1,000 puerperal years) and is strongly associated with cesarean delivery.

The risk of venous thromboembolism during pregnancy and puerperium depends on the type of thrombophilia and presence of additional risk factors. The risk of thromboembolism in antithrombin-deficient pregnant women is about 32% to 50% absent anticoagulant therapy, whereas the risk is lower in women with a protein C or S deficiency, 3% to 10% and 0% to -6%, respectively.[22,23] In these retrospective studies, women were either the probands or relatives of the probands, and they were included regardless of whether they had a previous thrombosis before pregnancy. Therefore, the calculated risks of thrombosis might be overestimated.[24] Despite the commonality of factor V Leiden, the actual risk of thromboembolism in asymptomatic pregnant women is low (0.2%).[25] In contrast, the asymptomatic pregnant carrier of the prothrombin mutation may have a clotting risk of 0.5%.[25]

The contribution of hyperhomocystinemia to thromboembolic events during pregnancy is unclear.[22] The pregnancy-related risk of thrombosis for combined factor V Leiden and prothrombin heterozygous mutations or homozygous factor V Leiden mutation has been studied in small groups; it is higher than in normal subjects or heterozygous patients.[24] In 21 women with both mutations, the relative risk (RR) was 9.2 (95% CI, 0.8–103) and for those homozygous for factor V Leiden, 41.3 (95% CI, 4.1–420).

■ The Tests

What is the purpose of the tests?

Detection of women at increased risk of venous thrombosis and the related complications of aberrant placental implantation.

What is the nature of the tests?

Both specific functional and/or immunologic tests are used for the detection of antithrombin, protein C, and protein S deficiencies. These genetic defects are too heterogeneous to seriously consider genetic testing as a routine diagnostic procedure. Over 120, 160, and 130 mutations have been described for antithrombin, protein C, and protein S, respectively.[1] In contrast, factor V Leiden and prothrombin mutations are always associated with the same genetic defect. Factor V causes thrombosis via the intermediate phenotype of APC resistance. This intermediate phenotype reflects the mutations effect on one of the cleavage sites in factor V. APC resistance is the poor anticoagulant response of plasma to addition of APC.

Hyperhomocystinemia is a graded risk factor, with the risk rising 40% for every 5-fmol/L increase in homocysteine.[26] These characteristics make homocysteine a relevant laboratory marker. Measurements of homocysteine before and after a methionine load increase the detection of metabolic abnormalities, although such provocative testing is more complex and costly.[27]

What are the implications of testing?

What does an abnormal test result mean? Antithrombin-deficient women have a higher incidence of pregnancy-related thrombosis than either protein C– or S–deficient women.[23] Decreased antithrombin activity, however, can also result from hepatic disease, acute use of heparin, disseminated intravascular coagulation (including preeclampsia), and nephrotic syndrome.[1] These patients are also at increased risk of thrombosis. Due to the nature of the test for protein C and S deficiency, arbitrary cutoff points are used, resulting in substantial percentages of false-positive and false-negative diagnoses. Second, vitamin K deficiency, hepatic disease, treatment with oral anticoagulants or oral contraceptives, pregnancy itself, and the presence of autoantibodies against protein C and S, respectively, decrease protein C and S concentrations. Although these patients also are at increased risk of thrombosis, the cause is acquired and not genetic. As a result, an abnormal test result during pregnancy may not necessarily reflect a genetic defect, whereas a normal result will rule it out.

Based on case–control studies, the risk of deep venous thrombosis in non-pregnant individuals appears increased five- to tenfold in heterozygous carriers of factor V Leiden, and some 80-fold in affected homozygotes.[28] Heterozygotes for the prothrombin 20210A allele have a two- to fivefold increase in thrombosis risk compared to unaffected subjects.[27]

A major clinical problem is that deficiencies in antithrombin, protein C, and protein S can coexist with other genetic abnormalities, synergistically increasing the risk of a venous thromboembolic event. For example, a nonpregnant person with an antithrombin deficiency alone has a 57% lifetime risk of thromboembolism, which increases up to 92% when combined with factor V Leiden.[27]

Women with antithrombin deficiency, who are homozygous for factor V Leiden or prothrombin mutation, or have a combined defect (factor V Leiden and prothrombin mutation), are at very high risk of thromboembolic events and require thromboprophylaxis throughout pregnancy and at least 6 weeks postpartum, even if they are asymptomatic. Women with or without a lesser thrombogenic, inherited thrombophilia but who experience a venous thrombotic event during pregnancy require anticoagulant therapy for the remainder of pregnancy and at least 6 weeks postpartum. For women with a lesser thrombophilia but no history of either a venous thrombosis or an adverse pregnancy outcome have a less than 1% risk of thrombosis and do not need thromboprophylaxis during pregnancy. Postpartum prophylaxis is, however, justified. There is no consensus regarding the treatment of a woman with a lesser thrombophilia and a history of an adverse pregnancy outcome. Therefore, thromboprophylaxis is not recommended in this circumstance and will not be until randomized trials have provided evidence. If hyperhomocystinemia is the sole coagulation defect, the woman should be placed on folic acid, vitamin B_6 or B_{12}, and supplementation. Which vitamins and dosages should be advised before and throughout pregnancy depends on the vitamin profile and the result of the methionine-loading test. Some investigators suggest the doses contained in the average prenatal vitamin supplement are adequate.

What does a normal test result mean? Women with a history of thrombosis outside of pregnancy, unassociated with identifiable or transient factors (e.g. immobilization after trauma), and who have a negative thrombophilia workup are unlikely to experience a recurrence. If none of the tests noted in "The Tests" are abnormal in a woman with a family history of venous thrombosis (first-degree relatives), it is reasonable to search for uncommon genetic coagulation defects such as dysfibrinogenemia (a normal or low fibrinogen level but a prolonged thrombin time, more than 20 mutations), increased factor IX or XI activities or an unidentified thrombophilia factor.[1] It is also possible that minor, undiscovered thrombophilias account for some cases of thromboses that occur in the absence of an identifiable, transient event.

What is the cost of testing?

The costs of thrombophilia detection are described in Table 26–2.

■ Conclusions and Recommendations

Fifty percent of women with a medical or family history of thrombosis have an identifiable thrombophilia and should be offered thrombophilia counseling and testing. Women who are compound heterozygotes are at especially high risk for a thrombotic event during pregnancy and the puerperium. The validity of other indications for screening unique to pregnancy is presently less clear. Because the results of these relatively small, poorly controlled studies are often conflicting, routine screening of women with poor pregnancy outcome including (severe) preeclampsia and intrauterine fetal death is not recommended and should be reserved for research purposes. After clear associations are established, randomized trials should be conducted to evaluate the effectiveness of thromboprophylaxis. Routine screening in the clinical setting can only be recommended if these interventions appear effective.

In the meantime, the optimal management of a pregnant women with a thrombophilia is based on expert opinion only. Until other evidence is available, we recommend women considered at very high risk of venous thromboembolism and pulmonary embolism, including those with antithrombin

Table 26–2 Costs and assay method of heritable, acquired, or both thrombophilias

Heritable	Costs, euros	Assay
Antithrombin deficiency	11.50	Activity
Protein C deficiency	23.00	Activity
Protein S deficiency	11.50	Activity
Factor V Leiden	11.50	DNA
Prothrombin 20210A	11.50	DNA
Complex/mixed		
Hyperhomocystinemia	23.00	Homocysteine levels ± DNA

deficiencies and thrombosis in their current pregnancy, use anticoagulation and antiembolic stockings throughout pregnancy and until at least 6 weeks postpartum. Women homozygous for factor V Leiden or prothrombin mutation or those with combined thrombophilias are considered high risk. Some clinicians may choose to initiate thromboprophylaxis at 24 weeks' gestation; however, we recommend using thromboprophylaxis with daily low-molecular–weight heparin (LMWH). from early pregnancy onward, up to at least 6 weeks postpartum.[21] Additional risk factors must be taken into account such as history of venous thrombosis, age of the mother, and immobilization during pregnancy.

For all women with thrombophilia and history of thrombosis, we recommend thromboprophylaxis for at least 6 weeks postpartum using (LMWH). In women with history of more than one personal thrombosis, with or without thrombophilia, we recommend thromboprophylaxis during pregnancy and at least 6 weeks postpartum. We recommend that women with thrombophilia (excluding those with antithrombin deficiency, homozygous for factor V Leiden, and/or prothrombin mutation or a combination of these mutations) but *no* personal history of thrombosis use thromboprophylaxis only postpartum. Breast feeding is compatible with LMWH.

■ Summary

1 ■ What Is the Problem that Requires Screening?

Inherited thrombophilia defines a group of disorders associated with an increased tendency to develop thrombosis. Pregnancy is an acquired state of hypercoagulability, and thrombophilias often manifest clinically (as thrombosis) during pregnancy. It is may be associated with poor pregnancy outcome.

a. What is the incidence/prevalence of the target condition?

Heritable thrombophilias are present in 50% of women with venous thromboembolism in pregnancy in the Western population.

b. What are the sequelae of the condition that are of interest in clinical medicine?

Preeclampsia. Preeclampsia is a pregnancy-specific disorder manifested by hypertension and proteinuria. The reported prevalence of pregnancy related hypertension ranges from 2%

Continued

to 35%. Evidence of a consistent, large effect of the factor V Leiden or prothrombin mutations on the risk of preeclampsia is lacking.

Intrauterine fetal death. Intrauterine fetal death rate occurs in approximately 0.5% of pregnancies after 20 weeks. Evidence of a consistent, large effect of thrombophilia on the risk of intrauterine fetal death is lacking.

Thrombosis. The risk of thromboembolism is about eight times higher in pregnancy (1%) than outside of pregnancy and is even further enhanced (about 25 times) in the puerperium. The risk of venous thromboembolism during pregnancy and puerperium depends on the type of thrombophilia and presence of additional risk factors. Despite the commonality of factor V Leiden, the actual risk of thromboembolism in asymptomatic pregnant women is low (0.2%).

2 ■ The Tests

a. What is the purpose of the tests?

To identify pregnancies at increased risk of venous thrombosis.

b. What is the nature of the tests?

Antithrombin, protein C, and protein S deficiencies are identified by specific and/or immunologic tests. Factor V Leiden and prothrombin mutations are single gene mutations.

c. What are the implications of testing?

1. What does an abnormal test result mean?

Due to the nature of the tests for antithrombin, protein C, and protein S deficiencies, an abnormal result obtained from testing during pregnancy or during periods of certain medication use (such as oral contraceptives) may not necessarily reflect a genetic defect. In contrast, carriers of the factor V Leiden and prothrombin allele mutations have an increased risk of thrombosis. Women considered at very high risk of venous thromboembolism include those with antithrombin deficiencies, homozygous for factor V Leiden mutation, and/or prothrombin mutation.

2. What does a normal test result mean?

A normal test rules out a known genetic defect associated with hypercoagulability.

d. What is the cost of testing?

The cost of combined testing of most common inherited thrombophilias is about 70 euros per test.

3 ■ Conclusions and Recommendations

Women with a medical or family history of thrombosis should be offered thrombophilia counseling and testing. The validity of other indications unique to pregnancy is presently less clear. As the results of these relatively small and poorly controlled studies are often conflicting, the routine testing of women with poor pregnancy outcome including (severe) preeclampsia and intrauterine fetal death is not recommended and should be reserved for research purposes. The following are recommendations:

Women with a history of thrombosis (outside of pregnancy), but *no* thrombophilia → thromboprophylaxis postpartum.

Women with antithrombin deficiency, homozygous for factor V Leiden and/or prothrombin mutation or a combination of these mutations → thromboprophylaxis during pregnancy and postpartum.

Women with a history of thrombosis, less thrombophilic factors → thromboprophylaxis postpartum.

Women with a history of recurrent thrombosis or during the current pregnancy *with or without* thrombophilia → thromboprophylaxis during pregnancy and postpartum.

Additional risk factors must be taken into account such as history of venous thrombosis, age of the mother, and immobilization during pregnancy

References

1. Seligsohn U, Lubetsky A. Genetic susceptibility to venous thrombosis. *N Engl J Med* 2001;344:1222–1231.
2. Greer IA. Thrombophilia: implications for pregnancy outcome. *Thromb Res* 2003;109:73–81.
3. Caprini JA, Glase CJ, Anderson CB, etal. Laboratory markers in the diagnosis of venous thromboembolism. *Circulation* 2004;109[Suppl 1]:I4–I8.
4. Bertina RM. Factor V Leiden and other coagulation factor mutations affecting thrombotic risk. *Clin Chem* 1997;43:1678–1683.

5. Bertina RM, Koeleman BP, Koster T, et al. Mutation in blood coagulation factor V associated with resistance to activated protein C. *Nature* 1994;369:64–67.
6. Poort SR, Rosendaal FR, Reitsma PH, et al. A common genetic variation in the 3'-untranslated region of the prothrombin gene is associated with elevated plasma prothrombin levels and an increase in venous thrombosis. *Blood* 1996;88:3698–3703.
7. Tripodi A, Mannucci PM. Laboratory investigation of thrombophilia. *Clin Chem* 2001;47:1597–1606.
8. Dekker GA. Blood pressure measurement in antenatal care. In: Wildschut HIJ, Weiner CP, Peters TJ, eds,. *When to Screen in Obstetrics and Gynecology*. London: Saunders, 1996:154–162.
9. Kosmas IP, Tatsioni A, Ioannidis JP. Association of Leiden mutation in factor V gene with hypertension in pregnancy and pre-eclampsia: a meta-analysis. *J Hypertens* 2003;21:1221–1228.
10. Morrison ER, Miedzybrodzka ZH, Campbell DM, et al. Prothrombotic genotypes are not associated with pre-eclampsia and gestational hypertension: results from a large population-based study and systematic review. *Thromb Haemost* 2002;87:779–785.
11. Martinelli I, Taioli E, Cetin I, et al. Mutations in coagulation factors in women with unexplained late fetal loss. *N Engl J Med* 2000;343:1015.
12. Dudding TE, Attia J. The association between adverse pregnancy outcomes and maternal factor V Leiden genotype: a meta-analysis. *Thromb Haemost* 2004;91:700–711.
13. Sarig G, Younis JS, Hoffman R, et al. Thrombophilia is common in women with idiopathic pregnancy loss and is associated with late pregnancy wastage. *Fertil Steril* 2002;77:342–347.
14. Martinelli I, Taioli E, Cetin I, et al. Mutations in coagulation factors in women with unexplained late fetal loss. *N Engl J Med* 2000;343:1015–1018.
15. Hefler L, Jirecek S, Heim K, et al. Genetic polymorphisms associated with thrombophilia and vascular disease in women with unexplained late intrauterine fetal death: a multicenter study. *J Soc Gynecol Investig* 2004;11:42–44.
16. Many A, Elad R, Yaron Y, et al. Third-trimester unexplained intrauterine fetal death is associated with inherited thrombophilia. *Obstet Gynecol* 2000;99:684–687.
17. Völzke H, Grimm R, Robinson DM, et al. Factor V Leiden and the risk of stillbirth in a German population. *Thromb Haemost* 2003;90:429–433.
18. Preston FE, Rosendaal FR, Walker ID, et al. Increased fetal loss in women with heritable thrombophilia. *Lancet* 1996;348:913–916.
19. Alfirevic Z, Roberts D, Martlew V. How strong is the association between maternal thrombophilia and adverse pregnancy outcome? A systematic review. *Eur J Obstet Gynecol Reprod Biol* 2002;101:6–14.
20. Gates S. Thromboembolic disease in pregnancy. *Curr Opin Obstet Gynecol* 2000;12:117–122.
21. McColl MD, Walker ID, Greer IA. The role of inherited thrombophilia in venous thromboembolism associated with pregnancy. *Br J Obstet Gynaecol* 1999;106:756–766.
22. Eldor A. Thrombophilia, thrombosis and pregnancy. *Thromb Haemost* 2001;86:104–111.
23. Greer IA. Thrombosis in pregnancy: maternal and fetal issues. *Lancet* 1999;353:1258–1265.
24. Conard J, Horellou MH, Samama MM. Inherited thrombophilia and gestational venous thromboembolism. *Semin Thromb Hemost* 2003;29:131–142.
25. Lockwood CJ. Inherited thrombophilias in pregnant patients: detection and treatment paradigm. *Obstet Gynecol* 2002;99:333–341.
26. Tripodi A, Mannucci PM. Laboratory investigation of thrombophilia. *Clin Chem* 2001;47:1597–1606.
27. Murin S, Marelich GP, Arroliga AC, et al. Hereditary thrombophilia and venous thromboembolism. *Am J Respir Crit Care Med* 1998;158:1369–1373.
28. van der Meer FJ, Koster T, et al. The Leiden Thrombophilia Study (LETS). *Thromb Haemost* 1997;78:631–635.

Screening for Autoimmune Diseases in Pregnancy

Lorin Lakasing

Catherine Williamson

Autoimmune diseases are usually most prevalent in women of childbearing age. The most common autoimmune disease during pregnancy is insulin dependent diabetes mellitus (see related material in Chapter 28). Other relatively common autoimmune conditions include thyroid disorders, systemic lupus erythematosus, and antiphospholipid syndrome. Less common conditions include autoimmune thrombocytopenia, rheumatoid arthritis, myasthenia gravis, and Addison's disease.

In general, the diagnosis of organ-specific autoimmune disorders (e.g., thyroid disease) and the monitoring of treatment are based on specific biochemical markers of organ function (e.g., serum thyroid hormone concentrations). In these conditions, the presence of autoantibodies simply confirms the autoimmune etiology of the disease. In non–organ-specific disease (e.g., systemic lupus erythematosus or antiphospholipid syndrome), the diagnosis relies on clinical features and the persistent presence of autoantibodies. Disease monitoring is largely based on clinical signs and symptoms, although less specific serologic markers such as complement may have a role. Thus, although the presence of autoantibodies can confirm the clinical suspicion of an autoimmune disease, autoantibodies are frequently present in asymptomatic individuals.[1] Screening for autoimmune diseases by autoantibody testing is fraught with difficulty, as 50% of individuals who subsequently develop autoimmune disease have autoantibodies present a median of 4.5 years before the clinical onset.[2] Although it has been suggested that quantification of autoantibodies can be used to monitor disease activity,[3] this is not always the case as autoantibodies vary greatly in their tissue affinity. Therefore, once the disease has been diagnosed, serial quantitative measurements of autoantibody concentrations are of little clinical value.[4] Finally, autoimmune diseases tend to coexist within individuals and in families. Thus, if a patient with one autoimmune condition develops clinical features that suggest another autoimmune disease, repeat autoantibody screening should be considered.

■ What Is the Problem that Requires Screening?

Thyroid disease.

Maternal hyper- or hypothyroidism, fetal and neonatal thyroid dysfunction (congenital thyroid disease secondary to either placental transfer of maternal autoantibodies or maternal treatment with antithyroid medication), and maternal postpartum thyroiditis.

What is the incidence / prevalence of the target condition?
Hyperthyroidism.

Hyperthyroidism affects 1/500 pregnant women.[5] Approximately half have a positive family history, and over 90% have Graves disease (thyroid-stimulating hormone [TSH] receptor–stimulating antibodies).

What are the sequelae of the condition that are of interest in clinical medicine?

Graves disease is characterized by clinical findings suggestive of hyperthyroidism and usually progressive exophthalmos. It is typically most active during the first trimester and puerperium,[6] with remission during the second and third trimesters allowing a reduction or even the discontinuation of maternal antithyroid medication in up to 30% of cases.[7] The frequency of complications during pregnancy is related to disease control with maternal hypertension, preterm birth, fetal growth restriction, and stillbirth being more common among women with inadequately treated disease either before or during pregnancy.[8] Thyroid storm is rare and usually occurs in women with untreated disease. This condition can cause congestive heart failure and pulmonary edema, and is life threatening unless immediate control is achieved using antithyroid medication, iodine, corticosteroids, beta-blockers, diuretics, and antiarrhythmic medications as required.

The fetus and neonate of women with Graves disease are at risk of thyroid dysfunction secondary to either transplacental transfer of maternal TSH receptor–stimulating antibodies (TSiG) or as a result of maternal treatment with antithyroid medication. Fetal thyrotoxicosis secondary to maternal autoantibodies is rare, although some studies report rates as high as 17% in neonates born to affected women.[9] This is likely to represent a reporting bias; a more realistic estimate is likely closer to 1%. Fetal thyrotoxicosis may present clinically with fetal tachycardia, intrauterine growth restriction, fetal goiter, and hydrops.[9] In contrast to fetal thyrotoxicosis, transient fetal/neonatal hyperthyroidism is more common affecting between 2% and 10%.[10] Both conditions are treated with commonly used antithyroid drugs (carbimazole and propylthiouracil) which cross the placenta and do not appear teratogenic. The previously reported association between carbimazole and aplasia cutis of the fetal scalp is not supported by more recent neonatal outcome data.[11,12] Fetal over treatment is common—biochemical hypothyroidism is detected in 10% to 20% of cases.[13] The long-term impact of sustained fetal hypothyroidism associated with maternal treatment remains unclear. Minor degrees of neonatal goiter occur in fewer than 2%, but this usually resolves within a few days and does not appear to have any acute clinical consequences.[13] Occasionally, large fetal goiters occur, and if undetected can cause fetal heart failure, death, obstructed labor and neonatal respiratory compromise.

■ The Tests

What is the purpose of the tests?

Blood tests and ultrasound assessment of the fetus, either alone or in combination with the following:

- Make the *de novo* diagnosis of maternal hyperthyroidism in pregnancy
- Monitor antithyroid medication in pregnancy and the puerperium
- Confirm that the disease is autoimmune in origin
- Diagnose fetal goiter
- Monitor fetal response to maternal medication
- Diagnose and monitor treatment of neonatal thyroid disorders

What is the nature of the tests?

Standard thyroid function tests are performed for the diagnosis of maternal and neonatal thyroid disease and for the monitoring treatment. These include TSH, free thyroxine (fT_4) and occasionally free triiodothyronine (fT_3). It is important not to use total T_4 or T_3 concentrations as the increased liver production of thyroid-binding globulin during pregnancy causes a significant increase in these values. These tests are enzyme-linked immunoassays (ELISAs), and most clinical laboratories have standard reference ranges for the nonpregnant population. Some maternity units have constructed pregnancy- and gestation-specific ranges due to small but potentially significant fluctuations in their concentrations during normal pregnancy. Maternal serum TSH concentrations decrease in early pregnancy as a result human chorionic gonadotrophin secretion. Later, there is a reduction in T_4 secretion and an increase in maternal TSH concentrations in the second and third trimesters due to positive feedback.

What are the implications of testing?

What does an abnormal test result mean? Abnormal thyroid function tests can confirm the diagnosis or suboptimal management of maternal hyperthyroidism. Medication may then be altered accordingly, and the testing repeated frequently to monitor the impact of therapeutic changes. It is important to note that while fT_3 and fT_4 concentrations change rapidly in response to changes in treatment, TSH concentrations may take weeks to change.[14] Inconsistent results may reflect poor compliance with medication, and borderline results may need to be repeated at close intervals. Biochemical test results should always be interpreted in light of the clinical history and examination.

For de novo diagnoses of maternal hyperthyroidism in pregnancy, propylthiouracil is the first line therapy since less placental transfer occurs compared to carbimazole. However, women stable on carbimazole therapy should not be changed to propylthiouracil. Radioiodine is contraindicated and surgery only very rarely necessary during pregnancy.

The presence of fetal/neonatal disease is strongly associated with the presence of maternal autoantibodies.[9] Thus, continued presence of maternal thyroid autoantibodies should be sought if not recently tested. Should the woman test negative, the fetus and neonate are at greatly reduced risk of maternal autoantibody mediated disease, and the level of fetal and neonatal surveillance can be decreased. Furthermore, maternal thyroid autoantibody screening is used to distinguish Graves disease from other causes of abnormal thyroid function tests in pregnancy (e.g., toxic nodular goiter, nonimmune thyroiditis, and in some cases of hyperemesis gravidarum).

What does a normal test result mean? A normal test result virtually eliminates the possibility of thyroid disease in pregnancy. Normal tests confirm the adequacy of treatment. If a pregnant woman is clinically euthyroid and has normal biochemistry, testing at 6- to 8-week intervals during pregnancy is usually sufficient. Of course, if there is any change in medication (e.g., reducing or discontinuing antithyroid medication), it is prudent to repeat the thyroid function tests 3 to 4 weeks later and to encourage the patient to report any symptoms early. A woman previously treated for Graves disease may be euthyroid, but still producing TSiG. The fetuses of these women are at risk of hyperthyroidism.

What is the Cost of Testing?

A maternal thyroid autoantibody screen currently costs approximately $28, and thyroid function tests (TSH, fT_4 and fT_3) cost approximately $17. Obstetric ultrasound examination costs approximately $250 per scan.

■ Conclusions and Recommendations

There is no need to routinely screen for maternal hyperthyroidism preconceptually or during pregnancy. Subclinical disease is uncommon, and adverse pregnancy outcome reflects mainly in undertreated disease. Women presenting with symptoms suggestive of hyperthyroidism and evolving exophthalmos at any time during pregnancy should be tested, and those with established disease should have regular thyroid function testing to monitor the adequacy of treatment.

Routine antenatal screening for fetal thyroid disease in women with hyperthyroidism who are TRH receptor–antibody positive is typically performed by ultrasound examination in the second trimester looking for goiter, and subsequent careful attention to the fetal heart rate during antenatal checks at later gestations.

The adequacy of this approach is unclear. In the event of fetal goiter, thyroid gland vascularity can be assessed by Doppler ultrasound examination.[15,16] Cordocentesis is advocated by some to determine fetal thyroid status before treatment.[17] Fetal thyrotoxicosis secondary to maternal autoantibodies is treated by increasing maternal antithyroid medication, and fetal hypothyroidism secondary to maternal antithyroid medication treated with intrauterine thyroid hormone administration.[18]

Neonatal thyroid disorders are routinely screened for in most developed countries 5 to 10 days postnatally. Treatment of neonatal thyrotoxicosis is symptom relief until circulating maternal autoantibodies disappear.

■ Summary

1 ■ **What Is the Problem that Requires Screening?**

Maternal hyperthyroidism, usually secondary to Graves disease.

a. What is the incidence/prevalence of the target condition?
1/500 pregnant women, of whom approximately half have a family history

b. What are the sequelae of the condition that are of interest in clinical medicine?
Sequelae reflect the severity of disease and the adequacy of treatment. Poorly controlled hyperthyroidism can lead to thyroid storm and substantial fetal thyroid abnormalities.

2 ■ **The Tests**

a. What is the purpose of the tests?
To identify and monitor abnormalities of thyroid function.

b. What is the nature of the tests?
The measurement of TSH, free T_4, and occasionally free T_3 using ELISA.

c. What are the implications of testing?
1. What does an abnormal test result mean?
Either identifies maternal hyperthyroidism or confirms suboptimal management of known disease.

Continued

■ **Summary—cont'd**

2. What does a normal test result mean?
   Either excludes disease or confirms the adequacy of treatment.

d. ***What is the cost of testing?***
   Maternal tests range between $50 and 100; fetal tests depend whether they are sonographic or invasive.

3 ■ **Conclusions and Recommendations**

Presently, there is no indication for the routine screening of pregnant women for hyperthyroidism.

■ What Is the Problem that Requires Screening?

Hypothyroidism.

What is the incidence / prevalence of the target condition?

Hypothyroidism affects approximately 1% of pregnant women.[19] Most cases of primary hypothyroidism are secondary to Hashimoto thyroiditis (thyroid peroxidase or antithyroglobulin autoantibodies), although women who previously had hyperthyroidism and were treated with radioiodine or thyroidectomy make a substantial contribution to the total.

What are the sequelae of the condition that are of interest in clinical medicine?

Although the older medical literature reported an association between maternal hypothyroidism and an increased risk of a adverse pregnancy outcomes including miscarriage,[20] congenital anomalies, hypertension, preterm delivery, fetal growth restriction, maternal anemia, and postpartum haemorrhage,[21] it is now clear appropriately treated maternal hypothyroidism is not associated with such complications. Two remaining areas of debate are the potential associations between thyroid peroxidase and antithyroglobulin autoantibodies with miscarriage[22] and gestational hypertension.[23]

Maternal thyroid peroxidase and antithyroglobulin autoantibodies cross the placenta but do not appear to affect fetal or neonatal thyroid function.[24] Congenital hypothyroidism is relatively common, affecting 1/3,500 newborns, and most are unrelated to maternal thyroid disease. More recently, the possibility that maternal hypothyroidism is associated with neurodevelopmental delay in older children has generated much interest. Adequate thyroid hormone is essential for normal fetal brain development,[25] and the association between severe untreated maternal hypothyroidism and reduced intelligence quotient (IQ) in children has been recognized for many decades.[26,27] However, even sub-clinical cases of maternal hypothyroidism (elevated TSH detected retrospectively in screened mid-trimester maternal serum samples) have were associated with neurodevelopmental delay and IQ scores 7 points lower than controls in 7- to 9-year-old children.[28] Other studies report similar associations between hitherto unrecognized or suboptimally treated hypothyroidism and neurodevelopmental delay in children,[29] and one prospectively conducted study suggested that optimizing maternal treatment with replacement thyroxine based on biochemical parameters in early gestation may reduce the incidence of impaired infant development.[30] Not surprisingly, these studies have prompted debate regarding screening and treatment of maternal biochemical hypothyroidism in early pregnancy or even pre-conceptually. The debate continues.

■ The Tests

What is the purpose of the tests?

Testing is used to make the de novo diagnosis of hypothyroidism in pregnancy and to monitor T_4 replacement in pregnancy and the puerperium

What is the nature of the tests?

Standard maternal thyroid function tests are performed as previously described. If a woman has hypothyroidism as a result of surgery or radioiodine therapy for Graves disease, an autoantibody screen should be obtained as the fetus may be as risk of autoimmune antibody mediated thyrotoxicosis if she still has TRH receptor stimulating autoantibodies.[31]

What are the implications of testing?

What does an abnormal test result mean? Abnormal thyroid function tests can confirm the diagnosis or identify suboptimal management of maternal hypothyroidism. T_4 replacement is the mainstay of treatment, and although there are many reports of increased T_4 requirements during gestation,[32] change in the T_4 dosage is rarely necessary in hypothyroid women well controlled pre-conceptually and in early pregnancy.

What does a normal test result mean? A normal test rules out hypothyroidism or confirms the adequate treatment of maternal hypothyroidism. If clinically euthyroid, testing need be repeated only once per trimester. Thyroid function tests should be repeated 3 to 4 weeks after any change in the T_4 dose.

What is the cost of testing?

The costs of thyroid antibody testing and thyroid functions tests are as previously noted (see page 282).

■ Conclusions and Recommendations

The need for routine preconceptual or early antenatal screening for maternal hypothyroidism has become controversial since its reported association with a decreased IQ in children born to affected mothers. Proponents of routine population-based antenatal screening have compelling arguments relating to the high prevalence of the condition, the high incidence of subclinical or suboptimally treated disease, the potentially serious effects on neurodevelopment in young children, and the eminently treatable nature of the condition.[33] A similar argument has been made for the screening of fetuses of women with Graves disease treated with antithyroid medications. However, careful analysis of the literature relating to child neurodevelopment highlight other contributory factors,[29] and in some cases problems occur in women who are already diagnosed but inadequately treated.[28] Thus it remains unclear whether the cost of implementing a screening program can be justified. Data from larger studies and from populations where such programs have been implemented are eagerly awaited.

There is no need to screen the fetus for thyroid dysfunction in cases of maternal hypothyroidism except when the mother is TRH receptor autoantibody positive as a result of previous Graves disease. All neonates are screened for congenital hypothyroidism and treated with replacement T_4 if required.

■ Summary

1 ■ What Is the Problem that Requires Screening?
Maternal hypothyroidism.

a. *What is the incidence/prevalence of the target condition?*
One percent of pregnant women.

b. *What are the sequelae of the condition that are of interest in clinical medicine?*

Sequelae reflect the severity of disease and the adequacy of treatment. There is growing evidence that maternal hypothyroidism is associated with compromised neurodevelopment of the child.

2 ■ The Tests

a. *What is the purpose of the tests?*

To identify and monitor abnormalities of thyroid function.

b. *What is the nature of the tests?*

The measurement of TSH, free T_4, and occasionally free T_3 using ELISA.

c. *What are the implications of testing?*

1. What does an abnormal test result mean?

Either identifies maternal hypothyroidism or confirms suboptimal management of known disease.

2. What does a normal test result mean?

Either excludes disease or confirms the adequacy of treatment.

d. *What is the cost of testing?*

Maternal tests range between $50 and $100.

3 ■ Conclusions and Recommendations

It remains unclear whether the cost of implementing a screening program for maternal hypothyroidism can be justified.

■ What Is the Problem that Requires Screening?

Postpartum thyroiditis.

What is the incidence / prevalence of the target condition?

This is a transient, subacute autoimmune condition with a wide variation in reported prevalence. Estimates range from 1.1% to 16.7% with a mean of 7.5%.[34]

What are the sequelae of the condition that are of interest in clinical medicine?

The clinical features are often vague including lethargy, irritability, agitation, amnesia, and generalized aches and pains. Postpartum thyroiditis often goes unrecognized. Typically, there are three phases: a thyrotoxic phase 1 to 3 months after delivery (destruction of thyroid tissue), a hypothyroid phase 3 to 8 months after delivery, and finally a euthyroid phase approximately 1 year after delivery. Although the condition is rarely serious, there is a 70% recurrence risk in future pregnancies[35] and about 5% develop permanent hypothyroidism annually.[36]

■ The Tests

What is the purpose of the tests?

Testing is used to diagnose maternal disease and to monitor T_4 replacement in the puerperium if necessary.

What is the nature of the tests?

Standard maternal thyroid function tests are performed as previously described.

What are the implications of testing?

What does an abnormal test result mean? This confirms maternal thyroid dysfunction in the puerperium. Treatment is begun if the woman is symptomatic, but it is likely the need for replacement will be temporary. Close surveillance is required so that treatment is not unnecessarily prolonged.

What does a normal test result mean? An initially normal test result 4 to 6 weeks postpartum may need to be repeated if the patient subsequently develops symptoms suggestive of hypothyroidism as the time course is variable. Postpartum thyroiditis is much more likely to occur in women who are screen positive for thyroid autoantibodies.

What is the cost of testing?

The costs of thyroid antibody testing and thyroid functions tests are as previously noted.

■ Conclusions and Recommendations

Although routine screening has been proposed,[35] there are no clear diagnostic criteria, many women require no treatment, and there is no evidence that early diagnosis and treatment improves the long-term outcome. Thus, routine postnatal screening is not recommended.[37]

■ Summary

1 ■ What Is the Problem that Requires Screening?

Postpartum thyroiditis.

a. *What is the incidence/prevalence of the target condition?*

Prevalence varies widely; a mean of 7.5% has been observed.

b. *What are the sequelae of the condition that are of interest in clinical medicine?*

The condition is rarely serious. Sequelae reflect the severity of disease and the adequacy of treatment.

2 ■ The Tests

a. *What is the purpose of the tests?*

To identify and monitor abnormalities of thyroid function.

b. *What is the nature of the tests?*

The measurement of TSH, free T_4, and occasionally free T_3 using ELISA.

c. *What are the implications of testing?*

1. What does an abnormal test result mean?

   Either identifies maternal hypothyroidism, or confirms suboptimal management of known disease.
2. What does a normal test result mean?

   Either excludes disease or confirms the adequacy of treatment.

d. *What is the cost of testing?*

Maternal tests range between $50 and $100.

3 ■ Conclusions and Recommendations

There is no indication for the routine screening of pregnant women for postpartum thyroiditis.

■ What Is the Problem that Requires Screening?

Systemic lupus erythematosus.

Systemic lupus erythematosus (SLE) with or without secondary antiphospholipid syndrome (APS) and maternal anti-Ro antibody–mediated fetal and neonatal congenital heart block.

What is the incidence / prevalence of the target condition?

SLE occurs in 1/1,000 women with 6% of these having coexistent autoimmune disease, most commonly secondary APS.[38]

What are the sequelae of the condition that are of interest in clinical medicine?

The clinical criteria for SLE are well established.[39] These have been updated to include newer serologic markers such as antiphospholipid antibodies (aPLs).[40] Several studies of pregnant women with SLE report an increased incidence of lupus "flare,."[41,42] especially in the puerperium,[43] although this remains an area of controversy.[44,45] Although cutaneous flares are common and may cause significant maternal discomfort, it is the renal "flares" or lupus nephritis that is associated with adverse pregnancy outcomes. This subgroup of women is at increased risk of miscarriage,[46] preeclampsia, fetal growth restriction, and preterm delivery.[47,48] The women with SLE who do worst are those with coexistent APS, since whether primary or secondary, APS is strongly associated with adverse pregnancy outcome (see APS section).

The presence of certain maternal autoantibodies, in particular anti-Ro (SSA) and, to a lesser extent, anti-La (SSB), are associated with the development of fetal and neonatal lupus syndromes in a minority of infants. Some 30% of women with SLE have these antibodies, but less than 10% of their neonates are affected.[49] The most serious fetal/neonatal condition is complete congenital heart block (CCHB), which occurs in 2% fetuses and can be detected in utero beginning at 18 weeks' gestation. CCHB is permanent and can cause fetal heart failure and death. Preterm birth is relatively common, and 70% of survivors require a pacemaker.[50] Although the recurrence risk was previously thought to be as high as 30%, more recent data indicate the risk is more in the range of 16%.[51] Less serious features of neonatal lupus syndrome include rash, hepatitis, pneumonitis, thrombocytopenia, and hemolysis. These conditions rarely require treatment and disappear during the neonatal period.

■ The Tests

What is the purpose of the test?

The main indications for testing during pregnancy are the following:

- *De novo* diagnosis of SLE in pregnancy
- Screening for "high-risk" subgroups of pregnant women with SLE
- Diagnosis of CCHB

What is the nature of the tests?

Immune serologic tests used in the diagnosis of SLE include antinuclear antibodies (ANAs), anti–double-stranded DNA (anti-dsDNA) antibodies and antibodies to extractable nuclear antigens (ENAs) of which anti-Ro and anti-La antibodies are the most clinically relevant.[38] ANA is detected by indirect immunofluorescence, and though a nonspecific marker of several other autoimmune diseases, is present in over 90% women with SLE. Anti-dsDNA is detected by immunoprecipitation and is more specific for SLE being present in 78% patients. Anti-Ro and anti-La are detected by counter immunoelectrophoresis and are present in 30% women with SLE.

Pregnant women with SLE who are known or considered to have lupus nephritis should undergo renal function testing: maternal serum urea and electrolytes, 24 hour urinary protein excretion, creatinine clearance and urinary albumin: creatinine ratio. Women suspected to have coexistent APS are offered tests for antiphospholipid antibodies as described in the APS section.

What are the implications of testing?

What does an abnormal test result mean? Positive immune serology may confirm the clinical suspicion of SLE and APS. The presence of anti-Ro or anti-La antibodies identifies those pregnancies requiring close fetal and neonatal surveillance. Immune serologic tests cannot be used to monitor maternal disease activity or as a basis to modify therapy. Those aspects of patient management are a matter of clinical judgment and experience. Abnormal maternal renal function tests identify a subgroup of women with SLE at higher risk of pregnancy complications.

What does a normal test result mean? The diagnosis of SLE is strongly weighted toward clinical features, so it is quite possible for seronegative women to fulfill the classification criteria for the disease. Women with negative tests for maternal autoantibodies anti-Ro or anti-La are not at risk of having a child with neonatal lupus syndromes. Similarly, normal renal function tests and a negative aPL screen indicate that these women with SLE are not at increased risk of adverse pregnancy outcome.

What is the cost of testing?

A standard immune serologic screen for the autoantibodies includes ANA at $25, anti-dsDNA at $32, and ENA at $39. Renal function tests include urea and electrolytes at $5, 24-hour urine collection for protein at $13.50, creatinine clearance at $14.00, and urinary albumen: creatinine ratio at $17.50. Obstetric ultrasound examination cost approximately $250 per scan.

■ Conclusions and Recommendations

It is not appropriate to screen for SLE during pregnancy as the condition is relatively rare, the diagnosis is based largely on clinical signs and symptoms, and, in the absence of renal involvement or coexistent APS, the outcome for pregnancy is generally good. However, all women with SLE should be screened for anti-Ro and anti-La antibodies, lupus nephropathy ("baseline" urea and electrolytes), and aPL antibodies, as these factors contribute to the risk of an adverse outcome. Women who test positive for anti-Ro or anti-La should be offered a targeted mid-trimester ultrasound examination of the fetus, including specialist fetal echocardiography and close monitoring of the fetal heart rate at later gestations. It is recommended that fetuses affected by CCHB are followed up by a fetal medicine specialist and delivered in a unit with pediatric cardiology services.

■ Summary

1 ■ What Is the Problem that Requires Screening?

Systemic lupus erythematosus.

a. What is the incidence/prevalence of the target condition?
One per 1,000 women with 6% having coexistent autoimmune disease, most commonly secondary APS.

b. What are the sequelae of the condition that are of interest in clinical medicine?
An increased risk of lupus flare, APS, and fetal congenital heart block. Women with SLE and coexistent APS have the highest risk of an adverse pregnancy outcome.

2 ■ The Tests

a. What is the purpose of the tests?
To identify women with SLE.

b. What is the nature of the tests?
Serologic tests including ANA, anti-dsDNA, and extractible nuclear antigens (anti-Ro, anti-La).

c. What are the implications of testing?

1. What does an abnormal test result mean?

   Positive immune serology may confirm the clinical suspicion of SLE and APS. The presence of anti-Ro or anti-La antibodies identifies those pregnancies requiring close fetal and neonatal surveillance.

2. What does a normal test result mean?

   The diagnosis of SLE is strongly weighted toward clinical features, so it is quite possible for seronegative women to fulfill the classification criteria for the disease.

d. What is the cost of testing?

A standard immune serological screen for the autoantibodies includes ANA at $25, anti-dsDNA at $32, and ENA at $39.

3 ■ Conclusions and Recommendations

It is not appropriate to screen for SLE during pregnancy as the condition is relatively rare, the diagnosis is based largely on clinical signs and symptoms, and in the absence of renal involvement or coexistent APS, the outcome for pregnancy is generally good. All women with SLE should be screened for anti-Ro and anti-La antibodies, lupus nephropathy (baseline urea and electrolytes) and aPL antibodies, as these factors contribute to the risk of an adverse outcome.

■ What Is the Problem that Requires Screening?

Antiphospholipid syndrome.

Maternal APS, which may be either primary or secondary to SLE or another connective tissue diseases.

What is the incidence / prevalence of the target condition?

APS occurs in approximately 1/700 women, although reported detection rates are increasing as clinicians have become more familiar with this condition. One problem estimating the exact prevalence of this condition is that unlike the clinical criteria for the diagnosis that are well defined,[52] the serologic diagnostic criteria vary greatly between units.[53,54] antiphospholipid antibodies are present at low titers in at least 2% of the population, particularly the elderly,[55] and they can be induced by infection, malignancy, stress, and drugs.[56] To overcome these difficulties, repeat testing is recommended at 6- to 8-week intervals, and only individuals with persistently high autoantibody titers are considered to have the disease. Unfortunately, laboratory assays for aPL are not internationally standardized, and despite considerable efforts,[57] different laboratories continue to use different cutoff titers in the categorization of low, moderate, or high levels of autoantibodies.[58] Until this issue is resolved, it is unlikely that the true prevalence of the disease will be established. Recognition of the problem is critical for any balanced interpretation of the literature.

What are the sequelae of the condition that are of interest in clinical medicine?

APS is an autoimmune acquired thrombophilia characterized by a combination of clinical features including arterial or venous thrombosis, thrombocytopenia, recurrent (three or more) first-trimester miscarriages and/or adverse pregnancy outcome, and persistently high titers of aPL antibodies. Pregnancy is a hypercoagulable state and pregnant women with APS are at even higher risk of thrombosis unless thromboprophylaxis or anticoagulation (as appropriate) is adequate.[59–61] Pregnancy may exacerbate preexisting maternal thrombocytopenia, and this may be further compounded by the aspirin and heparin commonly used in these women.

The association between APS and recurrent miscarriage is well known,[62–65] with second-trimester loss being particularly common.[66] The prospective fetal loss rate in primary APS is reported to be 50% to 75%.[67,68] Some studies suggest the loss rate in women with SLE and secondary APS may be as high as 90%,[69,70] although this is likely an overestimate. There is a high incidence of early-onset preeclampsia,[71–74] fetal growth restriction,[75,76] placental abruption,[77] and preterm delivery[78,79] in pregnancies that do not end in miscarriage or fetal loss. Because patients with APS are a heterogeneous group, the incidence of these complications varies greatly between units.[80–83] Mid-trimester uterine artery Doppler may be of some value identifying those women with APS who are likely to develop complications in pregnancy.[84–87] The main therapeutic options include aspirin, heparin, steroids and warfarin.[54]

■ The Tests

What is the purpose of the test?

The indications for testing are de novo diagnosis of APS in pregnancy and identification of the presence or absence of APS in high-prevalence groups (e.g., SLE).

What is the nature of the tests?

The two most common aPL antibodies of clinical significance are anticardiolipin antibodies (aCLs) and lupus anticoagulant (LA). The impact of normal pregnancy on the performance of these tests is poorly studied. Anticardiolipin antibodies are detected by ELISA, and isotype-specific reference sera allow quantification of IgG and IgM concentrations expressed as units of G phospholipid (GPL) and M phospholipid (MPL), respectively, where one unit represents the binding activity of 1 μg/mL of affinity purified aCL antibody. LA is identified in three stages.[88a] The first is the demonstration of an abnormal coagulation screen (either activated partial thromboplastin time [APTT], kaolin clotting time [KCT], or dilute Russell viper venom time [DRVVT]. The second is failure to correct the prolonged coagulation of the patient's plasma upon mixing with normal platelet poor plasma. The third is a confirmatory test demonstrating shortening or correction of the prolonged screening test upon addition of excess phospholipid. Some laboratories add a fourth stage, which involves the positive exclusion of other coagulopathies.

The frequent occurrence of false-positive results in the aCL ELISA hampers its application in identifying APS. One study highlighted some of the pitfalls of aPL antibody testing in clinical practice. The aCL ELISA commercially prepared anti–beta2-gylcoprotein 1 (β2-GP1) and antiphospholipid (APhL) assays were evaluated in the diagnosis of APS in 94 pregnant women who had spontaneous abortion and a group of 177 healthy blood donors. Most sera that were positive in the aCL ELISA were found to be false positives as 93%[27/29] of aCL-positive aborters and 67%[8,24] of aCL-positive healthy subjects were negative in the anti-β2-GP1assay.

What are the implications of testing?

What does an abnormal test result mean? The diagnosis is confirmed when a woman with a relevant clinical history has tests positive for aCL and/or LA on two separate occasions at least 6 weeks apart then. The IgG subfraction of aCL is able to cross into the fetoplacental circulation and although high concentrations of these particular antibodies have been eluted from placenta of women with aCL-positive sera,[89] the likelihood of a poor pregnancy outcome appears similar to women who test positive for IgM alone. Recurrent positive immune serology alone without a convincing clinical history does not confirm the diagnosis. It is wrong to label these women with a single first-trimester loss and positive serology as having APS and recommend treatment in a subsequent pregnancy that is potentially harmful[90] with no evidence of any benefit.

What does a normal test result mean? Negative immune serology confirms the absence of disease no matter how compelling the clinical findings may be. Clinicians should not "label" their patients with the diagnosis as it may lead to inappropriate interventions and has long-term consequences (e.g., regarding insurance policies), which are not to be taken lightly. It is, however, prudent to investigate thoroughly for other conditions that may have similar clinical manifestations to APS (e.g., certain congenital thrombophilias) or to test again some time later if further suspicious symptoms arise.

What is the cost of testing?

The approximate cost for aCL serology is $28 and for LA, it is $39. It is essential to test on two separate occasions if the first test is positive so this doubles the expense in these cases.

■ Conclusions and Recommendations

Routine testing for aPL in pregnancy is not advised as women who test positive but do not have clinical features of APS do not benefit from treatment.[91] However, testing is recommended in all women with a history of previous thrombosis, recurrent (three or more) miscarriage or previous adverse pregnancy outcome. Adequate maternal thromboprophylaxis, and where necessary full anticoagulation, may prevent life-threatening recurrent thrombosis, and from a pregnancy outcome perspective, APS is one of the few potentially treatable causes of recurrent pregnancy loss.[92,93] Once the diagnosis is established, women are offered treatments according to their clinical history.[53,54]

■ Summary

1 ■ What Is the Problem that Requires Screening?

APS either primary or secondary to SLE.

a. What is the incidence/prevalence of the target condition?
One per 700 women with reported detection rates increasing.

b. What are the sequelae of the condition that are of interest in clinical medicine?
Thrombosis, thrombocytopenia, and recurrent pregnancy loss.

2 ■ The Tests

a. What is the purpose of the tests?
To identify women with APS.

b. What is the nature of the tests?
Determination of anticardiolipins and lupus anticoagulant using a combination of ELISAs and clotting tests.

c. *What are the implications of testing?*

1. What does an abnormal test result mean?

The diagnosis is confirmed when a woman with a relevant clinical history has tests positive for aCL and/or LA on two separate occasions at least 6 weeks apart. Recurrent positive immune serology alone without a convincing clinical history does not confirm the diagnosis.

2. What does a normal test result mean?

Confirms the absence of APS.

d. *What is the cost of testing?*

Less than $100 per set of tests.

3 ■ Conclusions and Recommendations

Routine testing is not advised unless clinical features are present.

■ Miscellaneous Disorders

Autoimmune thrombocytopenia.

This condition occurs in 1/1,000 pregnancies and is characterized by antiplatelet antibodies. Pregnancy can exacerbate the maternal thrombocytopenia but treatment with corticosteroids and immunoglobulins ensures that maternal hemorrhagic complications are rare, although when they occur the results can be devastating.[94] Some 30% women will require treatment during pregnancy, especially predelivery, to minimize the risk of postnatal hemorrhage.[95] About 5% of neonates have platelet counts below $20 \times 10^9/L$, and about 1% have significant bleeding complications.[96] Some fetal medicine units perform third trimester ultrasound examination of the fetus in these pregnancies with a view to diagnosing intracranial bleeds and it is standard practice to avoid instrumental delivery. All neonates should be screened for thrombocytopenia immediately after delivery.

Rheumatoid arthritis.

Rheumatoid arthritis (RA) occurs in 1/2,500 pregnancies and is characterized by the presence of IgA autoantibodies to synovial joint membranes. Although 75% of women report improvement in symptoms in pregnancy, many remain severely symptomatic and 90% flare postpartum.[97,98] There are no recurrently reported adverse fetal or neonatal consequences[99] except in those rare cases where the women also have anti-Ro antibodies. It is therefore prudent to screen all pregnant women with RA for anti-Ro, and for those that test positive, to monitor the fetus and neonate as previously described.

Myasthenia gravis.

Myasthenia gravis (MG) occurs in 1/25,000 pregnancies and is characterized by autoantibodies to *N*-acetylcholine receptors. The maternal course is variable[100] and some report an association between MG and fetal growth restriction, premature rupture of membranes and subsequent preterm delivery.[101] Transient neonatal myasthenia occurs in 12% to 30% of infants, but is less common in thymectomized mothers.[100,102] Clinical features include floppiness, poor feeding, and respiratory distress. All infants born to women with MG should be observed closely as neonatal myasthenia may not be apparent until a few days after delivery and may require treatment with pyridostigmine.

Addison disease.

Addison disease occurs in less than 1/30,000 pregnancies and is characterized by autoantibodies to key enzymes involved in steroid biosynthesis. Women on adequate corticosteroid replacement therapy generally tolerate pregnancy well, although there are isolated reports of an association with fetal growth restriction.[103,104] It is appropriate to screen women with persistent vomiting and weight loss after 20 weeks' gestation for Addison disease by performing a short synacthen test.

Others.

Autoimmune hemolytic anemia, pemphigoid gestationalis, vitiligo, pernicious anemia, primary biliary cirrhosis, and chronic active hepatitis are all extremely rare autoimmune conditions that may be encountered in pregnancy.

References

1. Stone S, Langford K, Nelson-Piercy C, et al. Antiphospholipid antibodies do not a syndrome make. *Lupus* 2002;11:130–133.
2. Scofield RH. Autoantibodies as predictors of disease. *Lancet* 2004;363:1544–1546.
3. Guialis A, Patrinou-Georgoula M, Tsifetaki N, et al. Anti-5S RNA/protein (RNP) antibody levels correlate with disease activity in a patient with systemic lupus erythematosus (SLE) nephritis. *Clin Exp Immunol* 1994;95:385–389.
4. Sheldon J. Laboratory testing in autoimmune rheumatic diseases. *Best Pract Res Clin Rheumatol* 2004;18:249–269.
5. Burrow GN. The management of thyrotoxicosis in pregnancy. *N Engl J Med* 1985;313:562–565.
6. Amino N, Tanizawa O, Mori H, et al. Aggravation of thyrotoxicosis in early pregnancy and after delivery in Graves' disease. *J Clin Endocrinol Metab* 1982;55:395–401.

7. Mestman JH. Hyperthyroidism in pregnancy. *Clin Obstet Gynecol* 1997;40:45–64.
8. Millar LK, Wing DA, Leung AS, et al. Low birthweight and pre-eclampsia in pregnancies complicated by hyperthyroidism. *Obstet Gynecol* 1994;84:946–949.
9. Peleg D, Cada S, Peleg A, et al. The relationship between maternal serum thyroid-stimulating immunoglobulin and fetal and neonatal thyrotoxicosis. *Obstet Gynecol* 2002;99:1040–1043.
10. Laurberg P, Nygaard B, Glinoer D, et al. Guidelines for TSH receptor antibody measurement in pregnancy: results of an evidence based symposium organised by the European Thyroid Association. *Eur J Endocrinol* 1998;139;584–586.
11. Momotani N, Ito K, Hamada N, et al. Maternal hyper thyroidism and congenital malformation in the offspring. *Clin Endocrinol* 1984;20:695–700.
12. Wing DA, Millar LK, Cunnings PP, et al. A comparison of propylthiouricil versus methimazole in the treatment of hyperthyroidism in pregnancy. *Am J Obstet Gynecol* 1994;170:90–95.
13. Momotani N, Noh JY, Ishikawa N, et al. Effects of propylthiouracil and methimazole on fetal thyroid status in mothers with Graves' hyperthyroidism. *J Clin Endocrinol Metab* 1997;82:3633–3636.
14. Wiersinga WM. Thyroid hormone replacement therapy. *Horm Res* 2001;1:74–81.
15. Cohen O, Pinhas-Hamiel O, Sivan E, et al. Serial in utero ultrasonographic measurements of the fetal thyroid: a new complementary tool in the management of maternal hyperthyroidism in pregnancy. *Prenat Diagn* 2003;23:740–742.
16. Polak M, Le Gac I, Vuillard E, et al. Fetal and neonatal thyroid function in relation to maternal Graves' disease. *Best Pract Res Clin Endocrinol Metab* 2004;18:289–302.
17. Nachum Z, Rakover Y, Weiner E, et al. Graves' disease in pregnancy: prospective evaluation of a selective invasive treatment protocol. *Am J Obstet Gynecol* 2003;189:159–165.
18. Yanai N, Shveiky D. Fetal hydrops, associated with maternal propylthiouracil exposure, reversed by intrauterine therapy. *Ultrasound Obstet Gynecol* 2004;23:198–201.
19. Niswander KR, Gordon M. *Women and their Pregnancies.* Philadelphia: WB Saunders, 1972:246.
20. Greenman GW, Gabrielson MO, Flanders JH, et al. Thyroid dysfunction in pregnancy. Fetal loss and follow-up evaluation of surviving infants. *N Engl J Med* 1962;267:426–431.
21. Jones WS, Man EB. Thyroid function in human pregnancy. Premature deliveries and reproduction failure of pregnant women with low butanol extractable iodines. *Am J Obstet Gynecol* 1969;909–914.
22. Stagnaro-Green A, Glinoer D. Thyroid autoimmunity and the risk of miscarriage. *Best Pract Res Clin Endocrinol Metab* 2004;18:167–181.
23. Leung AS, Millar LK, Koonings PP, et al. Perinatal outcome in hypothyroid pregnancies. *Obstet Gynecol* 1993;348–353.
24. Fisher D. Fetal thyroid function: diagnosis and management of fetal thyroid disorders. *Clin Obstet Gynecol* 1997;40:25.
25. Karmarkar, MG, Prabarkaran D, Godbole MM. 5'monodeiodinase activity in developing human cortex. *Am J Clin Nutr* 1993;57:291S–294S.
26. Man EB, Holden RH, Jones WS. Thyroid function in human pregnancy VIII. Development and retardation of 4 year old progeny of euthyroid and hypothyroxinaemic women. *Am J Obstet Gynecol* 1971;109:12–19.
27. Man EB, Serunian SA. Thyroid function in human pregnancy, IX: development or retardation of 7 year old progeny of hypothyroxinaemic women. *Am J Obstet Gynecol* 1976;125:949–957.
28. Haddow JE, Palomaki GE, Allan WC, et al. Maternal thyroid deficiency during pregnancy and subsequent neuropsychological development of the child. *N Engl J Med* 1999;341:549–555.
29. Pop VJM, de Rooy HAM, van der Heide D, et al. Microsomal antibodies during gestation in relation to postpartum thyroid function and depression. *Acta Endocrinol* 1993;129:216–230.
30. Pop VJM, Brouwers EP, Vader HL, et al. Maternal hypothyroximaemia during pregnancy and subsequent child development: a 3 year follow-up study. *Clin Endocrinol* 2003;59:280–281.
31. Borras-Perez MV, Moreno-Perez D, Zuasnabar-Cotro A, et al. Neonatal hyperthyroidism in infants of mothers previously thyroidectomized due to Graves' disease. *J Pediatr Endocrinol Metab* 2001;14:1169–1172.
32. Brent GA. Maternal hypothyroidism: recognition and management. *Thyroid* 1999;9:661–665.

33. Allan WC, Haddow JE, Palomaki GE, et al. Maternal thyroid deficiency and pregnancy complications: implications for population screening. *J Med Screen* 2000;7:127–130.
34. Stagnaro-Green A. Postpartum thyroiditis. *Best Pract Res Endocrinol Metab* 2004; 18:303–316.
35. Lazarus JH, Ammari F, Oretti R, et al. Clinical aspects of recurrent postpartum thyroiditis. *Br J Gen Pract* 1997;47:305–308.
36. Othman S, Phillips DI, Parkes AB, et al. A long term follow-up of postpartum thyroiditis. *Clin Endocrinol* 1990;32:559–564.
37. Ball S. Antenatal screening of fetal autoantibodies. *Lancet* 1996;348:906–907.
38. Cevera R, Khamashta MA, Font J, et al. Systemic lupus erythematosus: clinical and immunologic patterns of disease expression in a cohort of 1,000 patients. *Medicine* 1993;72:113–124.
39. Tan EM, Cohen AS, Fries JF. The 1982 revised criteria for the classification of systemic lupus erythematosus. *Arthritis Rheum* 1982;25:1271–1277.
40. Hochberg MC. Updating the American College of Rheumatology revised criteria for the classification of systemic lupus erythematosus. *Arthritis Rheum* 1997;40:1725.
41. Lima F, Buchanan NMM, Khamashta MA, Kerslake S, Hughes GRV. Obstetric outcome in systemic lupus erythematosus. *Semin Arthritis Rheumat* 1995;25:184–192.
42. Khamashta MA, Ruiz-Irastorza G, Hughes GRV. Systemic lupus erythematosus flares during pregnancy. *Rheumatic Disease Clinics of North America* 1997;23:15–30.
43. Ruiz-Irastorza G, Lima F, Alves J, et al. Increased rate of lupus flare during pregnancy and the puerperium: a prospective study of 78 pregnancies. *Br J Rheumatol* 1996;35:133–138.
44. Lockshin MD. Pregnancy does not cause systemic lupus erythematosus to worsen. *Arthritis & Rheumatism* 1989;32:665–670.
45. Derksen R, Bruinse H, de Groot P, et al. Pregnancy in systemic lupus erythematosus: a prospective study. *Lupus* 1994;3:149–155.
46. Hayslett JP, Lynn RI. Effect of pregnancy in patients with lupus nephropathy. *Kid Internat* 1980;18:207–220.
47. Packman DK, Lam SS, Nicholls K, et al. Lupus nephritis and pregnancy. *Qu J Med* 1992;83:315–324.
48. Julkunen H, Kaaja R, Palosuo T, et al. Pregnancy in lupus nephropathy. *Acta Obstet Gynecol Scand* 1993;72:258–263.
49. Lee LA. Neonatal lupus: clinical features and management. *Paediatr Drugs* 2004;6:71–78.
50. Finkelstein Y, Adler Y, Harel L, et al. Anti-Ro (SSA) and anti-La (SSB) antibodies and complete congenital heart block. *Ann Med Interne* 1997;148:205–208.
51. Buyon JP, Hiebert R, Copel J, et al. Autoimmune-associated congenital heart block: demographics, mortality, morbidity and recurrence rates obtained from a national neonatal lupus registry. *J Am Coll Cardiol* 1998;31:1658–1666.
52. Wilson WA, Gharavi AE, Koike T, et al. International consensus statement on preliminary classification criteria for definite antiphospholipid syndrome. *Arthritis Rheum* 1999;42:1309–1311.
53. Branch DW, Khamashta MA. Antiphospholipid syndrome: obstetric diagnosis, management and controversies. *Obstet Gynaecol* 2003;101:1333–1344.
54. Derksen RHWM, Khamashta MA, Branch DW. Management of obstetric antiphospholipid syndrome. *Arthritis Rheum* 2004;50:1028–1039.
55. Harris EN, Spinnato JA. Should anticardiolipin tests be performed in otherwise healthy pregnant women? *Am J Obstet Gynecol* 1991;165:1272–1277.
56. Gharavi AE, Sammaritamo LR, Wen J, et al. Characteristics of human immunodeficiency virus and chlorpromazine induced antiphospholipid antibodies: effect of $\beta_2$glycoprotein-I on binding to phospholipid. *J Rheumatol* 1994;21:94–99.
57. Anonymous. Proceedings of the 6th International Symposium on Antiphospholipid Antibodies. Leuven, Belgium, 14-17th September 1994. *Lupus* 1994;3:207–364.
58. Nelson-Piercy C, Khamashta MA. Antiphospholipid antibodies: their clinical significance. *J Irish Coll Phys Surg* 1996;25:284–288.
59. Lima F, Khamashta MA, Buchanan NMM, Kerslake S, Hunt BJ, Hughes GRV. A study of sixty pregnancies in patients with the antiphospholipid syndrome. *Clin Exp Rheumatol* 1996;14:131–136.

60. Ringrose DK. Anaesthesia and antiphospholipid syndrome: a review of 20 patients. *Int J Obst Anaesth* 1997;6:107–111.
61. Levine JS, Branch DW, Rauch J. The antiphospholipid syndrome. *N Engl J Med* 2002;346: 752–763.
62. Julkunen H. Pregnancy in systemic lupus erythematosus. Contraception, fetal outcome and congenital heart block. *Acta Obst Gynecol Scand* 1994;73:517–520.
63. MacLean M, Cumming G, McCall F, et al. The prevalence of lupus anticoagulant and anticardiolipin antibodies in women with a history of first trimester miscarriages. *Br J Obstet Gynaecol* 1994;101:103–106.
64. Silver RM, Branch DW. Recurrent miscarriage: autoimmune considerations. *Clin Obstet Gynaecol* 1994;37:745–760.
65. Rai RS, Clifford K, Cohen H, et al. High prospective fetal loss rate in untreated pregnancies of women with recurrent miscarriage and antiphospholipid antibodies. *Hum Reprod* 1995;10:3301–3304.
66. Branch DW, Rodgers GM. Induction of endothelial cell tissue factor activity against sera from patients with antiphospholipid syndrome: a possible mechanism of thrombosis. *Am J Obstet Gynecol* 1993;168:206–210.
67. Lockwood CJ, Romero R, Feinberg RF, et al. The prevalence and biologic significance of lupus anticoagulant and anticardiolipin in a general obstetric population. *Am J Obstet Gynecol* 1989;161:369–373.
68. Perez MC, Wilson WA, Brown HL, et al. Anti-cardiolipin antibodies in unselected pregnant women in relationship to fetal outcome. *J Perinatol* 1991;11:33–36.
69. Branch DW, Scott JR, Kochenour NK. Obstetric complications associated with lupus anticoagulant. *N Engl J Med* 1985;313:1322–1326.
70. Lubbe WF, Butler WS, Palmer SJ, et al. Fetal survival after prednisolone suppression of maternal lupus anticoagulant. *Lancet* 1983;1:1361–1363.
71. Branch DW, Andres R, Digre KB, et al. The association of antiphospholipid antibodies with severe pre-eclampsia. *Obstet Gynecol* 1988;73:541–545.
72. Moodley J, Bhoola V, Duursma J, et al. The association of antiphospholipid antibodies with severe early-onset pre-eclampsia. *South Afr Med J* 1995;85:105–107.
73. Yasuda M, Takakuwa K, Tanaka K. Studies on the association between the anticardiolipin antibody and pre-eclampsia. *Acta Med Biol* 1994;42:145–149.
74. Dekker GA, de Vries JIP, Doelitzsch PM, et al. Underlying disorders associated with severe early-onset preeclampsia. *Am J Obstet Gynecol* 1995;173:1042–1048.
75. Pattison NS, Chamley LW, McKay EJ, et al. Antiphospholipid antibodies in pregnancy: prevalence and clinical associations. *Br J Obstet Gynaecol* 1993;100:909–913.
76. Yasuda M, Takakuwa K, Tokunaga A, et al. Prospective studies of the association between anticardiolipin antibody and outcome of pregnancy. *Obstet Gynecol* 1995;86:555–559.
77. Birdsall MA, Pattison NS, Chamley L. Antiphospholipid antibodies in pregnancy. *Aust N Z J Obstet Gynecol* 1992;32:328–330.
78. Kelly T, Whittle MJ, Smith DJ, et al. Lupus anticoagulant and pregnancy. *J Obstet Gynaecol* 1996;16:26–31.
79. Botet F, Romera G, Montagut P, et al. Neonatal outcome in women treated for the antiphospholipid syndrome during pregnancy. *J Perin Med* 1997;25:192–196.
80. Branch DW, Silver RM, Blackwell JL, et al. Outcome of treated pregnancies in women with antiphospholipid syndrome: an update of the Utah experience. *Obstet Gynecol* 1992;80: 614–620.
81. Granger KA, Farquharson RG. Obstetric outcome in antiphospholipid syndrome. *Lupus* 1997;6:509–513.
82. Backos M, Rai R, Baxter N, et al. Pregnancy complications in women with recurrent miscarriage associated with antiphospholipid antibodies treated with low dose aspirin and heparin. *Br J Obstet Gynaecol* 1999;106:102–107.
83. Huong DLT, Wechsler B, Blerty O, et al. A study of 75 pregnancies in patients with antiphospholipid syndrome. *J Rheumatol* 2001;28:2025–2030.
84. Kerslake S, Morton KE, Versi E, et al. Early Doppler studies in lupus pregnancy. *Am J Reprod Immunol* 1992;28:172–175.

85. Caruso A, De Carolis S, Ferrazzani S, et al. Pregnancy outcome in relation to uterine artery flow velocity waveforms and clinical characteristics in women with antiphospholipid syndrome. *Obstet Gynecol* 1993;82:970–976.

86. Venkat-Rahman N, Backos M, Teoh TG, et al. Uterine artery Doppler in predicting outcome in women with antiphospholipid syndrome. *Obstet Gynecol* 2001;98:235–242.

87. Bats AS, Lejeune V, Cynober E, et al. Antiphospholipid syndrome and second or third trimester fetal death: follow-up in the next pregnancy. *Eur J Obstet Reprod Biol* 2004;114:125–129.

88. Triplett D A. Many faces of lupus anticoagulants. *Lupus* 1998;7:S18–S22

88a. Smikle M, Wharfe G, Fletcher H, et al. Anticardiolipin, other antiphospholipid antibody tests and diagnosis of the antiphospholipid syndrome. *Hum Antibodies*. 2003;12:363–366.

89. Katano K, Aoki K, Ogasawara M, et al. Specific antiphospholipid antibodies (aPL) eluted from placentae of pregnant women with aPL-positive sera. *Lupus* 1995;4:304–308.

90. Dahlman TC. Osteoporotic fractures and the recurrence of thromboembolism during pregnancy and the puerperium in 184 women undergoing thromboprophylaxis with heparin. *Am J Obstet Gynecol* 1993;168:1265–1270.

91. Cowchock S, Reece EA. Do low-risk pregnant women with antiphospholipid antibodies need to be treated? *Am J Obstet Gynecol* 1997;176:1099–1100.

92. Kutteh WH. Antiphospholipid antibody-associated recurrent pregnancy loss: treatment with heparin and low-dose aspirin is superior to low-dose aspirin alone. *Am J Obstet Gynecol* 1996;174:1584–1589.

93. Rai R, Cohen H, Dave M, et al. Randomised controlled trial of aspirin and aspirin plus heparin in pregnant women with recurrent miscarriage associated with phospholipid antibodies (or antiphospholipid antibodies) *BMJ* 1997;314:253–257.

94. Chedraui PA, Hidalgo LA, San Miguel G. Fatal intracranial hemorrhage in a pregnant patient with autoimmune thrombocytopenic purpura. *J Perinat Med* 2003;31:526–529.

95. Webert KE, Mittal R, Sigouin C, et al. A retrospective 11-year analysis of obstetric patients with idiopathic thrombocytopenic purpura. *Blood* 2003;102:4306–4311.

96. Kelton JG. Idiopathic thrombocytopenic purpura complicating pregnancy. *Blood Rev* 2002;16:43–46

97. Thurnau GR. Rheumatoid arthritis. *Clin Obstet Gynecol* 1983;26:558–578.

98. Barrett JH, Brennan P, Fiddler M, et al. Does rheumatoid arthritis remit during pregnancy and relapse postpartum? Results from a nationwide study in the United Kingdom performed prospectively from late pregnancy. *Arthritis Rheum* 1999;42:1219–1227.

99. Nelson JL, Ostensen M. Pregnancy and rheumatoid arthritis. *Rheum Dis Clin North Am* 1997;23:195–212.

100. Djelmis J, Sostarko M, Mayer D, et al. Myasthenia gravis in pregnancy: report on 69 cases. *Eur J Obstet Gynecol Reprod Biol* 2002;104:21–25.

101. Hoff JM, Daltveit AK, Gilhus NE. Myasthenia gravis: consequences for pregnancy, delivery, and the newborn. *Neurology* 2003;61:1362–1366.

102. Morel E, Eymard B, Vernet-der Garabedian B, et al. Neonatal myasthenia gravis: a new clinical and immunologic appraisal on 30 cases. *Neurology* 1988;38:138–142.

103. Osler M. Addison's disease and pregnancy. *Acta Endocrinol* 1962;4:67.

104. O'Shaughnessy RW, Hackett KJ. Maternal Addison's disease and fetal growth retardation. A case report. *J Reprod Med* 1984;29:752–756.

28

Gestational Diabetes Mellitus

Seth C. Brody

■ What Is the Problem that Requires Screening?

Glucose intolerance, either new onset or first detected during pregnancy.[1,2]

What is the incidence/prevalence of the target condition?

Gestational diabetes is defined as glucose intolerance limited to pregnancy. It is, by definition, a retrospective diagnosis made after demonstrating normal glucose tolerance postpartum. Many women with preexisting diabetes are discovered during pregnancy and are often mislabeled as having gestational diabetes. Approximately 135,000 cases of gestational diabetes mellitus (GDM) are diagnosed annually in the United States.[1] It is likely that an unknown percentage of these women have overt rather than gestational diabetes. Low-risk groups have a prevalence of 1.4% to 2.8%,[3,4] whereas the prevalence ranges from 3.3% to 6.1% in high-risk populations.[4] Risk factors for developing GDM include increasing maternal age, family history of diabetes, and an increased pregravid body mass index (BMI).[5]

The prevalence of GDM varies depending on the criteria for diagnosis. In general, the World Health Organization (WHO) criteria identify twice as many women with GDM as the National Diabetes Data Group (NDDG) criteria; the American Diabetes Association (ADA) criteria give an intermediate prevalence (Table 28–1).[6,7]

What are the sequelae of the condition that are of interest in clinical medicine?

Most women with GDM have lower levels of maternal hyperglycemia than the type 1 or 2 diabetic patient. The additional risks of adverse health outcomes from these lower levels, detectable primarily by screening in the third trimester, and the magnitude of the benefit from treating that risk are presently uncertain.

| Table 28-1 | **Screening and diagnostic criteria for gestational diabetes mellitus** | | | |

	Reference Diagnostic Test – Glucose Tolerance Test: Cutpoints in Milligrams per deciliter (mg/dL)			**Screening**
Criteria glucose load	**National Diabetes Data Group**[a] **100 g**	**American Diabetes Association**[a] **100 g/75 g**	**World Health Organization**[b] **75 g**	**Glucose Challenge test, 50 g**
Glucose level:				
Fasting	105	95	≥126	—
1 h	190	180	—	130/140
2 h	165	155	≥ 140	—
3 h	145	140	—	—

[a]Two or more criteria must be met or exceeded for a positive diagnosis.
[b]One or more criteria must be met or exceeded for a positive diagnosis.
— Indicates glucose levels not used for the test indicated.

Markedly elevated maternal glucose levels most often occur in women with pregestational diabetes. These pregnancies are at higher risk of multiple complications affecting both the mother and fetus compared to women without diabetes. Current therapy improves outcomes for both mother and fetus in those with pregestational diabetes.[8]

Focusing on GDM, there are considerable problems determining the association between various degrees of GDM and adverse pregnancy outcomes. One problem is that we only have older studies of untreated GDM to help determine the association, performed at a time when obstetric practice was different from today's practice, or more recent studies in which all women received some treatment for GDM. Another problem is that some studies suggest[9–12] the risk of an adverse outcome increases with the degree of hyperglycemia, so that studies combining the few women with higher levels of hyperglycemia and the many women with lower levels may underestimate or even miss the association altogether. Thus, there is ample opportunity for positive and negative bias.

Offspring health outcomes. The literature is scant and mixed about whether untreated GDM is associated with increased perinatal mortality in the context of current obstetric care. Although older studies found an association,[13,14] more recent studies have not.[15–19] Perinatal mortality has declined in both non-GDM and GDM infants; it is a rare event in both groups.[15] For example, no stillbirths were seen in the three large studies including untreated women with GDM since 1985.[12,18,20] The lack of association between GDM and perinatal mortality in these recent studies may be attributable to the small size of the studies and concomitant lack of power to find small but real differences, the actual lack of an association, or improved obstetric care. It may also reflect the degree of hyperglycemia in the population studied.

Macrosomia is an intermediate outcome; the important adverse neonatal health outcomes linked to macrosomia are brachial plexus injury and clavicular fracture. The three most recent studies of untreated women with GDM[17–19] found that the percentage of macrosomic infants larger than 4,000 g was between about 19% and 29%, compared with the percentage in the general population of about 10%.[16,21–23] Still, most macrosomic infants are born to women without GDM.[24–28] The best, but still inadequate, data on untreated women with GDM reveal no difference in the rate of brachial plexus injury or clavicular fracture compared with the non-GDM population.[2,17,20,29–31] This too may be a reflection of the relative levels of hyperglycemia in the population studied as some studies suggest women with more severe hyperglycemia treated for GDM may have a 2% absolute increase in infant brachial plexus injury and 6% increase in infant clavicular fracture.[16,32] Although these outcomes are of concern, most brachial plexus injuries do not lead to permanent disability. The best studies show that 80% to 90% of brachial plexus injuries resolve by 1 year of life.[33–36] More than 95% of clavicular fractures heal within a few months without residual problems.[37–39]

Maternal obesity is a significant risk factor for macrosomia[40–42] and is an important potential confounder associated with GDM. And, although the association between GDM and fetal macrosomia persists after controlling for maternal weight, the magnitude of risk is diminished.[43,44]

GDM may be a risk factor for neonatal hypoglycemia. Studies among women with GDM find higher rates of hypoglycemia in their infants.[18] However, increased surveillance of infants of GDM women may significantly contribute to the increased prevalence. Furthermore, the magnitude of clinically important hypoglycemia is unclear.

The magnitude of any adverse health effects due to GDM and its potential association with preterm birth, hyperbilirubinemia, hypocalcemia, or polycythemia[2,18,22,45–49] is uncertain but likely to be small. The evidence relating to GDM and these outcomes is limited and the increased surveillance given to infants of women with GDM may again play a role.

Long-term implications suggested for the offspring of women diagnosed with GDM include an increased risk of impaired glucose tolerance, childhood obesity, and neuropsychological disturbances. These associations may well be true, but there are no large observational studies following a group of children of GDM mothers and a comparison group with non-GDM mothers for long enough to demonstrate whether any of these hypotheses are correct.[50–53]

Maternal health outcomes. Fetal macrosomia may lead to maternal trauma by increasing the risk of cesarean delivery[27,41,36,54–56] and the risk of third- and fourth-degree perineal lacerations.[34,57] Total cesarean delivery rates of 22%[58] to 30%[17] were reported in limited studies of unrecognized or untreated women with GDM, compared with a rate of about 17% for non-GDM women of the same populations.

Although there may be an association between GDM and increased cesarean delivery, much of the data is limited by a lack of adjustment for maternal obesity and by the impact of the diagnosis of GDM on clinical decision making. Some evidence suggests physicians are more likely to perform a cesarean delivery for women with GDM regardless of other indications.[17] For example, Naylor et al.[17] found that the cesarean delivery rates were 34% for women with treated GDM, about 30% for an untreated borderline GDM group (health care providers masked to results), and 20% for controls without GDM. The higher rate for the treated GDM group could not be attributed to macrosomia in light of the fact that macrosomia was 10% in both the GDM group and the control group. The increased risk of cesarean delivery among treated patients compared with controls persisted after adjustment for multiple maternal risk factors (adjusted odds ratio [OR], 2.1; 95% confidence interval [CI], 1.3–3.6).[17]

There is limited study of the rate of third- or fourth-degree lacerations in women with GDM. The one study that found a substantial percentage of GDM women who had such lacerations included only 16 subjects.[16] Another study found equally low rates among women with and women without GDM.[17]

Observational studies are inconclusive about the association of GDM and a higher risk of preeclampsia.[2,22,23,31,59–65] Data from untreated women with GDM[17] reveal a rate of preeclampsia that is similar to that for treated women and women in the non-GDM group.[66–69]

The diagnosis of GDM likely has long-term implications for mothers. Women with GDM have a higher risk of developing type 2 diabetes over the subsequent years.[70] However, the degree of glucose abnormality they develop remains to be quantified.[1]

■ The Tests

What is the purpose of the tests?

The purpose of the screening test, and subsequent reference diagnostic test, is to identify pregnant women who have glucose intolerance.

What is the nature of the tests?

Standard reference tests. No universally agreed reference test for the diagnosis of GDM exists. In the United States, the diagnostic test most commonly used consists of a 100-g 3-hour (3-h) oral glucose tolerance test (GTT) performed in the fasting state.[1,71] Two different U.S. groups have proposed competing diagnostic thresholds for this test (Table 28–1).[72,73] Outside of North America, the diagnosis of GDM is usually based on WHO criteria (Table 28–1), which uses a 75-g, 2-h oral GTT.[74,75]

There are concerns over the general reliability of the oral GTT. Harlass et al.[76] found that 23% of 64 unselected pregnant women who had had a positive screening test for GDM had inconsistent results between two different 100-g oral GTTs performed a week apart. The reproducibility of the oral GTT in nonpregnant groups was also questioned.[77–79]

Screening tests. The screening tests for GDM are evaluated against imperfect standards. Most studies on GDM screening strategies compare the results of one test with the results of another test (the reference diagnostic test) rather than examining how the test predicts adverse health outcomes. Some studies assess the association of the test with such intermediate outcomes as macrosomia rather than health outcomes such as brachial plexus injury.

In the United States, the 50-g, 1-h glucose challenge test (GCT) is the most commonly used screening test (right-hand panel of Table 28–1). The ADA and NDDG have recommended different criteria to define a positive screening test. If the 1-h GCT glucose value is above either 130 mg/dL[80] or 140 mg/dL,[72] then the woman is given the 100-g 3-h oral GTT for diagnosis. The 130 mg/dL and 140 mg/dL cutpoints of the 50-g 1-h GCT identify subgroups of 20% to 25% and 14% to 18%, respectively, of all pregnant women, depending on the presence of risk factors.[71] The 130-mg/dL GCT threshold identifies 90% and the 140-mg/dL threshold identifies 80% of all women with a positive 100-g 3-h oral GTT.[71]

False-positive results for the GCT are common in the general population. Fewer than one in five women with a positive GCT meet criteria for GDM on a full oral GTT.[81] Like other GTTs, therefore, the reliability of the GCT is questionable.[10]

The WHO approach to identifying women with GDM is to use a 75-g 2-h oral GTT as a single-step screening and diagnostic test. This approach classifies at least twice as many women as having GDM as the two-step approach, although the evidence is sparse about whether the one-step test is more or less predictive of adverse health outcomes than the two-step approach.[6,7]

Targeted versus universal screening. The efficiency of screening for GDM may be improved by restricting screening to women at higher risk ("targeted screening") rather than screening all women ("universal screening"). Some risk-factor–based screening strategies eliminate only 10% of pregnant women from being screened and improve screen efficiency only minimally.[1,82] In contrast, Naylor et al.[66] developed a scoring system in a study of targeted screening strategies that excluded nearly 35% of women from screening while detecting more cases of GDM than universal screening.

What are the implications of testing?

What does an abnormal test result mean? Women with an abnormal screen require diagnostic testing. Affected women may then receive counseling and diet therapy. Those with elevated glucose levels on diet therapy are started on hypoglycemic therapy. Both interventions seek to reduce adverse offspring and maternal health outcomes.

Ideally, a reference diagnostic test would be based on the threshold that identified a group at increased risk of developing disease-associated complications.[12] Abnormal values on both the 75-g 2-h[83,84] and 100-g 3-h[19,85,86] oral GTTs, using any of proposed criteria, are predictive of fetal macrosomia and, in some studies, preeclampsia as well. These associations are diminished or eliminated when adjustments are made for such potential confounders as pregravid weight, age, parity, and race. Although cesarean delivery rates are also directly associated with maternal hyperglycemia, the most careful study of this issue suggested that part of the increase in cesarean delivery can be attributed to the impact of the GDM diagnosis on physician decision making rather than an increase in macrosomia.[17] Thus, the thresholds for the current reference diagnostic tests do not clearly distinguish women at high risk from women at low risk of adverse maternal or fetal health outcomes.

No well-designed and conducted randomized controlled trial (RCT) of screening for GDM has been completed, and thus the evidence for screening is indirect. For screening to be effective, an intervention must be present that improves health outcomes. It is important to examine well-conducted RCTs of treatment for women with GDM as significant potential biases are inherent in observational evidence.

Several concepts are important in considering studies of the impact of tight glycemic control on the health outcomes of women with GDM. The first is that since the risk of at least some adverse health outcomes increase with the level of hyperglycemia, the potential absolute risk reduction is likely larger with higher glycemic levels. Yet, most women (70% or greater)[49,90] diagnosed have lower levels of hyperglycemia and are treated by diet alone; a minority of women have hyperglycemia deemed high enough to require insulin. Second, intensive treatment must produce a reasonable reduction in the glycemic level compared with conventional treatment (or no treatment) so that the hypothesis of improved glycemic control leading to better health outcomes can be tested. Third, the outcomes assessed are also important. Most studies focus on intermediate outcomes such as fetal macrosomia or chemical findings such as neonatal hypoglycemia. In the case of fetal macrosomia, only a small percentage of these cases lead to maternal or fetal trauma. In the case of chemical findings (e.g., glucose or bilirubin level), few studies report the percentage of abnormalities that require treatment; none clearly reassure the reader that any differences noted were not explainable by more intense surveillance of infants born to GDM women. Finally, interventions or outcomes that are dependent on clinician judgment (e.g., cesarean delivery rates) could be biased by knowledge of GDM status,[17] because few of the studies mask the obstetricians.[29,91]

No properly designed and conducted RCT has examined the benefit of universal or targeted screening for GDM compared to routine care without screening. The only RCT that examined the impact of different screening strategies had major methodologic flaws.[92] Retrospective studies comparing screened populations with unscreened control populations have also been flawed and had mixed results.[15,93] One ecologic study found no evidence that a program of universal screening compared with an area without such a program, reduced fetal macrosomia, cesarean delivery, or other diabetes-related complications.[94]

Few studies have examined the effectiveness of intensive compared with less-intensive glycemic control among women with GDM with lower levels of hyperglycemia. An overview of four trials with 612 women found no difference between diet and no therapy in adverse health outcomes.[95] An RCT conducted by Li et al.[29] reached similar conclusions.

Three RCTs[18,91,96] have compared intensive with less intensive glycemic control (achieving some glycemic separation) among women with GDM who had varying degrees of hyperglycemia, but who had a low mean entry fasting plasma glucose (FPG) or mean HbA1c. Two studies found statistically significant improvements in intermediate outcomes (e.g., large for gestational age [LGA] infants,[96] neonatal hypocalcemia[18]); however, none of these studies found clear differences in health outcomes between glycemic control groups.

Four other RCTs compared tight and less tight glycemic control among women with GDM with higher glycemic levels.[32,67,68,97] One trial achieved no difference in glycemic control between groups and found no difference in outcomes.[67] Two studies achieved small differences in glycemic control and both found no differences in the rate of fetal macrosomia.[32,68] One study found an absolute reduction in perinatal chemical abnormalities;[68] whereas the other found a reduction in cesarean deliveries not explained by fetal size.[32] These RCTs found no other health differences between groups. One study achieved a larger glycemic separation between groups (difference in mean glucose 24 mg/dL).[97] The infants of less intensively treated women had a higher mean birth weight plus higher rates of hypoglycemia and polycythemia. Although these differences were small and of uncertain clinical importance, they demonstrate the role hyperglycemia will play in determining the utility of any screening protocol.

de Veciana et al.[69] compared tight with less tight control among women with very high glycemic levels, some of whom likely had frank diabetes. They achieved a separation in glycemic control (Hb A1c difference of 1.6%) and found reductions in fetal macrosomia and neonatal hypoglycemia. Given the study population, however, this trial may have little relevance for the great majority of women detected with GDM who have lower levels of glycemia.

All these trials have too few participants to detect small differences among treatment groups in uncommon adverse health outcomes such as perinatal mortality and brachial plexus injury. They have even less power to determine if the health benefit is different for GDM women with high levels of hyperglycemia compared with lower levels. They provide a suggestion but insufficient evidence to prove that glycemic control improves health outcomes in this setting.

Several observational studies suggested improved intermediate or health outcomes with more intensive treatment of women with GDM.[17,30,83,98–103] Yet, the observed improvements may be attributable to factors other than glycemic control as the women in the treatment groups of these studies differ from women in the control groups in multiple ways (some known and some unknown) other than glycemic control. Many of these factors are also associated with the health outcomes of interest.

No completed study of women with GDM examined health outcomes among groups randomized to receive or not receive nonstress test (NST) or biophysical profile (BPP). Observational studies have found that using NSTs (with or without amniotic fluid index) or BPPs in women with GDM is associated with either absent or very low rates of stillbirth.[104–107] Small studies have found no stillbirths when delaying testing until 40 weeks' gestation in women with GDM with low levels of hyperglycemia (the majority).[107,108] Without appropriate control groups, we do not know whether the low rate of fetal death can be attributed to the additional procedures.[107] NSTs or BPPs have high false-positive rates,[104,105] and they may occasionally lead to interventions[107] that are unnecessary.

Ultrasound assessment of abdominal circumference was studied to allow improved targeting of insulin therapy to decrease fetal macrosomia and birth trauma. Three RCTs enrolled women with hyperglycemia into insulin therapy triggered by ultrasound abdominal circumference.[32,109,110] No study reported any important differences in health outcomes, but each lacked adequate power to detect such differences.

Recently, the Australian Study in Pregnant Women (ACHOIS) Trial Group reported results of a RCT comparing pregnancy outcomes in women with GDM receiving either routine prenatal care or treatment consisting of diet advice and insulin as indicated.[110a] A total of 1000 women participated. The prevalence of serious perinatal complications, a composite variable including death, shoulder dystocia, bone fracture and nerve palsy was reduced in the treatment arm (1% vs. 4%, RR adjusted for maternal age, race and parity 0.33, 95% CI 0.14-0.75). However, there were more labor inductions in the treatment group (RR 1.36, 95% CI 1.15-1.62), and more neonates from the treatment group were admitted to the nursery (RR 1.13, 95%CI 1.03-1.23). A similar trial is underway in the United States.

What does a normal test result mean? Because the glucose intolerance of GDM increases during pregnancy, screening is most commonly conducted between 24 and 28 weeks' gestation. Women who have normal testing at this time in gestation do not require further testing. However, this timing is not based on any evidence that it is the optimal period to identify the women who would benefit most from treatment. Determining the best time to screen involves examining the trade-off between the potential benefits of early screening (i.e., finding fewer women at higher risk and treating them for a longer time) and the potential benefits of later screening (i.e., finding a larger number of women at lower risk and treating them for a shorter time).[12]

Some studies suggest the additional women detected by the ADA criteria compared to the NDDG criteria have the same risk of macrosomia as those meeting the higher criteria.[19,87] Others note the risk of macrosomia in these additional GDM-classified women is predicted more by the degree of prepregnant obesity than by the level of hyperglycemia during pregnancy.[88] Some observers claim the adoption of the ADA criteria would increase the number of women with GDM by more than 50% while offering little opportunity to reduce the prevalence of fetal macrosomia.[89]

What is the cost of testing?

Precise evidence on the costs of screening and early treatment is lacking. Some studies examined the direct costs of screening and intensive management; others investigated approaches to improving efficiency by targeting screening or aggressive management toward women at highest risk.

Kitzmiller and colleagues[111] identified the direct costs of screening and intensive management of GDM from the perspective of managed care and subsequently reviewed studies examining aspects of the costs of treating women with GDM.[112] More than 50% of the costs involve surveillance measures such as NSTs, ultrasounds, and amnioceneses. Despite these analyses, there is no clear, generalizable study from the societal perspective of the additional total costs of screening and treating GDM compared with not screening.

Although many of these studies assume that intensive treatment of GDM will reduce cesarean deliveries, other evidence indicates that the reverse may often be true. Knowledge of the diagnosis of GDM by the obstetrician may lower the threshold for cesarean deliveries such that screening actually increases the cesarean rate, thus increasing costs.[17,109,111] If aggressive NSTs and BPPs are overly performed without a health benefit for many women with GDM, cost-effectiveness will be less favorable. Identification of GDM may needlessly increase false-positive NSTs or BPPs and rates of cesarean delivery (because of a lowered intervention threshold).[17,113] Additionally, obesity is a potential confounder in the literature on health care costs for women with GDM. Being moderately overweight is a risk factor for GDM; moreover, macrosomia and cesarean delivery are increased in obese mothers,[58,114-116] as are anesthetic and postoperative complications.[116]

Good information is lacking about the differences in health care costs between screened and nonscreened women. The cost-effectiveness of screening for GDM cannot be calculated with any confidence because the effectiveness of screening in improving health outcomes remains uncertain.

■ Conclusions and Recommendations

Screening and intensive treatment for GDM seeks to reduce both the maternal and neonatal morbidity that rises with increasing maternal glucose levels. Various screening strategies can detect women with different levels of hyperglycemia, but the threshold at which clinically important health outcomes begin to deteriorate by an important degree, given today's obstetric care, is presently uncertain.

There is no direct evidence comparing health outcomes in screened and unscreened groups. The direct evidence for the health outcomes of intensively treated women with GDM at various levels of maternal glycemia is limited, but the most recent study[110a] suggests current treatment of identified GDM improves perinatal short term outcome. The magnitude of any benefit of intensive treatment at various levels of glycemia associated with GDM is uncertain, but is likely to be greatest among those with the highest levels (i.e., usually treated with hypoglycemic agents), and small among the majority with lower glycemic levels (i.e., usually treated with diet and counseling). For women with GDM with lower levels of glycemia, the existing evidence does not show that dietary therapy improves important clinical outcomes compared with no diet therapy. About 70% or more of all women with GDM are in this group.

For women with GDM at the higher levels of glycemia, intensive treatment likely reduces macrosomia, an intermediate outcome. The extent to which this translates into reducing birth trauma is uncertain, but probably less than the reduction in macrosomia. The U.S. Preventative Task Force (USPSTF) made various assumptions and calculated the number of women needed to screen (NNS) to prevent one case of brachial plexus injury.[117,118] They assumed 4% of pregnant women have GDM,[1] that 30% have a high enough glycemic level to require insulin,[90] and that among these women, the macrosomia rate is reduced to the degree seen in a study showing the most significant reduction in parameter.[69] The NNS to prevent one brachial plexus injury in this scenario was about 8,900. When more generous assumptions of 6% GDM prevalence (high-risk group), 50% of women with GDM are treated with insulin, and that less than 4,000 g also benefit, the USPSTF determined that the NNS becomes 3,300 (best-case scenario). At least 80% of brachial plexus injuries resolve within the first year of life,[1,33,35,119] so an NNS estimate based on permanent brachial plexus injury, or one that included cesarean delivery rates or a lesser reduction in macrosomia, would be much larger.

Women with GDM have a higher risk of developing type 2 diabetes. However, the extent to which making this diagnosis in pregnancy leads to a health benefit for women later in life is uncertain. GDM may also have long-term implications for the offspring, such as increased risk of childhood obesity, glucose intolerance, or neuropsychological disturbances. Current studies on these potentially important issues are limited and mixed. Data are insufficient to show that routine screening will significantly influence these outcomes.

The evidence available on the costs of screening and intensive treatment is also limited. Costs are likely to rise due to the detection of GDM, which, in and of itself, may increase the probability of cesarean delivery. The detection of GDM often leads to multiple antenatal tests whose efficacies in GDM are unclear, and may increase the probability of a false-positive test leading to unnecessary procedures. Overall costs are likely to increase with little health benefit for the majority of women who have lower levels of hyperglycemia.

National groups have differed regarding their recommendations for GDM screening. The USPSTF found insufficient evidence to recommend for or against screening.[117,118] The Canadian Task Force on Preventive Health Care concluded in 1994 that the available evidence did not support a recommendation for universal screening, but a decision could be made on other grounds to screen.[120]

The ADA recommends screening all women at risk for GDM. This would mean screening women for GDM unless they are younger than 25 years, have normal body weight, are not a member of a high-risk ethnic group, have no first-degree relatives with diabetes, and have no personal history of glucose intolerance or poor obstetrical outcome.[73] Despite American College of Obstetrics and Gynecology (ACOG) acknowledging the weakness in the evidence,[1,24] a 2001 Practice Bulletin of the ACOG recommends a similar risk-based approach, but notes that since only a small percentage of women meet criteria for low risk, universal 50-g 1-h GCT screening may be a more practical approach.[1]

The issue of screening for GDM is a contentious one and the reason for this controversy is largely a lack of high-quality research addressing the central issues. This issue needs to be clarified with large RCTs that mask obstetric care and examine clinically important health outcomes.

■ Summary

1 ■ What Is the Problem that Requires Screening?

Glucose intolerance during pregnancy.

a. *What is the incidence/prevalence of the target condition?*

One percent to 6% depending on the diagnostic criteria, geographic location, and demographic profile.

b. *What are the sequelae of the condition that are of interest in clinical medicine?*

Sequelae may be long and short term. There is a six- to 18-fold increase in the likelihood of type 2 diabetes within 28 years. There is a higher prevalence of obesity, hyperlipidemia, atherosclerotic vascular disease, increased systolic blood pressure, and mortality in women who have had gestational diabetes. Maternal obesity is a significant risk factor for macrosomia and is an important confounder of GDM for this outcome. Whether the perinatal morbidity and/or mortality are altered by gestational diabetes in modern obstetrics remains unclear.

Potential long-term implications for the offspring of women with GDM include an increased risk of impaired glucose intolerance, childhood obesity, and neuropsychologic disturbances.

2 ■ The Tests

a. *What is the purpose of the tests?*

To identify glucose intolerance during pregnancy.

Continued

■ Summary—cont'd

b. *What is the nature of the tests?*

Screening tests: Neither history nor urine testing for glucose are effective. A 50-g glucose challenge with a blood sample obtained after 1 hour is common. There is controversy regarding the appropriate threshold value for diagnostic testing. Random blood testing is also effective.

Standard reference tests: Unclear whether a 100-g 3-hour oral glucose tolerance test (OGTT) or a 75-g 2-h OGTT is best. There is no consensus on the cutoffs.

c. *What are the implications of testing?*

1. What does an abnormal test result mean?

An abnormal screen indicates the woman should undergo diagnostic testing for gestational diabetes. The diagnosis of gestational diabetes is made when there are two abnormal values on the OGTT. It is assumed, but unproven, that treatment and surveillance will reduce both short-term and long-term maternal and perinatal morbidity.

2. What does a normal test result mean?

Women with a normal screen at 24 to 28 weeks' gestation do not require further testing.

d. *What is the cost of testing?*

Good information is lacking about the differences in health care costs between screened and nonscreened women. The cost-effectiveness of screening for GDM cannot be calculated with any confidence because the effectiveness of screening in improving health outcomes remains uncertain.

3 ■ Conclusions and Recommendations

Screening and intensive treatment for GDM seeks to reduce both the maternal and neonatal morbidity that rises with increasing maternal glucose levels. The issue of screening for GDM is a contentious one and the reason for this controversy is largely a lack of high-quality research addressing the central issues. This issue needs to be clarified with large RCTs that mask obstetric care and examine clinically important health outcomes.

References

1. ACOG Practice Bulletin. Clinical management guidelines for obstetrician-gynecologists. Number 30, September 2001. *Obstet Gynecol* 2001;98:525–538.
2. Magee MS, Walden CE, Benedetti TJ, et al. Influence of diagnostic criteria on the incidence of gestational diabetes and perinatal morbidity. *JAMA* 1993;269:609–615.
3. Moses RG, Moses J, Davis WS. Gestational diabetes: do lean young Caucasian women need to be tested? *Diabetes Care* 1998;21:1803–1806.
4. Marquette GP, Klein VR, Niebyl JR. Efficacy of screening for gestational diabetes. *Am J Perinatol* 1985;2:7–9.
5. Solomon CG , Willet WC, Carey VJ, et al. A prospective study of pregravid determinants of gestational diabetes mellitus. *JAMA* 1997;278:1078–1083.
6. Deerochanawong C, Putiyanun C, Wongsuryrat M, et al. Comparison of National Diabetes Data Group and World Health Organization criteria for detecting gestational diabetes mellitus. *Diabetologia* 1996;39:1070–1073.
7. Pettitt DJ, Bennett PH, Hanson RL, et al. Comparison of World Health Organization and National Diabetes Data Group procedures to detect abnormalities of glucose tolerance during pregnancy. *Diabetes Care* 1994;17:1264–1268.
8. Hunter DJS. *Diabetes in Pregnancy: Effective Care in Pregnancy and Childbirth.* Toronto: Oxford University Press, 1989:578–593.
9. Sermer M, Naylor DC, Gare DJ, et al. Impact of increasing carbohydrate intolerance on maternal-fetal outcomes in 3637 women without gestational diabetes: The Toronto Tri-Hospital Gestational Diabetes Project. *Am J Obstet Gynecol* 1995;173:146–156.
10. Sacks DA, Greenspoon JS, Abu-Fadil S, et al. Toward universal criteria for gestational diabetes: the 75-gram glucose tolerance test in pregnancy. *Am J Obstet Gynecol* 1995;172:607–614.
11. Langer O, Levy J, Brustman L, et al. Glycemic control in gestational diabetes mellitus—how tight is tight enough: small for gestational age vs. large for gestational age? *Am J Obstet Gynecol* 1989;161:646–653.
12. Naylor CD. Diagnosing gestational diabetes: is the gold standard valid? *Diabetes Care* 1989;12:565–572.
13. O'Sullivan JB, Gellis SS, Dandrow RV, Tenney BO. The potential diabetic and her treatment in pregnancy. *Obstet Gynecol* 1966;27:5683–5689.
14. Pettitt DJ, Knowler WC, Baird HR, et al. Gestational diabetes: infant and maternal complications of pregnancy in relation to third-trimester glucose tolerance in Pima Indians. *Diabetes Care* 1980;3:458–464.
15. Beischer NA, Wein P, Sheedy MT, et al. Identification and treatment of women with hyperglycaemia diagnosed during pregnancy can significantly reduce perinatal mortality rates. *Aust NZ J Obstet Gynaecol* 1996;36:239–247.
16. Adams KM, Li H, Nelson RL, et al. Sequelae of unrecognized gestational diabetes. *Am J Obstet Gynecol* 1998;178:1321–1332.
17. Naylor CD, Sermer M, Chen E, et al. Cesarean delivery in relation to birth weight and gestational glucose tolerance: pathophysiology or practice style? Toronto Tri-Hospital Gestational Diabetes Investigators. *JAMA* 1996;275:1165–1170.
18. Garner P, Okun N, Keely E, et al. A randomized controlled trial of strict glycemic control and tertiary level obstetric care versus routine obstetric care in the management of gestational diabetes: a pilot study. *Am J Obstet Gynecol* 1997;177:190–195.
19. Lu G, Rouse D, Dubard M, et al. The impact of lower threshold values for the detection of gestational diabetes mellitus. *Obstet Gynecol* 2000;95:S44.
20. Li DFH, Wong VCW, O'Hoy KMKY, et al. Is treatment needed for mild impairment of glucose in pregnancy? A randomized controlled trial. *Br J Obstet Gynaecol* 1987;94:851–854.
21. Ventura SJ, Martin JA, Curtin SC, et al. Births: final data for 1998. *Natl Vital Stat Rep* 2000;48:1–100.
22. Xiong X, Saunders LD, Wang FL, et al. Gestational diabetes mellitus: prevalence, risk factors, maternal and infant outcomes. *Int J Gynaecol Obstet* 2001;75:221–228.

23. Svare JA, Hansen BB, Molsted-Pedersen L. Perinatal complications in women with gestational diabetes mellitus. *Acta Obstet Gynecol Scand* 2001;80:899–904.

24. American College of Obstetricians and Gynecologists. Management of diabetes mellitus in pregnancy. 1994.

25. Gross TL, Sokol RJ, Williams T, et al. Shoulder dystocia: a fetal-physician risk. *Am J Obstet Gynecol* 1987;156:1408–1418.

26. McFarland LV, Raskin M, Daling JR, et al. Erb/Duchenne's palsy: a consequence of fetal macrosomia and method of delivery. *Obstet Gynecol* 1986;68:784–788.

27. Mondalou HD, Dorchester WL, Thorosian A, et al. Macrosomia: maternal, fetal, and neonatal implications. *Obstet Gynecol* 1980;55:420–424.

28. Sandmire HF, O'Halloin TJ. Shoulder dystocia: its incidence and associated risk factors. *Int J Gynaecol Obstet* 1988;26:65–73.

29. Li DF, Wong VC, O'Hoy KM, et al. Is treatment needed for mild impairment of glucose tolerance in pregnancy? A randomized controlled trial. *Br J Obstet Gynaecol* 1987;94:851–854.

30. Langer O, Rodriguez DA, Xenakis EM, et al. Arrendondo F. Intensified versus conventional management of gestational diabetes. *Am J Obstet Gynecol* 1994;170:1036–1046; discussion 1046–1047.

31. Casey BM, Lucas MJ, Mcintire DD, et al. Pregnancy outcomes in women with gestational diabetes compared with the general obstetric population. *Obstet Gynecol* 1997;90:869–873.

32. Kjos SL, Schaefer-Graf U, Sardesi S, et al. A randomized controlled trial using glycemic plus fetal ultrasound parameters versus glycemic parameters to determine insulin therapy in gestational diabetes with fasting hyperglycemia. *Diabetes Care* 2001;24:1904–1910.

33. Morrison JC, Sanders JR, Magann EF, et al. The diagnosis and management of dystocia of the shoulder. *Surg Gynecol Obstet* 1992;175:515–522.

34. Lipscomb KR, Gregory K, Shaw K. The outcome of macrosomic infants weighing at least 4500 grams: Los Angeles County + University of Southern California experience. *Obstet Gynecol* 1995;85:558–564.

35. Hardy AE. Birth injuries of the brachial plexus: incidence and prognosis. *J Bone Joint Surg Br* 1981;63-B:98–101.

36. Berard J, Dufour P, Vinatier D, et al. Fetal macrosomia: risk factors and outcome. A study of the outcome concerning 100 cases >4500 g. *Eur J Obstet Gynecol Reprod Biol* 1998;77:51–59.

37. Perlow JH, Wigton T, Hart J, et al. Birth trauma. A five-year review of incidence and associated perinatal factors. *J Reprod Med* 1996;41:754–760.

38. Oppenheim WL, Davis A, Growdon WA, et al. Clavicle fractures in the newborn. *Clin Orthop* 1990;250:176–180.

39. Chez RA, Carlan S, Greenberg SL, et al. Fractured clavicle is an unavoidable event. *Am J Obstet Gynecol* 1994;171:797–798.

40. Okun N, Verma A, Mitchell BF, et al. Relative importance of maternal constitutional factors and glucose intolerance of pregnancy in the development of newborn macrosomia. *J Matern Fetal Med* 1997;6:285–290.

41. Spellacy WN, Miller S, Winegar A, et al. Macrosomia: maternal characteristics and infant complications. *Obstet Gynecol* 1985;66:158–161.

42. Lucas MJ, Lowe TW, Bowe L, et al. Class A1 gestational diabetes: a meaningful diagnosis? *Obstet Gynecol* 1993;82:260–265.

43. Hod M, Bar J, Peled Y, et al. Antepartum management protocol: timing and mode of delivery in gestational diabetes. *Diabetes Care* 1998;21[Suppl 2]:B113–B117.

44. Sermer M, Naylor CD, Farine D, et al. The Toronto Tri-Hospital Gestational Diabetes Project: a preliminary review. *Diabetes Care* 1998;21:B33–B42.

45. Hod M, Rabinerson D, Peled Y. Gestational diabetes mellitus: is it a clinical entity? *Diabetes Reviews* 1995;3:602–613.

46. Ogata E. Perinatal morbidity in offspring of diabetic mothers. *Siabetes Reviews.* 1995;3:652–657.

47. Langer O, Conway D, Berkus M, et al. A comparison of glyburide and insulin on women with gestational diabetes mellitus. *N Engl J Med* 2000;343:1134–1138.

48. Langer O. Management of gestational diabetes. *Clin Obstet Gynecol* 2000;43:106–115.

49. Langer O. Maternal glycemic criteria for insulin therapy in gestational diabetes mellitus. *Diabetes Care* 1998;21:B91–B98.

50. Beischer NA, Wein P, Sheedy MT, et al. Maternal glucose tolerance and obstetric complications in pregnancies in which the offspring developed type I diabetes. *Diabetes Care* 1994;17:832–834.

51. Persson B, Gentz J, Moller E. Follow-up of children of insulin dependent (type I) and gestational diabetic mothers. Growth pattern, glucose tolerance, insulin response, and HLA types. *Acta Paediatr Scand* 1984;73:778–784.

52. Whitaker RC, Pepe MS, Seidel KD, et al. Gestational diabetes and the risk of offspring obesity. *Pediatrics* 1998;101:E9.

53. Vohr BR, McGarvey ST, Tucker R. Effects of maternal gestational diabetes on offspring adiposity at 4-7 years of age. *Diabetes Care* 1999;22:1284–1291.

54. Menticoglou SM, Manning FA, Morrison I, et al. Must macrosomic fetuses be delivered by cesarean section? A review of outcome for 786 babies greater than or equal to 4,500 grams. *Aust N Z J Obstet Gynaecol* 1992;32:100–103.

55. Rouse DJ, Owen J. Prophylactic cesarean delivery for fetal macrosomia diagnosed by means of ultrasonography: a Faustian bargain? *Am J Obstet Gynecol* 1999;181:332–338.

56. Lazer S, Biale Y, Mazor M, et al. Complications associated with the macrosomic fetus. *J Reprod Med* 1986;31:501–505.

57. el Madany AA, Jallad KB, Radi FA, et al. Shoulder dystocia: anticipation and outcome. *Int J Gynaecol Obstet* 1990;34:7–12.

58. Lu GC, Rouse DJ, Dubard M, et al. The effect of the increasing prevalence of maternal obesity on perinatal morbidity. *Am J Obstet Gynecol* 2001;185:845–849.

59. Joffe GM, Esterlitz JR, Levine RJ, et al. The relationship between abnormal glucose tolerance and hypertensive disorders of pregnancy in healthy nulliparous women. Calcium for Preeclampsia Prevention (CPEP) Study Group. *Am J Obstet Gynecol* 1998;179:1032–1037.

60. Suhonen L, Teramo K. Hypertension and pre-eclampsia in women with gestational glucose intolerance. *Acta Obstet Gynecol Scand* 1993;72:269–272.

61. Schaffir JA, Lockwood CJ, Lapinski R, et al. Incidence of pregnancy-induced hypertension among gestational diabetics. *Am J Perinatol* 1995;12:252–254.

62. Jensen DM, Sorensen B, Feilberg-Jorgensen N, et al. Maternal and perinatal outcomes in 143 Danish women with gestational diabetes mellitus and 143 controls with a similar risk profile. *Diabet Med* 2000;17:281–286.

63. Roach VJ, Hin LY, Tam WH, et al. The incidence of pregnancy-induced hypertension among patients with carbohydrate intolerance. *Hypertens Pregnancy* 2000;19:183–189.

64. Persson B, Hanson U. Neonatal morbidities in gestational diabetes mellitus. *Diabetes Care* 1998;21[Suppl 2]:B79–B84.

65. Lao TT, Tam KF. Gestational diabetes diagnosed in third trimester pregnancy and pregnancy outcome. *Acta Obstet Gynecol Scand* 2001;80:1003–1008.

66. Naylor CD, Sermer M, Chen E, et al. Selective screening for gestational diabetes mellitus. Toronto Tri-Hospital Gestational Diabetes Project Investigators. *N Engl J Med* 1997;337:1591–1596.

67. Persson B, Strangenberg M, Hansson U, et al. Gestational diabetes mellitus (GDM) comparative evaluation of two treatment regimens, diet versus insulin and diet. *Diabetes* 1985;11:101–105.

68. Nachum Z, Ben-Shlomo I, Weiner E, et al. Twice daily versus four times daily insulin dose regimens for diabetes in pregnancy: randomised controlled trial. *BMJ* 1999;319:1223–1227.

69. de Veciana M, Major CA, Morgan MA, et al. Postprandial versus preprandial blood glucose monitoring in women with gestational diabetes mellitus requiring insulin therapy. *N Engl J Med.* 1995;333:1237–1241.

70. O'Sullivan JB. Diabetes mellitus after GDM. *Diabetes.* 1991;40:131–135.

71. Metzger BE , Coustan DR. Summary and recommendations of the Fourth International Workshop-Conference pm gestational diabetes mellitus. *Diabetes Care* 1998;21:B161–B167.

72. National Diabetes Data Group. Classification and diagnosis of diabetes mellitus and other categories of glucose intolerance. *Diabetes* 1979;28:1039–1057.

73. American Diabetes Association. Gestational diabetes mellitus. *Diabetes Care* 2002;25:S94–S96.

74. World Health Organization. *Definition, Diagnosis and Classification of Diabetes Mellitus snd Its Complications.* Geneva: World Health Organization, 1999.

75. DeFronzo RA, Keen H. *International Textbook of Diabetes Mellitus.* New York: John Wiley and Sons, 1995.

76. Harlass FE, Brady K, Read JA. Reproducibility of the oral glucose tolerance test in pregnancy. *Am J Obstet Gynecol* 1991;164:564–568.

77. Troxler RG, Trabal JF, Malcolm CL. Interpretation of an abnormal glucose tolerance test encountered during multiphasic laboratory screening. *Aviat Space Environ Med* 1975;46:729–735.

78. McDonald GW, Fisher GF, Burnham C. Reproducibility of the oral glucose tolerance test. *Diabetes.* 1965;14:473–480.

79. Olefsky JM, Reaven GM. Insulin and glucose responses to identical oral glucose tolerance tests performed forty-eight hours apart. *Diabetes.* 1974;23:449–453.

80. Carpenter MW, Coustan DR. Criteria for screening tests for gestational diabetes. *Am J Obstet Gynecol* 1982;144:768–773.

81. Sermer M, Naylor CD, Gare DJ, et al. Impact of time since last meal on the gestational glucose challenge test: the Toronto Tri-Hospital Gestational Diabetes Project. *Am J Obstet Gynecol* 1994;171:607–616.

82. Williams CB, Iqbal S, Zawacki CM, et al. Effect of selective screening for gestational diabetes. *Diabetes Care* 1999;22:418–421.

83. Moses RG, Griffiths RD. Can a diagnosis of gestational diabetes be an advantage to the outcome of pregnancy? *J Society Gynecol Investig* 1995;2:523–525.

84. Conway DL, Langer O. Elective delivery of infants with macrosomia in diabetic women: reduced shoulder dystocia versus increased cesarean deliveries. *Am J Obstet Gynecol* 1998;178:922–925.

85. Canadian Task Force on the Periodic Health Examination. Screening for gestational diabetes mellitus. *Can Med Assoc J* 1992;147:435–443.

86. Coustan DR. Screening and testing for gestational diabetes mellitus. *Obstet Gynecol Clin North Am* 1996;23:125–136.

87. Sacks DA, Salim AF, Greenspoon JS, et al. Do the current standards for glucose intolerance testing in pregnancy represent a valid conversion of O'Sullivan's original criteria? *Am J Obstet Gynecol* 1989;161:638–641.

88. Rust OA, Bofill JA, Andrew ME, et al. Lowering the threshold for the diagnosis of gestational diabetes. *Am J Obstet Gynecol* 1996;175:961–965.

89. Schwartz ML, Ray WN, Lubarsky SL. The diagnosis and classification of gestational diabetes mellitus: Is it time to change our tune? *Am J Obstet Gynecol* 1999;180:1560–1571.

90. Landon MB, Gabbe ST, Sachs L. Management of diabetes mellitus and pregnancy: a survey of obstetricians and maternal-fetal specialists. *Obstet Gynaecol* 1978;51:306–310.

91. Bancroft K, Tuffnell DJ, Mason GC, et al. A randomised controlled pilot study of the management of gestational impaired glucose tolerance. *Br J Obstet Gynaecol* 2000;107:959–963.

92. Griffin ME, Coffey M, Johnson H, et al. Universal vs. risk factor-based screening for gestational diabetes mellitus: detection rates, gestation at diagnosis and outcome. *Diabet Med* 2000;17:26–32.

93. Santini DL, Ales KL. The impact of universal screening for gestational glucose intolerance on outcome of pregnancy. *Surg Gynecol Obstet* 1990;170:427–436.

94. Wen SW, Kramoer M, Joseph KS, et al. Impact of prenatal glucose screening on the diagnosis of gestational diabetes and on pregnancy outcomes. *Am J Epidem* 2000;152:1009–1014; discussion, 1015–106.

95. Tuffnell DJ, West J, Walkinshaw SA. Treatments for gestational diabetes and impaired glucose tolerance in pregnancy. *The Cochrane Database of Systematic Reviews* 2003, Issue 1. Art No: CD003395. DOI: 10.1002/14651858. CD003395.

96. Buchanan TS, Kjos SL, Montoro MN, et al. Use of fetal ultrasound to select metabolic therapy for pregnancies complicated by mild gestational diabetes. *Diabetes Care* 1994;17:275–283.

97. Langer O, Anyaegbunam A, Brustman L, et al. Management of women with one abnormal oral glucose tolerance test value reduces adverse outcome in pregnancy. *Am J Obstet Gynecol* 1989;161:593–599.

98. Shushan A, Ezra Y, Samueloff A. Early treatment of gestational diabetes reduces the rate of fetal macrosomia. *Am J Perinatol.* 1997;14:253–256.

99. Langer O, Brustman L, Anyaegbunam A, et al. The significance of one abnormal glucose tolerance test value on adverse outcome in pregnancy. *Am J Obstet Gynecol* 1987;157:758–763.

100. Gyves MT, Rodman HM, Little AB, et al. A modern approach to management of pregnant diabetics: a two-year analysis of perinatal outcomes. *Am J Obstet Gynecol* 1977;128:606–616.

101. Kalkhoff RK. Therapeutic results of insulin therapy in gestational diabetes mellitus. *Diabetes* 1985;34[Suppl 2]:97–100.

102. Drexel H, Bichler A, Sailer S, et al. Prevention of perinatal morbidity by tight metabolic control in gestational diabetes mellitus. *Diabetes Care* 1988;11:761–768.

103. Coustan DR, Imarah J. Prophylactic insulin treatment of gestational diabetes reduces the incidence of macrosomia, operative delivery, and birth trauma. *Am J Obstet Gynecol* 1984;150:836–842.

104. Johnson JM, Lange IR, Harman CR, et al. Biophysical profile scoring in the management of the diabetic pregnancy. *Obstet Gynecol* 1988;72:841–846.

105. Landon MB, Gabbe SG. Antepartum fetal surveillance in gestational diabetes mellitus. *Diabetes* 1985;34[Suppl 2]:50–54.

106. Girz BA, Divon MY, Merkatz IR. Sudden fetal death in women with well-controlled, intensively monitored gestational diabetes. *J Perinatol* 1992;12:229–233.

107. Kjos SL, Leung A, Henry OA. Antepartum surveillance in diabetic pregnancies: predictors of fetal distress in labor. *Am J Obstet Gynecol* 1995;173:1532–1539.

108. Landon MB, Gabbe SG. Fetal surveillance and timing of delivery in pregnancy complicated by diabetes mellitus. *Obstet Gynecol Clin North Am* 1996;23:109–123.

109. Buchanan TA, Kjos SL, Montoro MN, et al. Use of fetal ultrasound to select metabolic therapy for pregnancies complicated by mild gestational diabetes. *Diabetes Care* 1994;17:275–283.

110. Rossi G, Somigliana E, Moschetta M, Bottani B, Barbieri M, Vignali M. Adequate timing fetal ultrasound to guide metabolic therapy in mild gestational diabetes mellitus. *Acta Obstet Gynecol Scand* 2000;79:649–654.

110a. Crowther CA, Hiller JE, Moss JR, McPhee AJ, Jeffries WS, Robinson JS; Australian Carbohydrate Intolerance Study in Pregnant Women (ACHOIS) Trial Group. Effect of treatment of gestational diabetes mellitus on pregnancy outcomes. *N Engl J Med* 2005;352:2477-86. Epub 2005 Jun 12.

111. Kitzmiller JL, Elixhauser A, Carr S, et al. Assessment of costs and benefits of management of gestational diabetes mellitus. *Diabetes Care* 1998;21:B123–B130.

112. Kitzmiller JL. Cost analysis of diagnosis and treatment of gestational diabetes mellitus. *Clin Obstet Gynecol* 2000;43:140–153.

113. Coustan DR. Management of gestational diabetes mellitus: a self-fulfilling prophecy? *JAMA* 1996;275:1199–1200.

114. Sebire NJ, Jolly M, Harris JP, et al. Maternal obesity and pregnancy outcome: a study of 287,213 pregnancies in London. *Int J Obes Relat Metab Disord* 2001;25:1175–1182.

115. Baeten JM, Bukusi EA, Lambe M. Pregnancy complications and outcomes among overweight and obese nulliparous women. *Am J Public Health* 2001;91:436–440.

116. Galtier-Dereure F, Boegner C, Bringer J. Obesity and pregnancy: complications and cost. *Am J Clin Nutr* 2000;71:1242S–1248S.

117. *Screening for Gestational Diabetes Mellitus.* File Inventory, Systematic Evidence Review Number 26. February 2003. Agency for Healthcare Research and Quality, Rockville, MD. *http://www.ahrq.gov/clinic/prev/gdminv.htm.*

118. Brody S, Harris R, Lohr K. Screening for gestational diabetes: a summary of the evidence for the U.S. Preventive Services Task Force. *Obstet Gynecol* 2003;101:380–392.

119. Kolderup LB, Laros RK Jr, Musci TJ. Incidence of persistent birth injury in macrosomic infants: association with mode of delivery. *Am J Obstet Gynecol* 1997;177:37–41.

120. Beaulieu MD. Screening for gestational diabetes mellitus. In: Canadian Task Force on the Periodic Health Examination. *Canadian Guide to Clinical Preventive Health Care* Ottawa: Health Canada, 1994;16–23.

Screening for Low Birth Weight Using Maternal Height and Weight

Lambert H. Lumey

■ What Is the Problem that Requires Screening?

Low birth weight (<2,500 g).

What is the incidence/prevalence of the target condition?

The prevalence of low birth weight ranges from 5% to 10% in selected populations. The rate varies considerably by geographic region and by race, which is likely due in part to biologic differences and in part to the difficulties obtaining representative samples from well-defined populations. The proportion of infants weighing less than 2,500 g at birth in England and Wales in 1978 was 6.7%.[1]

Two data sources were used for this analysis of the association between maternal height and weight and infant size at birth. The first is from Amsterdam[2] and the second from California.[3] Both populations are relatively well defined and include adequate numbers of white, black, and Asian subjects.

For The Netherlands, all women delivering at three Amsterdam hospitals participating in the Gemeenschappelijke Verloskundige Registratie obstetric database (1972–1982) with pertinent information on the variables of interest were included. A secondary analysis was carried out using data originally assembled to evaluate risk factors in this population for perinatal mortality.[2] This population comprises Dutch women, black women mainly from Surinam and the Dutch Antilles, and Asian women mainly of Indian, Chinese, or Indonesian origin. About 30% of births in The Netherlands are planned home deliveries, and hospital births generally reflect a selection of at-risk pregnancies. There is universal health coverage in The Netherlands, and the selected population represents an urban population with a wide variety of economic and social characteristics deficient only in the extremes.

For the United States, women with pertinent information from the Child Health and Development Study (CHDS; 1959–1967) were included. A data tape was kindly provided by R. E. Christianson of the CHDS for secondary analyses. This population from the San Francisco East Bay area of California comprises white, black, and Asian members of the Kaiser Foundation Health Plan. In this prepaid medical insurance plan, comprehensive medical care is provided to members and their families who constitute an urban population with a wide variety of economic and social characteristics deficient only the in extremes.

What are the sequelae of the condition that are of interest in clinical medicine?

Perinatal mortality (PNM) and morbidity are markedly increased among low-birth-rate infants. In Amsterdam, 80% of PNM occurred in low-birth-weight infants who comprise only 7.8% of all births. In California, these figures are 65% and 6%, respectively.

■ The Tests

What is the purpose of the tests?

To identify a subgroup of women at increased risk of delivering a low birthweight infant.

What is the nature of the test?

Measurements of height and weight are commonly made during prenatal visits. These measurements are valid, accurate, and reliable when appropriate equipment is used. They have been used to identify women with an increased risk of delivering low-birth-rate infants since women of low height or weight are at increased risk of such adverse outcomes. In mothers with heights between 145 and 180 cm and mid-pregnancy weights between 35 and 80 kg in a large birth series from Aberdeen, Scotland, babies born to the shortest and lightest mothers were nearly 1kg lighter on average than those born to the tallest and heaviest mothers.[4] In Aberdeen, the effects of maternal height and weight on birth size were to some degree independent, with an prevalence of low birth weight of 4.1% among the heaviest 25% of primigravida at any given height compared with 9.6% in the lightest 25%.[5]

But while it is often useful to describe a clinical subpopulation by its mean height and weight, the effectiveness of prenatal measurements to accurately predict an increased risk of low birth weight for a given individual has not been satisfactory in the past.[3,6] Thus, the data from the Amsterdam and California populations were used to test the performance of these tests in predicting adverse outcomes with relatively extreme cutoff points: a very low height (<150cm or 59 inches) or a very low weight (<50 kg or 110lb). Test performances were examined separately for women of different ethnicity.

The efficacy of screening for low birth weight using low maternal height and weight are given in Tables 29–1 and 29–2. The number of subjects in the study group is listed first, and then the prevalence of a low-birth-rate pregnancy and finally the presumed risk factor (low height or weight). Also given as percentages are the sensitivity, specificity, and the positive and negative predictive values, together with likelihood ratios associated with positive and negative test results. These performance statistics are presented for the three ethnic groups, first separately, and then combined in the form of a weighted average. These analyses were repeated in a population of severely malnourished pregnant women during the Dutch famine of 1944 to 1945 using weight loss in pregnancy as the test criterion. Even weight loss during pregnancy performed no better as a predictor of an adverse pregnancy outcome than low maternal weight in this population (data not shown).[7]

What are the implications of testing maternal height as a screening test for low birth weight?

What does an abnormal test result mean? The overall sensitivity and positive predictive value of low maternal height as a screening test for low birth weight are very low (4% and 14%, respectively; Table 29–1). The sensitivity is highest among Asian women (17%), but the positive predictive value is highest in black women (about 20%). The likelihood ratio of a positive test result across all test populations is 2.0.

What does a normal test result mean? The specificity of a negative test is relatively high in all subgroups with a weighted average across populations of

Table 29–1	Screening for low birth weight (LBW) using low maternal height (<150 cm)						
	Whites		**Blacks**		**Asians**		
Population	**NL**	**US**	**NL**	**US**	**NL**	**US**	**All**
No.	17,435	10,422	1,405	3,795	1,670	629	35,356
Prevalence of LBW	7	5	9	10	10	7	7
Prevalence of height <150 cm	0.4	2	2	2	11	15	2
Sensitivity, %	1	5	5	5	16	17	4
Specificity, %	100	98	98	98	89	86	98
LR (pos)	—	2.5	2.5	2.5	1.5	1.2	2.0
LR (neg)	1.0	1.0	1.0	1.0	0.9	1.0	1.0
PPV, %	14	11	23	19	14	8	14
NPV, %	93	95	91	90	91	93	93

LBW, low birth weight; LR, likelihood ratio; NL, The Netherlands; NPV, negative predictive value; PPV, positive predictive value; US, United States.

Table 29-2 Screening for low birth weight using low maternal weight (<50 kg)

| Population | Whites | | Blacks | | Asians | | |
	NL	US	NL	US	NL	US	All
No.	18.151	11,730	1,295	4,083	1,544	699	37,502
Prevalence of LBW	7	5	10	10	10	7	7
Prevalence of weight <50 kg	2	7	7	5	28	40	6
Sensitivity, %	6	13	9	9	48	54	11
Specificity, %	98	94	93	96	74	61	95
LR (pos)	3.0	2.2	1.3	1.5	1.9	1.4	2.2
LR (neg)	1.0	0.9	1.0	0.9	0.7	0.8	0.9
PPV, %	19	10	12	18	17	10	16
NPV	93	95	90	91	93	95	93

LBW, low birth weight; LR, likelihood ratio; NL, The Netherlands; NPV, negative predictive value; PPV, positive predictive value; US, United States.

98%. The probability of low birth weight after a normal test result is 7%. However, the prevalence in the untested population is the same and the LR (neg) is approximately equal to 1.

What are the implications of testing maternal weight as a screening test for low birth weight?

What does an abnormal test result mean? The overall sensitivity and positive predictive values of low maternal weight as a screening test for low birth weight are low (11% and 16%; Table29–2). Sensitivity is highest among Asian women (50%), but the predictive value does not exceed 19% in any of the subgroups. The LR (pos) across all populations is 2.2.

What does a normal test result mean? The specificity of a negative test is relatively high in all subgroups and the weighted average across all populations is 95%. The probability of low birth weight after a normal test is 7%, which is the same as the prevalence of low birth weight in the untested population (LR(neg) is approximately 1).

What is the cost of testing?

The direct costs of height and weight measurements during prenatal visits are negligible given that measuring equipment is purchased once and used for years. Indirect costs include patient and staff time (maybe 90sec per visit) and waiting time (which can be considerable).

■ Conclusions and Recommendations

Neither low maternal height nor low maternal weight is an effective screening test to identify women at risk of a low-birth-rate child. The predictive values of a positive test for low birth weight are 14% and 16%, respectively. This means that only one out of six to seven women with a low height or weight actually delivers a low-birth-rate infant. Given the relatively low prevalence of low birth weight, even a doubling of risk (at the aggregate level) after positive test would not provide useful additional information for clinical practice. Normal test results also fail to provide useful information as the probability of an adverse outcome after a normal test is the same as the average prevalence of low birth weight (about 7%) in unscreened populations; all the LR (neg) values are close to 1.

Whereas the combined effect of low prepregnancy maternal weight and low weight gain in pregnancy on low birth weight may seem dramatic, the predictive value of both characteristics with respect to low birth weight among term births was only 6% in white women and 16% in black women in the study by Eastman and Jackson.[8] This is no higher than the positive predictive value of low maternal weight alone in our populations.

The measurement of maternal weight (or height) for the prediction of fetal growth abnormalities should be abandoned in the light of the evidence presented and because of other evidence revealing no benefit of weight measurements for individual screening or prediction of these or other adverse conditions.[9] It may still be desirable to document maternal height and weight at least once, preferably early in pregnancy to seek risk factors for other medical abnormalities.

■ Summary

1 ■ **What Is the Problem that Requires Screening?**

Low birth weight.

a. What is the incidence/prevalence of the target condition?

The prevalence of low birth weight ranges from 5% to 10% among populations.

b. What are the sequelae of the condition that are of interest in clinical medicine?

Perinatal mortality and morbidity is markedly increased among low-birth-rate infants.

2 ■ The Tests

a. What is the purpose of the tests?
To detect women at risk of delivery of a low-birth-rate infant.

b. What is the nature of the tests?
Measurement of maternal height and weight

c. What are the implications of testing?
1. What does an abnormal test result mean?
   One out of six to seven women with low height or weight actually have a low-birth-rate infant.
2. What does a normal test result mean?
   Normal tests do not provide useful information since the probability of an adverse outcome after a normal test is the same as the prevalence of low birth weight in unscreened populations.

d. What is the cost of testing?
The marginal costs are negligible.

3 ■ Conclusions and Recommendations

Screening for low birth weight cannot be achieved successfully with either low maternal height or low maternal weight as test criteria.

References

1. Office of Population Censuses and Surveys. Birthweight statistics. *Monitor DH3* 1980;81:4.
2. Doornbos JPR, Nordbeck HJ. Perinatal mortality. Obstetric risk factors in community of mixed ethnic origin in Amsterdam. Thesis. University of Amsterdam, 1985.
3. van den Berg BJ, Oechsli FW. Prematurity. In: Bracken MB, ed., *Perinatal Epidemiology*. New York: Oxford University Press, 1984.
4. Thomson AM, Billewicz, WZ, Hytten FE. The assessment of fetal growth. *J Obstet Gynaecol Br Commonw* 1968;75:903–916.
5. Thomson AM, Billewicz WZ. Nutritional status, maternal physique and reproductive efficiency. *Proc Nutr Soc* 1963;22:55–60.
6. Fortney JA, Whitehorne EW. The development of an index of high risk pregnancy. *Am J Obstet Gynec* 1982;143:501–508.
7. Lumey LH, Ravelli ACJ, Wiessing LG, et al. Dutch famine birth cohort study: design, validation of exposure, and selected characteristics of subjects after 43 years follow-up. *Paed Perinat Epidem* 1993;7:354–367.
8. Eastman NJ, Jackson E. Weight relationships in pregnancy, I: the bearing of maternal weight gain and pre-pregnant weight on birth weight in full tern pregnancies. *Obst Gyn Survey* 1968;23:1003–1025.
9. Chalmers I, Enkin M, Keirse MJNC, eds. *Effective Care in Pregnancy and Childbirth*. Oxford: Oxford University Press, 1989.

Fundal Height Measurement

Jeanne C. McDermott

■ What Is the Problem that Requires Screening?

A size-for-date discrepancy during pregnancy in the size of the uterine fundus.

What is the incidence/prevalence of the target condition?

The prevalence of intrauterine growth restriction (IUGR) when defined as birth weight below specified percentiles (variously 2.3 to 10) for gestational age ranges from 2.5% to 27% of births.[1,2] Estimates of IUGR rates are difficult in settings where gestational age is unknown or uncertain.

The prevalence of naturally occurring multiple fetal pregnancy ranges from a low of 0.43% of pregnancies in Japan up to about 1.2% in the United States and Scotland to 5.72% in Nigeria.[3] Assisted reproductive technologies have increased the rates of twin and higher order multiple fetal pregnancies in Western countries.[4,5] In the United States, the rate of twins in 2002 (3.1%) was 38% higher than 1990 and 65% higher than 1980. The rate of triplet and higher order multiple births has leveled off at 1.84% after a 400% increase between 1980 and 1998.[6]

Hydramnios complicates 0.2% to 1.6 % of pregnancies.[7]

A molar pregnancy occurs in 0.05% to 0.1% of pregnancies in the industrialized nations. It approaches 1% in areas of Asia.[8]

Erroneous dating is differentiated from unknown gestational age. Erroneous dating uses the stated last menstrual period for estimating gestational age, but that date does not result in an accurate estimate. The first day of the last

Disclaimer: This book chapter represents the personal views of the author and does not construe or imply any official National Institutes of Health, Department of Health and Human Services, or U.S. government policy.

menstrual period is traditionally used to establish the duration of gestation, although it is fraught with potential errors. Gestational age estimates based on the last menstrual period agree within 1 week of the best obstetric estimate (using all modalities including ultrasound) in only 60% of women.[9] Even among women with "certain dates," the range of error compared with ultrasound is up to 54 days.[10] Among women referred for an ultrasound examination because of suspected IUGR, over one third have their expected date of confinement recalculated.[11] Since the follicular phase of a cycle can be significantly longer than 14 days but not shorter than 6 to 7 days, most dating errors are over-rather than underestimates of the true gestational age.

Unknown gestational age due to unknown dates of last menstrual period is a frequently encountered problem in all antenatal care settings, but more often in resource-poor settings. For example, less than 8% of over 1,500 women in a study in Malawi were able to provide a date for their last menstrual period.[12] This problem is more serious in settings, such as Malawi, where ultrasound for dating and high-level obstetric and neonatal services are not readily available.

Low-birth-weight (LBW) babies are those with birth weight below 2,500 g, and include those at term but IUGR, preterm but without IUGR, and those who are both preterm and IUGR. LBW rate estimates range from 7% in the United States[13] to as high as 18% in Malawi[13] and 34% in India.[14]

Large babies with birth weights above 4,000 g are not as common as LBW, but still represent a high-risk group. While little prevalence data are available in many parts of the world, estimates of 6.5% to 10% are given for Europe.[15,16] In the United States, 9.1% of the live births in 2002 weighed more than 4,000 g.[6]

What are the sequelae of the condition that are of interest in clinical medicine?

The perinatal mortality rate associated with IUGR is four to eight times higher than that for the appropriately grown infant. Morbid events include fetal distress requiring cesarean delivery and neonatal hypoglycemia, hypocalcemia, hypothermia, polycythemia and long-term neurobehavioral problems.[1]

Both the mother and fetuses suffer increased morbidity and mortality in multiple fetal pregnancies. Perinatal[17] and neonatal[18] mortalities are four to five times higher for twins than singletons. The increased rate of death is due to all causes.[18] Maternal complications more common in women with a multiple fetal pregnancy include hyperemesis, preeclampsia, hydramnios, preterm rupture of membranes, preterm labor and delivery, cesarean delivery, and postpartum hemorrhage.[3]

Sequelae of hydramnios also affect both the mother and fetus. Hydramnios is often associated with fetal malformation. Depending on the presence or absence of associated conditions, the perinatal mortality rates range from 2.4% to over 60% when hydramnios is present.[19] Maternal complications include an increased risk of preeclampsia, respiratory compromise, cesarean delivery, preterm delivery, and postpartum hemorrhage.[7]

The most serious sequelae of molar pregnancy is the development of persistent gestational trophoblastic neoplasia in 15% to 20% of such pregnancies.

Other serious complications include hyperemesis gravidarum, preeclampsia, pulmonary embolization of trophoblastic tissue, and disseminated intravascular coagulation.[20]

Erroneous dating of the pregnancy may also lead to serious problems. Term fetuses misclassified as postterm may be subject to unnecessary and costly interventions such as antepartum fetal surveillance, induction of labor, and cesarean delivery for a failed induction. Preterm fetuses who are misclassified as term may be delivered without optimal management. Term pregnancies misclassified as preterm may be subject to unnecessary tocolysis. A postterm fetus misclassified as term may continue in utero without appropriate monitoring and result in a stillbirth (see also Chapter 20).

Unknown gestational age results in many of the same problems as erroneous dating with either over- or underutilization of appropriate interventions.

A LBW infant has a higher risk of mortality and morbidity than a normal-birth-weight infant, and this increased risk is due to the causes associated with IUGR and/or prematurity. LBW infants in the United States have 40 times the neonatal mortality as normal-birth-weight infants. This higher morbidity risk continues through childhood.[21]

Large babies (> 4,000 g) and their mothers are also at higher risk of poor outcome due to obstructed or protracted labor and delivery and the resulting birth trauma and operative deliveries. Mothers are more likely to suffer from postpartum hemorrhage.[16,22]

■ The Tests

What is the purpose of the tests?

In addition to the use of fundal height measurement to estimate gestational age and weight, serial measurements are used as a screening tool to monitor fundal growth. A fundal height measurement smaller than expected may indicate either IUGR or an error in the estimated gestational age. A large fundal height measurement may indicate macrosomia, multiple fetal pregnancy, hydramnios, molar pregnancy, or an error in dating. In addition, large variation in the growth of biologically normal fetuses may cause size for dates discrepancies.

What is the nature of the tests?

The uterine fundus is routinely measured to detect a discrepancy between the size and the estimated gestational age. A size for gestational age (size: date) discrepancy is one of the most common problems encountered in obstetrics. The possible explanations are many. In some instances, the discrepancy is detectable with a single measurement; in other cases, serial measurements are required.

Measurement issues. The measurement of fundal height is subject to many sources of variation. Although the current practice is to measure in centimeters above the symphysis pubis, the measurement was originally made in relation to several landmarks on the maternal abdomen. In addition to the normal, random variation inherent to any measurement, the conditions of fundal height measurement are usually not standardized. The measurement is affected by such factors as maternal position[23]; whether a tape measure or a pair of calipers are used[24,25]; whether the measurement is from the superior or inferior aspect of the pubic symphysis; whether the tape is curved around the uterus or held horizontally[25]; whether the measurement is made in the midline or to the superior fetal pole wherever it may lie; and whether the bladder is full.[26] Finally, serial measurements are graphed to aid the identification of any patterns as many become evident only after repeated screening.[27]

Criteria for an abnormal test. There is no consensus: below the 10th or above the 90th centile; more than 2 or 3 cm below or above the mean; 1 or 2 standard deviations (SDs) below or above the mean for gestation. In addition, a single abnormal measurement, two consecutive abnormal measurements, any three abnormal measurements, the percentage of all measurements that are abnormal (20%, 30%, or 40%), and the lack of growth for three successive measurements have all been used to define an abnormal fundal height. One practical rule of thumb is that the fundal height in centimeters is approximately equal to the gestational age in weeks between 20 and 31 to 36 weeks' gestation. Thereafter, most norms indicate that the rate of fundal height growth slows.

A number of countries have adopted a policy of one or two ultrasound examinations as part of routine prenatal care.[28] In the United States, most women undergo one or more "indicated" ultrasound examinations during pregnancy.[29] Even in settings with easily available ultrasound, a role still exists for the routine measurement of fundal height during each antenatal visit. Although the detection rates of multiple fetal pregnancies, molar pregnancies, and dating errors approach 100% with a mid–second-trimester ultrasound examination, serial fundal height measurements are still necessary to identify conditions that develop later in pregnancy such as IUGR and hydramnios. Several curves for normal fundal height have been developed.[30–40] The populations used to derive these norms tend to exclude women with pregnancy complications or who deliver small for gestational age infants. Opinion differs as to whether a single norm should be used for all populations,[41,42] whether separate norms should be used for developing countries,[43–46] or whether individual norms are needed for each local or institutional population.[39,47] One study examined the use of five commonly used curves in a U.S. population. The authors found large enough differences to conclude that providers should test the accuracy of any fundal height curve before adopting it into practice.[48]

The cutoff chosen to define abnormal fundal growth, along with the prevalence of IUGR in the population screened, will impact the calculated sensitivity, specificity, and positive and negative predictive values of the test.[49] Thus, the caregiver should set the cutoff at a level that provides acceptable false-negative and false-positive rates that do not overwhelm the clinical resources available to follow up women with a positive screen.[32]

Sensitivity, specificity, and predictive values of the test. Most studies that have formally evaluated fundal height measurement used IUGR as the outcome of interest (Table 30–1). Although a wide range of sensitivities is reported (partly the result of inconsistent definitions of abnormal), the sensitivity has centered around 65% and specificity around 90%. As would be expected, the positive predictive value varied, given that the prevalence of IUGR differed in the populations studied. The sensitivity of fundal height measurement to detect IUGR improves when the measurements are made by two or less caregivers rather than multiple (86% versus 42%), although this factor does not improve specificity or predictive power.[50]

The only randomized controlled trial (RCT) of fundal height measurement compared pregnancies in Denmark.[51] There were no differences between groups regarding the prediction of IUGR, the use of interventions or additional diagnostic procedures, or the condition of the newborn. However, other sophisticated screening tools such as ultrasound were routinely used. This was the only study eligible for inclusion in a recent Cochrane review in which the author concluded there was not enough evidence to evaluate the use of symphysis-fundal height measurement in antenatal care, but also opined "it would be unwise to abandon the use of symphysis-fundal height measurement unless a much larger trial likewise suggested that it is unhelpful."[52]

A few authors specifically evaluated fundal height measurement as a screening tool for multiple fetal pregnancies. Most studies report very high sensitivity of a "high" fundal height measurement (99%–100%),[26,53,54] although others report lower sensitivities between 50% and 76%.[40,55] Preterm delivery is one of the most common complications of a multiple fetal pregnancy, and an overdistended uterus is hypothesized to be a contributing cause. Two authors tested this hypothesis using fundal height measurements, but found no association between increased fundal height measurement and preterm labor among twin[56] and triplet[57] pregnancies.

Although no published studies have specifically evaluated the detection of hydramnios by fundal height measurement, authors typically refer to increased uterine size as a characteristic of hydramnios[7] and report a definite relationship between excessive amniotic fluid and fundal height.[58] Where documented, all cases of hydramnios had a fundal height measurement either more than 2 cm or 2 SD above the mean.[35,53] Several authors reported that increased uterine size in women with an IUGR fetus was due to hydramnios.[35,59,60]

Although review of the literature revealed no formal evaluation of the ability of fundal height measurement to ascertain molar pregnancies, authors report the uterine size is approximately 4 weeks larger than dates in 38% to 50% of molar pregnancies.[20]

Although several studies examined a single fundal height measurement for estimating gestational age,[12,61,62] the data necessary to evaluate sensitivity and specificity were not provided. Only two studies that examined single fundal height measurement for the detection of small babies included data for sensitivity and specificity: for IUGR infants in Brazil[63] and low-birth-weight infants in India (Table 30–2).[14]

Table 30–1 FHM as a screening tool for IUGR							
Reference	IUGR definition/prevalence	Population studied	Definition of + test	Sensitivity	Specificity	PPV	NPV
Westin, 1977 (35)	BW > 1 SD below mean Prevalence 11%	Sweden, N = 428	A. ≥ 3 cm below mean B. Static/falling FHM	A. 68% B. 52% A or B. 75%	A. 89% B. 95%	A. 44% B. 54%	A. 96% B. 95%
Belizan, 1978 (30)	BW < 10th centile Prevalence 32%	Guatemala, N = 139	< 10th centile × ≥ 1	86%	89%	79%	93%
Quaranta, 1981 (34)	BW < 10th centile Prevalence 30%	England, N = 138	Two consecutive/three isolated FHM < 10th centile	73%	79%	60%	88%
Wallin, 1981 (59)	BW ≥ 2 SD below mean Prevalence not stated	Sweden, N = 812 neonatal ward newborns	> 3 cm below mean × 2 or Threestatic, consecutive FHM	62%	88%	42%	94%
Rosenberg, 1982 (76)	BW < 10th centile Prevalence 6.6%	Scotland, N = 761	A. Two consecutive/three isolated FHM < 10th centile B. 20%, or C. 30%, or D. 40% FHMs <10th centile	A. 56% B. 61% C. 52% D. 48%	A. 85% B. 79% C. 92% D. 92%	A. 21% B. 17% C. 31% D. 30%	A. 96% B. 97% C. 96% D. 96%
Calvert, 1982 (32)	BW < 5th centile Prevalence 6.6% BW < 10th centile Prevalence 12%	England, N = 381	Applied: A. Westin criteria B. Belizan criteria C. Quaranta criteria	< 5th A. 72% B. 60% C. 36% < 10th A. 76% B. 64% C. 36%	< 5th A. 58% B. 76% C. 92% < 10th A. 60% B. 79% C. 94%	< 5th A. 11% B. 15% C. 24% < 10th A. 20% B. 29% C. 43%	< 5th A. 97% B. 96% C. 94% < 10th A. 95% B. 94% C. 92%
Cox, 1983 (33)	BW < 5th centile Prevalence 30% BW ≤ 10th centile Prevalence 48%	Ireland, N = 123	≥ Two FHM below 10th centile	< 5th 70% < 10th 58%	< 5th 87% < 10th 95%	< 5th 70% < 10th 92%	< 5th 87% < 10th 71%

Table 30-1   FHM as a screening tool for IUGR (Continued)

Reference	IUGR definition/prevalence	Population studied	Definition of + test	Sensitivity	Specificity	PPV	NPV
Cnattingius 1984 (77)	BW ≥ 2 SD below mean Prevalence 2.7%	Sweden, N = 527 women with IUGR risk factors	LOW (L): Last FHM ≥ 3 cm below the mean STATIC (S): Last three FHM same, but no FHM >2 cm below mean CATCHUP (C): One FHM > 3 cm below mean, but last < 3 cm below mean	L 50% S 7% C 29% L+C 79% L+C+S 86%	L 98% S 87% C 94% L+C 92% L+C+S 79%	L 39% S 1% C 12% L+C 21% L+C+S 10%	L 99% S 97% C 98% L+C 99% L+C+S 99.5%
Rogers, 1985 (78)	BW < 10 centile Prevalence 10.4% Lubchenko reference	England, N = 250	Westin definition	73%	92%	51%	97%
Tjon, 1985 (79)	Prevalence 8%	Lesotho, N = 122 hospital deliveries	(A) First FHM < 10th centile Belizan (B), Quaranta (C), Westin (D)	A. 40% B. 70% C. 56% D. 100%	A 96% B 84% C 93% D 49%	A 50% B 28% C 45% D 16%	A 95% B 97% C 95% D 100%
Linasmita, 1985 (60)	BW < 10th centile Prevalence 7%	Thailand, N = 257	Two consecutive/three isolated FHM < 10th centile.	61%	96%	55%	97%
Perrson, 1986 (40)	BW < 10th centile Prevalence 9%	Sweden, N = 2941	FHM > 2 SD below mean	27%	88%	18%	92%
Garde, 1986 (80)	BW < 10th centile Prevalence 32%	So. Africa, N = 92	Slope of FHM less than norm	85%	93%	87%	94%
Linasmita, 1986 (53)	BW < 10th centile Prevalence 7%	Thailand, N = 483	Two consecutive/three isolated FHM < 10th centile.	65%	96%	58%	97%
Okonofua, 1986 (81)	BW < 10th centile Prevalence 7%	London, N = 100	Two consecutive FHM < 10th centile	71%	85%	31%	98%
Pearce, 1987 (37)	BW < 10th centile Prevalence 14.3%	England, N = 200	FHM < 10th centile	76%	79%	36%	95%
Mathai, 1987 (2)	BW >1SD below mean Prevalence: at risk, 27%; low risk, 9%	India, at risk: N = 150 low risk: N = 208	>1 SD below mean	78%	88%	70%	92%

Study	Birthweight / Prevalence	Population	Criteria				
Fescina, 1987 (82)	BW < 10th centile Prevalence 38%	CLAP/PAHO Latin America, N = 100 high risk	FHM < 10th centile	56%	91%	80%	77%
Mathai, 1988 (83)	probably same as 1987 Prevalence 12.2%	India, low risk - N = 253	> 3 cm below mean	77%	79%	33%	96%
Azziz, 1988 (39)	BW < 10th centile Prevalence 14.6%	Washington DC N = 192	A. 1 FHM ≥ 1 SD below mean B. 2 FHM ≥ 1 SD below mean C. 3 FHM ≥ 1 SD below mean	A. 86% B. 75% C. 61%	A. 89% B. 95% C. 98%	A. 57% B. 72% C. 81%	A. 97% B. 96% C. 95%
Pattinson, 1988 (43)	BW < 10th centile Prevalence 14.4%	South Africa, N = 97	Two consecutive FHM < 10th centile, or three consecutive static FHM. Used Belizan (B), Quaranta (Q), Calvert (C) charts	B. 86% Q. 93% C. 93%	B. 89% Q. 51% C. 75%	B. 57% Q. 24% C. 38%	B. 97% Q. 98% C. 98%
Stuart, 1989 (84)	BW < 10th centile Prevalence A. General population, 7.6% B. Women with ≥ four FHMs, 7.2%	England, A. N = 1139 B. N = 319 ≥ 4	FHM < 10th centile	A. 51% B. 65%	A. 88% B. 88%	A. 26% B. 21%	A. 96% B. 97%
Norton, 1989 (85)	BW < 10th centile Prevalence 26%	Australia/NZ, N = 34	FHM < 10 centile	86%	85%	60%	96%
Pattinson, 1989 (50)	Criteria not stated Prevalence Group A: 14.1% Group B: 9.5%	South Africa, A = 97, B = 126	Two consecutive/ three isolated FHM < 10 centile	A. 86% B. 42%	A. 89% B 92%	A 57% B 36%	A 97% B 94%

Table continued on following page

Table 30–1	FHM as a screening tool for IUGR (Continued)						
Reference	IUGR definition/prevalence	Population studied	Definition of + test	Sensitivity	Specificity	PPV	NPV
Lindhard, 1990 (51)	BW < 10th centile Prevalence	Denmark, A. N = 804 B. N = 835	< 10th centile × ≥ 2 FHMs, or ≥ two consecutive FHM > 20% fall, or three static consecutive FHMs	A. 28% B. 48%	A. 97% B. 97%	A. 41% B. 47%	A. 94% B. 97%
Grover, 1991	BW > 1 SD below mean Prevalence 26%	India, N = 400	FHM > 1 SD below mean	81%	93%	84%	92%
Cronje, 1993	Dunn reference Prevalence 13.7%	South Africa, N = 314	≥ Two successive/ three isolated FHM <10th centile or three static consecutive FHM	42%	83%	28%	90%

BW=birth weight; FHM, fundal height measurement; IUGR, intrauterine growth restriction.

Table 30-2   Single FHM as a screening tool for IUGR or LBW baby in Labor

Reference	IUGR definition/prevalence	Population studied	Definition of positive test	Sensitivity	Specificity	PPV	NPV
Rondo, 2003 (63)	IUGR BW< 10th centile Williams Curve (1982) at 39 weeks' gestation Prevalence 6.3%	Brazil, $N = 366$	≤ 30 cm < 35 cm ≤ 33 cm	A. 17.4% B. 91.3% C. 60.8%	A. 99.1% B. 32.3% C. 78.7%	A. 57.1% B. 8.3% C. 16.1%	A. 94.7% B. 98.2% C. 96.8%
Mohanty, 1998 (14)	LBW ≦ 2.5 kg Prevalence 34.4%	India, $N = 151$	< 28 cm ≤ 32 cm < 30 cm	A. 51.9% B. 90.3% C. 76.9%	A. 95.9% B. 54.5% C. 77.7%	A. 87% B. 51% C. 64.5%	A. 79.1% B. 91.5% C. 86.5%

BW, birth weight; FHM, fundal height measurement; IUGR, intrauterine growth restriction; LBW, low birth weight.

Validity. Although it is not possible to directly measure the uterus, several investigators have compared tape measurements of the palpated fundal height with ultrasound measurements of the uterine fundus and/or fetus. Bagger et al.[64] observed a correlation of 0.86 between ultrasound and tape estimates of fundal height. The mean difference for five observers ranged from +0.49 to −1.97 cm. Another author found an even higher correlation at 0.96 with no differences by obesity or race in a U.S. population.[65] Engström et al.[66] found a mean absolute error of 1.25 cm, with a maximum error of 8.6 cm. Fifty-eight percent of the tape measurements were within 1 cm and 79% within 2 cm of the ultrasound estimates. Tape measurements of fundal height are affected by fetal presentation and uterine wall thickness. They are unaffected by maternal height, weight, body mass index, abdominal subcutaneous fat, parity, and fetal gestational age. However, one study found that clinicians' knowledge, as determined by their ability to see the markings on the tape measure and expected gestational age biased their fundal height measurements.[67]

Reliability/Reproducibility. Both intra- and interobserver problems with either reliability or reproducibility are described. Mean intraobserver differences of fundal height measurement range from 0.4 to 2.0 cm, with a maximum difference of 8.0 cm, whereas intraobserver SDs for repeated measures range from 0.8 to 1.35 cm, and coefficients of variation from 2.2 to 4.8%.[24,25,32,38,64,68] These errors are large enough to be clinically relevant.

Interobserver variation of fundal height measurement tends to be larger than the intraobserver variation. The mean difference in fundal height measurement between observers ranges from 0.5 to 4.0 cm, with a maximum difference of 13 cm. The SD of interobserver variation ranges from 0.7 to 3.6 cm, with reported coefficients of variation from 6.4 to 7.8%.[24,27,64,68–70] Beazley and Underhill[24] found that 85% of measurements were within 1.3 cm of those made by other observers, but Crosby and Engström[70] found that only 14% to 45% were within 2 cm.

Most studies use tape measures only. There is no difference in reliability among providers with different levels of training.[32,38] Nor is there any effect of gestational age on the reliability of the measurement.[64] The few studies that compare tape measurements with those obtained with pelvimetry calipers conclude that the caliper measurements are slightly more reproducible and give a smaller measurement.[24,25]

What are the implications of testing?

What does an abnormal test result mean? A discrepancy between uterine size and dates should trigger an ultrasound examination. Depending on the underlying cause, appropriate follow-up and clinical care for IUGR, multifetal pregnancy, hydramnios or molar pregnancy should be undertaken.

In labor, a fundal height measurement that is smaller or larger than expected for a singleton term fetus should trigger further assessment with palpation and other means that may be available. Referral to a higher level of care may be appropriate, based upon the conclusions after further assessment and the availability of the higher level of care.

What does a normal test result mean? Normal fundal height measurements are reassuring, especially when graphed and found to be increasing along the lines of normal growth curves. However, a normal fundal height measurement is not definitive evidence of fetal and maternal well-being. The caregiver must still use clinical judgment and continue to assess the pregnancy using those modalities accepted as appropriate care.

What is the cost of testing?

Fundal height measurement is among the least expensive tools in antenatal care requiring only a tape measure, a chart or, preferably, a fundal height graph to record the information, and knowledge of gestational age. The training required is minimal and the measurement itself takes less than a minute.

When a large size-for-dates discrepancy of unknown etiology is discovered, the first step is an ultrasound examination to document fetal biometry for gestational age and fetal growth, the number of fetuses, amniotic fluid volume, and fetal and placental abnormalities. The total charge for such an ultrasound varies considerable depending on the country (see Chapters 20 and 31 for more detailed information on ultrasound costs). Using the reimbursement schedule of the Centers for Medicare and Medicaid Services of the U.S. Department of Health and Human Services, the amount reimbursed ranges from $136 to $253. The number of ultrasound examinations ordered as a result of fundal height measurement screening reflects the prevalence and timing of ultrasound use in the population. Early, routine ultrasound examination will usually reveal multiple fetal pregnancies and molar pregnancies and resolve most date discrepancies.

The most prevalent condition identified by serial fundal height measurements is IUGR. If we assume an IUGR prevalence of 10%, a prevalence of hydramnios of 1%, a sensitivity of fundal height measurement for the diagnosis of IUGR of 60%, a sensitivity of fundal height measurement for the diagnosis of hydramnios of 100%, and a predictive value of a positive test of 50%, then approximately 13% of the population would be referred for ultrasound examination to evaluate fetal growth as a result of fundal height screening. At an average charge of $195 per ultrasound exam (based upon the U.S. reimbursement schedule), $2,535 would be spent per 100 women screened with fundal height measurement to identify six of the ten cases of IUGR and the one case of hydramnios. This would be $25 per woman screened and about $362 per positive detected. Once a definitive diagnosis is made, subsequent costs will depend on the particular condition found (for example IUGR, multiple fetal pregnancies).

Although policy makers are urged to use research findings in establishing policies, the impact of these policies on health care are rarely systematically evaluated in a rigorous manner. One study tried to prospectively evaluate the effect of a policy to use serially plotted fundal height measurements on a customized chart in antenatal care by community midwives in England in 1994 to 1995.[71] While more babies were identified as "at risk of" IUGR and LGA (larger than gestational age) by midwives who used the customized charts compared with those who used traditional abdominal palpation and recording, there was no difference in the outcomes between the two groups. Interestingly, although their detection rate was higher, the customized group had about the same number of referrals for ultrasounds as the traditional group, but significantly fewer visits to a specialist at a pregnancy assessment center and significantly fewer antenatal admissions. The authors interpreted these findings as possibly reflecting increased confidence in recognizing normal fetal growth for an individual fetus as a result of plotting the growth on the chart.

■ Conclusions and Recommendations

Fundal height measurement should continue be a routine part of antenatal care,[72] and it was included in the recent multicenter trial of a new model of antenatal care in Argentina, Cuba, Saudi Arabia, and Thailand based on components shown to improve outcomes.[73,74] It is one of the least expensive and simplest procedures/tests in the obstetric armamentarium. The increased use of ultrasound as a screening test in developed countries may alter the role of fundal height measurement. However, it remains an important and appropriate test in countries without universally available ultrasound and other high technology.

Fundal height measurement can effectively identify a size-for-dates discrepancy secondary to a variety of causes, with sensitivities ranging from about 65% (IUGR) to nearly 100% (twins and hydramnios). The cause of the discrepancy can be further evaluated using other tests.

The initial costs of fundal height measurement are exceptionally low, and with no reported risks. However, the charge for the follow-up ultrasound examination would average $23 per woman or about $325 per positive detected.

The effect of the diagnosis of a size-for-dates discrepancy on clinical management depends on the condition identified. Molar pregnancies should be terminated and the patient followed with serial human chorionic gonadotropin (hCG) measurements to search for persistent trophoblastic disease. A diagnosis of IUGR or hydramnios allows the possibility of close monitoring, treatment, and early delivery to minimize fetal and maternal compromise. Antenatal diagnosis of multiple fetal pregnancy allows the woman and her care provider to plan an optimal delivery strategy. Accurate dating of pregnancy prevents unnecessary intervention in falsely labeled preterm and, particularly, postterm pregnancies. Moreover, true preterm and postterm fetuses are more likely to receive appropriate management.

Even those who advocate routine antenatal ultrasound screening rarely recommend its use at every antenatal visit due to its labor-intensive nature and the high skill level required.[75] However, as the use of routine ultrasound becomes more widespread, researchers may wish to reevaluate the costs and benefits of the procedures. Until then, caregivers must rely on clinical suspicion, raised mainly by a size for dates discrepancy identified by fundal height measurement to appropriately order subsequent ultrasound tests.

■ Summary

1 ■ What Is the Problem that Requires Screening?

A size-for-dates discrepancy in the size of the uterine fundus during pregnancy.

a. What is the incidence/prevalence of the target condition?

- IUGR: 2.5% to 10% of births.
- Multiple fetal pregnancy: 0.43% to 5.72% of births
- Hydramnios: 0.2% to 1.6 % of pregnancies
- Molar pregnancy:0.05% to 0.1% of pregnancies in the West, 1% in areas of Asia
- Erroneous date: Only 40% are within 1 week
- LBW: 7% to 30%
- Neonate larger than 4,000 g: 6% to 10%
- Unknown gestational age: May be up to 92%

b. What are the sequelae of the condition that are of interest in clinical medicine?
Increased maternal and perinatal morbidity and mortality.

2 ■ The Tests

a. What is the purpose of the tests?
To detect a size-for-dates discrepancy or to estimate gestational age or fetal weight

b. What is the nature of the tests?
The measurement of the uterine fundal height.

Continued

■ **Summary—cont'd**

c. *What are the implications of testing?*

   1. What does an abnormal test result mean?

     Indicates that an ultrasound examination should be performed to determine the cause.

   2. What does a normal test result mean?

     Normal fundal height measurements are reassuring, especially when increasing along the lines of normal growth curves.

d. *What is the cost of testing?*

   At an average charge of $175 per ultrasound, $2,275 would be spent per 100 women screened with fundal height measurement to identify six of the ten cases of IUGR and the one case of hydramnios. This would be $23 per woman screened and about $325 per positive detected.

3 ■ Conclusions and Recommendations

1. The uterine fundus should be measured at each antenatal visit to screen for size-for-dates discrepancy even if ultrasound examination(s) have been performed.

2. The technique used for fundal height measurement should be as consistent as possible to improve the reproducibility and reliability of the test using as few providers per woman as possible.

3. Measurements should be routinely graphed and a definition of what is abnormal selected.

4. Research should be undertaken to identify the most appropriate definition of an abnormal test, whether population-based curves are necessary, and the role of fundal height measurement in settings where ultrasound is routinely performed.

References

1. Seeds JW. Impaired fetal growth: definition and clinical diagnosis. *Obstet Gynecol* 1984;64:303–310.
2. Mathai M, Jairaj P, Muthurathnam S. Screening for light-for-gestational age infants: a comparison of three simple measurements. *Br J Obstet Gynaecol* 1987;94:217–221.
3. Wenstrom KD, Gall SA. Incidence, morbidity and mortality, and diagnosis of twin gestations. *Clin in Perinatol* 1981;15:1–11.
4. Kiely Jl, Kiely M. Epidemiological trends in multiple births in the United States 1871–1998. *Twin Res* 2001 4:131–133.
5. Blondel B, Macfarlane A. Rising multiple maternity rates and medical management of subfertility: better information is needed. *Eur J Public Health* 2003;13:83–86.
6. Martin JA, Hamilton BE, Sutton PD, et al. Final data for 2002. *Natl Vital Stat Rep* 2003;52:10.

7. Cardwell MS. Polyhydramnios: a review. *Obstet Gynecol Survey* 1987;42:612–617.
8. Goldstein DP, Berkowitz RS. The management of molar pregnancy and gestational trophoblastic tumors. After Bagshawe KD: *Choriocarcinoma*. Baltimore, Williams & Wilkins Co, 1969, p.32 in *Gynecology Principals and Practice*, Kistner RW (ed), Chicago, Year Book Medical Publishers, Inc., 1986.
9. Goldenberg RL, Davis RO, Cutter GR, et al. Prematurity, postdates, and growth retardation: the influence of use of ultrasonography on reported gestational age. *Am J Obstet Gynecol* 1989;160:462–470.
10. Geirsson RT, Busby-Earle RMC. Certain dates may not provide a reliable estimate of gestational age. *Br J Obstet Gynaecol* 1991;98:108–109.
11. Whetham JCG, Muggah H, Davidson S. Assessment of intrauterine growth retardation by diagnostic ultrasound. *Am J Obstet Gynecol* 1976;125:577–580.
12. Verhoeff FH, Milligan P, Brabin BJ, et al. Gestational age assessment by nurses in a developing country using the Ballard method: external criteria only. *Ann Trop Ped* 1997;17:333–342.
13. Arias E, MacDorman MF, Strobino DM, et al. Annual summary of vital statistics-2002. *Pediatrics* 2003;112:1215–1230.
14. Mohanty C, Das BK, Mishra OP. Parturient fundal height as a predictor of low birth weight. *J. Trop Pediat* 1998; 44:222-4.
15. Wikström I, Bergström S, Bakketeig L, et al. Prediction of high birthweight form maternal characteristics, symphysis fundal height and ultrasound biometry. *Gynecol Obstet* 1993;35:25–33.
16. Jolly MC, Seibire NJ, Harris JP, et al. Robinson S. Risk factors for macrosomia and its clinical consequences: a study of 350,311 pregnancies. *Eur J Obstet Gynecol Reprod Biol* 2003; 111:9–1114.
17. Kiely JL. The epidemiology of perinatal mortality in multiple births. *Bull N Y Acad Med* 1990;66:618–637.
18. Kleinman JC, Fowler MG, Kessel SS. Comparison of infant mortality among twins and singletons: United States 1960 and 1983. *Am J Epidemiol* 1991;133:133–143.
19. Desmedt EJ, Henry OA, Beischer N. Polyhydramnios and associated maternal and fetal complications in singleton pregnancies. *Br J Obstet Gynaecol* 1990;97:1115–1122.
20. Kohorn EI. Molar pregnancy: presentation and diagnosis. *Clin Obstet Gynecol* 1984;27:181–191.
21. Kiely JL, Brett KM, Yu SY, et al. Low birth weight and intrauterine growth retardation. In: Wilcox LS, Marks JS, eds., *From Data to Action: CDC's Public Health Surveillance for Women, Infants and Children*. U.S. Department of Health and Human Services, 1994:p.185–202.
22. Raio L, Ghezzi D, Di naro E, et al. Perinatal outcomes of fetuses with birth weight greater than 4500 g: an analysis of 3356 cases. *Eur J Obstet Gynecol Reprod Biol* 2003;109:160–165.
23. Engström JL, Piscioneri LA, Low LK, et al. Fundal height measurement, 3: the effect of maternal position on fundal height measurements. *J Nurs Midwifery* 1993b;38:23–27.
24. Beazley JM, Underhill RA. Fallacy of the fundal height. *BMJ* 1970:404–406.
25. Engström JL, McFarlin BL, Sittler CP. Fundal height measurement, 2: intra- and interexaminer reliability of three measurement techniques. *J Nurs Midwifery* 1993a;38;17–22.
26. Engström JL, Ostrenga KG, Plass RV, et al. The effect of maternal bladder volume on fundal height measurements. *Br J Obstet Gynaecol* 1989;96:987–991.
27. Belizan JM, Villar J, Nardin JC. Poor predictive value of symphysial-fundal height when misused in clinical practice. *Am J Obstet Gynecol* 1990; 162:51348–51349.
28. Holzgreve W. Sonographic screening for anatomic defects. *Sem Perinat* 1990;14:504–513.
29. Ewigman BG, Crane JP, Frigoletto FD, et al, The RADIUS Study Group. Effect of prenatal .ultrasound screening on perinatal outcome. *N Engl J Med* 1993;329:821–827.
30. Belizan JM, Villar J, Nardin JC, et al. Diagnosis of intrauterine growth retardation by a simple clinical method: measurement of uterine height. *Am J Obstet Gynecol* 1978;131:643–646.
31. Williams RL, Creasy RK, Cunningham MD, et al. Fetal growth and perinatal viability in California. *Obstet Gynecol* 1982:59:624–632.
32. Calvert JP, Crean EE, Newcombe RG, et al. Antenatal screening by measurement of symphysis-fundus height. *BMJ* 1982;285:846–849.
33. Cox G, Walsh P, Stack J, et al. The value of fundal height measurement in prediction of fetal growth retardation. *Irish Med J* 1983;76:95–96.

34. Quaranta P, Currell R, Redman CWG. Prediction of small-for-dates infants by measurement of symphysial-fundal-height. *Br J Obstet Gynaecol* 1981;88:115–119.
35. Westin B. Gravidogram and fetal growth. *Acta Obstet Gynecol Scand* 1977;56:273–282.
36. Jimenez, JM, Tyson JE, Reisch JS. Clinical measures of gestational age in normal pregnancies. *Obstet Gynecol* 1983;61:438–43.
37. Pearce JM, Campbell S. A comparison of symphysis-fundal height and ultrasound as screening tests for light-for-gestational age infants. *Br J Obstet Gynaecol* 1987;94:100–104.
38. Rogers MS, Needham PG. Evaluation of fundal height measurement in antenatal care. *Aust N Z J Obstet Gynaecol* 1985;25:87–90.
39. Azziz R, Smith S. Fabro S. The development and use of a standard symphysial-fundal height growth curve in the prediction of small for gestational age neonates. *Int J Gynecol Obstet* 1988;26:81–87.
40. Persson B, Stangenberg M, Lunell NO, et al. Prediction of size of infants at birth by measurement of symphysis fundus height. *Br J Obstet Gynaecol* 1986;93:206–211.
41. Kiserud T. Fundal height growth in rural Africa. *Acta Obstet Gynecol Scand* 1986;65:713–715.
42. Medhat WM, Fahmy SI, Mortada MM, et al. Construction of a local standard symphis fundal height curve for monitoring intrauterine fetal growth. *J Egypt Pub Health Ass* 1991;LXVI:305–330.
43. Pattinson RC. Antenatal detection of small-for-gestational-age babies: choice of a symphysis-fundal growth curve. *S African Med J* 1988;74:282–283.
44. Challis K, Osman NB, Nystrom L, et al. Symphysis-fundal height growth chart of an obstetric cohort of 817 Mozambican women with ultrasound-dated singleton pregnancies. *Trop Med Intern Health* 2002;7:678–684.
45. Ogunranti JO, Fundal height in normal pregnant Nigerian women: anthropometric gravidogram. *Int J Gynecol Obstet* 1990;33:299–305.
46. Walraven GEL, Mkanje RJB, van Dongen PWJ, et al. The development of a local symphysis-fundal height chart in a rural area of Tanzania. *Eur J Obstet Gynecol* 1995;60:149–152.
47. Buhmann L, Elder WG, Hendricks B, et al. A comparison of Caucasian and Southeast Asian among uterine fundal height during pregnancy. *Acta Obstet Gynecol Scand* 1998;77: 521–526.
48. Engström JL, Work BA. Prenatal prediction of small and large-for-gestational age neonates. *J Obstet Gynecol Neonatal Nurs* 1992;21:486–495.
49. Goldenberg RL, Cutter GR, Hoffman HJ, et al. Intrauterine growth retardation: standard for diagnosis. *Am J Obstet Gynecol* 1989b;161:2271–2277.
50. Pattinson RC, Theron GB. Inter-observer variation in symphysis-fundus measurements. *S African Med J* 1989;76:621–622.
51. Lindhard A, Nielsen PV, Mouritsen LA, et al. The implications of introducing the symphyseal-fundal height-measurement: a prospective randomized controlled trial. *Br J Obstet Gynaecol* 1990;97:675–680.
52. Neilson JP. Symphysis-fundal height measurement in pregnancy [Cochrane Review]. In: *The Cochrane Library, Issue 2*. Chichester, UK: John Wiley & Sons, 2004.
53. Linasmita V. Serial symphysis-fundal height measurement of abnormal fetal growth. *J Med Assoc Thail* 1986;69:585–588.
54. Neilson JP, Verkuyl DAA, Bannerman C. Tape measurement of symphysis-fundal height in twin pregnancies. *Br J Obstet Gynaecol* 1988;95:1054–1059.
55. Smibert J. Some observations on the height of the fundus uteri in pregnancy. *Aust N Z J Obstet Gynaecol* 1962;8:125–131.
56. Rouse DJ, Skopec GS, Zlatnik FJ. Fundal height as a predictor of preterm twin delivery. *Obstet Gynecol* 1993;81:211–214.
57. Yokoyama Y. Fundal height as a predictor of early preterm triplet delivery. *Twin Res* 2002; 5:71–74.
58. Cabrol D, Landesman R, Muller J, et al. Treatment of polyhydramnios with prostaglandin synthetase inhibitor (indomethacin). *Am J Obstet Gynecol* 1987;157:422–426.
59. Wallin A., Gyllenswärd A, Westin B. Symphysis-fundus measurement in prediction of fetal growth disturbances. *Acta Obstet Gynecol Scand* 1981;60:317–323.
60. Linasmita V. Antenatal screening of small-for-gestational age infants by symphysial-fundal height measurement. *J Med Assoc Thai* 1985;68:587–591.

61. Faustin D, Gutierrez L, Gintautas J, et al. Clinical assessment of gestational age: a comparison of two methods. *J Nat Med Assoc* 1991; 83:425–429.
62. Andersson R, Bergstrom S. Use of fundal height as a proxy for length of gestation in rural Africa. *J Trop Med Hygiene* 1995;98:169–172.
63. Rondo PHC, Maia Filho NL, Valverde KK. Symphysis-fundal height and size at birth. *Int J Gynecol Obstet* 2003; 81:53–54.
64. Bagger PV, Eriksen PS, Secher NJ, et al. The precision and accuracy of symphysis-fundus distance measurements during pregnancy. *Acta Obstet Gynecol Scand* 1985;64:371–374.
65. Euans DW, Connor PD, Hahn RG, Rodney WM, Arheart KL. A comparison of manual and ultrasound measurements of fundal height. *J Fam Practice* 1995;40:233–236.
66. Engström JL, McFarlin BL, Sampson MB. Fundal height measurement, 4: accuracy of clinicians' identification of the uterine fundus during pregnancy. *J Nurs Midwifery* 1993c;38:318–323.
67. Engström JL, Sittler CP, Swift KE. Fundal height measurement, 5: the effect of clinician bias on fundal height measurements. *J Nurse Midwifery* 1994;39:130–141.
68. Pschera H, Söderberg G. Estimation of fetal weight by external abdominal measurements. *Acta Obstet Gynecol Scand* 1983;62:175–179.
69. Bailey SM, Sarmandal P, Grant JM. A comparison of three methods of assessing inter-observer variation applied to measurement of the symphysis-fundal height. *Br J Obstet Gynaecol* 1989;96:1266–1271.
70. Crosby ME, Engström JL. Inter-examiner reliability in fundal height measurement. *Midwives Chron Nurs Notes* 1989:254–256.
71. Gardosi J, Francis A. Controlled trial of fundal measurement plotted on customized antenatal growth charts. *Br J Obstet Gynaecol* 1999;106:309–317.
72. U.S. Public Health Service Expert Panel on the Content of Prenatal Care. *Caring for our Future: the Content of Prenatal Care.* Washington, DC: Public Health Service, Department of Health and Human Services, 1989.
73. Bergsjø P, Villar J. Scientific basis for the content of routine antenatal care, II: power to eliminate or alleviate adverse newborn outcomes; some special conditions and examinations. *Acta Obstet Gynecol Scand* 1997;76:15–25.
74. Villar J, Baaqeel H, Piaggio G, et al., for the WHO Antenatal Care Trial Research group. WHO Antenatal care randomized trail for the evaluation of a new model of routine antenatal care. *Lancet* 2001;357:1551–1564.
75. Editorial *BMJ* 1989;298:618.
   Anonymous
76. Rosenberg K, Grant JM, Tweedie I, Aitchison T, Gallagher F. Measurement of fundal height as a screening test for fetal growth retardation. *Br J Obstet Gynaecol* 1982 Jun;89(6):447–450.
77. Cnattingius S, Axelsson O, Lindmark G. Symphysis-fundus measurements and intrauterine growth retardation. *Acta Obstet Gynecol Scand* 1984;63(4):335–340.
78. Rogers MS, Needham PG. Evaluation of fundal height measurement in antenatal care. *Aust N Z J Obstet Gynaecol* 1985 May;25(2):87–90.
79. Tjon A, Ten WE, Kusin JA, De With C. Fundal height measurement as an antenatal screening method. *J Trop Pediat* 1985; 31:249–252.
80. Garde PM. Growth rate score to screen for intrauterine growth retardation. *Trop Doctor* 1986;15:71–74.
81. Okonofua FE, Ayangade SO, Chan RCW, O'Brien PMS. A prospective comparison of clinical and ultrasonic methods of predicting normal and abnormal fetal growth. *Int J Gynaecol Obstet* 1986;24:447–451.
82. Fescina RH, Martell M, Martinez G, Lastra L, Schwarcz R. Small for dates: evaluation of different diagnostic methods. *Acta Obstet Gynecol Scand* 1987;66:221–226.
83. Mathai M. Prediction of small-for-gestational-age infants using a specially calibrated tape measure. *Br J Obstet Gynaecol* 1988;95:313–314.
84. Stuart JM, Healy TJG, Sutton M, Swingler GR. Symphysis-fundul measurements in screening for small-for-dates infants: a community based study in Gloucestershire. *J R Coll Gen Pract* 1989;39:45–48.
85. Norton R. The prediction of intrauterine growth retardation in remote area aboriginal women using serial fundal-symphysial height measurements. *Aust NZ J Obstet Gynaecol* 1989;29:306–307.

31

Fetal Growth Restriction

Jason Gardosi

Kate Morse

Jill Wright

■ What is the Problem That Requires Screening?

Fetal growth restriction.

The effects of fetal growth restriction pervade all aspects of life and it is a universal aim to detect fetal growth restriction early. Yet current practice of fundal height measurement performs unsatisfactorily (see Chapter 30). Improvements in neonatal care and surveillance methods for the at-risk fetus place emphasis on enhanced screening and detection of antenatal growth problems.

What is the incidence/prevalence of the target condition?

There is no clear agreement on the definition of intrauterine growth restriction (IUGR). One definition is the "failure of the fetus to reach its growth potential." This begs the question as to what the individual's potential is, or said differently, what weight should a fetus be expected to reach at the end of a normal pregnancy? The prevalence of impaired fetal growth is dependent on the definition of birthweight below specified percentiles for gestational age and the population served (see also Chapters 29, 30, 32, and 37).

What are the sequelae of the condition that are of interest in clinical medicine?

Fetal growth is subject to constitutional/physiologic and pathologic factors. Whereas pathologically impaired growth can have a profound impact on all parts of the perinatal period, constitutionally small infants do not have an increased risk of stillbirth and neonatal death.[1] This important distinction is necessary to avoid unwarranted interference and intervention. The timely detection of pathologically impaired fetal growth is an essential prerequisite of good antenatal care because of its apparent links to perinatal morbidity and mortality[2] as well as adverse effects in childhood and later life.[3] There are many causes of growth restriction (Table 31–1), but about 80% to 90% of cases are associated with some form of placental dysfunction, a condition that is associated with inadequate placental development during the first and second trimesters. Recent studies highlight links between the antenatal, intrapartum, and postnatal periods.

Antenatal. Fetal growth restriction is associated with preterm labor,[4] suggesting that, in certain instances, early initiation of labor could be viewed as a feto–maternal adaptive response to allow escape from an unfavorable intrauterine environment.[5] This view is supported by preliminary evidence that, in some instances, the slowing of growth precedes the clinical manifestations of maternal hypertension in pregnancy and preeclampsia.[5] The corollary of a model of preterm labor as an adaptive response to growth restriction emerges when examining the cases where this escape mechanism fails. There is a clear association between IUGR and fetal demise. Many stillbirths are fetuses that failed to reach their growth potential.[6-8] Data from the U.K. Confidential Enquiries into Stillbirths and Deaths in Infancy suggest a strong link between smallness for gestational age and antepartum stillbirth.[2] Studies of large routinely collected databases in Sweden show that stillborn fetuses have a high chance of having been growth restricted before death.[1] Additional evidence comes from an analysis of stillbirths in Oslo, where 52% of "unexpected" antepartum fetal deaths, which yielded no postmortem findings, were fetal growth restricted (less than a tenth customized percentile).[9] Although fetal growth restriction is not in itself a "cause," it is a clinically relevant condition preceding stillbirth. A new classification system was developed to aid our understanding. Application of this method—called ReCoDe (Relevant Condition at Death, Table 31–2)—revealed that 57% of stillbirths previously considered "unexplained" according to standard Confidential Inquiries into Stillbirths and Infant Deaths (CESDI) classifications[2] fell into ReCoDe category A7 (fetal growth restriction).[10] It is apparent that a more clinically relevant classification system can allow for a better understanding of where priorities lie for instituting strategies for prevention.

Intrapartum. Diminished antenatal growth and small fetal size are also relevant in the intrapartum period. Small infants are more likely to develop fetal heart rate abnormalities and acidosis[11] (see related information in Chapter 37),

Table 31–1	**Pathologic associations of intrauterine growth restriction**
Fetal	Chromosomal, Potters, cardiac, etc. multifetal pregnancy
Maternal	Infections, hypertensive diseases, other medical conditions, socioeconomic deprivation, malnutrition, drugs, smoking
Placenta and cord	Bilobate; hemangioma, velamentous cord, single artery, placental insufficiency

Table 31-2   **The ReCoDe system**

A. Fetus	1. Lethal congenital anomaly
	2. Infection
	2.1 Chronic (e.g., TORCH)
	2.2 Acute
	3. Nonimmune hydrops
	4. Isoimmunization
	5. Fetomaternal hemorrhage
	6. Twin–twin transfusion
	7. Fetal growth restriction[1]
	8. Other
B. Umbilical cord	1. Prolapse
	2. Constricting loop or knot[2]
	3. Velamentous insertion
	4. Other
C. Placenta	1. Abruptio
	2. Previa
	3. Vasa previa
	4. Placental insufficiency/infarction[3]
	5. Other
D. Amniotic fluid	1. Chorioamnionitis
	2. Oligohydramnios[2]
	3. Polyhydramnios[2]
	4. Other
E. Uterus	1. Rupture
	2. Other
F. Mother	1. Diabetes
	2. Thyroid diseases
	3. Essential hypertension
	4. Hypertensive diseases in pregnancy
	5. Lupus/antiphospholipid syndrome
	6. Cholestasis
	7. Drug abuse
	8. Other
G. Intrapartum	1. Asphyxia
	2. Birth trauma
H. Trauma	1. External
	2. Iatrogenic
I. Unclassified	1. No relevant condition identified
	2. No information available

ReCoDe
Classification of stillbirths by Relevant Condition at Death
This system seeks to identify the conditions which existed at the time of death in utero.
The classification is based on the following principles:
1. Stillbirths are distinct from neonatal deaths and warrant their own classification.
2. There is hence no need for a subclassification according to gestation, as "prematurity" is not a relevant cause or condition for stillbirths.
3. There is no subclassification according to weight, but one related to fetal growth status, based on weight-for-gestation.
4. The classification emphasizes what went wrong, not necessarily "why." Hence, more than one category can be coded.
5. The hierarchy starts from conditions affecting the fetus and moves outwards, in simple anatomical categories (A–F), which are subdivided into pathophysiologic conditions.
6. The primary condition should be the highest on the list that is applicable to a case.

1. Defined as less than tenth customized weight-for-gestation percentile (centile calculator is available at *www.gestation.net/centile*).
2. If severe enough to be considered relevant.
3. Histologic diagnosis.

leading to the concept of "fetal reserve" where a well-grown fetus is better able to withstand the hypoxemic stress of labor.[12] A fetus with slow antepartum growth is more likely to require operative delivery for fetal distress and is more likely to be admitted to neonatal intensive care than one who has grown appropriately.[13] Recent guidelines for intrapartum monitoring in the United Kingdom suggest that intermittent auscultation is sufficient to monitor "low-risk" labor.[14] However, this presumes that "risk" can be reliably predicted. Most instances of growth restriction—and hence diminished fetal reserve—are unrecognized at the beginning of labor.

Postnatal. Neonatal morbidity and mortality are associated with fetal growth restriction.[1] The link between cerebral palsy and diminished fetal growth is also well known.[15,16] Interestingly, this link extends to fetal growth restriction at term only, whereas preterm infants with growth restriction do not have a higher risk of developing cerebral palsy than those born at similar preterm gestations without growth restriction.[17] Fetal growth restriction has also been described as having several delayed effects in adult life.[3]

■ The Tests

What is the purpose of the tests?

To detect pathologically impaired fetal growth. By distinguishing between constitutionally small infants and pathologically impaired growth, unnecessary interference and intervention for constitutional smallness can be avoided.

What is the nature of the tests?

Serial measurements of fundal height, supported by ultrasound estimation of fetal weight, are plotted on individually adjusted, customized antenatal charts to give an indication of the growth status of the fetus.[18]

Customized assessment of fundal height. It is recognized that only approximately a fourth of small-for–gestational age infants are detected antenatally.[19] In low-risk pregnancies, the rate is even lower, with detection only about 15%.[20,21] Therefore, detecting poor fetal growth in the *general* population requires a good screening test. Fundal height measurements are usually not well taught, not serially plotted, and often only recorded in a haphazard fashion against the number of weeks' gestation, under the (false) expectation that fundal height in centimeters should equal the week of pregnancy (see Chapter 30). In fact, fundal height varies with constitutional factors.[22] A controlled study in Nottingham[23] concluded that serial measurements of fundal height by well-trained midwives using a standard measurement technique, plotting on customized growth charts and applying clearly defined referral pathways significantly increased the detection of IUGR. Furthermore, the technique *decreased* the number of unnecessary referrals for hospital investigations, as normal measurements were more likely to fall within normal limits for that individual since the growth curves had been adjusted for constitutional variation.[23]

Customized assessment of fetal growth. Customized growth charts based on the estimated optimal fetal weight at term have been developed, taking into account variables that affect normal fetal growth, such as maternal height, weight in early pregnancy, parity, and ethnic origin. It is suggested that an estimated fetal weight below the tenth "customized" percentile is a better predictor of adverse pregnancy outcome than the fetal weight below the tenth percentile derived from traditional birthweight curves.[1] The method starts with the calculation of the optimal weight at term, using coefficients to adjust for constitutional variation. This requires accurate gestational age assessment, and adjustment for maternal height, weight in early pregnancy, parity, and ethnic origin. Pathologic factors that show significance in the analysis must be excluded (e.g., smoking) as the standard should calculate the growth potential (i.e., the optimum that can be achieved free from pathologic factors). Next, the growth curve to this optimal weight endpoint is delineated, using a "proportional" fetal growth function.[24,25] This avoids using a birthweight curve, as the latter is based on cross-sectional data, which, especially in the preterm period, are by definition derived from an abnormal, negatively skewed population. As there are an infinite number of possible combinations to produce an individual fetus' growth curve, the calculation requires a computer. The software (gestation-related optimal weight [GROW]) and associated percentile calculator is available for free download at *www.gestation.net*. Using customized percentiles allows the diagnosis of "fetal growth restriction"' to be made from weight at delivery, after adjusting for gestational age and the physiologic pregnancy characteristics. Receiver operating curves suggest that the tenth percentile is a suitable cutoff limit to detect those infants who will develop perinatal complications.[13] The change in estimated fetal weight over time is also a useful predictor of perinatal outcome.[26] Individually adjusted birthweight percentiles are more clearly associated with Apgar scores[18] and neonatal morphometry indices than unadjusted birthweight percentiles.[27,28] They also better reflect adverse pregnancy events, even across geographic boundaries. For example, small-for–gestational age defined by a customized standard derived from an English population has a better association with operative deliveries for fetal distress and admission to neonatal intensive care in a Dutch population than the local Dutch population standard.[29] Recent analysis of a large Swedish data set showed that small for gestational age defined by a customized birthweight percentile was more closely associated with stillbirths, neonatal deaths, or low Apgar scores (< 4) than the unadjusted population percentile.[1] Infants considered small by the general Swedish population standard but not by the customized standard did *not* have a larger risk of stillbirth, neonatal death, or low Apgar scores than the average-for–gestational age group (Figure 31–1). The inference from these

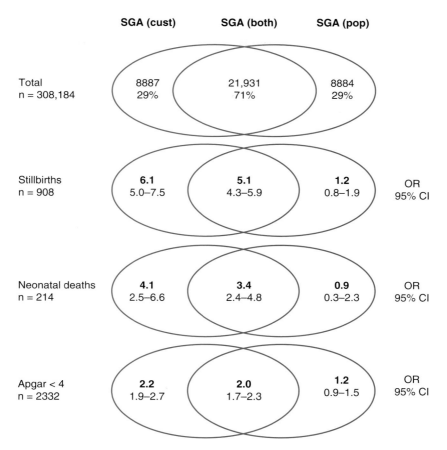

Figure 31-1   Association between small for gestational age (SGA) and adverse perinatal outcome in Swedish births 1992 to 1995. Outcomes: stillbirths, neonatal deaths, and low Apgars (< 4 at 5 minutes). Comparison between definition of SGA as lowest 10% of births by customized percentile (SGA_{cust}) and the lowest 10% by population-based percentile (SGA_{pop}), arranged in three categories: *1:* SGA by both methods; *2:* SGA by customized percentile only; and *3:* SGA by population centile only. Odds Ratios (ORs) and 95% confidence intervals are shown. Non-SGA $(_{cust\ and\ pop})$ was OR = 1.
(From Clausson B, Gardosi J, Francis A, et al. Perinatal outcome in SGA births defined by customised versus population based birthweight standards. *Br J Obstet Gynaecol* 2001;108:830–834.)

findings is that "customized" small for gestational age is equivalent to IUGR. Furthermore, this study confirms that small–normal fetuses are not at greater risk than normal size fetuses, and should be excluded when screening for fetal growth problems.

The calculation of customized percentiles requires the expected birthweight to be extrapolated backward into the antenatal period. Intrauterine weight standards are defined using a "proportionality growth curve."[30] Thus the optimal growth up to the previously calculated "term optimal weight" is delineated. Fetal weight curves reproduce differences between physiologic/ constitutional characteristics, in low-risk[31] and high-risk[32] populations. The use of fetal weight instead of individual scan biometry parameters (e.g., head and abdominal circumference, femur length) allows adjustment of normal intrauterine growth limits. It is clear that a large proportion of the population is misclassified if an unadjusted standard is used, and differences can be substantial.[29] Customized limits reduce false-positive "fetal growth restriction" in a normal population.[33] However, it is impossible to customize individual ultrasound scan parameters by multivariable analysis of all the nonpathologic factors that may influence fetal growth. Instead, the coefficients for adjustment are determined from large population-based birthweight databases and then applied to intrauterine growth curves for fetal weight.

Timing. Screening for fetal growth requires clearly delineated care pathways (Figure 31–2). All women should undergo fundal height measurements from 26 to 28 weeks' gestation using a standardized technique to reduce the degree of error (Figure 31–3).[34] The measurements are then plotted on a customized antenatal growth chart. Slowing of growth (dropping below an action line like the tenth percentile) would indicate the need for further investigations. Relative slowing within normal limits (e.g., a drop from say the 70th to the 20th percentiles in consecutive measurements) should also be a matter of concern. If IUGR is suspected, further investigation by ultrasound is recommended (Figure 31–2). The scan-based estimated fetal weight should be plotted using a second ordinate axis on the customized fundal height chart (Figure 31–4).

Ultrasound scanning at each antenatal visit has been suggested,[35] although routine third-trimester scans have failed to improve outcome.[36] It is also doubtful whether serial scanning in the entire population would prove cost-effective, or even be acceptable to expectant mothers. In pregnancies at risk of impaired fetal growth, serial ultrasound biometry will allow assessment of growth. In this context, both abdominal circumference (AC) and estimated fetal weight are useful indictors.[37]

There is a finite usefulness to the frequency of third-trimester scans: If the increment of a biometric parameter is approximately 5% per week, and the random error of a scan measurement in everyday use about 10% or more,[38] then more than fortnightly scans are not likely to give valuable information about true growth. In practice, therefore, we recommend that serial assessments of fetal biometry not be more frequent than every 2 to 3 weeks.

What are the implications of testing?

What does an abnormal test result mean? If the first fundal height measurement is below the tenth customized percentile, or if the rate of growth since a previous fundal height measurement is slow, excessive, or static, further investigations are recommended to assess fetal growth by means of ultrasound. If the sonographic estimated fetal weight is within the normal customized

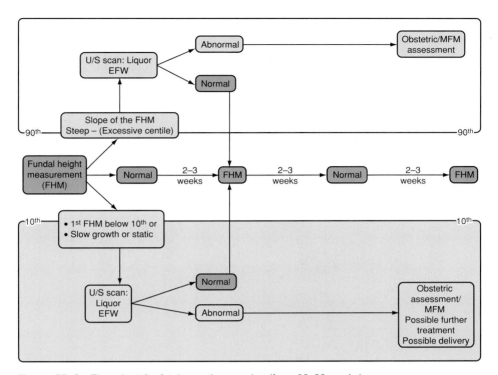

Figure 31-2 Flow chart for fetal growth screening (from 26–28 weeks)
U/S, ultrasound; *EFW*, estimated fetal weight; *FHM*, fundal height measurement; *MFM*, maternal fetal monitoring.

limits, standard, serial fundal height measurements are continued (Figure 31–2). However, if the estimated fetal weight is below the tenth customized percentile, or subsequent measurements show a slowing of growth with crossing of a customized percentile line, further investigations are recommended. These include assessment by Doppler flow velocimetry of the fetal vessels (see related information in Chapters 32 and 37). If the pregnancy continues, ultrasound biometry needs to be repeated fortnightly. Amniotic fluid volume is an integral part of the assessment.

It is often argued that separate plots of individual ultrasound parameters (e.g., head circumference and abdominal circumference) allow assessment of symmetry of growth failure. However, it is doubtful whether the distinction between symmetric and asymmetric growth failure adds any clinically useful information. In either case, further investigations are necessary—especially biophysical assessment by Doppler. If growth restriction is severe, assessment for chromosomal abnormality would need to be considered in both instances. The degree of deviation is more important than the symmetry between abdominal and head measurements. Studies comparing symmetric and asymmetric growth restriction have failed to demonstrate differences in etiology,[39] fetal

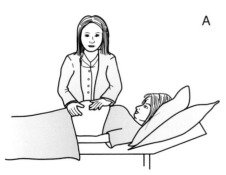

A

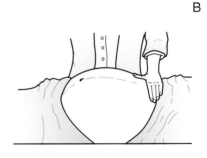

B

1. Mother semi-recumbent, with bladder empty.

2. Palpate to determine fundus with two hands.

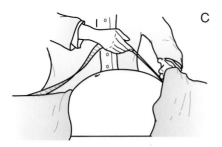

C

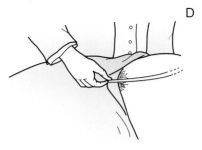

D

3. Secure tape with hand at top of fundus.

4. Measure to top of symphysis pubis.

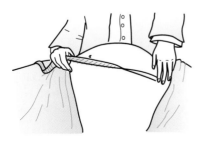

E

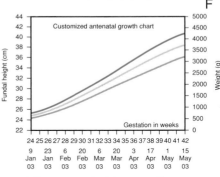

F

5. Measure along longitudinal axis of uterus, note metric measurement.

6. Plot on customized chart, record in notes.

Figure 31–3   Fundal height measurement.

acid-base status at time of cordocentesis,[40] neonatal morphometry,[41] and other indices of outcome.[42,43]

Doppler flow velocimetry has proven its value in defining the IUGR fetus[44] and is more useful than cardiotocogram (CTG) or biophysical profile scoring.[45] Regrettably, there is no satisfactory treatment of fetal growth problems in utero. Therefore, the timing of elective delivery is crucial and is different in every instance. The aim is not necessarily to increase birthweight at all cost, but to balance the (at-times) conflicting interests of increasing maturity and delivery from an unfavorable intrauterine environment, to allow achievement of the best possible outcome.

What does a normal test result mean? If the fundal height measurement is within the normal, customized limits, surveillance is continued with serial fundal height measurements every 2 to 3 weeks (Figure 31–2).

What is the cost of testing?

Information on the cost-effectiveness of this strategy is not available.

■ Conclusions and Recommendations

There is a problem with current screening for fetal growth. Only about a fourth of small-for–gestational age infants are detected antenatally,[19] and in low-risk pregnancies, the rate is even lower—about 15%.[20,21] A strategy to improve this situation must include better training in a standardized assessment of fundal height, plotting on individually "customized" charts, and appropriate care pathways for further assessment and delivery where indicated.

Individual adjustments of the weight limits for fetal growth are relevant for epidemiologic analysis and prospective assessment and to reduce false positives and therefore unnecessary interventions. They also help to identify those fetuses that are pathologically small. This should lead to improved detection and referral for further investigation of at-risk fetuses.

The role of ultrasound biometry here is to confirm or deny the suspicion of fetal growth problems on the basis of clinical examination (i.e., measurement of fundal height). If the estimated fetal weight is below the tenth customized percentile line, or if the rate of growth is slow and crosses centile lines, further investigation by Doppler is recommended.

However, although Doppler is of value in fetuses that are small-for–gestational age, it is less useful in predicting growth restriction or adverse outcome in the general population[37,46] (see related information in Chapter 32). This is consistent with the fact that the positive predictive value of any test depends on the prevalence of the condition being looked for (see Chapter 1). Diagnostic tests for fetal growth restriction need to be preceded by a good screening method, which is represented by fundal height measurement plotted on customized growth charts, combined with ultrasound estimation of fetal weight where indicated.[47]

A

CUSTOMIZED ANTENATAL GROWTH CHART
Mrs. Small (1 DOB: 01/01/75)

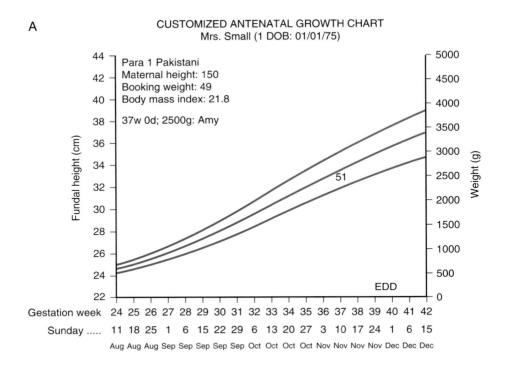

B

CUSTOMIZED ANTENATAL GROWTH CHART
Mrs. Small (1 DOB: 01/01/75)

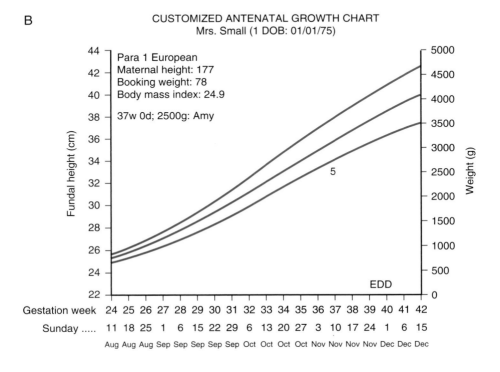

Figure 31-4 Two examples of customized fetal growth curves, printed out using gestation-related optimal weight (GROW; GROW.exe version 4.6.1; available at www.gestation.net). The charts can be used to plot previous baby weights and ultrasound estimated fetal weight(s) in the current pregnancy. Serial fundal height measurements can also be plotted. The graphs are adjusted to predict the optimal curve for each pregnancy, based on the variables which are entered (maternal height and weight, parity, ethnic group).
A: In the example, a baby born at 37 weeks' gestation weighing 2,500 g was within normal limits for Mrs. Small (51st percentile) but demonstrated intrauterine growth restriction (IUGR) for Mrs. Large (fifth percentile) as the latter's predicted optimal growth curve is steeper.
B: The pregnancy details entered are shown on the top left, together with the (computer-) calculated body mass index (BMI). The horizontal axis shows the day and month of each gestation week, calculated by the software on the basis of the estimated date of delivery (EDD) entered.

■ Summary

1 ■ What Is the Problem that Requires Screening?

Fetal growth restriction.

a. What is the incidence/prevalence of the target condition?

The prevalence of impaired fetal growth is dependent on the definition of birthweight below specified percentiles for gestational age and the population served and depends on factors such as the rate of smoking in pregnancy. About 80% to 90% of cases with impaired fetal growth are associated with some form of placental dysfunction.

b. What are the sequelae of the condition that are of interest in clinical medicine?

Recent studies have highlighted links in the antenatal (e.g., preterm labor, stillbirth), intrapartum (e.g., fetal distress, metabolic acidosis), and postnatal periods (e.g., cerebral palsy).

2 ■ The Tests

a. What is the purpose of the tests?

To detect pathologically impaired fetal growth.

Continued

■ **Summary—cont'd**

b. *What is the nature of the tests?*

Serial measurement of fundal height, supported by ultrasound estimation of fetal weight, where indicated. Fundal height measurements and ultrasound findings are plotted on individually adjusted, customized antenatal charts to give an indication of the growth status of the fetus. Receiver operating curves suggest that the tenth percentile is a suitable cutoff limit to detect those infants who will develop perinatal complications.

c. *What are the implications of testing?*

1. What does an abnormal test result mean?

If the first fundal height measurement is below the tenth customized percentile or if the rate of growth since a previous fundal height measurement is slow, excessive, or static, ultrasound investigations are recommended to assess fetal weight. If the estimated fetal weight is below the tenth customized percentile, further investigations are recommended including Doppler flow velocimetry. Unfortunately, there is no satisfactory treatment of fetal growth problems in utero. Therefore, the timing of elective delivery is most crucial.

If the estimated fetal growth, as assessed by ultrasound, is within the normal customized limits standard, serial fundal height measurements are continued (Figure 31–2).

2. What does a normal test result mean?

If the fundal height measurement is within the normal, customized limits, surveillance is continued with serial fundal height measurements every 2 to 3 weeks.

d. *What is the cost of testing?*

Fundal height measurements are cost-effective as they can be integrated into antenatal assessment and the use of individual charts reduces false positives and hence unnecessary intervention.

3 ■ **Conclusions and Recommendations**

Fetal growth restriction can be defined as the failure of a fetus to reach its growth potential. The potential varies in individual pregnancies and should be adjusted to improve the accuracy of assessment, which is done using customized antenatal growth charts.

The charts are used for fetal growth screening and assessment, through serial fundal height measurement and with clear pathways for further evaluation as indicated, including ultrasound biometry and Doppler flow. Individually adjusted or "customized" growth curves and birthweight percentiles have a better association with Apgar scores and neonatal morphometry indices and better reflect adverse perinatal events, such as operative deliveries for fetal distress and admission to neonatal intensive care. Furthermore, customized limits reduce false-positive diagnoses of "fetal growth restriction" in a normal population.

References

1. Clausson B, Gardosi J, Francis A, et al Perinatal outcome in SGA births defined by customised versus population based birthweight standards. *Br J Obstet Gynaecol* 2001;108: 830–834.
2. Maternal and Child Health Consortium. CESDI 8th Annual Report: Confidential Enquiry of Stillbirths and Deaths in Infancy, 2001. www.cemach.org.uk.
3. Barker DJP. Long term outcome of retarded fetal growth. In: Divon MY, ed. *Clinical Obstetrics and Gynecology*. Philadelphia: Lippincott-Raven, 1997: 853–863.
4. Tamura RK, Sabbagha RE, Depp R, et al. Diminished growth in fetuses born preterm after spontaneous labor or rupture of membranes. *Am J Obstet Gynecol* 1984;148:1105–1110.
5. Gardosi J, Kady SM, Francis A. Fetal growth, maturity and preterm birth. In: Critchley H, Bennett P, Thornton S, eds. *Preterm Birth*. London: *Royal College of Obstetrics and Gynaecology*, 2004.
6. Gardosi J, Mul T. Mongelli M, et al. Analysis of birthweight and gestational age in antepartum stillbirths. *Br J Obstet Gynaecol* 1998;105:524–530.
7. Kady SM, Gardosi J. Perinatal mortality and fetal growth restriction. In: Arulkumaran S, Gardosi J, eds. *Best Practice and Research in Clinical Obstetrics and Gynaecology*. New York: Elsevier, 2004:397–410.
8. Gardosi J, Badger S, Tonks A, et al. Unexplained stillbirth: an investigation of clinically relevant conditions at the time of fetal death. *Am J Obstet Gynecol* 2003;189:6:S353.
9. Froen F, Gardosi J, Thurman A, et al. Restricted fetal growth in sudden intrauterine unexplained death. *Acta Obstet Gynecol Scand* 2004;83:801–807.
10. Gardosi J. Antepartum stillbirths and strategies for prevention. In: Edwards G, ed. *Adverse Outcomes in Maternity Care: Baby Lifeline*. New York: Elsevier, 2004.
11. Low JA. Fetal asphyxia during the intrapartum period in intrauterine growth retarded infants. *Am J Obstet Gynecol* 1972;113:351–357.
12. Low J. Metabolic acidosis and fetal reserve. In: Gardosi J, ed. *Intrapartum Surveillance*. London: Bailliere Tindall, 1996:211–224.
13. de Jong CLD, Francis A, vanGeijn HP, et al. Fetal growth rate and adverse perinatal events. *Ultrasound Obstet Gynecol* 1998;13:86–89.
14. The use and interpretation of cardiotocography in intrapartum fetal surveillance: clinical guidelines. London: National Institute of Clinical Excellence, 2001.
15. Uvebrant P, Hagberg G. Intrauterine growth in children with cerebral palsy. *Acta Paediatr* 1992;81:407–412.
16. Jarvis S, Gilianaia SV, Torrioli M-G, et al. Cerebral palsy and intrauterine growth in single births: European collaborative study. *Lancet* 2003;362:1106–1111.

17. Jacobsson B, Francis A, Hagberg G, et al. Cerebral palsy is strongly associated with severe intrauterine growth restriction in term but not in preterm cases. *Am J Obstet Gynecol* 2003; 189[Suppl]: S74.

18. Gardosi J, Chang A, Kalyan B, et al. Customised antenatal growth charts. *Lancet* 1992;339: 283–287.

19. Hepburn M, Rosenberg K. An audit of the detection and management of small-for-gestational age babies. *Br J Obstet Gynaecol* 1986;93:212–216.

20. Kean LH, Liu DT. Antenatal care as a screening tool for the detection of small for gestational age babies in the low risk population. *J Obstet Gynaecol* 1996;16:77–82.

21. Backe B, Nakling J. Effectiveness of antenatal care: a population based study. *Br J Obstet Gynaecol* 1993;100:727–732.

22. Mongelli M, Gardosi J. Symphysis-Fundus Height and Pregnancy Characteristics in Ultrasound-Dated Pregnancies. *Obstet Gynecol* 1999;94:591–594.

23. Gardosi J, Francis A. Controlled trial of fundal height measurement plotted on customised antenatal growth charts. *Br J Obstet Gynaecol* 1999;106:309–317.

24. Gardosi J, Mongelli M, Wilcox M, et al. An adjustable fetal weight standard. *Ultrasound Obstet Gynecol* 1995;6:168–174.

25. Gardosi J. The application of individualised fetal growth curves. *J Perinatal Med* 1998;26: 137–142.

26. Chang TC, Robson SC, Spencer JA, et al. Prediction of perinatal morbidity at term in small fetuses: comparison of fetal growth and Doppler ultrasound. *Br J Obstet Gynaecol* 1994;101:422–427.

27. Sanderson DA, Wilcox MA, Johnson IR. The individualized birth weight ratio: a new method of identifying intrauterine growth retardation. *Br J Obstet Gynaecol* 1994;101:310–314.

28. Owen P, Farrell T, Hardwick JCR, et al. Relationship between customised birthweight centiles and neonatal anthropometric features of growth restriction. *Br J Obstet Gynaecol* 2002;109:658–662.

29. de Jong CLD, Gardosi J, Dekker GA, et al. Application of a customised birthweight standard in the assessment of perinatal outcome in a high risk population. *Br J Obstet Gynaecol* 1998;105:531–535.

30. Gardosi J, Mongelli M, Wilcox M, et al. An adjustable fetal weight standard. *Ultrasound Obstet Gynecol* 1995;6:168–174.

31. Mongelli M, Gardosi J. Longitudinal study of fetal growth in subgroups of a low risk population. *Ultrasound Obstet Gynecol* 1995;6:340–344.

32. de Jong CLD, Gardosi J, Baldwin C, et al. Fetal weight gain in a serially scanned high-risk population. *Ultrasound Obstet Gynecol* 1998;11:39–43.

33. Mongelli M, Gardosi J. Reduction of false-positive diagnosis of fetal growth restriction by application of customized fetal growth standards. *Obstet Gynecol* 1996;88:844–848

34. Engstrom JL, Sittler CP. Fundal height measurement, 1: techniques for measuring fundal height. *J Nurse-Midwifery* 1993;38:5–16.

35. Sim D, Beattie RB, Dornan JC. Evaluation of biophysical assessment in high risk pregnancy to assess ultrasound parameters suitable for screening in the low risk population. *Ultrasound Obstet Gynecol* 1993;3:11–17.

36. Jahn A, Razum O, Berle P. Routine screening for intrauterine growth retardation in Germany: low sensitivity and questionable benefit for diagnosed cases. *Acta Obstet Gynecol Scand* 1998;1977:43–48.

37. Chang TC, Robson SC, Boys RJ, et al. Prediction of the small for gestational age infant: Which ultrasonic measurement is best? *Obstet Gynecol* 1992;80:1030–1037.

38. Dalsgaard L, Wiberg N, Dragsted N. Quality control of ultrasound weight estimation in a central hospital. *Ugeskrift for Laeger* 2002;164:2280–2283.

39. Todros T, Piazzotta CLP. Body proportionality of the small-for-date fetus: is it related to aetiological factors? *Early Human Develop* 1996;45:1–9.

40. Blackwell SC, Moldenhauer J, Redman M, et al. Relationship between the sonographic pattern of intrauterine growth restriction and acid base status at the time of cordocentesis. *Arch Gynecol Obstet* 2001;13:191–193.

41. Colley NV, Tremble JM, Henson GL, et al. Head circumference/abdominal circumference ratio, ponderal index and fetal malnutrition. Should head circumference/abdominal circumference ratio be abandoned? *Br J Obstet Gynaecol* 1991;98:524–527.

42. Kramer MS, Olivier M, McLean FH, et al. Impact of intrauterine growth retardation and body proportionality on fetal and neonatal outcome. *Pediatrics* 1990;86:707–713.

43. Lin C, Su S, River P. Comparison of associated high-risk factors and perinatal outcome between symmetric and asymmetric fetal intrauterine growth retardation. *Am J Obstet Gynecol* 1991;164:1535–1542.

44. Alfirevic Z, Nielson JP. Doppler ultrasonography in high risk pregnancies: systematic review with meta-analysis. *Am J Obstet Gynecol* 1995;172:1379–1387.

45. Soothill PW, Ajayi RA, Campbell S, et al. Prediction of morbidity in small and normally grown fetuses by fetal heart rate variability, biophysical profile score and umbilical artery Doppler studies. *Br J Obstet Gynaecol* 1993;100:742–745.

46. Chien PF, Arnott N, Gordon A, et al. How useful is the uterine artery Doppler flow velocimetry in the prediction of pre-eclampsia, intrauterine growth retardation and perinatal death? An overview. *Br J Obstet Gynaecol* 2000;107:196–208.

47. Royal College of Obstetricians and Gynaecologists. The investigation and management of the small-for-gestational age fetus. *RCOG Green Top Guideline* No. 31, 2002.

32

Doppler Velocimetry for the Detection of Intrauterine Growth Restriction

Sicco A. Scherjon

■ What Is the Problem that Requires Screening?

Intrauterine growth restriction (IUGR).

IUGR is a major clinical problem. Although the phrases "IUGR" and "small for gestational age" (SGA) are often used interchangeably, they are not the same. The phrase "IUGR" denotes a fetus that is likely to have experienced intrauterine nutritional deprivation, resulting in a reduction of fetal growth velocity. If severe, the fetus is also likely to experience chronic hypoxemia. Only half of the SGA infants are really growth restricted by objective criteria postnatally.

What is the incidence/prevalence of the target condition?

Several definitions based on birth weight (less than the 2.3, fifth, or tenth percentile, or a birth weight 2 SD below the mean birth weight for gestational age) are commonly used to define both IUGR and SGA. A birth weight below the tenth percentile means that 10% of newborns in the population are by definition growth restricted. As SGA is often used as a proxy for IUGR, SGA defined only on the basis of birth weight is a heterogeneous group consisting of neonates born growth restricted, infants with chromosomal abnormalities,[1] and normal, healthy, but small infants. Individual growth curves are preferred during pregnancy, particularly ones based on the population served and adjusted for ethnicity, maternal height, parity, and fetal sex.[2] The difference between the actual birth weight and the predicted birth weight based on several maternal characteristics and fetal sex is an alternative definition of IUGR.[3] Definitions of IUGR such as the Ponderal Index or skinfold thickness identify IUGR neonates more accurately than birth weight,[4] but are more complicated to perform.

What are the sequelae of the condition that are of interest in clinical medicine?

More than a third of structurally normal infants who die in utero are IUGR. Besides stillbirth, IUGR is also associated with an increased risk of neonatal death, fetal distress, and other adverse outcomes, especially if IUGR is defined using customized standards.[3,5-7] Chapter 37 includes a detailed discussion of screening for fetal distress in IUGR using Doppler velocimetry and will not be discussed here. The Ponderal Index is an independent predictor of neonatal morbidity, whether the infant is below or above the tenth percentile of the growth curve.[4] IUGR newborns are at increased risk of compromised neurodevelopment; both minor neurological dysfunction and lower developmental scores are more common.[8-12] Consistent with the "fetal origin of adult disease" hypothesis,[13] adults who are born growth restricted have an increased risk of developing in later life diabetes, and vascular diseases such as myocardial infarction, cerebrovascular accident (CVA), hyperlipidemia, and hypercoagulopathies.

■ The Tests

What is the purpose of the tests?

To detect IUGR.

What is the nature of the tests?

Doppler ultrasonography permits the noninvasive measurement of blood flow velocity, which is in turn a reflection of downstream resistance to flow. Because the measurement of velocity is dependent on the angle of insonation, a variety of angle-independent indices are used that combine systolic, diastolic, and mean velocities (Figure 32–1).

The angle under which velocities are recorded is critical for the measurement of absolute velocities, such as used in venous Doppler studies and for the

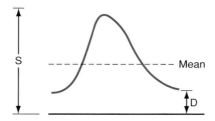

Figure 32–1 Flow Velocity waveform.
The waveform is characterized by three different indices as proposed by three different authors: S/D = S/D ratio (Stuart et al., Fetal blood velocity wave forms in normal pregnancy. *Br J Obstet Gynaecol* 1980;87: 780–785); (S-D)/S = resistance index (RI) (Pourcelot, 1974); (S-D)/mean = pulsatility index (PI) (Gosling and King, 1975).

screening of fetal anemia. In general, the angle of insonation should be less than 60 degrees. If this angle is too large, especially in cases of mild placental insufficiency, incorrect low and even absent velocities may be recorded in the diastolic phase of the waveform.

Two basic types of Doppler technology are used in obstetrics. Continuous wave (CW) has the advantage of requiring less expensive and less complicated equipment. It can be used when simultaneous visualization of the targeted vessel is not required (e.g., the umbilical artery and the uterine arteries), although it is rarely used in the screening setting any longer. Pulsed Doppler (PD) in combination with ultrasound imaging is obligatory when the targeted vessel must be visualized (e.g., the fetal aorta, the cerebral vessels, and when venous Doppler studies are performed). The indices obtained with CW and PD instrumentation are comparable.[14] Color PD imaging facilitates the examination by shortening the time to identify the vessel; as a result, the success rate is increased.[15] A ratio between the umbilical and cerebral artery indices (U/C ratio)[16] may be used to illustrate the hemodynamic redistribution of blood flow to the brain associated with IUGR secondary to placental dysfunction.

Reliability and technology assessment. The location of the vessel affects the Doppler measurement.[17,18] For example, resistance to flow through the uterine artery is lower on the placental side of the uterus compared to the non-placental side. Thus, it is common practice to take the mean of the measurements from the two uterine arteries. The resistance to flow in the umbilical artery is lowest at the placental and highest on the fetal cord origin. As a result, it is customary to measure the umbilical artery resistance in a free-floating mid segment of the cord. Fetal breathing and movement also affect the Doppler measurements, which should be made during fetal apnea and in the absence of fetal movements. The reliability is improved if the mean of three to six waveforms is used.[19,20] Examiner experience and equipment variation have only minor impact on reproducibility.[21–23]

What are the implications of testing?

What does an abnormal test result mean? An elevated Doppler resistance index in the setting of sonographic parameters consistent with SGA is indicative of uteroplacental dysfunction. The most characteristic change of the flow velocity waveform in the umbilical artery and the descending aorta of the IUGR fetus is a reduction and even loss or reversal of the end-diastolic velocities. As a result, the Doppler resistance indices are increased. Several gestational age–dependent normative curves [16,24–29] have been published: indices either above the 95th percentile[30] or 2 SDs above the mean[31] are usually considered abnormal. The umbilical and the uterine artery resistance indices are inversely proportional,[32] whereas the resistance indices of the middle cerebral artery are directly proportional to the fetal PO_2.[33] Abnormal velocities in the inferior vena cava are also associated with fetal acidemia and hypercapnia.[34]

Diastolic velocities should be considered as a continuum. As the index of peripheral vessels rise, both the severity of the growth restriction and hypoxemia increase [32, 35-37] (Figure 32–2). The presence of a diastolic notch is considered the most severe abnormality in the uterine artery. The subjective assessment of the presence of a diastolic notch is comparable to more objective methods and is a better predictor of adverse neonatal outcome than measurement of indices of resistance, although the screen positive rate is higher.[38,39] The reversal of end-diastolic flow is the most extreme waveform abnormality in the umbilical artery.

Venous Doppler studies. Characteristic changes in fetal velocity waveforms seen in IUGR pregnancies are apparent not only in arteries but also in the veins. The deterioration of fetal hemodynamic function is progressive. Abnormal umbilical artery Doppler studies precede abnormalities in the U/C ratio and in venous vessels as the umbilical vein,[40] the ductus venosus,[41] and the inferior vena cava[42] (see also Chapter 37). The ductus venosus is an important regulator of the distribution of well-oxygenated blood returning from the placenta to the right atrium.[43] An increase in ductal shunting, bypassing the liver and providing a higher proportion of the highly oxygenated blood through the foramen ovale to the left atrium and by this to the heart and the brain, is characteristically seen in the IUGR fetus. Even during severe IUGR, this adaptive mechanism maintains normal absolute flow through the ductus venosus to

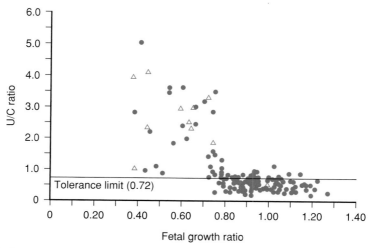

Figure 32–2 The association between the umbilical/cerebral (U/C) ratio and fetal growth restriction.
In cases of moderate/severe growth restriction (i.e., fetal growth below the 80%) a rising U/C ratio is seen. In all cases of intrauterine death (*open triangle*), except in one case associated with an intrauterine fetal infection, the U/C ratio appeared to be above the tolerance limit. Filled circles show liveborn infants.
U/C ratio: umbilical pulsatility index/cerebral pulsatility index.

organs vital for fetal survival. The changes in venous indices, indicative of fetal heart failure, provide a more refined assessment of the fetal condition (e.g., impending fetal mortality) when IUGR is present.[44] The potential benefits of the optimal timing of the delivery of these high risk fetuses need further evaluation[45,46] (see related material in Chapter 37).

The value of a test such as Doppler velocimetry for IUGR can be expressed in terms of likelihood ratios (see Chapter 1). Likelihood ratios can be used to compute post-test probabilities from (pretest) prevalences, via the odds ratios (Table 32–1).

In general, uteroplacental artery Doppler performs the worst as a screen for IUGR in studies where the prevalence of IUGR exceeds the 5%, whereas the fetal cerebral artery—especially the U/C ratio—performs the best. There are no substantial differences among likelihood ratios in studies where the prevalence of IUGR is below 5%. Use of the Ponderal Index rather than birth weight to diagnose IUGR does not alter Doppler test performance.[47] The ultrasonic estimate of fetal weight is superior to Doppler for the diagnosis of low birth weight.[48]

Doppler indices may be elevated weeks or even months before IUGR is clinically detectable. The placentas of newborns with abnormal flow velocity waveforms often show obliteration of tertiary stem villi, a finding consistent with abnormal trophoblastic invasion.[49–51] Growth-restricted fetuses with

Table 32–1   Test characteristics of maternal and fetal vessels in a high-risk population for the prediction of IUGR.

Artery	Sens, %	Spec, %	LR^pos	LR^neg	PPV, %	NPV, %	Prev, %	Posttest probability Pos test, %	Posttest probability Neg test, %
Utero placental	49.5	77.0	2.3	0.64	47.9	74.3	10	20	7
							40	61	30
Umbilical	59.1	83.4	5.0	0.49	63.8	77.4	10	36	5
							40	77	25
Aorta	49.1	78.4	4.7	0.67	71.2	59.4	10	34	7
							40	76	31
Cerebral	50.9	89.0	12.9	0.55	79.2	71.8	10	59	6
							40	90	27
U/C ratio	69.2	89.2	17.3	0.34	78.3	75.7	10	66	4
							40	92	19

Numbers given in this table were calculated from more than 75 studies, and more than 10,000 patients, in which sufficient details were given to be able to calculated test characteristics.
IUGR, intrauterine growth restriction; sens, sensibility to predict IUGR; spec, specificity to predict IUGR; LR^pos, likelihood ratio for a positive test result; LR^neg, likelihood ratio for a negative test result; PPV, positive predictive value of the test; NPV, negative predictive value of the test; prev, prevalence of IUGR in the population; pos test, positive test; neg test, negative test; U/C ratio, ratio of the umbilical pulsatility index to cerebral pulsatility index.

absent end-diastolic velocity (AEDV) are consistently hypoxemic and/or acidemic compared with gestational-age corrected norms for the fetuses of nonlaboring women.[32,52-55] The same cannot be said when diastolic flow is still present. Although several studies report the reappearance of diastolic velocities (up to 30%), this is a relatively rare event in settings of severe IUGR where diastolic flow is absent in all sections of the umbilical cord and where there is decreased middle cerebral artery resistance. Reappearance of diastolic velocities is a sign of severe fetal compromise and is only found in the presence of abnormal venous flow.[56] There is no physiologic explanation for a decrease in resistance observed in the umbilical artery absent either resolving placentitis of pharmacologic therapy. Nevertheless, umbilical artery Doppler studies should not be used as the sole and definite argument for the immediate delivery of a preterm fetus (see Chapter 37).[57-60]

Hypoxemia/acidemia in the umbilical cord blood at delivery is less common when the elevated umbilical artery pulsatility index (PI) of an SGA pregnancy is associated with normal fetal heart rate testing (4%). The likelihood of hypoxemia at delivery increases to over 60% if the fetal heart rate pattern is abnormal.[55] Flow velocity waveform abnormalities occur earlier than abnormalities in fetal heart rate variability.[61,62] A low cerebral artery PI may precede an abnormal fetal heart rate pattern by weeks or even months.[63] Decreased cerebral resistance is often associated with an elevated resistance in the descending aorta or the umbilical artery.[64] This "brain sparing," defined as a raised U/C ratio, identifies the fetus whose IUGR is likely to be based on uteroplacental dysfunction severe enough to impede oxygen delivery.[35] This organ-sparing effect also occurs in the coronary circulation of the fetal heart.[65] In some studies of SGA fetuses, umbilical artery velocimetry was a better predictor of perinatal distress than either measurement of the abdominal circumference or the Biophysical Profile Score.[66] Further fetal artery Doppler studies are of no clinical value when the findings of umbilical artery studies in fetuses with suspected IUGR are normal.[67]

The application of umbilical artery Doppler velocimetry in observational studies is associated with a decrease in the number of labor inductions and operative deliveries for fetal distress in pregnancies with an SGA fetus,[68-70] whereas in six randomized clinical trials (RCTs), reductions in antenatal admissions (odds ratio [OR] 0.56; 95% confidence interval [CI], 0.43-0.72), number of labor inductions (OR, 0.78; CI, 0.63-0.96), elective deliveries (OR, 0.73;CI, 0.61-0.88) and cesarean deliveries (OR, 0.78; CI, 0.65-0.94) were found.[71] Based on meta-analysis of four RCTs, the systematic use of umbilical artery Doppler in unselected or low risk pregnancies does not have an effect on perinatal mortality, antenatal hospitalization, obstetric outcome and perinatal morbidity.[72] However, an unexpected abnormal umbilical artery Doppler waveform at the 20- to 22-week anomaly scan might be clinically relevant.

The published RCTs of routine Doppler ultrasound in either general obstetric populations or in high-risk pregnancies and the potential effects on pregnancy outcome are summarized in Table 32–2 and Table 32–3.

Table 32-2   Evaluation of screening for intrauterine growth restriction using doppler velocimetry

Study	Risk population	Screening Outcome
Davies et al.,[76]	General obstetric population	Higher PM in study group; no reduction in antenatal admissions
Omzigt et al.,[77]	University population	No effect on antenatal or neonatal admissions; no obstetric management effect; PM halved
Whittle et al.,[78]	Unselected population	No difference in antenatal and neonatal admissions or neonatal morbidity
Mason et al.,[100]	Low risk	No effect on obstetric intervention rates and short term neonatal mortality
Newnham et al.,[31]	Medium risk	Prediction of intrauterine growth restriction
Trudinger et al.[73]	High risk	No effect on interventions; less fetal distress in labor; No effect on neonatal morbidity
Newnham et al.,[75]	High risk	No effect on neonatal morbidity or obstetric management
Tyrell et al.,[101]	High risk	Lower gestational age at delivery; lower rate of low Apgar scores; no increase in obstetrical interventions
Almstrom et al.,[68]	SGA pregnancies	Less monitoring, fewer antenatal admissions, Fewer inductions and fewer emergency cesarean deliveries
Pattinson et al.,[70]	High risk	AEDV in control group showed more stillbirths; Doppler group had fewer antenatal and neonatal admissions
Johnstone et al.,[97]	High risk	No reduction in admissions, FHR testing, interventions; no reduction in PM
Nienhuis et al.,[81]	High risk	No reduction in admissions; reduction in duration of hospitalization
Haley et al.,[102]	High risk	Reduction in the use of hospital resources and hospital admissions; No effect on induction rates or cesarean delivery rates

AEDV, absent end diastolic velocities; FHR, fetal heart rate; IUGR, intrauterine growth restriction; PM, perinatal mortality; SGA, small for gestational age.

Screening studies. The routine use of Doppler has no effect on gestational age at delivery or the rates of labor induction or cesarean delivery, including elective sections. Neither neonatal intensive care nor medium care nursery admissions are altered.[73–78] It should, however, be noted that the response to abnormal testing is rarely standardized.

Studies of both high-risk and low-risk pregnancies have failed to show any improvement in perinatal outcome with the addition of Doppler velocimetry.[73,75,76]

Table 32-3 **Effects of Doppler-indicated interventions (aspirin or hospital admission) on pregnancy outcome with abnormal Doppler findings**

Study	Risk population	Intervention	Outcome
Nienhuis et al.,[81]	University population	Doppler indication for antenatal admission	Reduction of admissions; no effect on neonatal outcome
Omzigt et al.,[77]	University population	Doppler indication for antenatal admission	No reduction in antenatal or neonatal admissions
Trudinger et al.,[85]	Raised umbilical artery S/D Raised uterine artery	Aspirin (150 mg/d)	Increased BW in study group
Subtil et al.,[103]	RI or Persistent notching (bilateral)	Aspirin (100 mg/d)	No reduction in severe IUGR or perinatal deaths
McCowan et al.,[89]	Raised umbilical artery RI (24–36 wk)	Aspirin (100 mg/d)	No increase in birth weight
Goffinet et al.,[88]	Raised uterine artery D/S ratio or a notch	Aspirin (100 mg/d)	No effect on IUGR, birth weight or perinatal morbidity
Harrington et al.,[90]	Raised uterine artery RI and/or a persisting notch	Aspirin SR (100 mg/d)	No effect on IUGR, birth weight

BW: birthweight

Surprisingly, the perinatal mortality rate and the prevalence of low Apgar scores in the Doppler group was in one study four times higher in the low-risk population of normally formed fetuses compared with the control group where no Doppler was performed.[75,76] It may be that normal Doppler findings provide false reassurance to clinicians and pregnant women.[79] In the other studies of high-risk pregnancies, the routine use of Doppler screening was associated with a reduction in the frequency of low Apgar scores and a reduction in serious neonatal morbidity.[74] With the exclusion of congenital malformations, perinatal mortality was reduced by a third compared to the control group, mainly because there were fewer stillbirths.[77,78] Although the performance of Doppler ultrasound as a diagnostic test in a high-risk population seems better compared with low-risk populations, the seemingly inconsistent findings between studies should not be too surprising as IUGR can result from different pathologies that may defy the use of a single test. The use of this test as a screening method in a low-risk population might be unfavorable as it will result in 100 normal pregnant women being alarmed unnecessarily for the detection of only two or three IUGR cases.[80]

Hospital admission in intrauterine growth restriction. In some countries, it is common practice to routinely hospitalize a woman whose fetus is suspected of being growth restricted for bed rest and fetal monitoring. Thus, the ability to predict the absence of IUGR could theoretically lead to a more selective maternal hospitalization and a reduction in unnecessary fetal monitoring and interventions.[81] Although several studies suggested this may be true,[68,82] these consequences were not supported by the findings of RCTs.[76,77,81]

Bed rest. The return of end-diastolic velocities after these were initially recorded as being absent is associated with a better pregnancy outcome than pregnancies where they do not return. One possible explanation for the apparently better outcome is a gain in pregnancy duration. However, the prevalence of IUGR (defined as a birth weight below the tenth percentile) is also lower,[59,83] which suggests that the initial assessment of absent end diastolic flow was likely to have been erroneous, perhaps due to the angle of insonation. Some note a decrease in umbilical artery resistance in half of the women with bedrest. This decrease in resistance is associated with both an increase in birth weight and a decrease in the risk of fetal distress and perinatal death.[84] A lack of improvement after the initiation of bed rest is claimed by some to identify the category of women that may benefit from more intensive surveillance.

Aspirin. Trudinger et al.[85] observed in a randomized trial that maternal aspirin (150 mg per day) was associated with increased birth weight and placental weight of fetuses with an elevated umbilical artery systolic/diastolic (S/D) ratio. Unfortunately, the sample was small, and a larger, similar trial by Newnham et al.[86] in IUGR fetuses with an elevated umbilical artery resistance index could not demonstrate a benefit of aspirin (100 mg per day). Early (12–14 weeks) use of aspirin in women at high risk of preeclampsia and/or IUGR with uterine artery abnormalities failed to reduce the prevalence of IUGR in blinded, controlled trials.[87] There is also no decrease in IUGR when the aspirin is started comparatively late in pregnancy (17–24 weeks and even later) [88–90] The first study was criticized because the treatment was started at a time when many women would be expected to develop normal flow patterns. In contrast, the second set of studies were begun after placentation was presumably completed (see also Chapter 35).

Fetal distress. Antepartum identification of the pregnancy at increased risk of an adverse perinatal outcome remains an obstetric challenge. Although some Doppler screening studies report a decrease in perinatal mortality (especially the stillbirth rate) in the Doppler group, none reveal the expected, concomitant effect on obstetric management or reduction in interventions.[70,73,77,78] In a meta-analysis, Alfirevic and Neilson[91] concluded that there was a 38% reduction of perinatal mortality, with a concomitant decrease in antenatal admissions, inductions of labor and cesarean sections for fetal distress in high-risk pregnancies. The apparent benefit of Doppler measurements on perinatal mortality was no longer present after adjusting for congenital abnormalities and birth weights less than 1,000 g.[77] Pattinson et al.[70] reported that the clinical actions triggered by the Doppler studies were associated with a reduction in both hospital days (antenatal and neonatal) and the risk of fetal distress in fetus considered SGA. The knowledge of AEDV has also been associated with an improvement in fetal survival. In high-risk pregnancies, umbilical Doppler studies are predictive of fetal distress,[92] although the nonstress test (NST) may be superior.[93] One should consider explanations for a nonreactive NST other than fetal distress when the Doppler studies are normal, such as a prolonged quiet sleep or the maternal ingestion of a drug acting on the nervous system.

In one observational study, fetuses with abnormal uteroplacental fetal velocity waveforms and normal birth weights were more likely to develop perinatal complications.[94] In another, abnormal Doppler velocimetry was associated with a poor fetal or neonatal outcome when the intrapartum fetal heart rate tracing suggested fetal distress.[95] However, the use of intrapartum Doppler velocimetry in low-risk pregnancies as a screening test in the latent phase of labor failed to predict subsequent fetal distress.[96] This may be because of the high frequency of umbilical cord compression as a cause of fetal distress during labor.

What does a normal test result mean? A normal umbilical artery Doppler indicates a normal trophoblastic invasion and conversion of the maternal spiral arteries to low resistance vessels. The fetus is not hypoxemic. Diastolic flow rises with advancing gestational age in both the maternal and fetal arteries. Normal umbilical artery velocimetry is not associated with an abnormal Biophysical Profile. A normal Doppler ultrasound excludes IUGR secondary to uteroplacental dysfunction (Table 32–1). This is perhaps its greatest virtue. Fetuses who are SGA with normal umbilical artery velocimetry are at no greater risk of developing fetal distress than those who are appropriately grown.[61,69]

What is the cost of testing?

Doppler studies can be conducted for little additional cost if an ultrasound examination is already being performed. The charge for the umbilical artery velocimetry is currently about $25 per test. The cost of a Doppler examination as part of a screening program can be estimated at around $50. If screening is performed in a low-risk population whose IUGR prevalence is below 10%, the cost of identifying one IUGR fetus is over ten times more than if the same technique is used in a high-risk population (IUGR prevalence of 30%) (Tables 32–4 and 32–5). Table 5 reflects a theoretic mixed risk population similar to Omzigt et al. [77] The percentage of women tested and the number of Doppler measurements are also extracted from this study.

The potential harmful consequences of routine Doppler ultrasound screening include false reassurance and overtreatment. The need for further testing is only increased in the abnormal Doppler group (i.e., biophysical profile testing).[74] Doppler screening does not decrease the use of fetal heart rate testing, ultrasound, or fetal blood sampling during labor.[75,76] In high-risk pregnancies,

Table 32-4   Economic evaluation of Doppler screenings programs for intrauterine growth restriction

Screening program	Total cost (10,000 screened), $	Cost per patient Screened, $	Cost per positive screened fetus, $	Cost per IUGR fetus Identified, $
Prevalence < 10%	500.000	50	545	3163
Prevalence > 10%	500.000	50	166	287
Mixed-risk population[1]	337.033	25	151	266

[1]Using a risk classification (see Table 32–5) and as defined by Omzigt et al. (ref. 77)
IUGR: intrauterine growth restriction

Table 32-5   Resources required for Doppler screening for intrauterine growth restriction

Pregnancy risk (% of the population)	Women tested, %	Measurement per woman tested	IUGR, %
High (40)	69	3.8	40
Medium (30)	30	1.8	15
Low (30)	29	1.7	6

IUGR, intrauterine growth restriction.

Doppler screening has been associated with increased fetal monitoring.[97] It is possible that the finding of a normal umbilical artery resistance index could lead to a more conservative management and actually reduce the need for intervention in some SGA pregnancies.[98] In addition, although only an impression of a change in the cascade of fetal testing has been observed after the introduction of Doppler velocimetry by some investigators, most note an increase in the use of other testing modalities.

■ Conclusions and Recommendations

Doppler measurements of fetal and maternal arterial resistances are rapid and noninvasive. As such, it is attractive as a potential screening test for IUGR secondary to uteroplacental dysfunction. A major problem in screening for IUGR is the absence of a "gold standard."

The benefits of routine Doppler ultrasound screening in practice are limited in terms of improving perinatal outcome measures. Doppler of the umbilical or uterine artery cannot be used as a screening test for the detection of IUGR in low-risk populations[80] but is most likely of value in a high-risk population.[91] The current best application of Doppler velocimetry to obstetrics is as part of the overall testing process to aid the identification of the SGA fetus (i.e., small because of uteroplacental dysfunction and thus at high risk of hypoxemia/acidemia). It may be appropriate to reassess the application of Doppler ultrasound to the screening of IUGR fetuses should there be further developments in management options.

Doppler analysis of fetal hemodynamics allows health care providers to shift their focus from the fetus with clinically insignificant SGA to the fetus with SGA secondary to fetoplacental dysfunction and hypoxemia. The U/C ratio is a better criterion of placental dysfunction than ultrasound biometric measurements.[99] Doppler studies of fetal vessels may thus provide useful information for the supervision of high-risk pregnancies complicated by IUGR.

■ Summary

1 ■ What Is the Problem that Requires Screening?
Intrauterine growth restriction (IUGR).

a. What is the incidence/prevalence of the target condition?
Most definitions are unfortunately based on a birth weight centile. Definitions of IUGR such as the Ponderal Index, skin-fold thickness, or neonatal upward crossing of centile growth curves are more accurate in their identification of IUGR, but more complicated to perform than the measurement of birth weight. A major problem with any single physical measurement as a definition of IUGR is that there are many causes of an SGA fetus other than IUGR.

b. What are the sequelae of the condition that are of interest in clinical medicine?
Fetal distress, depression at birth, compromised neurodevelopment, adult diseases, and perinatal death.

2 ■ The Test
a. What is the purpose of the tests?
To detect IUGR.

Continued

■ Summary—cont'd

b. ***What is the nature of the tests?***
Doppler velocimetry of maternal and fetal vessels. Continuous wave (CW), although less expensive and less complicated, is used less and less. Pulsed wave (PD) is now used on a routine basis, although it is only obligatory when the vessel of interest has to be visualized. The use of color Doppler technique reduces the time needed for the identification of vessels and is essential if vessels are investigated which are not part of a routine Doppler examination (e.g., in a research setting).

c. ***What are the implications of testing?***
1. What does an abnormal test result mean?
   An elevated Doppler resistance index in the setting of sonographic parameters consistent with SGA is consistent with uteroplacental dysfunction. There is an inverse relationship between the resistance index in either the umbilical or uterine arteries and fetal PO_2. Unfortunately, randomized controlled trials of Doppler screening for IUGR have failed to change outcome beneficially.
2. What does a normal test result mean?
   Normal umbilical artery velocimetry is not associated with an abnormal biophysical profile. Doppler ultrasound can also be used to exclude IUGR secondary to uteroplacental dysfunction. Fetuses who are SGA with normal umbilical artery velocimetry are at no greater risk of developing fetal distress than are appropriately grown fetuses.

d. ***What is the cost of testing?***
The cost per case identified of Doppler screening for IUGR depends on the prevalence of IUGR in the population screened. In most RCTs, Doppler screening has led to the increased use of other fetal surveillance tests independent of the population studied, without an improvement in outcome.

3 ■ Conclusions and Recommendations

Doppler measurements of fetal and maternal arterial resistances are rapid and noninvasive; they are attractive as a potential screening test for IUGR secondary to uteroplacental dysfunction. Unfortunately, the benefits of routine Doppler ultrasound screening in practice have been at best limited. Doppler is not useful as a screening test for IUGR in low-risk pregnancies. It is most possibly of value in a high-risk pregnancy. The current best application of Doppler velocimetry in obstetrics is as part of the overall testing process to aid the identification of the SGA fetus, small because of uteroplacental dysfunction.

References

1. Snijders RJM, Sherrod C, Gosden CM, et al. Fetal growth retardation: associated malformations and chromosomal abnormalities. *Am J Obstet Gynecol* 1993;168:547–555.
2. Mongelli M, Gardosi J. Reduction of false-positive diagnosis of fetal growth restriction by application of customized growth standards. *Obstet Gynecol* 1996;88:844–848.
3. Sanderson DA, Wilcox MA, Johnson IR. The individualised birthweight ratio: a new method of identifying intrauterine growth retardation. *Br J Obstet Gynaecol* 1994;101:310–314.
4. Villar J, deOnis M, Kestler E, et al. The differential neonatal morbidity of the intrauterine growth retardation syndrome. *Am J Obstet Gynecol* 1990;163:151–157.
5. Clausson B, Gardosi J, Francis A, et al. Perinatal outcome in SGA births defined by customised versus population based birthweight standards. *Br J Obstet Gynaecol* 2001;108:830–834.
6. McIntire DD, Bloom SL, Caseay BM, et al. Birth weight in relation to morbidity and mortality among newborn infants. *N Engl J Med* 1999;340:1234–1238.
7. Kramer MS, Olivier M, McLean FH, et al. Determinants of fetal growth and body proportionality. *Pediatrics* 1990;86:18–26.
8. Hadders-Algra M, Touwen BCL. Body measurements, neurological and behavioral development in six-year-old children born preterm and/or small-for-gestational-age. *Early Hum Dev* 1990;22:1–13.
9. Martikainen MA. Effects of intrauterine growth retardation and its subtypes on the development for the preterm infant. *Early Hum Dev* 1992;28:7–17.
10. Ounsted MK, Moar VA, Scott A. Children of deviant birthweight at the age of seven years: health, handicap, size and developmental status. *Early Hum Dev* 1984;9:323–340.
11. Teberg AJ, Walther FJ, Pena IC. Mortality, morbidity and outcome of the small for gestational age infant. *Semin Perinatol* 1988;12:84–94.
12. Kok JH, den Ouden AL, Verloove-Vanhorick SP, et al. Outcome of very preterm small for gestational age infants: the first nine years of life. *Br J Obstet Gynaecol* 1988;105:162–168.
13. Barker DJP. Fetal origin of coronary disease. *BMJ* 1995;311:171–174.
14. Gudmundsson S, Fairlie F, Lingman G, et al. Recording of blood flow velocity waveforms in the uteroplacental and umbilical circulation: reproducibility study and comparison of pulsed and continous wave Doppler ultrasonography. *J Clin Ultrasound* 1990;18:97–101.
15. Noordam MJ, Heydanus R, Hop WCJ, et al. Doppler colour flow imaging of fetal intracerebral arteries and umbilical artery in the small for gestational age fetus. *Br J Obstet Gynaecol* 1994;101:504–508.
16. Wladimiroff JW, VanDenWijngaard JAGW, Degani S, et al. Cerebral and umbilical arterial blood flow velocity waveforms in normal and growth-retarded pregnancies. *Obstet Gynecol* 1987;69:705–709.
17. Maulik D, Yarlagadda AP, Youngblood JP, et al. Components of variability of umbilical arterial Doppler velocimetry: a prospective analysis. *Am J Obstet Gynecol* 1989;160:1406–1412.

18. Mehalek KE, Rosenberg J, Berkowitz GS, et al. Umbilical and uterine artery flow velocity waveforms: effect of sampling site on Doppler ratios. *J Ultrasound Med* 1989;8:171–176.
19. Spencer JAD, Price J. Intraobserver variation in Doppler ultrasound indices of placental perfusion derived from different numbers of waveforms. *J Ultrasound Med* 1989;8:197–199.
20. Spencer JAD, Price J, Lee A. Influence of fetal breathing and movements on variability of umbilical Doppler indices using different numbers of waveforms. *J Ultrasound Med* 1991;10:37–41.
21. Nienhuis SJ, VanVught JMG, Hoogland HJ, et al. Interexaminer variability study of fetal velocity waveforms. *Gynecol Obstet Invest* 1988;25:152–157.
22. Tessler FN, Kimme-Smith C, Sutherland ML, et al. Inter- and Intra-observer variability of Doppler peak velocity measurements: an in-vitro study. *Ultrasound Med Biol* 1990;16:653–657.
23. Scherjon SA, Kok JH, Oosting H, et al. Intra-observer and inter-observer reliability of the pulsatility index calculated from pulsed Doppler flow velocity waveforms in three fetal vessels. *Br J Obstet Gynaecol* 1993;100:134–138.
24. Arduini D, Rizzo G, Mancuso S, et al. Longitudinal assessment of blood flow velocity waveforms in the healthy human fetus. *Prenat Diagn* 1987;7:613–617.
25. Woo JSK, Liang ST, Lo RLS, et al. Middle cerebral artery Doppler flow velocity waveforms. *Obstet Gynecol* 1987;70:613–616.
26. McCowan LM, Ritchie K, Mo LY, et al. Uterine artery flow velocity waveforms in normal and growth retarded pregnancies. *Am J Obstet Gynecol* 1988;158:499–504.
27. Cameron A, Nicholson S, Nimrod C, et al. Duplex ultrasonography of the fetal aorta, umbilical artery, and placental arcuate artery throughout normal human pregnancy. *J Can Assoc Radiol* 1989;40:145–149.
28. Arstrom A, Eliasson A, Hareide JH, et al. Fetal blood velocity waveforms in normal pregnancies: a longitudinal study. *Acta Obstet Gynecol Scand* 1989;68:171–178.
29. Bahlmann F, Reinhard I, Krummenauer F, et al. Blood flow velocity waveforms of the fetal middle cerebral artery in a normal population: reference values from 18 weeks to 42 weeks of gestation. *J Perinat Med* 2002;30:490–501.
30. VanVugt JMG. Validity of umbilical artery blood velocimetry in the prediction of intrauterine growth retardation and fetal compromise. *J Perinat Med* 1991;19:15–20.
31. Newnham JP, Patterson LL, James IR, et al. An evaluation of the efficacy of Doppler flow velocity waveform analysis as a screening test in pregnancy. *Am J Obstet Gynecol* 1990;162:403–410.
32. Weiner CP. The relationship between the umbilical artery systolic/diastolic ratio and umbilical blood gas measurements in specimens obtained by cordocentesis. *Am J Obstet Gynecol* 1990;162:1198–1202.
33. Rizzo G, Capponi A, Arduini D, et al. The value of fetal arterial, cardiac and venous flows in preciting pH and blood gases measured in umbilical blood at cordocentesis in growth retarded fetuses. *Br J Obstet Gynaecol* 1995;102:963–969.
34. Rizzo G, Capponi A, Talone PE, et al. Doppler indices form inferior vena cava and ductus venosus in predicting pH and oxygen tension in umbilical blood at cordocentesis in growth-retarded fetuses. *Ultrasound Obstet Gynecol* 1996;7:401–410
35. Divon MY, Girz BA, Lieblich R, et al. Clinical management of the fetus with markedly diminished umbilical artery end-diastolic flow. *Am J Obstet Gynecol* 1989;161:1523–1527.
36. Scherjon SA. Smolders-deHaas H, Kok JH, et al. The "brain-sparing" effect: antenatal cerebral Doppler findings in relation to neurologic outcome in very preterm infants. *Am J Obstet Gynecol* 1993;169:169–175.
37. Soregaroli M, Bonera R, Danti L, et al. Prognostic role of umbilical artery Doppler velocimetry in growth-restricted fetus. *J Mat Fetal Neonat Med* 2002;11:199–203.
38. Bower S, Kingdom J, Campbell S. Objective and subjective assessment of abnormal uterine artery Doppler flow velocity waveforms. *Ultrasound Obstet Gynecol* 1998;12:260–264.
39. Papageorghiou AT, Yu CKH, Bindra R, et al. Multicenter screening for pre-eclampsia and fetal growth restriction by transvaginal uterine artery Doppler at 23 weeks of gestation. *Ultrasound Obstet Gynecol* 2001;18:441–449.
40. Ferrazzi E, Rigano S, Bozzo M, et al. Umbilical vein blood flow in growth restricted fetuses. *Ultrasound Obstet Gynecol* 2000;16:432–438.

41. Rizzo G, Capponi A, Arduini D, et al. Ductus venosus velocity waveforms in appropriate and small for gestational age fetuses. *Early Hum Dev* 1994;39:15–26.

42. Rizzo G, Arduini D, Romanini C. Inferior vena cava flow velocity waveforms in appropriate- and small-for-gestational-age fetuses. *Am J Obstet Gynecol* 1992;166:1271–1280.

43. Bellotti M, Pennati G, De Gasperi C, et al. Simultaneous measurement of umbilical venous, fetal hepatic, and ductus venosus blood flow in growth-restricted human fetuses. *Am J Obstet Gynecol* 2004;190:1347–1358.

44. Hofstaetter C, Gudmundsson S, Hansmann M. Venous Doppler velocimetry in the surveillance of severely compromised fetuses. *Ultrasound Obstet Gynecol* 2002; 20:333–339.

45. Gramelinni D, Piantelli G, Verrotti C, et al. Doppler velocimetry and non stress test in severe fetal growth restriction. *Clin Exp Obstet Gynecol* 2001;28:33–39.

46. Ritter S, Jörn H, Weiss C, et al. Importance of ductus venosus Doppler assessment for fetal outcome in cases of intra uterine growth restriction. *Fetal Diagn Therapy* 2004;19:348–355.

47. Sijmons EA, Reuwer PJHM, Van Beek E, et al. The validity of screening for small-for-gestational-age and low-weight-for-length infants by Doppler ultrasound. *Br J Obstet Gynaecol* 1989;96:557–561.

48. Chang TC, Robson SC, Spencer JAD, et al. Identification of fetal growth retardation: comparison of Doppler waveform indices and serial ultrasound measurements of abdominal circumference and fetal weight. *Obstet Gynecol* 1993;82:230–236.

49. Giles WB, Trudinger BJ, Cook CM. Fetal umbilical artery flow velocity-time waveforms in twin pregnancies. *Br J Obstet Gynaecol* 1985;92:490–497.

50. Arabin B, Siebert M, Jimenez E, et al. Obstetrical characteristics of a loss of end-diastolic velocities in the fetal aorta and/or umbilical artery using Doppler ultrasound. *Gynecol Obstet Invest* 1988;25:173–180.

51. Lin S, Shimizu I, Suehara N, et al. Uterine artery Doppler velocimetry in relation to trophoblast migration into the myometrium of the placental bed. *Obstet Gynecol* 1995;85:760–765.

52. Hackett GA, Nicolaides KH, Campbell S. Doppler ultrasound assessment of fetal and uteroplacental circulations in severe second trimester oligohydramnios. *Br J Obstet Gynaecol* 1987;94:1074–1077.

53. Nicolaides KK, Bilardo CM, Soothill PW, et al. Absence of end diastolic frequencies in the umbilical artery: a sign of fetal hypoxia and acidosis. *BMJ* 1988;297:1026–1027.

54. Al-Ghazali WH, Chapman MG, Rissik JM, et al. The significance of absent end-diastolic flow in the umbilical artery combined with reduced fetal cardiac output estimation in pregnancies at high risk for placental insufficiency. *J Obstet Gynaecol* 1990;10:271–275.

55. Pardi G, Cetin I, Marconi AM, et al. Diagnostic value of blood sampling in fetuses with growth retardation. *N Engl J Med* 1993;328:692–696.

56. Rowlands DJ, Vyas SK. Longitudinal study of fetal middle cerebral artery flow velocity waveforms preceding fetal death. *Br J Obstet Gynaecol* 1995;102:888–890.

57. Johnstone FD, Haddad NG, Hoskins P, et al. Umbilical artery Doppler flow velocity waveform: the outcome of pregnancies with absent end diatolic flow. *Eur J Obstet Gynec Reprod Biol* 1988;28:171–178.

58. Wenstrom KD, Weiner CP, Williamson RA. Diverse maternal and fetal pathology associated with absent diastolic flow in the umbilical artery of high-risk fetuses. *Obstet Gynecol* 1991;77:374–378.

59. Bell JG, Ludomirsky A, Bottalico J, et al. The effect of improvement of umbilical artery absent end-diastolic velocity on perinatal outcome. *Am J Obstet Gynecol* 1992;167:1015–1020.

60. GRIT Study Group. A randomised trial of timed delivery for the compromised preterm fetus: short term outcomes and Bayesian interpretation. *Br J Obstet Gynaecol* 2003;110:27–32.

61. Pattinson R, Dawes G, Jennings J, et al. Umbilical artery resistance index as a screening test for fetal well being, I: prospective revealed evaluation. *Obstet Gynecol* 1991;78:353–358.

62. Soothill PW, Ajayi RA, Campbell S, et al. Prediction of morbidity in small and normally grown fetuses by fetal heart rate variability. biophysical profile score and umbilical artery Doppler studies. *Br J Obstet Gynaecol* 1993;100:742–725.

63. Arduini D, Rizzo G, Romanini C. Changes of pulsatility index from fetal vessels preceding the onset of late decelerations in growth-retarded fetus. *Obstet Gynecol* 1992;79:605–610.

64. Wladimiroff JW, Tonge MM, Stewart PA, et al. Severe intrauterine growth retardation; assessment of its origin from fetal arterial flow velocity waveforms. *Eur J Obstet Gynaecol Reprod Biol* 1986;22:23–28.

65. Baschat AA, Gembruch U, Reiss I, et al. Demonstration of fetal coronary blood flow by Doppler ultrasound in relation to arterial and venous flow velocity waveforms and perinatal outcome—the "heart-sparing effect." *Ultrasound Obstet Gynecol* 1997; 9:362–372.

66. James DK, Parker MJ, Smoleniec JS. Comprehensive fetal assessment with three ultrasonographic characteristics. *Am J Obstet Gynecol* 1992;166:1486–1495.

67. Madazli R, Uludag S, Ocak V. Doppler assessment of umbilical artery, thoracic aorta and middle cerebral artery in the management of pregnancies with growth restriction. *Acta Obstet Gynecol Scand* 2001;80:702–707.

68. Almstrom H, Axelson O, Cnattingius S, et al. Comparison of umbilical-artery velocimetry and cardiotocography for surveillance of small-for-gestational-age fetus. *Lancet* 1992;340:936–940.

69. Baschat AA, Weiner CP. Umbilical artery Doppler screening for the detection of the small fetus in need of antepartum surveillance. *Am J Obstet Gynecol* 2000;182:154–158.

70. Pattinson RC, Norman K, Odendaal HJ. The role of Doppler velocimetry in the management of high risk pregnancies. *Br J Obstet Gynaecol* 1994;101:114–120.

71. Westergaard HB, Langhoff-Roos J, Lingman G, et al. A critical appraisel of the use of umbilical artery Doppler ultrasound in high risk pregnancies: use of meta-analyses in evidence-based obstetrics. *Ultrasound Obstet Gynecol* 2001;17:466–476.

72. Goffinet F, Paris-Llado J, Nisand I, et al. Umbilical artery Doppler velocimetry in unselected and low risk pregnancies: a review of randomized controlled trials. *Br J Obstet Gynaecol* 1997;104:425–430.

73. Trudinger BJ, Giles WB, Cook CM, et al. Umbilical artery flow velcity waveforms in high-risk pregnancy: randomised clinical trail. *Lancet* 1987;188–190.

74. Tyrrell SN, Lilford RJ, MacDonald HN, et al. Randomized comparison of routine vs highly selective use of Doppler ultrasound and biophysiacal scoring to investigate high risk pregnanacies. *Br J Obstet Gynaecol* 1990;97:909–916.

75. Newnham JP, O'Dea MRA, Reid KP, et al. Doppler flow velocity waveform analysis in high risk pregnancies: a randomized controlled trial. *Br J Obstet Gynaecol* 1991;98:956–963.

76. Davies JA, Gallivan S, Spencer JAD. Randomised controlled trial of Doppler ultrasound screening of placental perfusion during pregnancy. *Lancet* 1992;340:1299–1303.

77. Omzigt AWJ, Reuwer PJGH, Bruinse HW. A randomized controlled trial on the clinical value of umbilical Doppler velocimetry in antenatal care. *Am J Obstet Gynecol* 1994;170:625–634.

78. Whittle MJ, Hanretty KP, Primrose MH, et al. Screening for the compromised fetus: A randomized trial of umbilical artery velocimetry in unselected pregnancies. *Am J Obstet Gynecol* 1994;170:555–559.

79. Bewley S, Cooper D, Campbell S. Doppler investigation of uteroplacental blood flow resistance in the second trimester: a screening study for pre-eclampsia and intra-uterine growth retardation. *Br J Obstet Gynaecol* 1991;98:871–879.

80. Todros T, Ferrazzi E, Arduini D, et al. Performance of Doppler ultrasonography as a screening test in low risk pregnancies. *J Ultrasound Med* 1995;14:343–348.

81. Nienhuis SJ, Vles JSH, Gerver WJM, et al. Doppler ultrasonography in suspected intrauterine growth retardation: a randomized clinical trial. *Ultrasound Obstet Gynecol* 1997;9:6–13.

82. Ruissen CJ, Nienhuis SJ, Hoogland HJ, et al. Cost effectiveness of a Doppler based policy of intrauterine growth retardation: a randomized controlled trial. *J Matern Fetal Invest* 1991;1:126.

83. Brar HS, Platt LD. Antepartum improvement of abnormal umbilical artery velocimetry: does it occur? *Am J Obstet Gynecol* 1989;160:36–39.

84. Sengupta S, Harrigan JT, Rosenberg JC, et al. Perinatal outcome following improvement of abnormal umbilical artery velocimetry. *Obstet Gynecol* 1991;78:1062–1066.

85. Trudinger BJ, Cook CM, Thompson RS, et al. Low-dose aspirin therapy improves fetal weight in umbilical placental insuffucency. *Am J Obstet Gynecol* 1988;159:681–685.

86. Newnham JP, Godfrey M. Walters B, et al. Low dose aspirin for the treatment of fetal growth restriction: a randomized controlled trial. *Proceedings of the Combined New Zealand and Australian Perinatal Society*, Auckland, abstract 87, 1995.

87. Vainio M, Kujansuu E, Iso-Mustajarvi M, et al. Low dose acetylsalicylic acid in prevention of pregnancy-induced hypertension and intrauterine growth retardation in women with bilateral uterine artery notches. *Br J Obstet Gynaecol* 2002;109:61–167.
88. Goffinet F, Aboulker D, Paris-Llado J, et al. Screening with a uterine Doppler in low risk pregnant women followed by low dose aspirin in women with abnormal results: a multicenter randomized controlled trial. *Br J Obstet Gynaecol* 2001;108:510–518.
89. Mc Cowan LM, Harding J, Roberts A, et al. Administration of low-dose aspirin to mothers with small for gestational age fetuses and abnormal umbilical artery Doppler studies to increase birthweight: a randomized double-blind controlled trial. *Br J Obstet Gynaecol* 1990;106:647–651.
90. Harrington K, Kurdi W, Aquilina J, et al. A prospective management study of slow-release aspirin in the palliation of uteroplacental insufficiency predicted by uterine artery Doppler at 20 weeks. *Ultrasound Obstet Gynecol* 2000;15:13–18.
91. Alfirevic Z and Neilson JP. Doppler ultrasonography in high risk-pregancies: systematic review with meta-anaysis. *Am J Obstet Gynecol* 1995;172:1379–1387.
92. Maulik D, Yarlagadda P, Youngblood JP, et al. The diagnostic efficacy of the umbilical arterial systolic/diastolic ratio as a screening tool: a prospective blinded study. *Am J Obstet Gynecol* 1990;162:1518–1525.
93. Devoe LD, Gardner P, Dear C, et al. The diagnostic values of concurrent nonstress testing, amniotic fluid measurment, and Doppler velocimetry in screening a general high-risk population. *Am J Obstet Gynecol* 1990;163:1040–1048.
94. Bower S, Schuchter K, Campbell S. Doppler ultrasound screening as part of routine antenatal screening: prediction of pre-eclampsia and intrauterine growth retardation. *Br J Obstet Gynaecol* 1993;100:989–994.
95. Ogunyemi D, Stanley R, Lynch R, et al. Umbilical artery velocimetry in predicting perinatal outcome with intrapartum fetal distress. *Obstet Gynecol* 1992;80:377–380.
96. Sarno AP, Brar HS, Phelan JP, et al. Intrapartum Doppler velocimetry, amniotic fluid volume, and fetal heart rate as predictors of subsequent fetal distress. *Am J Obstet Gynecol* 1989;161:1508–1514.
97. Johnstone FD, Prescott R, Hoskins P, et al. The effect of the introduction of umbilical artery Doppler recordings to obstetric practice. *Br J Obstet Gynaecol* 1993;100:733–741.
98. Burke G, Stuart B, Crowley P, et al. Is intrauterine growth retardation with normal umbilical artery blood flow a benign condition? *BMJ* 1990;300:1044–1045.
99. Bilardo CM, Nicolaides KH, Campbell S. Doppler measurements of fetal and uteroplacental circulations: relationship with venous blood gases measured at cordocentesis. *Am J Obstet Gynecol* 1990;162:115–120.
100. Mason GC, Lilford RJ, Porter J, Nelson E, Tyrell S. Randomised comparison of routine versus highly selective use of Doppler ultrasound in low risk pregnancies. *Br J Obstet Gynaecol* 1993;100:130–133.
101. Tyrell SN, Lilford RJ, Macdonald HN, et al. Randomized comparison of routine vs highly selective use of Doppler ultrasound and biophysical scoring to investigate high risk pregnancies. *Br J Obstet Gynaecol* 1990;97:909–916.
102. Haley J, Tuffnell DJ, Johnson N. Randomised controlled trial of cardiotocography versus umbilical artery Doppler in the management of small for gestational age fetuses. *Br J Obstet Gynaecol* 1997;104:431–435.
103. Subtil D, Goeusse P, Houfflin-Debarge V, et al. Randomised comparison of uterine artery Doppler and aspirin (100 mg) with placebo in nulliparous women: the Essai Regional Aspirine Mere-Enfant study (Part 2). *BJOG* 2003;110:485–491.

33

Preterm Delivery

Jay D. Iams

David N. Hackney

■ What Is the Problem that Requires Screening?

Preterm delivery (PTD) is defined as delivery before 37 and after 20 weeks' estimated gestational age from the last menstrual period. Some reports use "viability" as the lower threshold, variably defined as 22 to 24 weeks' gestation. Other reports use 34 to 37 weeks' gestation as the upper threshold because most infants delivered between 34 and 37 weeks' gestation have normal outcomes.

Preterm labor (PTL) is defined as regular contractions accompanied by cervical change between 20 and 37 weeks' gestation. Contractions alone do not fulfill the definition of preterm labor, as these commonly occur prior to 37 weeks.[1] Estimates of cervical "change" have poor reproducibility until the effacement is 80% and dilation is 3 cm.

Low-birth-weight (LBW) and very low–birth-weight (VLBW) infants are defined as weighing less than 2500 and less than 1500 g, respectively. LBW infants are not necessarily preterm, but may instead be term infants with significant intrauterine growth restriction (IUGR).

Preterm births may be "indicated" or "spontaneous." Indicated preterm deliveries occur as the result of perceived maternal or fetal complications, such as fetal growth restriction or severe preeclampsia. Spontaneous preterm births occur without a clear precipitating cause, usually through the onset of contractions, "cervical insufficiency," or preterm premature rupture of the membranes (PPROM). The focus of this chapter is spontaneous preterm birth.

What is the incidence/prevalence of the target condition?

The prevalence of preterm births (<37 weeks) in the United States was 12.1% in 2002.[2] This represents approximately 480,000 deliveries a year. Not included in this figure are the losses occurring before 20 weeks. Neonates delivered before 32 weeks' gestation experience the greatest morbidity and mortality and account for 1.96% of births.[2] The LBW rate rose from 7.7% to 7.8% from 2001 to 2002, the highest level reported in more than three decades.[2]

The percent of VLBW infant births was 1.46% in 2002, compared with 1.44% for the previous year.[2] The prevalence of PTD, LBW, and VLBW has steadily increased since the 1980's.[2] This rise is thought to result from two trends: the increasing occurrence of multiple gestations secondary to increased use of assisted reproduction technologies,[3] and an increased number of medically indicated preterm births.

What are the sequelae of the condition that are of interest in clinical medicine?

Infants delivered preterm account for a disproportionate percentage of neonatal morbidity and mortality. Surviving preterm infants, especially those born before 32 weeks or less than 1,500, suffer the high rates of intraventricular hemorrhage, chronic lung disease (i.e., bronchopulmonary dysplasia), necrotizing enterocolitis, and retinopathy of prematurity, among other illnesses.[4] Twenty-three percent of infants delivered at 25 weeks' estimated gestational age or less during 1995 in the United Kingdom alive at a 30-month follow-up suffered from a severe disability.[5] Even survivors who lack major morbidities often suffer learning disabilities and have lower rates of high school graduation.[6]

■ The Tests

What is the purpose of the tests?

To detect women at high risk of preterm delivery.

An ideal screening test for preterm delivery would be inexpensive and non-invasive, with sufficiently high sensitivity to warrant interventions should the test results return positive. There are two major obstacles to screening low-risk women: low negative and positive predictive values (PPVs) and the inability of most interventions to prevent PTD. For example, a history of PTD carries a two- to fourfold increased risk of recurrent preterm birth, yet has a weak positive predictive value because most of these women still deliver a subsequent pregnancy at term.[7,8] More comprehensive analyses of risk may be individually useful but also lack accuracy. The best clinical risk assessment system that could be developed from data collected during the National Institute of Child Health and Human Development (NICHD) Maternal Fetal Medicine Unit (MFMU) Network Preterm Prediction Study of 2,929 women had positive predictive values of only about 30%.[9] Among laboratory tests for preterm birth in that study,[9] a positive fetal fibronectin (fFN) in asymptomatic pregnant women was significantly associated with an increased risk of preterm birth before 32 and 35 weeks,[10] but the sensitivities were low (38% and 21%, respectively).

The second major problem that precludes widespread PTD screening even with the availability of an ideal screening test is the lack of successful intervention strategies should a screening test result return as positive. Although various infections have been implicated in the etiology of PTD, and the treatment of asymptomatic bacterial vaginosis in high-risk populations decreased rates of PTD in some studies,[11] benefit was not demonstrated in a large study of low risk women with bacterial vaginosis.[12] Treatment of asymptomatic *Trichomonas vaginalis* infections has also proven not to be fruitful,[13] as have outpatient daily uterine contraction monitoring,[14,15] bed rest,[16] intravenous (IV) hydration,[17,18] and tocolysis.[19–21] Intensive patient education and increased nursing contact have also been studied in randomized trials and found to be ineffective.[15,22] Data concerning the benefit of cervical cerclage are conflicting.[23–25] For these reasons the American College of Obstetricians and Gynecologists has stated that *"Screening for risk of preterm labor by means other than historic risk factors is not beneficial in the general obstetric population."*[26]

Recent reports of randomized placebo-controlled trials using progesterone supplementation to prevent preterm birth are encouraging but not yet definitive.[27,28] The NICHD MFMU Network studied weekly injections of 250 mg of 17 α-hydroxyprogesterone caproate and found a significant decrease in PTD before 37 weeks' gestation (36.3% in the treatment group versus 54.9% of placebo patients) with corresponding improvements in neonatal outcomes.[27] Women were enrolled in these trials primarily because of a history of preterm delivery. The use of progesterone in women with positive PTD screening tests such as a short cervix or positive fetal fibronectin was not evaluated. Weekly injections were started between 16 and 20 weeks' gestation, before some screening tests are available. However, a report from Brazil described the initiation of treatment as late as 25 to 26 weeks' gestation and yet still demonstrated fewer births before 34 weeks.[28] Thus, the most effective time to initiate progesterone therapy is not clear, nor is it known whether there is a gestational age beyond which it is not effective. If, for example, a woman without a prior PTD is discovered to have a dramatically decreased cervical length at 28 weeks' gestation, there is no current evidence to support the use of progesterone.

What is the nature of the test?

Fetal fibronectin. fFN is a glycoprotein that exists normally between the placenta or membranes and the uterine wall[29] and plays a structural role. It is not normally present in the vagina or cervix between 22 and 34 weeks, and its presence during those times indicates a disruption of the amniotic–decidual interface. The "onco–fetal domain" serves to differentiate it from other fibronectins and can be detected by the monoclonal antibody FDC-6.[30] In the United States, the Food and Drug Administration (FDA) approved an fFN test using an enzyme-linked immunosorbent assay (ELISA) in 1995 and later approved a more rapid test using a Dacron swab. A level of 50 ng/mL is the best threshold for a "positive" test.[29]

fFN is abundant in amniotic fluid and is present in the endocervix or vaginal fluid of virtually 100% of women with ruptured membranes.[29] In fact a negative fFN test makes the diagnosis of PPROM highly unlikely, if not impossible.

Fetal fibronectin is also present in maternal blood, and false-positive results are common with vaginal bleeding.

Samples may be collected from the posterior fornix of the vagina or cervical canal; the manufacturer recommends the former. The fFN swab must be obtained before the cervix is examined. Women should not have had a digital or ultrasound examination or intercourse within 24 hours,[31] and cervical dilation should be less than or equal to 3 cm. The presence of a cervical cerclage is not a contraindication to the measurement of fFN.[32] Testing is optimally performed between 22 and 34 weeks' gestation, because for results before 22 weeks the test may be physiologically positive, and after 34 weeks management for preterm labor is not typically aggressive.

What are the implications of testing?

The significance of a positive fFN in a woman between 24 and 34 weeks of gestation depends on the whether the woman is symptomatic. The fibronectin test was approved by the FDA as a screening test in asymptomatic pregnant women at 24 weeks, but has not been widely used because there is no intervention available for women who test positive. The sensitivity of fFN at 24 weeks in the Preterm Prediction Study to predict delivery before 35 weeks was 23%[10]; it was 40% to predict birth before 34 weeks in a recent meta-analysis of studies in asymptomatic women.[33] In the Preterm Prediction Study analysis limited to women with a prior PTD, 45% to 50% of women with a positive test for fFN at 22-24 weeks delivered before 35 weeks estimated gestational age.[7] That number increased to 65% in women who had both a positive fFN and a cervical length of <25mm, but the sensitivity of combined testing was very low.[7] In a subsequent study conducted in women with a prior PTD, the sensitivity of a fFN to identify women who would deliver before 35 weeks was 18.9% at 22-24 weeks' gestation with a positive predictive value of 35%, and 21.4% at 27-28 weeks with a PPV of 30%[34] (Table 33–1). Such performance values are far below optimal for a screening test.

What does an abnormal test result mean? An asymptomatic woman with a positive fFN has a higher risk of PTD than an untested woman or one with a negative result, but the clinical utility depends on the availability, effectiveness, cost, and risk of an intervention to prevent or reduce the morbidity of prematurity. Because a positive fibronectin test was also linked to an increased risk of perinatal infection,[35] investigators attempted to treat these patients with antibiotics. Unfortunately, the prevalence of PTD was not decreased in 703 women with a positive fFN between 21 and 25 weeks' gestation who were enrolled and randomized to receive either metronidazole and erythromycin or placebo; in fact, the PTD rate was *increased* in the treated group.[36] *There is currently no intervention that is known to reduce the risk or consequences of preterm birth after a positive fFN test.* The American College of Obstetricians and Gynecologists[8] does not recommend fFN as a screening test for preterm birth.

Table 33–1   **Performance of Tests Predicting Preterm Birth**

Test	Week of Gestation at Time of Testing		
	22-24	27-28	31-32
	Percent		
Maximal nighttime contraction frequency ≥4/hr			
Sensitivity	8.6	28.1	27.3
Specificity	96.4	88.7	82.0
Positive predictive value	25.0	23.1	11.3
Negative predictive value	88.3	91.1	93.0
Maximal daytime contraction frequency ≥4/hr			
Sensitivity	0	12.9	13.6
Specificity	98.4	93.9	84.9
Positive predictive value	0	20.0	7.1
Negative predictive value	87.0	90.2	92.1
Cervicovaginal fibronectin ≥50 ng/ml			
Sensitivity	18.9	21.4	41.2
Specificity	95.1	94.5	92.5
Positive predictive value	35.0	30.0	30.4
Negative predictive value	89.4	91.6	95.2
Cervical length ≤25 mm			
Sensitivity	47.2	53.6	82.4
Specificity	89.2	82.2	74.9
Positive predictive value	37.0	25.0	20.9
Negative predictive value	92.6	94.1	98.1
Bishop score ≥4[1]			
Sensitivity	35.1	46.4	82.4
Specificity	91.0	77.9	61.8
Positive predictive value	35.1	18.8	14.7
Negative predictive value	91.0	92.9	97.8

[1]The Bishop score is a composite measure of cervical length, dilatation, position, consistency, and the degree of descent (station) of the presenting part of the fetus. The results indicate the degree of readiness for labor; values from 0 to 4 indicate not ready for labor, and values from 9 to 13 indicate ready for labor.

What does a normal test result mean? Asymptomatic pregnant women with a negative fFN have a very low chance of PTD, but screening asymptomatic women with fFN is not recommended. A negative test might in rare instances provide reassurance about the risk of preterm birth (e.g., when there is increased anxiety about the chance of preterm birth despite a normal clinical examination). The fFN test has been used in women with symptoms to improve the specificity of diagnosis.[37,38] In this setting, the test has clinical value if clinicians use a negative result to exclude the diagnosis of preterm labor and avoid overtreatment.

What is the cost of testing?

The laboratory assay costs vary but are usually between $100 and $200. When used in women with symptoms of preterm labor, the cost of fFN testing depends almost entirely on the care algorithm applied. If a practitioner is willing to act upon a negative FFN result and not hospitalize or transfer a patient being triaged for preterm labor, then the cost saving from the test is substantial.[39,40] However, the test only adds cost without benefit if clinicians choose not to avoid treatment following a negative result.[41] When a care protocol is followed, the cost of the test is weighed against money saved by having avoided false positive diagnosis and unnecessary hospitalization. In the absence of such a protocol, fFN is not cost-effective.

The cost of use in asymptomatic women is not easily calculable without an appropriately effective and safe intervention. In rare cases, a negative test may provide a rationale to avoid or defer other even more costly testing for preterm birth, such as ambulatory uterine activity monitoring.

What is the nature of the test?

Manual examination of the cervix. The cervical examination, well known to all practitioners of obstetrics, involves the placement of two gloved fingers in the patient's vagina followed by manual palpation of the cervix. The Bishop's score[42] consists of the sum of five components that are each given 0 to 3 points (Table 33–2). It was originally designed to assess the likelihood of a successful labor induction for women at term, although its use in PTD screening has since been evaluated.[34,43,44] A "cervical score" has also been used to evaluate the risk of PTD. One obtains the score by subtracting the cervical length in centimeters, measured by digital examination along the lateral vaginal fornix, from the cervical dilation in centimeters (e.g., a cervix that is 3 cm long and not dilated at all yields a score of +3; a cervical length of 1 cm with 3 cm dilation yields a score of –2). Scores of +1 or less have been associated with an increased risk of preterm birth.[43,44]

Station is the distance of the fetal presenting part (not actually the cervix per se) from the ischial spine. A presenting part at the spine is said to be at "zero station," with negative and positive numbers assigned to positions more cephalad and caudad, respectively. Physicians describe station in either thirds or centimeters. In the United States, since 1988, the American College of Obstetricians and Gynecologists has endorsed the use of centimeters over thirds for operative vaginal deliveries. Regardless of which grading system is used, physicians should designate it appropriately (i.e., +1/3 for a station one third of the distance distal from the spine, as opposed to just "+1").

Table 33–2 **The Bishop's Score**				
Points Assigned	**0**	**1**	**2**	**3**
Dilation	0	1–2	3–4	5–6
Effacement	0%–30%	40%–50%	60%–70%	80%
Station	–3	–2	–1 or 0	+1 or +2
Consistency	Firm	Medium	Soft	
Position	Posterior	Mid	Anterior	

Cervical dilation is measured at the internal os. The external os is less reliable since it is often patulous at baseline in multigravid patients. If a finger cannot be passed through the external os, then the cervix is "closed," even though the internal os cannot truly be assessed. It is difficult to determine the presence of funneling based on the digital examination of a closed cervix. Trials using simulated models have demonstrated substantial interexaminer variation of 1 cm.[45,46]

Effacement represents the total length of the cervix from the external to the internal os. It can either be expressed as the total length in centimeters or as a percentage of normal length. Because the beliefs about "baseline" cervical lengths vary widely among physicians, the use of centimeters provides more uniformity.[47] Even when a consistent definition is used, interexaminer differences vary by 20% to 30%.[48] If the external os allows passage of a finger, then this length can be palpated directly. If the external os is closed, the length of the cervix must be estimated through palpation alongside the cervix into the lateral fornix. These estimates are limited because only a variable portion of the cervix lies distal to the vaginal fornix. This explains the poor correlation seen between digital estimations of effacement and ultrasound measurements of length.[48]

What are the implications of testing?

Although the results of digital examination of the cervix can be related to the risk of preterm birth,[50–52] a prospective randomized trial of such examinations failed to show any effect on the rate of preterm delivery.[53] This may reflect the poor reproducibility of the examination,[48] or because examiners were focused more on dilation than on effacement, consistency (soft vs. firm) and station. These later features are actually more strongly correlated with the risk of premature delivery than is dilation.[54] When logistic regression was applied, manual examination of the cervix to create a Bishop score was almost as predictive as endovaginal sonography for the prediction of PTD (see Table 33–1).[34]

What does an abnormal test result mean? Although an effaced or soft cervix can suggest an increased risk of PTD in asymptomatic women, there have been no interventions shown to decrease the risk of preterm birth in such women.[53] The discovery of a significantly dilated or effaced (3 cm or more and/or 100% effacement) cervix in a woman remote from term has been treated with an "emergent" cerclage. Studies of this technique have included relatively few patients and reports of effectiveness vary widely.[55,56] Contraindications include active labor or cervical change, bleeding, rupture of the membranes, evidence of chorioamnionitis, or fetal anomalies. Extensive counseling is required. The woman should be made aware that the effect of cerclage on a pregnancy that would otherwise be lost, might be only to prolong it long enough so the infant survives but suffers major morbidities. The indications and technique of emergent cervical cerclage are beyond the scope of this chapter.

What does a normal test result mean? A long, firm, and closed cervix provides some reassurance for the pregnant woman who wishes to travel in late pregnancy. The clinician should remember, however, that effacement begins at the internal os and is best detected on digital examination by softness and thinning of the lower uterine segment, not dilation.

What is the cost of testing?

The cost of digital examination derives primarily from the time spent by the physician or nurse–midwife interaction.

What is the nature of the test?
Transvaginal ultrasound measurement of cervical length. The cervix can be imaged with ultrasound through a transabdominal, translabial, or transvaginal approach. A full maternal bladder is required for adequate transabdominal visualization, but will also compresses the cervix, resulting in poorly reproducible measurements.[57] Endovaginal sonography is performed with an empty bladder and provides clear images of the cervix without compression of the cervix. A translabial approach is almost as good in patients for whom the placement of a transvaginal probe may pose risk (e.g., PPROM or placenta previa), although some authors believe it is not necessary.[58]

Transvaginal ultrasound is the most accurate and reliable modality. The probe is placed in the anterior fornix and sagittal views are measured, as in Figure 33–1. Applying pressure against the cervix with the probe may enhance cervical visualization, but care must be taken to avoid compression. Thus, the goal is to apply the least amount of pressure on the probe while still visualizing the entire cervical canal. Excessive pressure is likely when the anterior–posterior

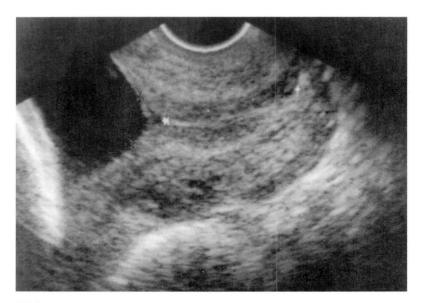

Figure 33-1   Cervical length measurement—normal.

dimension of the anterior lip of the cervix is smaller then that of the posterior lip, as in Figure 33–2. Once an adequate view has been obtained, the length of the canal is measured from the internal to the external os. Multiple separate recordings should be obtained, and the "shortest best" measurement used.[59] At the conclusion of the study, fundal or suprapubic pressure can be applied to look for funneling of the cervix.

What are the implications of testing?

What does an abnormal test result mean? As cervical function is increasingly understood as a relative rather than absolute measurement,[59] the definition of "abnormal" cervical length has become a threshold that varies with the clinical circumstances. Cervical length in mid pregnancy is normally distributed and is associated with the risk of preterm birth Figure 33–3.[59] In a study of 2,915 women whose cervical length was measured at 22 to 24 weeks' gestation, the median length was 35 mm, with 30 mm representing the 25th percentile, 26 mm the tenth percentile, 20 mm the fifth percentile, and 13 mm the first percentile. The relative risk of spontaneous PTD before 35 weeks' gestation at the tenth percentile was sixfold higher than the risk for the reference population, whose cervical length was above the 75th percentile.[59] The actual risk of PTD before 35 weeks for women with a cervical length at or below the tenth percentile is about 18% in a general obstetric population,[59] and 37% in a high-risk population.[34] Thus, a cervical length of 25 mm in asymptomatic women at 22 to 24 weeks' gestation has been used as a threshold in clinical practice[60] and in research studies.[23–25,61]

The appropriate management of asymptomatic, low-risk women who are discovered to have a short cervix is unclear. The sensitivity and positive

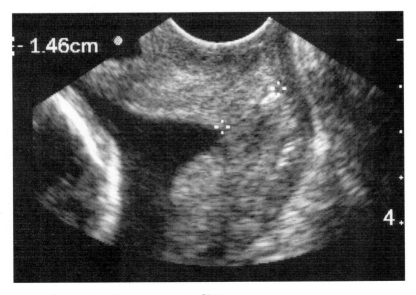

Figure 33-2 Cervical length measurement—Short.

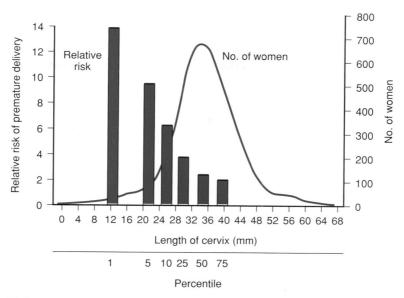

Figure 33-3 Distribution of subjects among percentiles for cervical length measured by transvaginal ultrasonography at 24 weeks of gestation (*solid line*) and relative risk of spontaneous preterm delivery before 35 weeks of gestation according to percentiles for cervical length (*bars*). The risks among women with values at or below the first, fifth, tenth, 25th, 50th, and 75th percentiles for cervical length are compared with the risk among women with values above the 75th percentile.

predictive value of this test in a general obstetric population are both low.[62] Widespread screening of such women will place them at risk for potentially morbid interventions such as cervical cerclage, or long term tocolysis or bed rest, neither of which have demonstrable benefits. Thus, the American College of Obstetricians and Gynecologists does not recommend transvaginal ultrasound for surveillance in normal pregnancy.[26,60]

Endovaginal sonographic measurement of cervical length in women with risk factors for preterm birth, such as prior PTD or multifetal gestation, has been studied extensively as a test to quantify risk of PTD and to choose appropriate candidates for cervical cerclage. The risk of preterm birth rises as cervical length in mid pregnancy declines in women with a prior preterm birth and in women with multifetal pregnancies. To date, the primary value of these findings has been to reassure at-risk women who have a long cervix that their risk is less than expected, and thereby to avoid unnecessary interventions. Successful interventions to decrease the risk of PTD for women with clinical risk factors who have a short cervix have not been identified. Studies of cerclage have been mixed but the largest randomized trial concluded cerclage was of no benefit of cerclage in this cohort.[23-25,63 64] There are no studies of interventions such as progesterone supplementation conducted in women with a short cervix. The predictive value of cervical funneling has varied in large studies[59,65] and is not considered as reliable as the residual length itself.

What does a normal test result mean? The risk of PTD decreases with increasing cervical length.[59] A normal test result can be helpful in women with symptoms of possible preterm labor to exclude that diagnosis when cervical length is more than 30 mm (the 25th percentile)[66,67] and in women with twins to avoid restriction of physical activity when the cervical length is more than 35 mm (the 50th percentile).[68]

What is the cost of testing?

In addition to basic ultrasound equipment, the cost of transvaginal ultrasound probes is usually thousands of dollars. Physician fees will vary. A technology such as transvaginal ultrasound is likely to be cost-effective only when practitioners use it to avoid unnecessary, expensive interventions.

■ Conclusions and Recommendations

A screening test for preterm labor/delivery with adequate sensitivity and specificity and for which there is a suitable intervention should the test be positive does not yet exist. Screening for asymptomatic bacterial vaginosis in low risk women has no impact on the rate of PTD[12] and its role in high-risk women is uncertain. We do not screen for bacterial vaginosis in our high-risk patients, but do treat women with symptoms.

The primary utility of fFN is in the triage of patients presenting with acute preterm labor symptoms, where a negative test result can avoid unnecessary interventions. Because the appropriate management of an asymptomatic or low risk patient with a positive fFN is unclear, its use as a general screening test outside of experimental trials is discouraged.

Manual examination of the cervix is often unable to detect subtle, early changes in the internal os, and thus lacks adequate sensitivity. When gross cervical effacement or dilation is detected on manual examination, it is often too late for interventions other than emergency cerclage, which is of uncertain value. Earlier, subtler changes in the internal os can be detected through endovaginal sonography, but the appropriate intervention is again not clear.

While transvaginal cervical length measurements should not be used as a universal screening tool for preterm birth, it may provide useful information in two scenarios. In the first, among women with a prior preterm birth, a normal cervical length between 22 and 24 weeks' gestation would offer reassurance they are unlikely to have a recurrence. In the second, women who present to the labor suite with symptoms of preterm labor but no definitive evidence of cervical change can also be reassured that they are not in labor if their cervical length is normal.

Finally, a history of preterm delivery is a historical test that identifies women who may benefit from supplemental progesterone.[27,28] The value of progesterone supplementation in other populations has not yet been determined.

■ Summary

1 ■ What Is the Problem that Requires Screening?

Preterm birth.

a. What is the incidence/prevalence of the target condition?

Three percent to 12 % of all births are preterm, with large social and geographic variation.

b. What are the sequelae of the condition that are of interest in clinical medicine?

Infants delivered preterm account for a disproportionate percentage of neonatal morbidity and mortality. Surviving preterm infants, especially those born before 32 weeks or those weighing less than 1,500 g, suffer the high rates of intraventricular hemorrhage, chronic lung disease (i.e., bronchopulmonary dysplasia), necrotizing enterocolitis, and retinopathy of prematurity, among other illnesses.

2 ■ The Tests

a. What is the purpose of the tests?

To identify women at high risk of delivering preterm.

b. What is the nature of the tests?

Measurement of fetal fibronectin from the cervix, manual, or transvaginal examination of the maternal cervix.

c. What are the implications of testing?

1. What does an abnormal test result mean?

   A fetal fibronectin between 22 and 24 weeks' gestation has a PPV of 35% for preterm birth. The corresponding figure for a transvaginal measurement of cervical length of 25 mm is 37%. Thus, a woman with either a positive fetal fibronectin or a sonographically short cervix between 22 and 24 weeks'

Continued

> ■ **Summary—cont'd**
>
> gestation has a likelihood of preterm birth similar to a woman who has experienced a prior preterm birth preceded by preterm premature rupture of the membranes.
>
> 2. What does a normal test result mean?
> A fetal fibronectin between 22 and 24 weeks' gestation has a negative predictive value of 89% for preterm birth. The corresponding figure for a transvaginal measurement of cervical length more than 25 mm is 93%. Thus, a woman with normal values is unlikely to deliver preterm.
>
> d. *What is the cost of testing?*
> Measurement of fFN or transvaginal cervical length is likely to be cost-effective only when practitioners use them to avoid unnecessary, expensive interventions.
>
> 3 ■ **Conclusions and Recommendations**
>
> A screening test for preterm labor/delivery with adequate sensitivity and specificity and for which there is a suitable intervention should the test be positive does not yet exist.

References

1. Moore TR, Iams JD, Creasy RK, et al. Diurnal and gestational patterns of uterine activity in normal human pregnancy. *Obstet Gynecol* 1994;83:517–523.
2. Martin JA, Hamilton BE, Sutton PD, et al. Births: final data for 2002. *National Vital Statistics Reports* 2002;52:16.
3. Bergh T, Ericson A, Hillensjo T, et al. Deliveries and children born after in-vitro fertilization in Sweden 1982-95: a retrospective cohort study. *Lancet* 1999;354:1579–1585.
4. El-Metwally D, Vohr B, Tucker R. Survival and neonatal morbidity at the limits of viability in the mid 1990's: 22 to 25 weeks. *Pediatrics* 2000;137:616–622.
5. Wood NS, Marlow N, Costeloe K, et al. Neurologic and developmental disability after extremely preterm birth. *N Engl J Med* 2000;343:378–384.
6. Hack M, Flannery DJ, Schluchter M, et al. Outcomes in young adulthood for very-low-birth-weight infants. *N Engl J Med* 2002;346:149–157.
7. Iams, JD, Goldenberg RI, Mercer BM, et al. Preterm Prediction Study: recurrence risk of spontaneous preterm birth. *Am J Obstet Gynecol* 1998;178:1035–1040.
8. Adams MM, Elam-Evans LD, Wilson HG, et al. Rates of and factors associated with recurrence of preterm delivery. *JAMA* 2000;283:1591–1596.
9. Mercer BM, Goldenberg RI, Das A, et al. The preterm prediction study: a clinical risk assessment system. *Am J Obstet Gynecol* 1996;174:1885–1893.
10. Goldenberg RL, Mercer BM, Meis PJ, et al. The preterm prediction study: fetal fibronectin testing and spontaneous preterm birth. *Obstet Gynecol* 1996;87:643–648.

11. Hauth JC, Goldenberg RL, Andrews WW, et al. Reduced incidence of preterm delivery with metronidazole and erythromycin in women with bacterial vaginosis. *N Engl J Med* 1995;333:1732–1736.

12. Carey JC, Klebanoff MA, Hauth JC, et al. Metronidazole to prevent preterm delivery in pregnant women with asymptomatic bacterial vaginosis. *N Engl J Med* 2000;342:534–540.

13. Klebanoff MA, Carey JC, Hauth JC, et al. Failure of metronidazole to prevent preterm delivery among pregnant women with asymptomatic *Trichomonas vaginalis* infection. *N Engl J Med* 2001;345:487–493.

14. Collaborative Home Uterine Monitoring Study (CHUMS) Group. A multicenter randomized controlled trial of home uterine monitoring: active versus sham device. *Am J Obstet Gynecol* 1995;173:1120–1127.

15. Dyson DC, Danbe KH, Bamber JA, et al. Monitoring woman at risk for preterm labor. *N Engl J Med* 1998;338:15–19.

16. Goldenberg RL, Cliver SP, Bronstein J, et al. Bed rest in pregnancy. *Obstet Gynecol* 1994; 84:131–136.

17. Pircon RA, Strassner HT, Kirz DS, et al. Controlled trial of hydration and bed rest versus bed rest alone in the evaluation of preterm uterine contractions. *Am J Obstet Gynecol* 1989;161:775–779.

18. Guinn DA, Goepfert AR, Owen J, et al. Management options in women with preterm uterine contractions: a randomized clinical trial. *Am J Obstet Gynecol* 1997;177:814–818.

19. Higby K, Xenakis EM, Pauerstein CJ. Do tocolytic agents stop preterm labor? A critical and comprehensive review of efficacy and safety. *Am J Obstet Gynecol* 1993;168:1247–1259.

20. Macones GA, Berlin M, Berlin JA. Efficacy of oral beta-agonist maintenance therapy in preterm labor: a meta-analysis. *Obstet Gynecol* 1995;85:313–317.

21. Ramsey PS, Rouse DJ. Magnesium sulfate as a tocolytic agent. *Semin Perinatol* 2001;25:236–247.

22. Collaborative Group on Preterm Birth Prevention. Multicenter randomized controlled trial of a preterm birth prevention program. *Am J Obstet Gynecol* 1993;169:352–365.

23. Rust OA, Atlas RO, Jones KJ, et al. A randomized trial of cerclage versus no cerclage among patients with ultrasonographically detected second trimester preterm dilation of the internal os. *Am J Obstet Gynecol* 2000;183:830–835.

24. Althuisius SM, Dekker GA, Hummel P, et al. Final results of the Cervical Incompetence Prevention Randomized Cerclage Trial (CIPRACT): therapeutic cerclage with bed rest versus bed rest alone. *Am J Obstet Gynecol* 2001;185:1106–1112.

25. To MS, Alfirevic Z, Heath VC, et al. Cervical cerclage for prevention of preterm delivery in women with short cervix: randomized controlled trial. *Lancet* 2004;363:1849–853.

26. ACOG. Assessment of risk factors for preterm birth. *Obstet Gynecol* 2001;98:709–716.

27. Meis PJ, Klebanoff M, Thom E, et al. for the NICHD MFMU Network. Prevention of recurrent preterm birth by 17 alpha-hydroxyprogesterone caproate. *N Engl J Med* 2003;348:2379–2385

28. da Fonseca EB, Bittar RE, Carvalho MHB, et al. Prophylactic administration of progesterone by vaginal suppository to reduce the incidence of spontaneous preterm birth in women at increased risk: a randomized placebo-controlled double-blinded study. *Am J Obstet Gynecol* 2003;188:419–424.

29. Lockwood CJ, Senyei AE, Dische R, et al. Fetal Fibronectin in cervical and vaginal secretions as a predictor of preterm delivery. *N Engl J Med* 1991;325:669–674.

30. Matsuura H, Hakomori S. The oncofetal domain of fibronectin defined by monoclonal antibody FDC-6: its presence in fibronectins from fetal and tumor tissues and its absence from normal adult tissues and plasma. *Proc Natl Acad Sci U S A* 1985;82:6517–6521.

31. McKenna DS, Chung K, Iams JD. Effect of digital examination on the expression of fetal fibronectin. *J Repro Med* 1999;44:796–800.

32. Roman AS, Rebarber AR, Sfakianaki AK, et al. Vaginal fetal fibronectin as a predictor of spontaneous preterm delivery in the patient with cervical cerclage. *Am J Obstet Gynecol* 2003;189:1368–1372.

33. Leitich H, Kaider A. Fetal fibronectin-how useful is it in the prediction of preterm birth? *Br J Obstet Gynaecol* 2003;110[Supp]:66–70.

34. Iams JD, Newman RB, Thom EA, et al for the NICHD MFMU Network. Frequency of uterine contractions and the risk of spontaneous preterm delivery. *N Engl J Med* 2002;346:250–255.
35. Goldenberg RL, Thom E, Moawad AH, et al. The preterm prediction study: fetal fibronectin, bacterial vaginosis, and peripartum infection. *Obstet Gynecol* 1996;87:656-60.
36. Andrews WW, Sibai BM, Thom EA, et al. for the NICHD MFMU Network. Randomized clinical trial of metronidazole plus erythromycin to prevent spontaneous preterm delivery in fetal fibronectin-positive women. *Obstet Gynecol* 2003;101:847–855.
37. Iams JD, Casal D, McGregor JA, et al. Fetal fibronectin improves the accuracy of diagnosis of preterm labor. *Am J Obstet Gynecol* 1995;173:141–145.
38. Peaceman AM, Andrews WW, Thorp JM, et al. Fetal fibronectin as a predictor of preterm birth in patients with symptoms: a multicenter trial. *Am J Obstet Gynecol* 1997;177:13–18.
39. Joffe GM, Jacques D, Bemis-Heys R, et al. Impact of the fetal fibronectin assay on admissions for preterm labor. *Am J Obstet Gynecol* 1999;180:581–586.
40. Giles W, Bisits A, Knox M, et al. The effect of fetal fibronectin testing on admissions to a tertiary maternal-fetal medicine unit and cost savings. *Am J Obstet Gynecol* 2000;182:439–442.
41. Grobman WA, Welshman EE, Calhoun EA. Does fetal fibronectin use in the diagnosis of preterm labor affect physician behavior and health care costs? *Am J Obstet Gynecol* 2004;191:235–240.
42. Bishop EH. Pelvic scoring for elective induction. *Obstet Gynecol* 1964;24:266–268.
43. Neilson JP, Verkuyl DA, Crowther CA, et al. Preterm labor in twin pregnancies: prediction by cervical assessment. *Obstet Gynecol* 1988;72:719–723.
44. Newman RB, Godsey RK, Ellings JM, et al. Quantification of cervical change: relationship to preterm delivery in the multifetal gestation. *Am J Obstet Gynecol* 1991;165:264–269.
45. Truffnell DJ, Johnson N, Bryce F, et al. Simulation of cervical changes in labour: reproducibility of expert assessment. *Lancet* 1989;2:1089–1090.
46. Phelps JY, Higby K, Smyth MH, et al. Accuracy and intraobserver variability of stimulated cervical dilation measurements. *Am J Obstet Gynecol* 1995;173:942–945.
47. Holcomb WL, Smeltzer JS. Cervical effacement: variation in belief among clinicians. *Obstet Gynecol* 1991;78:43–45.
48. Stubbs TM, Van Dorsten P, Miller MC. The preterm cervix and preterm labor: relative risks, predictive values and change over time. *Am J Obstet Gynecol* 1986;155:829–834.
49. Sonek JD, Iams JD, Blumenfeld M, et al. Measurement of cervical length in pregnancy: comparison between vaginal ultrasonography and digital examination. *Obstet Gynecol* 1990;76:172–175.
50. Bouyer J, Papiernik E, Dreyfus J, et al. Maturation signs of the cervix and prediction of preterm birth. *Obstet Gynecol* 1986;68:209–214.
51. Papiernik E, Bouyer J, Collin D, et al. Precocious cervical ripening and preterm labor. *Obstet Gynecol* 1989;67:238–242.
52. Blondel B, le Coutour X, Kaminski M, et al. Prediction of preterm delivery: is it substantially improved by routine vaginal examinations? *Am J Obstet Gynecol* 1989;162:1042–1048.
53. Buekens P, Alexander S, Boutsen M, et al. Randomized controlled trial of routine cervical examinations in pregnancy. European Community Collaborative Study Group on Prenatal Screening. *Lancet* 1994;344:841–844.
54. Copper RL, Goldenberg RL, Davis RO, et al. Warning symptoms, uterine contractions, and cervical examination findings in women at risk of preterm delivery. *Am J Obstet Gynecol.* 1990;162:748–754.
55. Aarts JM, Brons JTJ, Bruinse HW. Emergency cerclage: a review. *Obstet Gynecol Surv* 1995;50:459-469.
56. Olatunbosun OA, al-Nuaim L, Turnell RW. Emergency cerclage compared with bedrest for advanced cervical dilation during pregnancy. *Int Surg* 1995;80:170–174.
57. Mason GC, Maresh MJ. Alterations in bladder volume and the ultrasound appearance of the cervix. *Br J Obstet Gynaecol* 1990;97:457–458.
58. Carlan SJ, Richmond LB, O'Brien WF. Randomized trial of endovaginal ultrasound in preterm premature rupture of the membranes. *Obstet Gynecol* 1997;89:458–461.

59. Iams JD, Goldenberg RL, Meis PJ, et al. and the NICHD MFMU Network. The length of the cervix and the risk of spontaneous premature delivery. *N Engl J Med* 1996;334:567–572.
60. ACOG2003 Practice Bulletin No. 48. Cervical Insufficiency.
61. Owen J, Iams JD, Hauth JC. Vaginal sonography and cervical incompetence. *Am J Obstet Gynecol* 2003;188:586–596.
62. Iams JD, Goldenberg RL, Mercer BM, et al. The Preterm Prediction Study: Can low-risk women destined for spontaneous preterm birth be identified? *Am J Obstet Gynecol* 2001;184: 652–655.
63. To MS, Alfirevic Z, Heath VC, et al. Fetal Medicine Foundation Second Trimester Screening Group. Cervical cerclage for prevention of preterm delivery in women with short cervix: randomised controlled trial. *Lancet* 2004;363:1849–1853.
64. Drakeley A, Roberts D, Alfirevic Z. Cervical cerclage for prevention of preterm delivery: meta-analysis of randomized trials. *Am J Obstet Gynecol* 2003;102:621–627.
65. Owen J, Yost N, Berghella V, et al. Mid-trimester endovaginal sonography in women at high risk for spontaneous preterm birth. *JAMA* 2001;286:1340–1348.
66. Iams JD, Paraskos J, Landon MB, et al. Cervical sonography in preterm labor. *Obstet Gynecol* 1994;84:40–46.
67. Gomez R, Galasso M, Romero R, et al. Ultrasonographic examination of the uterine cervix is better then cervical digital examination as a predictor of the likelihood of premature delivery in patients with preterm labor and intact membranes. *Am J Obstet Gynecol* 1994;171:956–964.
68. Imseis HM, Albert TA, Iams JD. Identifying twin gestations at low risk for preterm birth with a transvaginal ultrasonographic cervical measurement at 24 to 26 weeks' gestation. *Am J Obstet Gynecol* 1997;177:1149–1155.

Preeclampsia: Blood Pressure, Weight Gain, and Edema

Peter von Dadelszen

Thomas R. Easterling

■ What Is the Problem that Requires Screening?

The preeclampsia–eclampsia syndrome.

What is the incidence/prevalence of the target condition?

Preeclampsia complicates 2% to 5% of pregnancies and is most common in nulliparous women and women with underlying vascular or renal diseases.

What are the sequelae of the condition that are of interest in clinical medicine?

Preeclampsia is a multisystem disease whose etiology remains unclear and whose only definitive treatment is delivery. Preeclampsia remains one of the two most common causes of maternal death in the developed world.[1,2] It is the most common cause of iatrogenic preterm birth. In the United States, preeclampsia results annually in 1,200 infant deaths and costs more than $7.5 billion, of which $4.11 billion is for infant illness and $0.41 billion for ongoing pediatric sequelae.[3,4]

Preeclampsia has both maternal and fetal manifestations; however, it is usually defined by its clinical manifestations: hypertension (blood pressure [BP] >140/90 mm Hg) and proteinuria (>0.3 g per 24 hours or dipstick criteria [2+], used most often clinically) that appear at more than 20 weeks' gestation and regress after pregnancy. The *maternal syndrome* of preeclampsia is more complex than hypertension alone.[5] Preeclampsia is believed associated with abnormal placentation characterized by incomplete invasion of maternal spiral arterioles by fetal cytotrophoblast.[6] Human placentation is unique in that the cytotrophoblast invades the spiral arterioles and replaces maternal endothelium resulting in local vasodilation and increased maternal blood flow into the intervillous space. The price paid for increased perfusion is the exposure of circulating maternal immune elements to foreign, fetal tissue (Figure 34–1).

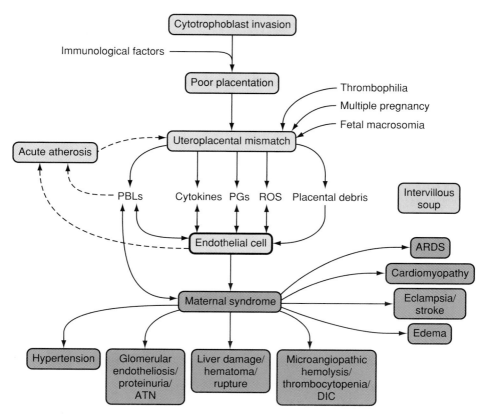

Figure 34-1 The pathogenesis of preeclampsia.
In this model of preeclampsia, the maternal syndrome develops from a number of alternative pathways leading to uteroplacental mismatch, whereby the fetoplacental demands outstrip the maternal circulatory supply. In response to the mismatch, and probably due in part to recurrent ischemia–reperfusion injury within the intervillous (maternal blood) space of the placenta and accelerated placental apoptosis, a "soup" of endothelium-damaging substrates is released with resulting endothelial cell activation and consequent development of the maternal syndrome of preeclampsia. Some elements of the soup, namely activated peripheral blood leukocytes, can cause direct end-organ damage. There is cross-talk between elements of the soup (not illustrated) (modified from von Dadelszen P, Magee LA, Lee SK, et al. Activated protein C in normal human pregnancy and pregnancies complicated by severe preeclampsia: a therapeutic opportunity? *Crit Care Med* 2002;30:1883–1892). *ARDS,* acute respiratory distress syndrome; *ATN,* acute tubular necrosis; *DIC,* disseminated intravascular coagulation; *PBLs,* peripheral blood leukocytes; *PGs,* eicosanoids; *ROS,* reactive oxygen species.

Injury and/or activation of endothelialized cytotrophoblast may initiate a maternal immune response to foreign fetal tissue and the exportation of activated maternal leukocytes, humoral agents, or cellular debris into the maternal circulation. The impact of these factors on a vulnerable maternal endothelial environment is believed to result in the end-organ manifestations of preeclampsia. Many of these physiologic changes begin weeks to months before the clinical manifestations of preeclampsia. Therefore, assessing clinical markers of these physiological changes may provide an opportunity to predict women who will develop preeclampsia.

■ The Tests

The prediction of preeclampsia is largely guided by clinical impression rather than evidence-based criteria determined by pregnancy outcome. Ideally, the development of a disease prediction model for preeclampsia will be predicated on the prospective development of a complete database of women at risk of the condition (by historical criteria), some of who will develop preeclampsia in the index pregnancy. Pregnancy is associated with changes in tests of coagulation,[7] placental hormones and factors,[8] host response to infectious agents,[9] and cardiovascular adaptations[10] compared with the normal ranges established among nonpregnant men and women. Often, abnormalities are defined by results that lie outside the normal range for nonpregnant individuals. However, it is possible that quantitative variations of cardiovascular or other parameters, either singly or together, may be important in determining preeclampsia risk. This is consistent with the notion that normal ranges for various factors are based on the mean and standard deviation (SD) of values obtained from healthy or unhealthy nonpregnant individuals. "Abnormality" is present only in a statistical sense and says nothing about its relationship with associated adverse outcomes or which point treatment does more good than harm.[11] For example, computer models of soluble factors have been generated[12] in an attempt to measure the "thrombi-generation potential" of a patient's blood. Unfortunately, these have not been proven to predict thrombotic risk in humans.

Blood pressure.

BP will be discussed as a discrete entity and by examination of its components, cardiac output and peripheral vascular resistance.

What is the purpose of the tests?

To identify women at increased risk of developing preeclampsia.

What is the nature of the tests?

BP measurement is a core component of antenatal assessment for all pregnancies. Hypertension in pregnancy is defined by peaks in BP: two measurements 6 hours apart, taken in a semirecumbent position. Korotkoff phase V is used to designate diastolic BP (dBP).[13] It is essential an appropriate-sized blood pressure cuff be used, as a small cuff will overestimate the blood pressure in obese women. Although there are no guidelines, the serial measurement of BP in pregnancy is prudent, as it would address much of the inaccuracy of office BP measurement.

As in the nonpregnant patient, up to 25% of patients with mild office hypertension (i.e., dBP of 90–104 mm Hg) have repeated normal BP measurements at home.[14] Two prospective studies concluded that only 43% to 65% of pregnant women with clinic BP above 140/90 mm Hg remain hypertensive upon serial measurements in obstetric day units.[15,16] More important,, women with sustained elevation of BP have more severe hypertension and more frequent perinatal complications, such as small-for-gestational age (SGA) infants. Assessing white coat hypertension improves specificity in terms of screening for preeclampsia, but at risk of reducing sensitivity. The recognition of white-coat hypertension focused attention on the use of ambulatory BP monitoring in pregnancy. Compared with office measurements, 24-hour and daytime ambulatory BP values more closely relate to abnormal pregnancy outcomes (severe hypertension, preterm delivery, cesarean delivery, SGA infants, and admission to neonatal intensive care,[15–17] just as they are to adverse cardiovascular outcomes outside of pregnancy.[18–21]

Second-trimester blood pressure. Second-trimester BP measurement has been assessed for its ability to predict preeclampsia, in response to the recognition that women destined to develop preeclampsia often do not have the normal midtrimester fall in their BP.[22] Both mean arterial pressure (MAP; dBP + [pulse pressure/3]) and systolic BP (sBP) have been assessed.

Devices available for ambulatory monitoring. Out-of-office BP measurements can be made by either 24-hour ambulatory or home devices. Each approach has advantages and disadvantages. Twenty-four–hour ambulatory devices provide information about daytime and nighttime BP values, but such studies are costly to perform, inconvenient for women, and not widely available. On the other hand, there are few home BP devices that meet the standards for reliability and accuracy.[23] Many devices become less accurate over time, and women must be trained by a qualified health care professional. Even then, there may be biased self-reporting of BP values.[24]

An important consideration in pregnancy is that only a few 24-hour ambulatory (e.g., Spacelabs 90207; Hawthorne, CA) and home BP (e.g., Omron 705C; Shaumburg, IL) monitoring devices meet published criteria for reliability in pregnancy. Only one (an inflationary oscillometric device) has done so for preeclampsia, for which deflationary oscillometric devices repeatedly underestimated BP.[25] There are no randomized controlled trials (RCTs) to support the use of ambulatory or home BP monitoring during pregnancy. The American guidelines make no recommendations about ambulatory monitoring.[26] The current Canadian pregnancy hypertension guidelines also make no specific recommendations about the use of ambulatory or home BP monitoring, although they acknowledge that home BP measurement is practiced in some Canadian centers.[27] The Australasia pregnancy hypertension guidelines state that automated devices and ambulatory BP are not ready for routine use.[13]

What are the implications of testing?

What does an abnormal test result mean? The sensitivity of second-trimester MAP in identifying women at increased risk of preeclampsia varies with the threshold of blood pressure used. In general, a second-trimester MAP above 85 mm Hg has a 48% sensitivity for identifying women at risk of preeclampsia; unfortunately, the positive predictive value (PPV) is only 5%.[22] A midtrimester sBP of 120 to 134 mm Hg has a sensitivity of 18% and a PPV of 13% for identifying women at risk of preeclampsia.[22]

What does a normal test result mean? The specificity of second-trimester MAP in identifying women at increased risk of preeclampsia varies with the threshold used. In general, a second-trimester MAP below 85 mm Hg has an 80% specificity for the identification of women not at risk of preeclampsia, and a negative predictive value (NPV) of 99%.[22] Midtrimester sBP of below 120 mm Hg has a specificity of 91% and an NPV of 93% for identifying women not at risk of preeclampsia.[22]

Third-trimester blood pressure. More significant elevations of blood pressure in the third trimester do seem to predict the development of preeclampsia. In a cohort of 748 women who developed gestational hypertension (BP = 140/90 mm Hg) between 24 and 35 weeks' gestation, Barton et al.[28] observed that 46% subsequently developed preeclampsia and 9.6% developed severe preeclampsia. About one half with gestational hypertension before 32 weeks' gestation developed preeclampsia. Of importance, the prevalences of low birth weight, very low birth weight, and thrombocytopenia was increased among those who progressed to preeclampsia.[28] These findings are identical to an international cohort study of 305 women presenting with mild nonproteinuric hypertension before 34 weeks' gestation.[29] The development of proteinuria was associated with an earlier gestational age at delivery, lower birth weight, and an increased incidence of small-for-gestational age newborns.[29]

What does an abnormal test result mean? The development of hypertension remote from term in the third trimester identifies a cohort of women at significant risk. Potential interventions include more frequent maternal and fetal surveillance or treatment of maternal hypertension, while balancing concerns for the maternal condition and fetal growth. The efficacy of these interventions is not established, leaving the clinician to make reasonable choices based on individual patients and available data.

What does a normal test result mean? The relevant studies do not report on the outcomes of the "screen-negative" group, those women who failed to develop gestational hypertension. Therefore, we cannot make conclusions regarding the negative predictive value of the test.

Cardiac output.

What is the purpose of the tests?

To identify women at increased risk of developing preeclampsia. Easterling et al.[30,31] report that the manipulation of maternal hemodynamics using atenolol, furosemide, and hydralazine in women deemed at high risk reduces the prevalence of preeclampsia from 18% to 3.8%). This reduced prevalence may have been at the expense of lower fetal growth, consistent with current meta-analyses and meta-regression analyses that included RCTs in which atenolol was used.[32-34] Treatment of hypertension modestly reduced fetal growth, 185 g per 10 mm Hg reduction in MAP.[33,34] The observed growth reduction was associated with atenolol only and was unrelated to the timing of initiation. Magee et al.[32] confirmed the reduction in prevalence of severe maternal hypertension and proteinuria, but there was no change in gestational age at delivery. Easterling et al.[30,31] concluded that an excessive reduction in cardiac output lead to decreased fetal growth. The balance between maternal and perinatal risks will remain unclear at least until the completion of the CHIPS (Control of Hypertension In Pregnancy Study) trial, for which recruitment is complete.

What is the nature of the tests?

Cardiac output (CO) is measured by Doppler technique.[10,30] The aortic diameter is measured using A-mode ultrasound and a cross-sectional area (CSA) calculated. A time–velocity curve is generated by insonating the ascending aorta from the suprasternal notch using continuous-wave Doppler. The integral of the time–velocity curve is the distance the blood has traveled during systole. The product of the time–velocity curve integral and the CSA is the stroke volume (SV). SV times heart rate (HR) gives CO.

The first, prospective study of 179 nulliparous women examined at 22 to 25 weeks' gestation.[6] The prevalence of preeclampsia in this cohort was 5.0%. The CO of women who developed preeclampsia was higher than those who did not develop preeclampsia over the course of pregnancy. These results were confirmed in a larger study by Bosio et al.[35] Based on these studies, the threshold of abnormality for maternal CO is above 7.4 L per minute before 24 weeks' gestation 1.0 SD above the mean for gestational age).

In a prospective study conducted within the framework of a RCT of 511 nulliparous women, 4.3% developed preeclampsia.[30] Maternal CO above 7.4 L per minute (+1.0 SD) again predicted later preeclampsia.

What are the implications of testing?

What does an abnormal test result mean? Women with a CO above 7.4 L per minute have an increased risk of developing preeclampsia (52% sensitivity, PPV 16%).[30]

What does a normal test result mean? Women with a normal CO have a low risk of developing preeclampsia (75% specificity, negative predictive value (NPV) 95%).[30]

Peripheral vascular resistance.

What is the purpose of the tests?

To identify women at increased risk of developing preeclampsia.

What is the nature of the tests?

Total peripheral resistance (TPR), which is calculated from the MAP and maternal CO, where TPR is equal to 80 times MAP/CO.

What are the implications of testing?

What does an abnormal test result mean? Taylor[36] concluded that the onset of preeclampsia was associated with a full, but constricted vascular bed. The change from a hyperdynamic state to one of increased TPR was coincident with the onset of clinical symptoms preeclampsia in most cases. However, others found that an increased TPR was a late finding of preeclampsa.[30,35,37] Once hypertension occurs remote from term, high TPR predicts both an earlier gestational age at delivery and lower birthweight percentile.[37] In women with hypertension at 28 weeks, TPR above 1,150 dynes/sec/cm^{-5} is associated with a birthweight percentile of 18.7% ± 19.9%.

What does a normal test result mean? A normal TPR (<1,150) increases the likelihood of a normal outcome and is associated with a higher birthweight percentile of 38.8% ± 32.3% compared with women with a high TPR ($p = 0.003$). An abrupt change in TPR, a so-called crossover, is associated with a high (37.5%) perinatal mortality rate compared with those who did not cross over (7.9%, $p = 0.01$).[37]

Weight gain.

Weight gain is a part of the standard assessment of pregnancy health. It is determined by the prepregnancy weight, caloric balance in pregnancy, and accumulation of intravascular and extravascular water. The measurement is variously described in pounds or kilograms over the whole of pregnancy or within defined epochs.

What is the purpose of the tests?

To identify women at increased risk of developing preeclampsia.

What is the nature of the tests?

The measurement of maternal weight is part of routine prenatal care and preeclampsia is more frequent in obese women.[36,38,39]

What are the implications of testing?

What does an abnormal test result mean?

Excessive weight gain: Excessive weight gain is associated with edema and hypertension,[38] but not necessarily the full spectrum of preeclampsia.[38] Maternal prepregnancy obesity is a more powerful predictor of later preeclampsia than is excessive weight gain during pregnancy.[38] Rhodes[40] examined the weight gain patterns (12–20 weeks' gestation) of women who developed eclampsia ($n = 29$), mild preeclampsia ($n = 46$), moderate preeclampsia ($n = 42$), severe preeclampsia ($n = 25$), and normal pregnancy ($n = 50$). Women who developed eclampsia were more likely at normal weight prepregnancy, but had no net gain. Women who developed mild or moderate preeclampsia were heavier prepregnancy, but had either no net gain or 10-lb (4.5-kg) gain, respectively. Those women destined to develop severe preeclampsia were of normal prepregnancy weight but gained 3 lb (1.4 kg). Women with a normal pregnancy gained 10 lb (4.5 kg).

Excessive weight gain is variably described in the published series. Taylor[41] observed that maternal weight of more than 2.5 lb/inch height occurred in 84% of women with normal pregnancy and 16% of women with preeclampsia. From these data, he derived a "toxemia chart"' using an upper weight gain limit and concluded that weight gain crossing the line identified those who were more likely to develop preeclampsia.

While weight gain above the 90th percentile is more often associated with pregnancy hypertension (16% excessive weight gain) compared with normotensive pregnancy (10% excessive weight gain), there is a large degree of overlap between groups.[42] Although mean maternal weight gain is greater from 20 weeks' onward in women who develop hypertension, only 9.6% of the variation in average weekly weight gain could be predicted by the development of hypertension.[43] Using a similar approach of deriving weight gain percentiles, Theron and Thompson[44] also concluded weight gain was not discriminatory for the prediction of later preeclampsia.

Excessive weight gain, defined as more than 1 kg/week (>2.2 lb/week), has a sensitivity of 44%, a specificity of 76.4%, a PPV of 6.6%, and an NPV of 97.4%.[45] Weight gain of more than 1.25 lb/week (0.57 kg) between weeks 20 and 30 is associated with a 34% risk of subsequent sustained pregnancy hypertension. Weight gain of more than 8 to 12 lb (> 3.6–5.5 kg) from 20 to 30 weeks' pregnancy has a sensitivity between 53% (12 lb [5.4 kg]) and 85% (8 lb [3.6 kg]) for identifying women at risk of preeclampsia, and a PPV between 7% (8 lb [3.6 kg]) and 10% (10 [4.5 kg] or 12 lb [5.4 kg]).[22]

What does a normal test result mean?

Maternal weight gain below 8 [3.6 kg]) to 12 lb [5.4 kg] has a specificity ranging between 25 (8 lb [3.6 kg]) and 66 (12 lb

[5.4 kg]) for identifying women not at risk of preeclampsia, and a NPV of about 95%.[22] Given that the prevalence of preeclampsia is about 2% to 5%, this is not a reassuring NPV.

Edema.

Edema is the demonstrable presence of excessive subcutaneous fluid.

What is the purpose of the tests?

To identify women at increased risk of developing preeclampsia.

What is the nature of the tests?

Peripheral edema is physiologic in pregnancy.[46] Although increased capillary permeability and extracellular fluid volume accumulation are well identified in preeclampsia,[47] these changes do not differ between women with and without edema.[47]

What are the implications of testing?

What does an abnormal test result mean? In a World Health Organization (WHO) study of 15,476 pregnancies in Southeast Asia, the most efficient strategy to screen for increased antenatal diastolic hypertension, preeclampsia, and of eclampsia was to use the presence of edema and/or proteinuria.[48] However, in MacGillivray's 1961 series,[49] generalized edema was present in only 14% of women with labile BP in pregnancy and 21% of women with elevated BP in pregnancy.

What does a normal test result mean? The absence of peripheral edema does not mean no risk of preeclampsia,[49] because "dry toxemia" (i.e., manifestations of preeclampsia in the absence of peripheral edema) has historically been considered to be at increased risk of maternal complications.

What is the cost of testing?

There are no cost-effectiveness studies.

■ Conclusions and Recommendations

The measurement of cardiac output in women with preexisting hypertension has led to interventions associated with a reduced rate of diagnosis of the clinical syndrome of preeclampsia but at the expense of reduced fetal growth velocity. The applicability of this approach is limited by the availability of appropriate technology and the training required for its use. The balance of benefit versus potential for growth reduction is dependent on the magnitude of maternal risk and the degree of reduced growth velocity.

Although the lack of a second trimester fall in BP, an abnormal increase in maternal weight gain, and excessive edema are all associated with increased risk for the later development of preeclampsia, these tests have insufficient specificity, sensitivity, PPV, and NPV to be useful in clinical practice.

Based on the current evidence, the practitioner is best advised to ensure that the BP is elevated during serial office measurements before diagnosing hypertension and initiating antihypertensive therapy. The role of ambulatory devices remains unclear. Women with new-onset, gestational hypertension arising before 32 weeks' gestation are at increased risk of developing preeclampsia. Prepregnancy hypertension is also a risk factor for preeclampsia, especially when the hypertension is associated with proteinuria. Women in these two groups should be followed frequently with surveillance for maternal and fetal well-being.

■ Summary

1 ■ What Is the Problem that Requires Screening?
Preeclampsia syndrome.

a. What is the incidence/prevalence of the target condition?
Two percent to 5% of all pregnant women.

b. What are the sequelae of the condition that are of interest in clinical medicine?
Preeclampsia is a leading cause of maternal mortality and the most common cause of iatrogenic preterm birth.

2 ■ The Tests

a. What is the purpose of the tests?
To identify women at increased risk of preeclampsia.

b. What is the nature of the tests?
Measurement of BP under standardized conditions, CO, peripheral vascular resistance, weight gain, and the assessment of edema.

Continued

■ **Summary—cont'd**

c. *What are the implications of testing?*

1. What does an abnormal test result mean?

An elevated MAP in the first trimester is suggestive of chronic hypertension. In the second trimester, the PPV of an elevated MAP (85 mm Hg) for preeclampsia ranges from 5% to 13%. About one half of women who develop gestational hypertension between 24 and 32 weeks' gestation subsequently develop preeclampsia.

A CO above 7.5 L/minute has a PPV for preeclampsia of 16%.

A TPR above 1,150 is poor predictor of preeclampsia.

Edema is poor predictor of preeclampsia.

2. What does a normal test result mean?

A normal MAP (< 85 mm Hg) in the second trimester has an NPV of 99%.

A CO below 7.4 L/minute has an NPV for preeclampsia of 95%.

A normal TPR (< 1,150 dynes/sec/cm^{-5}) is reassuring.

Edema is a normal finding of pregnancy.

d. *What is the cost of testing?*

There are no cost effectiveness studies.

3 ■ Conclusions and Recommendations

The measurement of cardiac output in women with preexisting hypertension has led to interventions associated with a reduced rate of diagnosis of the clinical syndrome of preeclampsia, but at the expense of reduced fetal growth velocity. The practitioner is best advised to ensure that the BP is elevated during serial office measurements before diagnosing hypertension and initiating antihypertensive therapy. The role of ambulatory devices remains unclear. Women with new-onset, gestational hypertension arising before 32 weeks' gestation are at increased risk of developing preeclampsia.

References

1. Health Canada. Special report on maternal mortality and severe morbidity in Canada: enhanced surveillance: the path to prevention. Ottawa, Minister of Public Works and Government, 2004.

2. National Institute for Clinical Excellence. *Why Women Die. Report on Confidential Enquiries into Maternal Deaths in the United Kingdom, 1997–1999.* London, RCOG Press, 2001.

3. CDC (US). Preeclampsia. Available at http://www.cdc.gov.nchs. 2002.

4. Preeclampsia Foundation. Preeclampsia. Available at http://www.preeclampsia.org. 2002.

5. Roberts JM, Redman CWG. Pre-eclampsia: more than pregnancy-induced hypertension. *Lancet* 1993;341:1447–1451.

6. Khong TY, De Wolf F, Robertson WB, et al. Inadequate maternal vascular response to placentation in pregnancies complicated by pre-eclampsia and by small-for-gestational age infants. *Br J Obstet Gynaecol* 1986;93:1049–1059.

7. Baker PN, Cunningham FG. Platelet and coagulation abnormalities. In: Lindheimer MD, Roberts JM, Cunningham FG, eds. *Chesley's Hypertensive Disorders of Pregnancy.* Stamford: Appleton and Lange, 1999:349–373.

8. Knight M, Redman CWG, Linton EA, et al. Shedding of syncytiotrophoblast microvilli into the maternal circulation in pre-eclamptic pregnancies. *Br J Obstet Gynaecol* 1998;105:632–640.

9. von Dadelszen P, Magee LA, Krajden M, et al. Levels of antibodies against cytomegalovirus and *Chlamydophila pneumoniae* are increased in early onset pre-eclampsia. *Br J Obstet Gynaecol* 2003;110:725–730.

10. Easterling TR, Benedetti TJ, Schmucker B, et al. Maternal hemodynamics in normal and preeclamptic pregnancies: a longitudinal study. *Obstet Gynecol* 1990;76:1061–1069.

11. Gehlbeck SH. Interpretation: distributions, averages and the normal. In: Gehlbeck SH, ed. *Interpreting the Medical Literature: Practical Epidemiology for Clinicians.* New York: MacMillan Publishing, 1988:97–111.

12. Adams TE, Everse SJ, Mann KG. Predicting the pharmacology of thrombin inhibitors. *J Thromb Haemost* 2003;1:1024–1027.

13. Brown MA, Hague WM, Higgins J, et al. The detection, investigation and management of hypertension in pregnancy: full consensus statement. *Aust N Z J Obstet Gynaecol* 2000;40:139–155.

14. Pickering TG, James GD, Boddie C, et al. How common is white coat hypertension? *JAMA* 1988;259:225–228.

15. Bellomo G, Narducci PL, Rondoni F, et al. Prognostic value of 24-hour blood pressure in pregnancy. *JAMA* 1999;282:1447–1452.

16. Hermida RC, Ayala DE. Prognostic value of office and ambulatory blood pressure measurements in pregnancy. *Hypertension* 2002;40:298–303.

17. Penny JA, Halligan AW, Shennan AH, et al. Hypertension in pregnancy: which method of blood pressure measurement is most predictive of outcome? *Am J Obstet Gynecol* 1998;178:521–526.

18. Appel LJ, Stason WB. Ambulatory blood pressure monitoring and blood pressure self-measurement in the diagnosis and management of hypertension. *Ann Intern Med* 1993;118:867–882.

19. Millar JA, Isles CG, Lever AF. Blood pressure, "white-coat" pressor responses and cardiovascular risk in placebo-group patients of the MRC Mild Hypertension trial. *J Hypertens* 1995;13:175–183.

20. Perloff D, Sokolow M, Cowan R. The prognostic value of ambulatory blood pressure monitoring in treated hypertensive patients. *J Hypertens Suppl* 1991;9:S33–S39.

21. Verdecchia P, Porcellati C, Schillaci G, et al. Ambulatory blood pressure. An independent predictor of prognosis in essential hypertension. *Hypertension* 1994;24:793–801.

22. Friedman SA, Lindheimer MD. Prediction and differential diagnosis. In: Lindheimer MD, Roberts JM, Cunningham FG, eds. *Chesley's Hypertensive Disorders in Pregnancy.* Stamford: Appleton and Lange; 1999:201–227.

23. O'Brien E, Petrie J, Littler W, et al. An outline of the revised British Hypertension Society protocol for the evaluation of blood pressure measuring devices. *J Hypertens* 1993;11:677–679.

24. Mengden T, Hernandez Medina RM, et al. Reliability of reporting self-measured blood pressure values by hypertensive patients. *Am J Hypertens* 1998;11:1413–1417.

25. Golara M, Jones C, Randhawa M, et al. Inflationary oscillometric blood pressure monitoring: validation of the OMRON-MIT. *Blood Press Monit* 2002;7:325–328.

26. Report of the National High Blood Pressure Education Program Working Group on High Blood Pressure in Pregnancy. *Am J Obstet Gynecol* 2000;183:S1–S22.

27. Helewa ME, Burrows RF, Smith J, et al. Report of the Canadian Hypertension Society Consensus Conference: 1. Definitions, evaluation and classification of hypertensive disorders in pregnancy. *CMAJ* 1997;157:715–25.

28. Barton JR, O'Brien JM, Bergauer NK, et al. Mild gestational hypertension remote from term: progression and outcome. *Am J Obstet Gynecol* 2001;184:979–983.

29. Magee LA, von Dadelszen P, Bohun CM, et al. Serious perinatal complications of non-proteinuric hypertension: an international, multicentre, retrospective cohort study. *J Obstet Gynaecol Can* 2003;25:372–382.

30. Easterling TR, Brateng D, Schmucker B, et al. Prevention of preeclampsia: a randomized trial of atenolol in hyperdynamic patients before onset of hypertension. *Obstet Gynecol* 1999;93:725–733.

31. Easterling TR, Carr DB, Brateng D, et al. Treatment of hypertension in pregnancy: effect of atenolol on maternal disease, preterm delivery, and fetal growth. *Obstet Gynecol* 2001;98:427–433.

32. Magee LA, Ornstein MP, von Dadelszen P. Fortnightly review: management of hypertension in pregnancy. *BMJ* 1999;318:1332–1336.

33. von Dadelszen P, Ornstein MP, Bull SB, et al. Fall in mean arterial pressure and fetal growth restriction in pregnancy hypertension: a meta-analysis. *Lancet* 2000;355:87–92.

34. von Dadelszen P, Magee LA. Fall in mean arterial pressure and fetal growth restriction in pregnancy hypertension: an updated metaregression analysis. *J Obstet Gynaecol Can* 2002;24:941–945.

35. Bosio PM, McKenna PJ, Conroy R, et al. Maternal central hemodynamics in hypertensive disorders of pregnancy. *Obstet Gynecol* 1999;94:978–984.

36. Taylor JB. "Saturovolaemia": a new concept in the aetiology of toxaemia of pregnancy. *J Roy Coll Gen Practit* 1970;20:129–136.

37. Easterling TR, Benedetti TJ, Carlson KC, et al. The effect of maternal hemodynamics on fetal growth in hypertensive pregnancies. *Am J Obstet Gynecol* 1991;165:902–906.

38. Hohn N, Junge S. The relationship of maternal obesity, excessive weight gain in pregnancy and pre-eclampsia. *Geburtshilfe Frauenheilkd* 1979;39:1079–1082.

39. Sibai BM, Ewell M, Levine RJ, et al. Risk factors associated with preeclampsia in healthy nulliparous women: the Calcium for Preeclampsia Prevention (CPEP) Study Group. *Am J Obstet Gynecol* 1997;177:1003–1010.

40. Rhodes P. The significance of weight gain in pregnancy. *Lancet* 1962;i:663–665.

41. Taylor JB. On predicting the onset of toxaemia of pregnancy. *J Roy Coll Gen Practit* 1969;18:156–163.

42. Dawes MG, Grudzinskas JG. Repeated measurement of maternal weight during pregnancy. Is this a useful practice? *Br J Obstet Gynaecol* 1991;98:189–194.

43. Dawes MG, Grudzinskas JG. Patterns of maternal weight gain in pregnancy. *Br J Obstet Gynaecol* 1991;98:195–201.

44. Theron GB, Thompson ML. The usefulness of weight gain in predicting pregnancy complications. *J Trop Paediatr* 1993;39:269–272.

45. De Muylder X. Is it worth weighing pregnant women in a developing country? *Arch Gynecol Obstet* 1992;251:65–68.

46. MacGillivray I, Campbell DM. The relevance of hypertension and oedema in pregnancy. *Clin Exp Hypertens* 1980;2:897–914.

47. Brown MA, Zammit VC, Lowe SA. Capillary permeability and extracellular fluid volumes in pregnancy-induced hypertension. *Clin Sci (Lond)* 1989;77:599–604.

48. Could oedema and proteinuria in pregnancy be used to screen for high risk? The WHO Collaborative Study of Hypertensive Disorders of Pregnancy. *Paediatr Perinat Epidemiol* 1988;2:25–42.

49. MacGillivray I. Hypertension in pregnancy and its consequences. *J Obstet Gynaecol Brit Cmwlth* 1961;68:557–69.
50. von Dadelszen P, Magee LA, Lee SK, et al. Activated protein C in normal human pregnancy and pregnancies complicated by severe preeclampsia: a therapeutic opportunity? *Crit Care Med* 2002;30:1883–1892.

35

Uterine Artery Doppler as Screening Tool for Preeclampsia

Antoinette C. Bolte

Gustaaf A. Dekker

■ What Is the Problem that Requires Screening?

Preeclampsia syndrome.

Preeclampsia is a pregnancy complication defined by new-onset hypertension and proteinuria. Obstetric hypertension is defined as a blood pressure of at least 140/90 mm Hg. However, the diagnostic criteria and classification of hypertensive disorders during pregnancy are not uniform. There has been progress unifying the classification, and the major consensus statements agree on most the terminology.[1-3] Two extremes of the diagnostic spectrum take either a "restrictive" or an "inclusive" approach. The restrictive criteria require both an elevation of blood pressure defined as 140 mm Hg systolic or 90 mm Hg diastolic in a women who was normotensive before 20 weeks' gestation plus proteinuria of 300 mg/24 hours.[1] The inclusive approach assumes that preeclampsia is a multisystem disorder, and diagnosis of preeclampsia is based on symptoms and signs in the organs commonly affected in this condition.[2] Although the restrictive criteria can be used for research purposes, the inclusive approach is more useful in clinical practice.

What is the incidence/prevalence of the target condition?

Reported prevalence of preeclampsia in an unselected population is dependent on the diagnostic criteria used and ranges from 0.5% for severe preeclampsia to 2% to 5% overall.[4]

What are the sequelae of the condition that are of interest in clinical medicine?

There is a relationship between preeclampsia and defective placentation. Endovascular trophoblast invasion is shallow compared to normal pregnancy, and physiologic changes in the spiral artery vessel wall are for the great part absent. The same pathologic changes are observed in placentas of small-for-dates neonates.[5] This association has led to the suggestion that some cases of fetal growth restriction differ from preeclampsia only in the maternal response to a shared placental pathology.

Preeclampsia is a major cause (15%–25%) of maternal mortality in developed countries[6–8] and associated with high perinatal mortality and morbidity rates primarily due to iatrogenic preterm birth. Screening for preeclampsia and treatment of women at risk is motivated by the chance of preventing maternal and fetal complications. However, women with mild or late-onset disease have pregnancy outcomes similar to normotensive pregnancy[9,10] and the results of preeclampsia-prevention trials have been disappointing.[11] Primary prevention is presently impossible, as the cause of preeclampsia proves elusive (see also Chapter 34).

■ The Tests

Uterine artery Doppler waveform analysis.

What is the purpose of the tests?

To identify women at risk of developing preeclampsia.

What is the nature of the tests?

The Doppler principle is used to measure the flow velocity and resistance through blood vessels. It is based on the fact that the frequency of ultrasound waves changes when they are reflected off a moving surface. The difference between the emitted and reflected frequencies, the frequency shift, is determined by the velocity at which the target is moving. If the angle between the direction of the emitted wave and the direction of movement of a column of blood is known, the velocity of the blood can be calculated on the basis of the frequency shift. The velocity of blood flowing in a given vessel reflects the resistance to flow in the vessels that are downstream to the vessel under investigation. Commonly used Doppler indices[1] include systolic/diastolic ratio (A/B ratio),[2] resistance index (RI; systolic–diastolic)/systolic),[3] pulsatility index (PI; systolic–diastolic)/mean velocity). Flow velocity waveforms change with gestational age.[12]

A successful pregnancy requires adequate placental perfusion for the necessary exchange of substances between maternal and fetal circulation. Blood flows to the uterus via two uterine arteries. The uterine arteries divide into the arcuate arteries, which after branching into radial arteries, continue in the direction of the endometrial surface taking a corkscrew appearance and are now called "spiral" arteries. The spiral arteries too undergo marked physiologic change. The trophoblast penetrates the spiral arteries in the decidua and upper third of the myometrium, replacing the endothelium and disrupting muscular and elastic elements. As a result, the spiral arteries are converted into saclike structures, the uteroplacental arteries that accommodate the intervillous space blood supply and are unresponsive to circulating pressor agents. It is suggested that the trophoblast migrates into the maternal vessels in waves. Initially, the spiral arteries of the decidua are altered, and ultimately, those in the myometrium are altered by 20 to 22 weeks.

These pregnancy adaptations are necessary for low resistance in the uteroplacental circulation.[13] Failure or only partial adaptation at the level of the spiral arteries is implicated in several complications of pregnancy including preeclampsia and intrauterine growth restriction (IUGR).[4] The resulting abnormal uteroplacental blood flow leads to the measurement of the uterine artery velocity waveform as a method to screening for this complication.[14,15] Nonpregnant and first-trimester uterine artery blood flow velocity waveforms are characterized by a low end-diastolic velocities and an early diastolic notch. The persistence of a diastolic notch beyond 24 weeks' gestation is associated with inadequate trophoblast invasion.[16] High resistance patterns on Doppler interrogation are closely associated with impaired trophoblastic migration when assessed by placental bed biopsies.[17] Thus, an screening abnormal test is characterized by an abnormal flow velocity ratio or the presence of an early diastolic notch.

The results of Doppler ultrasound studies of the uteroplacental circulation typically conducted at mid pregnancy (22–26 weeks) reveal considerable variation that may be well explained by methodologic differences.[18] Many of the earlier controversies relate to differences with regard to (a) ultrasound technique used; (b) pregnancy-related factors such as gestational age, sampling site, or placental location; (c) the use of dichotomous parameters or calculated indices with different cutoff values; (d) exams performed by a limited number of researchers or in routine care setting with multiple investigators; (e) the inclusion of unselected low- or high-risk populations; and (f) different definitions of obstetric hypertensive disorders. Continuous-wave and pulsed-wave Doppler with and without color Doppler have all been used. No differences in performance were demonstrated among them.[19] However, screening was usually performed by a small number of researchers in these studies, and it can be anticipated that the combination of pulsed wave technique with visualization by color Doppler in a routine clinical setting will have higher reproducibility.

The normal range for the indices used to measure the uterine artery waveform is influenced by several variables. Indices decrease with increasing gestation from 16 to 24 weeks.[20,21] The resistance indices are lower in the arcuate or subplacental arteries than in the uterine arteries.[20,22] To standardize sample site and increase reproducibility the use of flow velocity waveforms obtained with pulsed wave Doppler at the crossing of the uterine artery with the external iliac artery is recommended.

There is a relationship between placental position and uterine artery Doppler indices. Indices are lower at placental than at nonplacental sites,[20,22,23] These differences are particularly striking in the second trimester, when differences of up to 50% may occur between observations from nonplacental and placental sites in the arcuate and uterine arteries.[23] An abnormal placental-side uterine artery waveform is a better screening test for preeclampsia than the nonplacental-side.[24-26] The predictive value of the test is extremely low in women with a fully lateral placenta.[24]

Abnormal waveform is described as the presence of either high impedance in form of high PI, RI, A/B ratio, or the presence of a notch in one or both uterine arteries or a combination of both. The optimal method for defining an abnormal uterine artery flow velocity waveform (resistance index, pulsatility index, systolic to end-diastolic ratio, systolic to early-diastolic ratio, persistence of an early diastolic notch) is uncertain.[27,28] A combination of bilateral early diastolic notching with any of the velocimetric indices improves the detection of women who subsequently develop preeclampsia.[25,26,29,30]

The presence of a notch is generally assessed subjectively, which has raised questions as to the reproducibility of the method. Several methods of notch quantification are proposed, with varying results as to the usefulness of these for the prediction preeclampsia in either high- or low-risk population.[26,28,29,31-33] Measuring the resistance index and pulsatility index requires additional waveform measurements and calculations, where notch assessment is a subjective dichotomous parameter. Agreement between observers for detection of the presence or absence of an early diastolic notch is reported to be good,[32,34] or very good (Kappa statistic, 0.81; 95% confidence interval [CI], 0.48–1.0)[35] even in a routine setting with multiple operators.

Although longitudinal uterine artery flow patterns or two-stage measurements perform better predicting preeclampsia than a single measurement,[24,36,37] a one-stage test at 20 weeks is better suited for screening purposes if the effect of preventive therapy is taken into account.

What are the implications of testing?

Chien et al.[19] performed a systematic review of 27 observational studies involving 12,994 women to evaluate the clinical usefulness of Doppler analysis of the uterine artery waveform for the prediction of preeclampsia, IUGR, and perinatal death (Table 35–1). Most studies focus on the relationship between abnormal uterine artery flow velocity waveforms and adverse perinatal outcome; fewer studies address specifically identifying mothers at high risk of hypertensive disorders.

The likelihood ratios for the prediction of preeclampsia in low-risk women were heterogeneous and could not be adequately explained using sensitivity analyses involving study subgroups.[19] The pooled likelihood ratios from all the analyses in the high-risk group were homogeneous. The authors of this systematic review concluded that uterine artery Doppler flow waveform ratio with or without presence of a diastolic notch has limited diagnostic accuracy in predicting preeclampsia. The presence of a diastolic notch alone in low-risk population also has limited predictive value and further investigation as a screening tool in high-risk population is required.[19]

Table 35–1	**Systematic review of abnormal uterine artery Doppler ultrasound in prediction of preeclampsia**					
Population	**No. of studies**	**Pooled likelihood ratio**			**Post-test probability**	
		LR⁺	**LR⁻**	**Pre-test probability %**	**Positive test %**	**Negative test %**
High risk						
FWV±notch	11	2.8	0.8	9.8	23.5	7.8
notch alone	1	20.2	0.2	5.8	55.6	1.1
Low risk						
FWV±notch	11	6.4	0.7	3.5	18.8	2.5
notch alone	3	6.8	0.7	3.0	17.7	2.2

FVW ± notch, abnormal flow velocity waveform ± diastolic notch; LR, likelihood ratio

Table 35–2 contains the results of studies published after the meta-analysis of Chien et al.[19] All studies were performed in the second trimester using color flow pulsed Doppler; the sampling site was where the uterine and external iliac artery crossed. Including bilateral notches in the definition of the screen positive nearly doubled the screen-positive rate, but only marginally improves sensitivity.[38,39] As the RI values increase in a high-risk population, the proportion of pregnancies with notches also increase significantly.[35] Harrington et al.[40] included only multiparous women with high-risk factors and noted that abnormal flow patterns at 20 weeks' gestation identified the vast majority of women who subsequently developed complications secondary to uteroplacental dysfunction. Normal uterine artery Doppler studies in these high-risk women confers a risk of an adverse outcome similar to that of women with an uncomplicated obstetric history. Chien et al.[19] concluded that uterine artery Doppler assessment has limited diagnostic accuracy in predicting preeclampsia, and these later studies, although more uniform methodologically, did not perform better, meaning their performance is moderate at best. But as noted by Dekker and Sibai,[41] the impact can still be large enough to be important to the woman and her obstetrician.

What does an abnormal test result mean? An abnormal uterine artery waveform mid pregnancy indicates the woman is at increased risk for the development of either preeclampsia or fetal growth restriction. In low-risk pregnancy, the positive predictive value (PPV) approximates 18% (albeit with considerable heterogeneity across studies), whereas in high-risk groups it ranges from 24% to 56%. An abnormal test can be used as a screening tool to stratify level of antenatal care.

The question that remains is whether there is an effective intervention that changes outcome once a group at high risk has been identified? Numerous

Table 35-2 Prediction of preeclampsia by uterine artery doppler waveform

N	Doppler/ sampling site	GA weeks	Abnormal test	Preeclampsia (%)	Screen + (%)	sens	spec	ppv	npv	RR 95%CI	Ref.
High risk population											
116	Color PW	22–24	Bi notch	32 (27.5%)	17 (17%)	29	86	47	74	RR 2.5 (1.2–5.3) (LR+ 2.1)	35
144	Color PW/ crossing	24	RI ≥ 0.58	36 (25%)	63 (44%)	77.8	67.7	44.4	90.1	Significant LR+ 2.4	37
170	Color PW/ crossing	19–21	Bi+RI>0.55 Uni+RI>0.65	20 (11.8%)	49 (28.8%)	95.0%	80.0%	38.8%	99.2%	OR 75.0 (9.8–590.5) LR+ 4.9	40
Low risk population											
322	Color PW/ crossing	22–28	Any notch	19 (5.9%)	58 (18%)	36.8	83.2	12.1	95.5	RR2.7 (1.1–6.5) (LR+ 2.2)	45
458	Color PW/ crossing	19–21	Bi+RI>0.55 Uni+RI>0.65	2 (0.4%)	41 (9.0%)	50	91.2	2.1	99.8	OR 10.4 (0.6–169.4) LR+ 5.7	40
Unselected population											
946	Color PW/ crossing	19–21	Bi + RI>0.55	21 (2.2%)	117 (12.4)	61.9	88.7	11.1	99.0	OR12.8 (5.3–30.8) (LR+ 5.4)	30
1757	Color PW/ crossing	23	PI > 1.45	65 (3.7%)	89 (5.1%)	35.5	96	25.8	97.5	(LR+ 8.9)	38

LR^{pos} as given in text or (LR^{pos}) calculated as (sens) /(1-spec). GA, gestational age; sens, sensitivity; spec, specificity; ppv, positive predictive value; npv, negative predictive value; RR, relative risk; LR, likelihood ratio; PW, pulsed wave Doppler; RI, resistance index.

randomized trials evaluating the effect of aspirin on the prevalence of preeclampsia in women identified as being high risk by uterine Doppler waveform analysis. Many were underpowered and most conclude that aspirin failed to have an effect. The report by Yu et al.[42] is noteworthy as the study was appropriately powered. In that study, 560 women with abnormal uterine artery Doppler waveforms were randomized to 150 mg aspirin or placebo. There was no effect on the prevalence of preeclampsia or growth restriction.

One might argue that screening at 20 to 22 weeks' gestation is too late for intervention to be effective. Vaino et al.[43] conducted a randomized double blind, placebo controlled trial in a high-risk population. In that study, 120 women underwent transvaginal color Doppler ultrasound investigation at 12 to 14 weeks of gestation. Bilateral notches were found in 90 women of whom 45 were allocated aspirin and 45 allocated placebo. Bilateral notching had sensitivity, specificity, PPV, and negative predictive value (NPV) of 83%, 45%, 27.4%, and 92.8%, respectively, in predicting preeclampsia. Aspirin use was associated with a statistically significant reduction in the risk of preeclampsia (4.7% vs. 23.3%; RR = 0.2; 95% Cl, 0.05–0.86). The recurrence rate of preeclampsia was 14.3 in the aspirin group and 33.3% in the placebo group RR 0.48 (95% CI, 0.13–1.75). The prevalence of preeclampsia did not differ significantly between women in the aspirin group and the women without bilateral notches who were excluded from randomization. Others report a similar efficiency with first-trimester screening.[44] Thus, aspirin may reduce the risk of preeclampsia in high-risk women with early abnormal Doppler waveforms when started at 12 to 14 weeks' gestation. This finding requires further validation.

What does a normal test result mean? Women with normal uterine artery waveforms are unlikely to develop preeclampsia.[30,45] All studies confirm the high NPV of the test, which identifies a population at low-risk of preeclampsia. They range from 96% to 100% (Table 35–2). In high-risk women, the NPV ranges from 74% to 99%. The addition of color Doppler imaging of the uterine arteries at the time of the routine 20-week anomaly scan may be of use in determining the type and level of antenatal care offered[30] and minimize unnecessary interventions.[45] In general, normal uterine artery Doppler studies in high-risk women confer a risk of adverse outcome similar to that of women with an uncomplicated obstetric history.[40]

What is the cost of testing?

Few good-quality economic evaluations and primary cost studies of ultrasound screening are available. Bricker et al.[46] published a systemic review of the clinical and cost effectiveness, and women's views of ultrasound screening in pregnancy. Routine scanning in the second trimester was shown to be relatively cost-effective. Routine Doppler ultrasound in pregnancy has not been shown to be of benefit.[46] The resource use and costs associated with routine obstetric ultrasound and follow-up tests were assessed from both the U.K. National Health Service (NHS) and women's perspectives. Bottom-up and top-down costing of NHS resources were performed using questionnaires and diaries to record staff time associated with procedures. Questionnaires were used to assess women's costs of attending the antenatal ultrasound scans. Routine antenatal ultrasound scans at Liverpool Women's Hospital cost the NHS between £14 and £16 per scan. The costs to women, their families and their employers were estimated at between £9 and £15 per scan, depending on assumptions about the opportunity costs of time when not in paid employment and costs to employers of women who were in paid employment. Accurate estimates of costs to the NHS associated with routine antenatal ultrasound scanning are substantially lower than those cited in much of the literature. Costs to women are very similar to NHS costs.[47]

An analysis was made of the cost effectiveness of Doppler ultrasonography in high-risk pregnancies in Denmark. The cost-effectiveness analysis was based on results from a meta-analysis on clinical effects, patient costs, immediate health care costs, and costs per "saved" perinatal death. Incremental health care costs were estimated to be 13.5 million DKK (approximately 1.8 million euros) with patients costs set at zero. The cost of avoiding one perinatal death was estimated to be 1 million DKK (approx. 134,000 euros) would seem reasonable. In view of the paucity of available cost and effects data and the sensitivity of the results to changes in the assumptions made, more reliable information is needed before a decision can be made regarding the organization of Doppler ultrasonography for high-risk pregnancies.[48] Clinicians, women, and health planners should decide if Doppler ultrasound is justified, where in high-risk pregnancies a normal result can be reassuring and reduce a woman's anxiousness.

■ Conclusions and Recommendations

Doppler ultrasound scanning of the uterine arteries is a noninvasive, well-tolerated, and rapidly performed technique for assessing resistance to flow within the uteroplacental circulation. The use of flow velocity waveforms obtained with pulsed wave Doppler at the crossing of the uterine artery with the external iliac artery is recommended to standardize the sample site and increase reproducibility. The addition of color Doppler imaging of the uterine arteries at the time of the routine 20-week dating/anomaly scan may be of use in determining the type and level of antenatal care that is offered to women. In obstetric units where such a routine scan is already offered, the addition of uterine artery Doppler assessment would have little additional resource implications.

Clearly, normal uterine Doppler signals can be used to reassure women or help stratify their obstetric care. The weight of evidence forces the conclusion that low dose aspirin initiated after 20 weeks' gestation does not alter either the prevalence of preeclampsia or intrauterine growth restriction. It may be that screening followed by treatment with aspirin before 14 weeks' gestation is effective, but this needs confirmation.

■ Summary

1 ■ What Is the Problem that Requires Screening?

Preeclampsia syndrome.

a. What is the incidence/prevalence of the target condition?
Two percent to 5% of all pregnant women.

b. What are the sequelae of the condition that are of interest in clinical medicine?
Preeclampsia is one of the most common causes of maternal mortality and the most common cause of iatrogenic preterm birth.

2 ■ The Tests

a. What is the purpose of the tests?
To identify women at increased risk of preeclampsia.

b. What is the nature of the tests?
Uterine artery Doppler waveform analysis performed variably in the first or second trimesters.

c. What are the implications of testing?
1. What does an abnormal test result mean?
   An abnormal uterine artery waveform mid pregnancy indicates the woman is at increased risk for the development of either preeclampsia or fetal growth restriction. In low-risk pregnancy, the PPV approximates 18% (albeit with considerable heterogeneity across studies), while in high-risk groups it ranges from 24% to 56%.
2. What does a normal test result mean?
   Women with normal uterine artery waveforms are unlikely to develop preeclampsia. All studies that identified a population at low risk of preeclampsia confirm the high NPV of the test: They range from 96% to 100% (Table 35–2). In high-risk women, the NPV ranges from 74% to 99%.

d. What is the cost of testing?

Although the identification of a high-risk group is of value in stratifying care and allocating resources, a definitive cost benefit analysis awaits confirmation that there is an effective therapeutic intervention.

3 ■ Conclusions and Recommendations

Normal uterine Doppler signals can be used either to reassure women or help stratify their obstetric care. The weight of evidence forces the conclusion that low-dose aspirin initiated after 20 weeks' gestation does not alter either the prevalence of preeclampsia or intrauterine growth restriction. It may be that screening followed by treatment with aspirin before 14 weeks' gestation is effective, but this needs confirmation.

References

1. Report of the National High Blood Pressure Education Program Working Group on High Blood Pressure in Pregnancy. *Am J Obstet Gynecol* 2000;183:S1–S22.
2. Brown MA, Hague WM, Higgins J, et al. The detection, investigation and management of hypertension in pregnancy: full consensus statement. *Aust N Z J Obstet Gynaecol* 2000;40: 139–155.
3. Brown MA, Lindheimer MD, de Swiet M, et al. The classification and diagnosis of the hypertensive disorders of pregnancy: statement from the International Society for the Study of Hypertension in Pregnancy (ISSHP). *Hypertens Pregnancy* 2001;20:IX–XIV.
4. Saftlas AF, Olson DR, Franks AL, et al. Epidemiology of preeclampsia and eclampsia in the United States, 1979-1986. *Am J Obstet Gynecol* 1990;163:460–465.
5. Khong TY, De Wolf F, Robertson WB, et al. Inadequate maternal vascular response to placentation in pregnancies complicated by pre-eclampsia and by small-for-gestational age infants. *Br J Obstet Gynaecol* 1986;93:1049–1059.
6. Berg CJ, Chang J, Callaghan WM, Whitehead SJ. Pregnancy-related mortality in the United States, 1991-1997. *Obstet Gynecol* 2003;101:289–296.
7. Schuitemaker N, van Roosmalen J, Dekker G, et al. Confidential enquiry into maternal deaths in The Netherlands 1983-1992. *Eur J Obstet Gynecol Reprod Biol* 1998;79:57–62.
8. Lewis G, Drife J. Why mothers die: a report on confidential enquiries into maternal deaths in the United Kingdom 1994-1996. 1998. London, HMSO.
9. Buchbinder A, Sibai BM, Caritis S, et al. Adverse perinatal outcomes are significantly higher in severe gestational hypertension than in mild preeclampsia. *Am J Obstet Gynecol* 2002; 186:66–71.
10. Hauth JC, Ewell MG, Levine RJ, et al. Pregnancy outcomes in healthy nulliparas who developed hypertension. Calcium for Preeclampsia Prevention Study Group. *Obstet Gynecol* 2000;95: 24–28.

11. Sibai BM. Prevention of preeclampsia: a big disappointment. *Am J Obstet Gynecol* 1998;179: 1275–1278.

12. Detti L, Mari G, Cheng CC, et al. Fetal Doppler velocimetry. *Obstet Gynecol Clin North Am* 2004;31:201–214.

13. Jauniaux E, Jurkovic D, Campbell S, et al. Doppler ultrasonographic features of the developing placental circulation: Correlation with anatomic findings. *Am J Obstet Gynecol* 1992;166: 585–587.

14. Campbell S, Diaz-Recasens J, Griffin DR, et al. New doppler technique for assessing uteroplacental blood flow. *Lancet* 1983;1:675–677.

15. Steel SA, Pearce JM, Chamberlain G. Doppler ultrasound of the uteroplacental circulation as a screening test for severe pre-eclampsia with intra-uterine growth retardation. *Eur J Obstet Gynecol Reprod Biol* 1988;28:279–287.

16. Eyck vJ, Reuwer PJ. Foetale en uteroplacentaire circulatie. In: Stoutenbeek Ph, Vugt van JM, Wladimiroff JW, eds. *Echoscopie in de Gynaecologie en Obstetrie.* Utrecht: Bunge, 1997:170–177.

17. Lin S, Shimizu I, Suehara N, et al. Uterine artery Doppler velocimetry in relation to trophoblast migration into the myometrium of the placental bed. *Obstet Gynecol* 1995;85:760–765.

18. Chappell L, Bewley S. Pre-eclamptic toxaemia: the role of uterine artery Doppler. *Br J Obstet Gynaecol* 1998;105:379–382.

19. Chien PF, Arnott N, Gordon A, et al. How useful is uterine artery Doppler flow velocimetry in the prediction of pre-eclampsia, intrauterine growth retardation and perinatal death? An overview. *Br J Obstet Gynaecol* 2000;107:196–208.

20. Bewley S, Campbell S, Cooper D. Uteroplacental Doppler flow velocity waveforms in the second trimester: a complex circulation. *Br J Obstet Gynaecol* 1989;96:91040–1046.

21. Pearce JM, Campbell S, Cohen-Overbeek T, et al. References ranges and sources of variation for indices of pulsed Doppler flow velocity waveforms from the uteroplacental and fetal circulation. *Br J Obstet Gynaecol* 1988;95:248–256.

22. Oosterhof H, Aarnoudse JG. Ultrasound pulsed Doppler studies of the uteroplacental circulation: the influence of sampling site and placenta implantation. *Gynecol Obstet Invest* 1992;33: 75–79.

23. Low JA. The current status of maternal and fetal blood flow velocimetry. *Am J Obstet Gynecol* 1991;164:1049–1063.

24. Antsaklis A, Daskalakis G, Tzortzis E, et al. The effect of gestational age and placental location on the prediction of pre-eclampsia by uterine artery Doppler velocimetry in low-risk nulliparous women. *Ultrasound Obstet Gynecol* 2000;16:635–639.

25. Aquilina J, Barnett A, Thompson O, et al. Comprehensive analysis of uterine artery flow velocity waveforms for the prediction of pre-eclampsia. *Ultrasound Obstet Gynecol* 2000;16:163–170.

26. North RA, Ferrier C, Long D, et al. Uterine artery Doppler flow velocity waveforms in the second trimester for the prediction of preeclampsia and fetal growth retardation. *Obstet Gynecol* 1994;83:378–386.

27. Aardema MW, Lander M, Oosterhof H, et al. Doppler ultrasound screening predicts recurrence of poor pregnancy outcome in subsequent pregnancies, but not the recurrence of PIH or preeclampsia. *Hypertens Pregnancy* 2000;19:281–288.

28. Irion O, Masse J, Forest JC, et al. Prediction of pre-eclampsia, low birthweight for gestation and prematurity by uterine artery blood flow velocity waveforms analysis in low risk nulliparous women. *Br J Obstet Gynaecol* 1998;105:422–429.

29. Becker R, Vonk R, Vollert W, et al. Doppler sonography of uterine arteries at 20-23 weeks: risk assessment of adverse pregnancy outcome by quantification of impedance and notch. *J Perinat Med* 2002; 30:388–394.

30. Kurdi W, Campbell S, Aquilina J, et al. The role of color Doppler imaging of the uterine arteries at 20 weeks' gestation in stratifying antenatal care. *Ultrasound Obstet Gynecol* 1998;12: 339–345.

31. Aardema MW, De Wolf BT, Saro MC, et al. Quantification of the diastolic notch in Doppler ultrasound screening of uterine arteries. *Ultrasound Obstet Gynecol* 2000;16:630–634.

32. Bower S, Kingdom J, Campbell S. Objective and subjective assessment of abnormal uterine artery Doppler flow velocity waveforms. *Ultrasound Obstet Gynecol* 1998;12:260–264.

33. Ohkuchi A, Minakami H, Sato I, et al. Predicting the risk of pre-eclampsia and a small-for-gestational-age infant by quantitative assessment of the diastolic notch in uterine artery flow velocity waveforms in unselected women. *Ultrasound Obstet Gynecol* 2000;16:171–178.

34. Farrell T, Chien PF, Mires GJ. The reliability of the detection of an early diastolic notch with uterine artery Doppler velocimetry. *Br J Obstet Gynaecol* 1998;105:1308–1311.

35. Coleman MA, McCowan LM, North RA. Mid-trimester uterine artery Doppler screening as a predictor of adverse pregnancy outcome in high-risk women. *Ultrasound Obstet Gynecol* 2000; 15:7–12.

36. Harrington K, Cooper D, Lees C, et al. Doppler ultrasound of the uterine arteries: the importance of bilateral notching in the prediction of pre-eclampsia, placental abruption or delivery of a small-for-gestational-age baby. *Ultrasound Obstet Gynecol* 1996;7:182–188.

37. Parretti E, Mealli F, Magrini A, et al. Cross-sectional and longitudinal evaluation of uterine artery Doppler velocimetry for the prediction of pre-eclampsia in normotensive women with specific risk factors. *Ultrasound Obstet Gynecol* 2003;22:160–165.

38. Albaiges G, Missfelder-Lobos H, Lees C, et al. One-stage screening for pregnancy complications by color Doppler assessment of the uterine arteries at 23 weeks' gestation. *Obstet Gynecol* 2000;96:559–564.

39. Papageorghiou AT, Yu CK, Bindra R, et al. Multicenter screening for pre-eclampsia and fetal growth restriction by transvaginal uterine artery Doppler at 23 weeks of gestation. *Ultrasound Obstet Gynecol* 2001;18:441–449.

40. Harrington K, Fayyad A, Thakur V, et al. The value of uterine artery Doppler in the prediction of uteroplacental complications in multiparous women. *Ultrasound Obstet Gynecol* 2004;23: 50–55.

41. Dekker G, Sibai B. Primary, secondary, and tertiary prevention of pre-eclampsia. *Lancet* 2001; 357:209–215.

42. Yu CK, Papageorghiou AT, Parra M, et al. Randomized controlled trial using low-dose aspirin in the prevention of pre-eclampsia in women with abnormal uterine artery Doppler at 23 weeks' gestation. *Ultrasound Obstet Gynecol* 2003;22:233–239.

43. Vainio M, Kujansuu E, Iso-Mustajarvi M, et al. Low dose acetylsalicylic acid in prevention of pregnancy-induced hypertension and intrauterine growth retardation in women with bilateral uterine artery notches. *Br J Obstet Gynaecol* 2002;109:161–167.

44. Martin AM, Bindra R, Curcio P, et al. Screening for preeclampsia and fetal growth restriction by uterine artery Doppler at 11-14 weeks of gestation. *Ultrasound Obstet Gynecol* 2001;18:583–586.

45. Phupong V, Dejthevaporn T, Tanawattanacharoen S, et al. Predicting the risk of preeclampsia and small for gestational age infants by uterine artery Doppler in low-risk women. *Arch Gynecol Obstet* 2003;268:158–161.

46. Bricker L, Garcia J, Henderson J, et al. Ultrasound screening in pregnancy: a systematic review of the clinical effectiveness, cost-effectiveness and women's views. *Health Technol Assess* 2000;4: 161–193.

47. Henderson J, Bricker L, Roberts T, et al. British National Health Service's and women's costs of antenatal ultrasound screening and follow-up tests. *Ultrasound Obstet Gynecol* 2002;20: 154–162.

48. Westergaard HB, Sorensen J, Langhoff-Roos J. Illustrative estimates of costs and effects of the use of Doppler ultrasonography in high-risk pregnancies. *Int J Technol Assess Health Care* 2003; 19:624–631.

36

Preeclampsia and Uric Acid

Antoinette C. Bolte

Gustaaf A. Dekker

■ What Is the Problem that Requires Screening?

Preeclampsia.

Preeclampsia is a multisystem disorder of unknown etiology.

What is the incidence/prevalence of the target condition?

The "preeclampsia–eclampsia syndrome" is defined as hypertension new to pregnancy manifesting after 20 weeks' gestation associated with new onset of proteinuria that resolves after delivery. The reported prevalence of hypertensive disorders in pregnancy ranges from 2% to 35% depending on the diagnostic criteria used and the population studied.[1] The reported prevalence of preeclampsia in an unselected population is dependent on the diagnostic criteria and ranges from 0.5% for severe preeclampsia to 2% to 5% overall.[2]

What are the sequelae of the condition that are of interest in clinical medicine?

Preeclampsia is a leading cause of maternal and perinatal morbidity and mortality in developing and developed countries.[3] For details on the sequelae, see Chapter 34.

■ The Tests

Measurement of serum uric acid.

What is the purpose of the tests?

The prediction of preeclampsia.

What is the nature of the tests?

Uric acid is a biochemical marker for preeclampsia. The question is whether the uric acid measurement can be used as screening test for the disorder. Although a small amount of uric acid is derived from the diet, the greatest proportion results from tissue breakdown. Approximately three fourths of the circulating uric acid is excreted by the kidney; the remaining part is excreted by the gastrointestinal tract.

Uric acid levels are significantly reduced during pregnancy (2.5–4 mg/dL) compared with nonpregnant norms (4–6 mg/dL). During late gestation, uric acid rises toward nonpregnant values. Alterations in the renal handling of uric acid are responsible for the pronounced decrease in serum uric acid during the first 20 weeks of gestation, its gradual increase in the latter part of pregnancy,[4,5] and its further increase with pregnancy-induced hypertension.[6] The diurnal variation in serum uric acid concentration may be as high as 40%.[6] As with many biochemical parameters, increases over time are often the best indicator; significant hyperuricemia is repeatedly reported as more than 5.9 mg/dL (>350 fmol/L).[7]

Hyperuricemia may result from renal and extrarenal factors. Uric acid concentration is increased over normal pregnant values in established preeclampsia. The increase precedes and exceeds that based on the reduction in glomerular filtration rate associated with preeclampsia.[8] Altered renal handling of uric acid is an important cause of hyperuricemia in preeclampsia. Renal tubular pathophysiology, an early feature of preeclampsia, results in a reduced renal clearance of uric acid and thus increased plasma uric acid levels. Later in the development of the disease, glomerular function becomes impaired about the time proteinuria appears.[9] A significant association exists between hyperuricemia and the severity of the histologic finding of "glomerular endotheliosis" on antepartum percutaneous renal biopsies.[10,11] However, it is unlikely that reduced renal clearance explains the rise in uric acid observed before any clinical manifestation of the disease.[4]

Oxidative stress is defined as an imbalance between the level of oxidants and antioxidants. For more than a decade, it has been associated with the development of preeclampsia. Xanthine dehydrogenase/oxidase (XDH/XO) is thought a key enzyme of purine catabolism. The two enzyme forms (XDH/XO) and the products of their reactions are often referred to as "xanthine oxidoreductase" (XOR) activity. XOR produces uric acid. With XDH, the conversion of purines to uric acid is coupled with the reduction of nicotinamide adenine dinucleotide (NAD) to NADH, and the oxidase (XO) form of the enzyme metabolizes xanthine and hypoxanthine to uric acid with production of hydrogen peroxide and superoxide. Superoxide generation may in preeclampsia be related to maternal oxidative stress. With hypoxia and in response to several cytokines, XOR synthesis increases and the conversion of the enzyme to its XO form is enhanced.[12] Preeclampsia is characterized by multiorgan dysfunction with reduced perfusion of all affected organs. Uric acid, a product of the XOR pathway, may reflect a response to placental ischemia/reperfusion, and as such, hyperuricemia may be indirectly associated with free radical generation.[13] Of note, XDH enzymatic activity (i.e., the physiologic isoform of this enzyme) also generates uric acid. Early reports failed to demonstrate XOR activity in human placenta.[14] However, more recent research showed that XOR enzyme activity is present in the human placenta and it is substantially elevated at the maternal–fetal interface in preeclampsia.[12,15]

Metabolic syndrome, or "syndrome X," defined by insulin resistance, hypertension, obesity, and dyslipidemia, contributes to be the development of atherosclerosis and has been associated with preeclampsia. Hyperuricemia is one of the classic features of the metabolic syndrome. Hyperinsulinemia secondary to insulin resistance reduces uric acid clearance, leading to the hyperuricemia. In addition, visceral fat accumulation increases uric acid synthesis via activation of triglyceride synthesis. Despite numerous epidemiologic and experimental studies into the effect of uric acid on the vascular injury, there is no direct evidence that uric acid per se damages blood vessels.[16] It may be that the hyperuricemia reflects an attempt to mitigate against vascular damage by other counter mechanisms.[17]

For many years, uric acid (or more correctly, urate when measured at physiologic pH), was considered a waste product of purine metabolism without physiologic value. However, urate is itself a potent antioxidant with radical scavenging and reducing activities. At physiologic concentrations, urate is an especially strong antioxidant for water-soluble free radicals. However, it is ineffective against lipid-soluble free radicals, and forms potent free radicals when oxidized.[18] Urate protects against reperfusion damage. Urate prevents oxidative inactivation of endothelial enzymes (e.g., cyclooxygenase, angiotensin converting enzyme) and preserves the ability of endothelium to mediate vascular dilation in the face of oxidative stress.[17] Elevated serum uric acid is associated with established cardiovascular risk factors such as hypertension, diabetes mellitus, hyperlipidemia and obesity. It is unclear whether uric acid has a damaging or protective effect in these circumstances.[19] Another possibility is that the breakdown of the nuclear-rich syncytiotrophoblast might increase the formation of uric acid from purine catabolism. However, no association was found between uric acid levels and placental pathology in preeclamptic pregnancies.[20] Thus, while there are many theories or potential explanations for the increased uric acid during preeclampsia, the exact mechanism and role of uric acid in preeclampsia remains unknown.

In support of the hypothesis that an imbalance between antioxidants and oxidants has a role in the pathogenesis of preeclampsia, significantly decreased first trimester uric acid excretion in a 24-hour urine sample was shown in nulliparous women who later developed preeclampsia.[21] Further, the uric acid increase in the second half of normal pregnancy parallels the rise of total antioxidant capacity.[4,5,13]

Established preeclampsia. The first report of increased maternal uric acid concentrations in preeclampsia/eclampsia was published in 1917.[22] Subsequently, Lancet and Fisher[23] were among the first to note a positive association between serum urate levels and the severity of the hypertension. This association between serum urate levels and clinical severity as well as poor fetal prognosis has since been reported by many investigators.[6,9,24–30] However, others concluded that uric acid levels, although significantly elevated in women with preeclampsia compared with those of normotensive pregnant women, were not good prognostic indicators of the severity of the maternal or fetal complications.[31–36] They found no relation between serum urate level and the outcome of the pregnancies, and concluded that management could not be based on uric acid levels as a single predictive value. Nor was a weekly change (increase of 20 μmol/L) found to be of any use.[32]

Predicting preeclampsia. Despite the fairly large number of reports dealing with uric acid in patients diagnosed with preeclampsia, less information is available on the predictive value of uric acid serum concentration. The results of some longitudinal studies of normotensive pregnant women[4,7,37–42] but not of others,[5,40,41] suggest that an increased serum uric acid is an early sign of preeclampsia.

Two cross-sectional studies concluded that women who subsequently develop preeclampsia had significantly higher uric acid levels at 24 weeks'[42] and 29 weeks' gestation,[43] whereas a third at 28 weeks' gestation could not confirm the findings.[44] These studies included nulliparous and multiparous women and women at low risk, high risk, or mixed risk, which could explain some of the contradictory findings. However, the overall conclusion from these studies is that uric acid is a poor predictor of preeclampsia in asymptomatic women and is thus not clinically useful as a screening test for preeclampsia.[3,5,37,40,41,44–47]

A number of studies tested the utility of serum uric acid measurements to differentiate various hypertensive diseases of pregnancy.[7,36,40,44,48] Uric acid may be helpful in diagnosing superimposed preeclampsia in women with chronic hypertension. Lim et al.[33] observed a sensitivity of 54% and specificity of 78% and a positive likelihood ratio of 2.5 for serum uric acid levels of 5.5 mg/dL or greater. This increases the posttest probability to nearly 40% given the incidence of superimposed preeclampsia in women with chronic hypertension approximates 25%.[36]

Perhaps its greatest clinical use is a confirmatory marker for established preeclampsia. Hypertensive women with normal uric acid levels are unlikely to have the preeclampsia/eclampsia syndrome. However, there is considerable overlap between normal, hypertensive, and preeclamptic uric acid levels. It is important to take into account the gestational age in making an interpretation due to the changes observed in normal pregnancy. Restoration to normal levels occurs rapidly in the postpartum period of preeclamptic women, generally within the first week.

What are the implications of testing?

What does an abnormal test result mean? Serum uric acid concentration is a useful confirmatory marker for established preeclampsia[3,5,23,25–28,33,34,48,49]

In women with chronic hypertension, an elevation of serum uric acid level identifies those with an increased likelihood of having superimposed preeclampsia.[33] However, no particular uric acid value can be given above which to advise delivery. Women with mild hypertension and hyperuricemia are at increased risk of developing the preeclampsia syndrome. It may be prudent to observe these women more closely. As yet there is no evidence that the determination of uric acid levels can be used to predict the later development of preeclampsia.

What does a normal test result mean? A low uric acid concentration is of some use in excluding preeclampsia because of the relatively high negative predictive value and specificity.[42,43,48] However, there is no easy applicable cutoff value as levels depend on gestational age, are sensitive to diurnal variation and can be influenced by some drugs (increased by low-dose aspirin and antibiotics; decreased by allopurinol). A woman with mild hypertension and a normal uric acid level is unlikely to develop the preeclampsia syndrome.

What is the cost of testing?

Uric acid measurement is an inexpensive test and readily available test. Price of uric acid test is € 1.55 (price in The Netherlands) and AUS $8 (Australia). Testing can be performed during a scheduled antenatal visit. No cost-effectiveness analysis has been performed.

■ Conclusions and Recommendations

The preeclampsia syndrome can only be treated by delivery, and any benefit of pharmacologic secondary prevention is controversial.[1] However, increased surveillance might affect the outcome of pregnancies identified as high risk, and there is evidence of a preclinical stage. Dysfunctional placentation occurs in early gestation, whereas the clinical signs and symptoms of preeclampsia become apparent only later.[3] Prevention of preeclampsia requires knowledge of the early pathophysiologic mechanisms, methods for their early detection and a way to correct them. Hyperuricemia is said to be an early feature of preeclampsia, and in some subgroups, low dose aspirin may be effective prophylaxis.

Serum uric acid concentration is a useful marker of preeclampsia; serum uric acid is a poor predictor of future preeclampsia in an apparently healthy woman.[49] For women with chronic hypertension, it is useful for the identification of those with superimposed preeclampsia where such information may lead to enhanced antenatal surveillance.

■ Summary

1 ■ What Is the Problem that Requires Screening?

Preeclampsia syndrome.

a. What is the incidence/prevalence of the target condition?
Two to three percent depending on criteria and the population studied.

b. What are the sequelae of the condition that are of interest in clinical medicine?
Preeclampsia is a leading cause of maternal mortality and is the number one cause of iatrogenic preterm birth.

2 ■ The Tests

a. What is the purpose of the tests?
To identify pregnancies at high risk of preeclampsia.

b. What is the nature of the tests?
Measurement of serum uric acid.

c. What are the implications of testing?
1. What does an abnormal test result mean?
   Women with new-onset hypertension plus hyperuricemia are at increased risk of developing preeclampsia. Women with chronic hypertension who experience an exacerbation associated with hyperuricemia are at increased risk of developing superimposed preeclampsia. It may be prudent to increase the level of surveillance for these women.
2. What does a normal test result mean?
   Women with hypertension but normal uric acid levels are unlikely to develop preeclampsia.

d. What is the cost of testing?
No cost-effective analysis has been performed.

Continued

■ **Summary—cont'd**

3 ■ **Conclusions and Recommendations**

Serum uric acid concentration is a useful marker of preeclampsia; serum uric acid is a poor predictor of future preeclampsia in an apparently healthy woman. For women with chronic hypertension, it is useful for the identification of those with superimposed preeclampsia where such information may lead to enhanced antenatal surveillance.

References

1. Sibai BM. Preeclampsia-eclampsia. *Curr Prob Obstet Gynecol Fertil* 1990;13:3–45.
2. Saftlas AF, Olson DR, Franks AL, et al. Epidemiology of preeclampsia and eclampsia in the United States, 1979-1986. *Am J Obstet Gynecol* 1990;163:2460-465.
3. Dekker GA. Prevention of preeclampsia. In: Sibai BM, ed. *Hypertensive Disorders in Women.* Philadelphia: WB Saunders, 2001:61–84.
4. Chappell LC, Seed PT, Briley A, et al. A longitudinal study of biochemical variables in women at risk of preeclampsia. *Am J Obstet Gynecol* 2002;187:127–136.
5. Fay RA, Bromham DR, Brooks JA, et al. Platelets and uric acid in the prediction of preeclampsia. *Am J Obstet Gynecol* 1985;152:1038–1039.
6. Hill LM. Metabolism of uric acid in normal and toxemic pregnancy. *Mayo Clin Proc* 1978;53:743–751.
7. Blackburn S. *Maternal, Fetal and Neonatal Physiology: a Clinical Perspective,* 2nd ed. St. Louis: Saunders, 2003.
8. Redman CW, Beilin LJ, Bonnar J. Renal function in preeclampsia. *J Clin Pathol Suppl (R Coll Pathol)* 1976;10:91–94.
9. Conrad KP, Lindheimer MD. Renal and cardiovascular alterations. In: Lindheimer MD, Roberts JM, Cunningham FG, eds. *Chesley's Hypertensive Disorders in Pregnancy.* Stamford: Appleton & Lange, 1999:263–326.
10. Pollak VE, Nettles JB. The kidney in toxemia of pregnancy: a clinical and pathologic study based on renal biopsies. *Medicine* 1960;39:469–526.
11. Nochy D, Birembaut P, Hinglais N, et al. Renal lesions in the hypertensive syndromes of pregnancy: immunomorphological and ultrastructural studies in 114 cases. *Clin Nephrol* 1980;13:155–162.
12. Many A, Hubel CA, Fisher SJ, et al. Invasive cytotrophoblasts manifest evidence of oxidative stress in preeclampsia. *Am J Pathol* 2000;156:321–331.
13. Chappell LC, Seed PT, Kelly FJ, et al. Vitamin C and E supplementation in women at risk of preeclampsia is associated with changes in indices of oxidative stress and placental function. *Am J Obstet Gynecol* 2002;187:777–784.
14. Hayashi TT, Baldridge RC, Olmsted PS, et al., Purine nucleotide catabolism in placenta. *Am J Obstet Gynecol* 1964;88:470–478.
15. Many A, Westerhausen-Larson A, Kanbour-Shakir A, et al. Xanthine oxidase/dehydrogenase is present in human placenta. *Placenta* 1996;17:361–365.
16. Conen D, Wietlisbach V, Bovet P, et al. Prevalence of hyperuricemia and relation of serum uric acid with cardiovascular risk factors in a developing country. *BMC Public Health* 2004;4:19.
17. Becker BF. Towards the physiological function of uric acid. *Free Radic Biol Med* 1993;14:615–631.
18. Sevanian A, Davies KJ, Hochstein P. Serum urate as an antioxidant for ascorbic acid. *Am J Clin Nutr* 1991;54[Suppl]:1129S–1134S.

19. Waring WS, Webb DJ, Maxwell SR. Uric acid as a risk factor for cardiovascular disease. *QJM* 2000;93:707–713.
20. Lee IS, Hsu CD. Placental pathologies are not associated with hyperuricemia in preeclamptic pregnancies. *Conn Med* 1999;63:459–461.
21. de Jong CL, Paarlberg KM, van Geijn HP, et al. Decreased first trimester uric acid production in future preeclamptic patients. *J Perinat Med* 1997;25:347–352.
22. Slemons JM, Bogert LJ. The uric acid content of maternal and fetal blood. *J Biol Chem* 1917;32:63–69.
23. Lancet M, Fisher IL. The value of blood uric acid levels in toxaemia of pregnancy. *J Obstet Gynaecol Br Emp* 1956;63:116–119.
24. Sagen N, Haram K, Nilsen ST. Serum urate as a predictor of fetal outcome in severe pre-eclampsia. *Acta Obstet Gynecol Scand* 1984;63:71–75.
25. Redman CW, Beilin LJ, Bonnar J, et al. Plasma-urate measurements in predicting fetal death in hypertensive pregnancy. *Lancet* 1976;1:370–373.
26. Voto LS, Illia R, Darbon-Grosso HA, et al. Uric acid levels: a useful index of the severity of preeclampsia and perinatal prognosis. *J Perinat Med* 1988;16:123–126.
27. Liedholm H, Montan S, Aberg A. Risk grouping of 113 patients with hypertensive disorders during pregnancy, with respect to serum urate, proteinuria and time of onset of hypertension. *Acta Obstet Gynecol Scand Suppl* 1984;118:43–48.
28. Schuster E, Weppelmann B. Plasma urate measurements and fetal outcome in preeclampsia. *Gynecol Obstet Invest* 1981;12:162–167.
29. Varma TR. Serum uric acid levels as an index of fetal prognosis in pregnancies complicated by pre-existing hypertension and pre-eclampsia of pregnancy. *Int J Gynaecol Obstet* 1982;20:401–408.
30. Wakwe VC, Abudu OO. Estimation of plasma uric acid in pregnancy induced hypertension (PIH). Is the test still relevant? *Afr J Med Med Sci* 1999;28:155–158.
31. Witlin AG, Saade GR, Mattar F, et al. Risk factors for abruptio placentae and eclampsia: analysis of 445 consecutively managed women with severe preeclampsia and eclampsia. *Am J Obstet Gynecol* 1999;180:322–329.
32. Calvert SM, Tuffnell DJ, Haley J. Poor predictive value of platelet count, mean platelet volume and serum urate in hypertension in pregnancy. *Eur J Obstet Gynecol Reprod Biol* 1996;64:179–184.
33. Lim KH, Friedman SA, Ecker JL, et al. The clinical utility of serum uric acid measurements in hypertensive diseases of pregnancy. *Am J Obstet Gynecol* 1998;178:1067–1071.
34. Williams KP, Galerneau F. The role of serum uric acid as a prognostic indicator of the severity of maternal and fetal complications in hypertensive pregnancies. *J Obstet Gynaecol Can* 2002;24:628–632.
35. Sibai BM, Anderson GD, McCubbin JH. Eclampsia, II: clinical significance of laboratory findings. *Obstet Gynecol* 1982;59:153–157.
36. Odendaal HJ, Pienaar ME. Are high uric acid levels in patients with early pre-eclampsia an indication for delivery? *S Afr Med J* 1997;87:213–218.
37. Hanisch CG, Pfeiffer KA, Schlebusch H, et al. Adhesion molecules, activin and inhibin-candidates for the biochemical prediction of hypertensive diseases in pregnancy? *Arch Gynecol Obstet* 2004; 270:110–115.
38. Mello G, Parretti E, Cioni R, et al. Individual longitudinal patterns in biochemical and hematological markers for the early prediction of pre-eclampsia. *J Matern Fetal Neonatal Med* 2002;11:93–99.
39. Redman CW, Williams GF, Jones DD, et al. Plasma urate and serum deoxycytidylate deaminase measurements for the early diagnosis of pre-eclampsia. *Br J Obstet Gynaecol* 1977; 84:904–908.
40. Salako BL, Odukogbe AT, Olayemi O, et al. Serum albumin, creatinine, uric acid and hypertensive disorders of pregnancy. *East Afr Med J* 2003;80:424–428.
41. Masse J, Forest JC, Moutquin JM, et al. A prospective study of several potential biologic markers for early prediction of the development of preeclampsia. *Am J Obstet Gynecol* 1993;169:501–508.

42. Jacobson SL, Imhof R, Manning N, et al. The value of Doppler assessment of the uteroplacental circulation in predicting preeclampsia or intrauterine growth retardation. *Am J Obstet Gynecol* 1990;162:110–114.
43. Paternoster DM, Stella A, Mussap M, et al. Predictive markers of pre-eclampsia in hypertensive disorders of pregnancy. *Int J Gynaecol Obstet* 1999;66:237–243.
44. Weerasekera DS, Peiris H. The significance of serum uric acid, creatinine and urinary microprotein levels in predicting pre-eclampsia. *J Obstet Gynaecol* 2003;23:17–19.
45. Conde-Agudelo A, Lede R, Belizan J. Evaluation of methods used in the prediction of hypertensive disorders of pregnancy. *Obstet Gynecol Surv* 1994;49:210–222.
46. Merviel P, Ba R, Beaufils M, et al. Lone hyperuricemia during pregnancy: maternal and fetal outcomes. *Eur J Obstet Gynecol Reprod Biol* 1998;77:145–150.
47. O'Brien WF. Predicting preeclampsia. *Obstet Gynecol* 1990;75:445–452.
48. Grunewald C. Biochemical prediction of pre-eclampsia. *Acta Obstet Gynecol Scand Suppl* 1997; 164:104–107.
49. Conde-Agudelo A, Belizan JM, Lede R, et al. Prediction of hypertensive disorders of pregnancy by calcium/creatinine ratio and other laboratory tests. *Int J Gynaecol Obstet* 1994; 7:285–286.

Fetal Hypoxia

Caterina M. Bilardo

Ahmet Alexander Baschat

Gerard H. A. Visser

■ What Is the Problem that Requires Screening?

Fetal hypoxia.

Fetal hypoxia is a general term defining oxygen deficiency in the fetal tissues. It is considered an ominous condition because decreased cellular oxygenation may impair fetal organ function and development. Hypoxemia is low blood oxygen (O_2) content. The risk of stillbirth and/or irreversible fetal damage increases when hypoxemia progresses to acidemia as the underlying disease process deteriorates beyond tolerability. As such, fetal hypoxemia is a predisease state whose severe and irreversible sequelae may be preventable by intervention.

What is the incidence/prevalence of the target condition?

Placental dysfunction, as a potential cause of fetal hypoxia, is a relatively common problem, affecting about one third of all cases of intra uterine growth restriction (IUGR) or about 3% of all pregnancies.[1,2] The prevalence of intrauterine hypoxia as a result of placental dysfunction varies from 50% to 80% of IUGR fetuses with absent end-diastolic flow in the umbilical artery.[3,4]

What are the sequelae of the condition that are of interest in clinical medicine?

Chronic hypoxemia may cause IUGR, stillbirth, and long-term neurodevelopmental, cardiovascular, and endocrine compromise.

Diagnosis of fetal hypoxia. There are two tools to directly diagnose fetal hypoxemia (and by inference tissue hypoxia). Beginning in the early 1980s, cordocentesis allowed the direct measurement of fetal blood gases under normal and pathological circumstances.[5] By this technique, it is possible to diagnose hypoxemia when the fetal pO_2 is more than 2 SDs below the normal range.[6] Fetal blood gas measurement at cordocentesis of normal fetuses revealed that similar to animals, the unperturbed human fetus grows and develops at a lower oxygen level than the mother.[6–8] Fetal pO_2 decreases progressively with advancing gestation, while O_2 is maintained by an increasing hemoglobin concentration.[2] The second direct method to diagnose fetal hypoxemia is to obtain a scalp sample during labor or an umbilical cord venous/arterial sample at birth. However, hypoxemia diagnosed at birth is not in itself related to neonatal mortality and morbidity.[9] It is the metabolic component of the fetal acidemia (base deficit and bicarbonate) that best predicts neonatal outcome.[9]

Several mechanisms may be responsible for the onset of fetal hypoxia:

1. Reduced placental perfusion due to impaired uteroplacental circulation. This leads to a progressive decrease in fetal arterial O_2 due to low pO_2 (hypoxemic hypoxia);
2. Reduced fetal arterial blood O_2 due to reduced oxygen carrying ability of fetal blood (low hemoglobin concentration = anemic hypoxemia) as in Rhesus isoimmunization or other causes of fetal anemia;
3. Reduced blood flow to the fetal tissues (ischemic hypoxia), as in the case of poor cardiac output, placental abruption, acute cord accident, or umbilical cord compression intrapartum.

Hypoxia from any cause leads to a conversion from aerobic to anaerobic metabolism, producing less energy and more lactate. The increasing lactate and progressive decrease in pH may lead to fetal death. Although we address the hypoxia secondary to placental dysfunction in this chapter, the basic physiology is similar regardless of the cause if present long enough for fetal adaptation to occur.

Pathophysiology of fetal hypoxia/acidemia. In mild placental dysfunction, the fetus compensates for intervillous hypoxia by increasing the fractional O_2 extraction. Only when uterine oxygen delivery falls below a critical value (0.6 mmol/min/kg in the ovine fetus) is fetal oxygen uptake and placental glucose transfer reduced.[10] Pancreatic insulin responses are blunted with the onset of fetal hypoglycemia, allowing gluconeogenesis from hepatic glycogen stores.[11–14] A proportion of the fetal glucose and lactate is used for placental nutrition. Since fetal hepatic glycogen stores are minimal, persistent or increasing nutrient deficit leads to worsening hypoglycemia, and the ability of the fetus to maintain oxidative metabolism and placental nutrition becomes limited. Down-regulation of active placental transport and the requirement that the fetus mobilize other energy sources has widespread metabolic consequences. Limitation of amino acid transfer depletes branched chain and other essential amino acids and triggers the breakdown of endogenous muscle protein for gluconeogenic aminoacids.[15–17] Simultaneously, lactate accumulates because of the limited capacity for oxidative metabolism.

Overall placental transfer capacity for fatty acids remains unaltered unless there is considerable loss of placental substance. However, transport mechanisms selectivity may suffer, especially those for essential fatty acids. Fetal free fatty acid and triglyceride levels rise due to reduced utilization. Consequently, there is a failure to accumulate adipose stores. In this setting of advanced malnutrition, the liver metabolizes most of the accumulating lactate, but the fetal brain and heart also switch their primary nutrient source from glucose to lactate and ketones.[18] Cardiac metabolism can remove up to 80% of the circulating fetal lactate.[19,20]

Acid-base balance is maintained as long as acid production is matched by sufficient buffering capacity of fetal hemoglobin and an adequate removal rate. Metabolic compromise progresses through degrees of severity that have been documented by umbilical blood sampling (cordocentesis) in human fetuses. Hypoglycemia and hypoxemia occurs first with decreased levels of essential amino acids. As placental dysfunction worsens, increasing hypoxemia and lactate production are exponentially related to the severity of the acidemia. Overt hypoaminoacidemia, hypercapnia, hyperlactic acidemia, and hypertriglyceridemia accompany the development of acidemia.[17,21–23] The glycine/valine ratio and the level of ammonia are increased in the amniotic fluid, providing additional markers of protein energy malnutrition.[24,25] Metabolic deterioration is associated with elevated transaminases suggestive of hepatic dysfunction and may be precipitated by a marked decline in umbilical venous blood flow to the liver secondary to excessive shunting at the level of the ductus venosus.[26,27] Fetuses who manifest IUGR in the third trimester are more likely to have less severe metabolic and acid-base disturbance and only subtle changes in lipid metabolism.[28]

Fetal hypoxia in the setting of placental dysfunction is commonly associated with iatrogenic preterm delivery of an IUGR newborn. Such perinates display variable degrees of the metabolic derangement. In response to a low pO_2, the fetus redistributes its circulation in such a way that the vital organs are preferentially perfused (brain, heart, adrenal gland) at the expense of less critical organs.[29]

The hemodynamic changes occurring in both chronically hypoxic animal and human fetuses, result in an asymmetric growth, whereby splanchnic and subcutaneous fat accumulation is reduced while cerebral development is relatively spared.[29] These compensatory/adaptive mechanisms allow the fetus to survive a hostile environment. The range of manifestations reflects the balance between compensatory and decompensatory responses. The consequences of nutrient shortage with successful compensation may remain largely subclinical, only to be unmasked by its restrictive effect on the normally exponential fetal growth in the second to third trimesters. In these instances, vascular manifestation can be less pronounced and physical characteristics more apparent. A decrease in adipose tissue or abnormal body proportions at birth may be the only evidence. The neonatal prognosis is usually favorable should the fetus reach a reasonable gestational age and delivery occur when the hypoxia is only marginal. However, compensatory mechanisms may prove inadequate or counterproductive should the placental dysfunction become pronounced and permanent fetal damage or stillbirth ensues. When the hypoxemia/acidemia is severe and the fetus delivered at very prematurely, the likelihood of neonatal death and long-term sequelae are high. Fetal acidemia and major neonatal complications have a major impact on subsequent neurodevelopment, while the combinations of fetal and neonatal deaths determine the overall perinatal mortality.[30] These fetuses are prone to multiorgan failure, intracranial hemorrhage, respiratory distress syndrome, necrotizing enterocolitis, bronchopulmonary dysplasia, clotting disorders, and disturbed endocrine homeostasis.[31–33] Long-term sequelae may be observed in infancy should the infant survive the early neonatal period. Suboptimal growth, reduced school performance, and concentration disturbances are common problems.[34] Research into the fetal origin of maternal disease has revealed a hostile intrauterine environment is associated with the development in adulthood of cardiovascular diseases and endocrine disturbances.[35]

The effects of fetal hypoxemia, placental dysfunction, and iatrogenic interventions are difficult to separate. It appears that fetal hypoxemia has few measurable effects. Possible explanations for the short- and long-term outcomes associated with progressive deterioration include the following. During fetal life, progression to acidemia is a stronger determinant of long-term neurodevelopmental outcome than the existence of hypoxia alone. The accompanying decompensation can have three important consequences. First, there may be irreversible fetal organ damage. Second, there may be a stillbirth or a preterm delivery as a result of the medical decision. Third, the neonate is at additional risk of complication once delivered. This risk is determined by liabilities that persist as a consequence of the fetal condition, the transition to extrauterine life and the gestational age related risk of complications. In summary, the sequelae that may arise from placental dysfunction are diverse as they extend from fetal life into adulthood.

■ The Tests

What is the purpose of the tests?

The purposes of the available tests are as follows:

1. To detect conditions predisposing to fetal hypoxia,
2. To detect the presence of fetal hypoxia and the fetal response to it.

What is the nature of the tests?

There is no single test used to screen for fetal hypoxemia. Effective detection requires a combination of tests that seek evidence of the fetal adaptive responses to hypoxemia. The tests available seek physical, cardiovascular, and behavioral manifestations of fetal hypoxemia utilizing various techniques of ultrasound. Two-dimensional (2D) ultrasound methods include fetal biometry, amniotic fluid quantification, and an evaluation of fetal activity (body and breathing movements). Color and pulsed Doppler techniques are used to evaluate the maternal and fetal circulations. Continuous wave Doppler is used to record the fetal heart rate pattern (cardiotocography [CTG]). Information derived from visual or computerized analysis with respect to baseline frequency, short- and long-term variability, and presence of decelerations and accelerations are differently related to the state of fetal oxygenation. The biophysical profile score (BPS) analyzes dynamic fetal variables (movement, tone, breathing movement, heart rate reactivity) and amniotic fluid volume.[36] The number and complexity of the screening and diagnostic techniques available for the prediction or diagnosis of fetal hypoxia require that they be addressed separately.

Screening for conditions predisposing to fetal hypoxia—fetal growth restriction. Fetal growth restriction (IUGR) is a physical sign rather than a singular disease (also see Chapters 29–32 for related information).

A wide range of conditions is associated with IUGR (Figure 37–1). In some, IUGR may be the only sign of the underlying condition, whereas in others, IUGR is accompanied by abnormalities in several organ systems. Infections and maternal diseases such as chronic renal disease, hypertension, collagen vascular disease and thrombophilia, and socioeconomic factors such as smoking, malnutrition and drug use are also commonly associated with IUGR, presumably by altering either placental function or development.

The many underlying etiologies and presentations of fetal growth restriction require the diagnostic approach be directed by information obtained from the maternal history as well as an evaluation of fetal, placental and amniotic fluid characteristics. The accurate identification of those fetuses truly at risk of

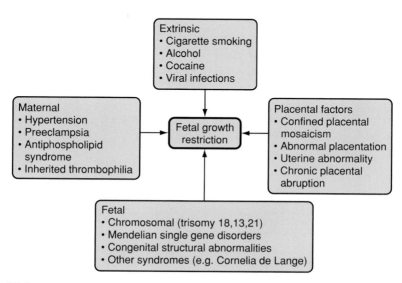

Figure 37-1 This figure shows the principle causes and most common conditions that are associated with fetal growth restriction.

hypoxemia and adverse outcome requires the exclusion of normoxic small fetuses who are otherwise normally grown, and those fetuses whose IUGR is due to an underlying condition not amenable to intervention even if associated with hypoxemia (Figure 37–2). Among the latter include aneuploidy (especially trisomies 18, 13, and 21), skeletal dysplasia, nonaneuploid syndromes and viral infection. Overall, fetal abnormalities (both chromosomal and/or anatomic) and abnormal placental vascular development in the fetal and/or maternal compartments are responsible for the vast majority of IUGR in singleton pregnancies.[37-41] Suspicion of suboptimal growth can be clinical (e.g., shorter than expected symphysis–fundal height) (see related material in Chapter 30), but the test with the highest accuracy and greatest ability to define the severity of growth restriction is fetal biometry by ultrasound investigation in the second/third trimester of pregnancy (see related material in Chapter 31).

■ The Test

Fetal 2D ultrasound examination.

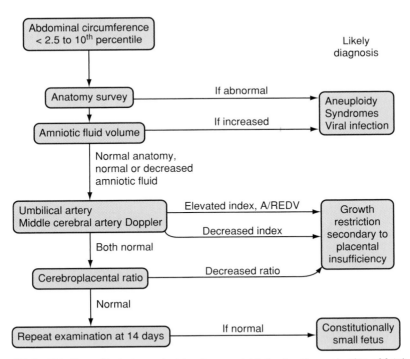

Figure 37–2   This figure illustrates a decision tree model following the evaluation of fetal anatomy, amniotic fluid volume, and umbilical and middle cerebral artery Doppler. The most likely clinical diagnosis is presented on the right-hand side. A high index of suspicion for aneuploidy, viral and nonaneuploid syndrome needs to be maintained. *IUGR*, intrauterine growth restriction.

What are the purposes of the tests?

To assess fetal growth by biometric measurements and to semiquantitate amniotic fluid volume.

What is the nature of the tests?

Two-dimensional ultrasound, usually performed using real-time equipment, can provide important information to diagnose IUGR, identify fetal anomalies and/or markers for aneuploidies, and inspect the placenta and assessment of amniotic fluid volume.

The diagnosis of suboptimal fetal growth requires accurate dating of the pregnancy (see related material in Chapter 20). An estimated date of confinement (EDC) is based on the last menstrual period when the sonographic estimate of gestational age is within the predictive error (typically 7 days in the first trimester, 10–11 days in the second trimester, and 21 days in the third trimester). Once the EDC is set, it should not be changed. It is important to use appropriate reference ranges derived from uncomplicated pregnancies delivered at term. Individualized reference ranges of growth potential that consider maternal, ethnic and fetal variables provide the most accurate reference.[42]

What are the implications of testing?

What does an abnormal test result mean? Biometric parameters below the fifth to tenth percentiles are generally considered to indicate suboptimal growth. Abdominal circumference (AC) reflects liver size, the major site of fetal glycogen storage. It is the single best measurement with the highest sensitivity and negative predictive value for the detection of IUGR.[43–45] Its sensitivity is further enhanced (up to 85%) by serial measurements at least 14 days apart (21 days in third trimester).[46] The most accurate AC is the smallest technically accurate directly measured circumference obtained at the level of the hepatic vein between fetal respirations.[47] Using a reference range based on healthy women delivering appropriately nourished neonates at term, an AC below the tenth percentile for gestational age is consistent with IUGR. The 2.5 percentile is more appropriate if tables derived from a cross-sectional population including small, appropriately grown, preterm, and term newborns are used.[48] Compared with the AC, the biparietal diameter, head circumference and transverse cerebellar diameters are poor tools for the detection of IUGR. This is in part due to the inherent physiologic variation in skull shape[49] and the relative sparing of head growth when there is placental dysfunction.[50] Concurrent measurement of the head circumference, AC, and femur length allows calculation of the sonographically estimated fetal weight. An estimated weight below the tenth percentile for gestation has a lower sensitivity than the AC (85% vs. 98%), but a higher positive predictive value (51% vs. 36%)[45] or IUGR.

It is important to establish the cause once the diagnosis of IUGR is made. The amniotic fluid volume should be assessed along with a complete fetal anatomic survey. Amniotic fluid volume in the late second to third trimester is primarily dependent on urine production. Placental dysfunction and fetal hypoxia may cause fetal oliguria and consequently oligohydramnios. However, the accuracy of ultrasound for the assessment of actual amniotic fluid volume is poor.[51] Further, amniotic fluid volume is a poor screening tool for the prediction of IUGR and fetal acidemia.[52,53] Nonetheless, an assessment of amniotic fluid volume by any method (four-quadrant Amniotic Fluid Index (AFI) and maximum vertical pocket), especially if performed serially, provides an important diagnostic as well as prognostic tool. In the setting of IUGR, excess amniotic fluid volume suggests the possibility of aneuploidy or fetal infection,[39] whereas normal or decreased amniotic fluid is compatible with placental dysfunction, aneuploidy, or infection. IUGR is likely to be placental-based when associated with normal fetal anatomy, normal or low amniotic fluid volume, a small AC measurement, an elevated umbilical artery (UA) Doppler index, and/or a decreased cerebroplacental (umbilical artery/cerebral artery [U/C] Doppler ratio (see below).[54–56] However, it is the combination of fetal biometry with Doppler that is best for the identification of the small fetus at risk for fetal hypoxia from placental dysfunction.[57–60] The complementary use of these two ultrasound imaging modalities is necessary whenever IUGR is suspected.

What does a normal test result mean? Fetal size above the tenth percentile associated with normal amniotic fluid all but eliminates the presence of IUGR at the time of the examination. Normal biometry does not exclude the possibility that IUGR may develop in the future (see Doppler).

What is the cost of the test?

The cost of testing is that of a fetal scan: about 30 minutes for biometry and a complete anatomic survey. The cost of ultrasound equipment varies with the sophistication from € 30,000 to € 150,000. Personnel costs vary according to the educational level of the operator (ultrasonographer, midwife, or medical staff).

Placental dysfunction. Placental ysfunction (insufficiency) is the primary condition predisposing to fetal hypoxia. The term dysfunction recognizes there may be single gene disorders that interfere with transport of nutritional factors but not respiratory gas exchange. Understanding the importance of gestational epochs allows insight into how placental dysfunction may manifest.

Pathophysiology of uteroplacental dysfunction: In the first trimester, the cytotrophoblast migrates to form anchoring sites and establish placental adherence to the decidua. Subsequent vascular connections between the

maternal circulation and the intervillous space are established through angiogenesis. From this point on, nutrient and oxygen delivery are sufficient to meet the demands of the growing trophoblast and the embryo.[61,62] Increasing synthetic activity results in the appearance of several secretory products in the maternal circulation (e.g., human chorionic gonadotrophin and placental lactogen). At a placental level, several paracrine signaling substances appear (e.g., nitric oxide, endothelin, myometrial quiescent factor). Active cellular transport systems for major nutrient classes (glucose, amino acids, and fatty acids) differentiate. The villous trophoblast provides a nutrient-exchange interface and consists of a maternal microvillus and fetal basal layer.[63] The onset of fetal cardiac activity allows the active distribution of substances between fetus and placenta and completes the functionality of the fetoplacental unit. Oxygen and nutrients are taken up and distributed to the fetus via the umbilical vein. By the second trimester, trophoblast invasion into the maternal spiral arteries results in a progressive loss of musculoelastic media, first in the decidual, then the myometrial portions of these vessels.[64] There is progressive thinning of the villous trophoblast down to 4 μm by the 16th week and a rapid increase in villous surface area until 26 weeks.[65] Concurrently, intermediary and terminal villi form in the fetal compartment as the main sites of exchange.[66] An exponential rise in fetal cardiac output elevates villous blood flow and increases the capacity for fetal substrate uptake. As a result of these developments, high-capacitance–low-resistance vascular compartments are established on both sides of the placenta.[67-70] The placenta grows significantly in size along a sigmoid growth curve. Nutrient transport capacity rises sufficiently to promote an exponential fetal growth spurt and differentiation of organ systems.

The third trimester is characterized by ongoing organ differentiation. The increase in fetal size is typically due to longitudinal growth plus the accumulation of essential body stores. These stores serve as a nutrient reservoir during neonatal life, when food intake may provide inconstant amounts of essential substrate. For example, the relative amount of fetal body fat increases to almost 20% of body weight in the third trimester. This fat provides essential fatty acids necessary for the maintenance of myelination and retinal function.[71,72]

Mechanisms of placental dysfunction: The precise mechanisms by which specific diseases affect placental function are still under investigation. In *maternal hypertensive disorders*, increased syncytial knot formation suggests premature placental aging and apoptosis. Occlusive vasculopathy, which is most pronounced in women with *antiphospholipid syndromes*, affects the maternal and fetal placental circulations.

Placental causes may decrease placental blood flow, or alter transport mechanisms and cellular homeostasis at the placental level. Of the possible etiologies, conditions that interfere with placental vascular development account most pregnancies complicated by IUGR.[73] Suboptimal maternal adaptation to pregnancy early in the first trimester coupled with deficient nutrient delivery pose limitations at all levels of placental function. If the trophoblast invasion remains confined to the decidual portion of the myometrium, maternal spiral and radial arteries fail to undergo the physiologic transformation into low resistance vessels.[74–76] Defective trophoblastic invasion[77] and inadequate maternal vascular response to placentation may both lead to IUGR.[74] The local balance of production of vasoactive substances is impaired leading to vasospasm in the small arterioles of the uteroplacental compartment as well as of other systemic vascular beds. An abnormal increase in the systemic vasopressor response impairs maternal renal function and increases total peripheral resistance.[78] Activated or injured endothelial cells lose their ability to maintain vascular integrity, causing increased vascular permeability, platelet thrombosis, and increased vascular tone. This further aggravates the vasospasm in the small arterioles of the uteroplacental compartment as well as other systemic vascular beds.[79] Subsequent damage to the vascular wall promotes an atherosis-like occlusive process in the small arteries.[80–83] With progressive vascular occlusion, fetoplacental flow resistance is increased throughout the vascular bed and eventually, the metabolically active placental mass is reduced. With progression of disease, local placental ischemia and necrosis occurs.

■ The Test

Doppler investigation of the maternal circulation.

What is the purpose of the tests?

To identify pregnancies at risk of placental dysfunction, IUGR. and hypoxia.

What is the nature of the tests?

Doppler ultrasound allows for the noninvasive study of blood flow through the uteroplacental and fetal circulations[84] (see related material in Chapter 32). In this instance, we focus on the uterine artery. Most techniques use combined color and pulsed Doppler investigation measure uterine artery flow above the level where it crosses the external iliac artery. The sample gate is placed in the vessel lumen, and a continuous, low-resistance arterial flow pattern recorded. Normal ranges for angle-independent parameters of Doppler measurement of uterine artery resistance are published. Investigations are performed as early as in the late first trimester, at 20 weeks, or at 22 to 24 weeks. Systolic-to-diastolic ratio (S/D), resistance index (RI), pulsatility index (PI), and presence of early diastolic notch are used alone or in combination to establish a normal uteroplacental circulation. The impedance to flow in the uterine arteries decreases with gestation in normal pregnancy, reflecting the trophoblastic invasion of the spiral arteries and their conversion in low-resistance vessels. Defective or delayed trophoblastic invasion can be suspected as early as 12 to 14 weeks when there is an early, diastolic notch in the Doppler waveform. Persistence of high-resistance flow patterns and "notching" beyond 24 weeks is consistent with failure of normal physiologic adaptation to pregnancy.[76,85,86]

What are the implications of testing?

What does an abnormal test result mean? Increased impedance in the uterine arteries is associated with an increased risk of the subsequent development of preeclampsia, IUGR, and perinatal death. S/D ratios above 2.18 at 18 weeks, RI above 0.58 at 18 to 24 weeks, PI above the 95th centile at 22 to 24 weeks, or the presence of notches have all been defined as abnormal. Screen positive rate varies from 5% to 13% according to the gestation and the criterion used. In women with increased uterine artery impedance, the positive likelihood ratio (LR[pos]) for the subsequent development of preeclampsia approximates 6.[87] Abnormal uterine artery Doppler is a better predictor of severe than mild disease.[88,89] The LR[pos] of abnormal uterine artery impedance for the development of IUGR is 3.7.[87] The sensitivity is also higher for severe early-onset than for late-onset IUGR. The data on the prediction of intrauterine death are limited and vary considerably in sensitivity. Pooled estimates suggest the LR[pos] for subsequent fetal or perinatal death in women with increased impedance to flow in the uterine arteries is 2.4. First-trimester studies confirm the trend found in the second trimester, although their sensitivities are even lower. Yet, the theoretic advantage of earlier identification is the potential of enhancing the efficacy of prophylactic interventions.[89,90]

What does a normal test result mean? A normal test result has a high negative predictive value for subsequent IUGR and preeclampsia. Women with normal impedance to flow in the uterine arteries have a negative likelihood ratio (LR[neg]) of 0.5 and 0.8 for the development of preeclampsia and IUGR, respectively. The LR[neg] ratio of a normal result for perinatal death was 0.8.[87]

What is the cost of the test?

The cost is moderate, as it requires an additional 5 to 10 minutes scanning time during the routine fetal ultrasound examination. It is unlikely a pathologic uterine artery flow pattern identified at 20 to 24 weeks will normalize; study repetition is therefore unnecessary.

Screening for fetal hypoxemia.

Doppler investigations. There are two nonexclusive study sites: (a) the umbilical and fetal arterial circulation and (b) the fetal central venous circulation. Fetal circulatory responses to placental dysfunction can be subdivided into early and late.[91,92]

Early Doppler changes: Reduced umbilical venous blood flow volume[93] and increased multigate-measured placental blood flow resistance[94] are the earliest Doppler signs of disturbed fetal villous perfusion. Umbilical artery end-diastolic velocity decreases and the Doppler resistance indices increase when some 30% of the fetal villous vessels are abnormal.[95] Absent or even reversal of umbilical artery end-diastolic velocity may occur when 60% to 70% of the villous vascular tree has been damaged.[96] Increasing abnormal umbilical flows indicate increased risk of hypoxemia and acidemia proportional to the severity of the Doppler abnormality.[97,98] The initial circulatory responses are in part passive and due to the effects of placental afterload on the distribution of fetal cardiac output and in part due to active organ autoregulation. Elevated placental blood flow resistance increases right ventricular afterload. Due to the parallel arrangement of the fetal circulation, this shifts cardiac output away from the right side of the heart. The result is a relative increase in left-sided cardiac output.[99,100] Consequently, blood (and nutrient) supply to the upper part of the body by the left ventricle increases. The ratio of Doppler indices in umbilical and cerebral arteries (cerebroplacental Doppler ratio [U/C]) declines because of this redistribution of cardiac output.[101] In addition, cerebral blood flow can be enhanced during periods of perceived hypoxemia by an endothelium mediated decrease in cerebral blood flow resistance, which manifests as a decrease in the Doppler index of the cerebral vessels ("brain sparing").[102] Fetuses who show these early Doppler changes are at increased risk of hypoxemia, whereas the pH is usually in the normal range.[103–105] Concurrently, blood flow resistance in peripheral pulmonary arteries,[106] celiac axis,[107] mesenteric vessels,[108,109] renal,[110,111] and femoral and iliac arteries[112] may be elevated. Individual vital organs such as the adrenal glands[113] and spleen[114] may show enhanced blood flow. The overall impact of these adaptations is the distribution of well-oxygenated blood to the heart and brain and preferential streaming of descending aortic blood flow to the placenta for reoxygenation. Such circulatory abnormalities are associated with elevations of endothelin, vasoactive intestinal peptide, vasopressin, and renin-angiotensin levels.[115–117] A decrease in the thromboxane to prostacyclin ratio provides additional evidence of endothelial dysfunction, while elevations in NO production may indicate a compensatory response.[118,119]

Late Doppler changes generally accompany further metabolic deterioration and reflect declining forward cardiac function and aberrant organ autoregulation. Increasing venous Doppler indices are the hallmark of advancing circulatory deterioration since they document the inability of the heart to accommodate venous return.[120] The venous flow velocity waveform is triphasic, and consists of systolic and diastolic peaks (the S- and D-wave, respectively) that are generated by the descent of the atrioventricular (AV) ring during ventricular systole and passive diastolic ventricular filling, respectively. The sudden increase in right atrial pressure with atrial contraction in late diastole causes a variable amount of reverse flow producing a second trough after the D wave (the a-wave). In extreme cases, atrial pressure waves may be transmitted all the way back into the free umbilical vein producing pulsatile flow At this stage, ductus venosus shunting away from the liver can compromise hepatic perfusion and impairs organ function. Marked increases in blood lactate and transaminases, as well as sudden compensatory hepatic artery vasodilatation as a secondary source of hepatic blood flow, are reported under these conditions.[26,27,121]

When the increased metabolic demands of cardiac work cannot be met, myocardial dysfunction occurs. A rise in atrial natriuretic peptide (ANP) concurrent with the elevation in venous Doppler indices is probably a compensatory mechanism to regulate blood volume.[122,123] When forward cardiac function declines past a gestational age-dependent minimum, coronary vasodilatation becomes exaggerated in an effort to recruit all the available coronary blood flow reserve.[124] If this fails to support myocardial nutrition sufficiently, the cardiac dysfunction becomes critical and the downward spiral toward death begins. Cardiac dilatation with holosystolic tricuspid regurgitation and loss of cerebral autoregulation (normalizing cerebral Doppler indices) are indicative of a loss of cardiovascular homeostasis.[125] If the fetus remains undelivered, spontaneous late decelerations of the fetal heart rate and stillbirth ensue.[126,127]

■ The Tests

Doppler studies of the fetal arterial system.

What is the purpose of the tests?

To assess the severity of placental dysfunction for diagnostic and prognostic prediction of fetal compromise.

What is the nature of the tests?

The most common test used in clinical practice to identify fetal compromise secondary to placental dysfunction is a Doppler study of the umbilical artery flow velocity profile. A free umbilical cord loop far from the fetal and placental insertions is interrogated by continuous or pulsed Doppler ultrasound. Most current ultrasound equipment allows concurrent use of color and pulsed Doppler ultrasound techniques. Waveform analysis includes classifying end-diastolic velocity into positive, absent, or reversed. Angle independent indices are used for clinical Doppler waveform analysis. Of these, the PI offers the advantage of a smaller measurement error, narrower reference limits and the possibility of ongoing numerical analysis even when end-diastolic velocity is absent.[128,129] Serial measurements are recommended as intrafetal variation may be misleading. Only serial investigations can confirm deterioration trends.

Another index frequently used is the U/C ratio between umbilical artery PI as index of vasoconstriction in the placenta and the middle cerebral artery PI (MCAPI) as an index of vasodilation in the fetal brain ("brain sparing" in reaction to falling pO_2 levels). Abnormal umbilical artery flow alone or in combination with Doppler evidence of brain sparing is observed in fetuses who are found to be hypoxemic at cordocentesis.[4,62,98,117]

What are the implications of testing?

What does an abnormal test mean? An abnormal test result is defined as an umbilical artery angle independent index above the 95th percentile or either absent or reduced end-diastolic velocity flow. The neonatal mortality rate in such fetuses is 5% to 18% when the venous Doppler indices are normal. However, randomized trials and meta-analyses each conclude that the use of umbilical artery Doppler in suspected IUGR results in a considerable reduction in perinatal mortality and iatrogenic intervention, since documentation of placental vascular insufficiency effectively separates constitutionally small fetuses from those who might benefit from intervention (e.g., delivery).[130–132]

In observational studies, the relationship between abnormal Doppler velocimetry and perinatal death is very strong.[133] A systematic review from the Cochrane database included 11 randomized trials.[55] The use of Doppler ultrasound in high-risk pregnancies to assess umbilical artery waveforms (without controlling for the clinical response) was associated with a 29% reduction in overall perinatal mortality; the 95% confidence interval ranged from "no effect" to a 50% reduction of perinatal mortality. Although no individual index of perinatal mortality revealed a statistically significant effect, each suggested a reduction. The integration of Doppler ultrasound appears to reduce the likelihood of an antepartum hospital admission and of elective cesarean delivery or induction of labor. Another critical appraisal of umbilical artery Doppler in high-risk pregnancies was recently published.[56] Thirteen randomized controlled trials (RCTs) were identified using Medline, Embase, and the Cochrane Library. Of these, six studies included pregnancies with well-defined suspected IUGR and/or hypertensive disease of pregnancy. In contrast, the remaining seven included a wide variety of high-risk pregnancies (general-risk studies). The well-defined studies revealed a marked reduction in antenatal hospital admission (odds ratio [OR], 0.56; confidence interval [CI], 0.43–0.72), induction of labor (OR, 0.56; CI, 0.73–0.96), elective delivery (OR, 0.73; CI, 0.61–0.88) and cesarean delivery (OR, 0.78; CI, 0.65–0.94). It was determined at audit that more perinatal deaths in the well-defined studies were avoided if Doppler velocimetry was used (rate of avoidable deaths in controls 50% vs. 20% in study group, $p<0.0005$). In fetuses with IUGR due to placental dysfunction presenting before 34 weeks' gestation, the umbilical artery Doppler waveform is frequently abnormal. However, after this gestational age the umbilical artery Doppler waveform may be normal with hypoxemia present. At the same time, cerebral artery Doppler responses to placental dysfunction still occur.[59,134] Since the relationship between placental and cerebral blood flow resistance remains altered under these circumstances, the U/C ratio may be abnormal in fetuses with mild placental disease.[57,135] After 34 weeks' gestation, a decrease in either the middle cerebral artery Doppler index or the U/C ratio should heighten one's suspicion for IUGR even if the umbilical artery blood flow is normal. Once the sonographic diagnosis of IUGR is confirmed, close surveillance of the fetus should be instituted based on the severity of the maternal and/or fetal condition

What does a normal test result mean? A normal test result means that the IUGR is not the result of clinically detectable poor placentation, and fetal hypoxemia can effectively be excluded.[98]

■ The Tests

Doppler investigation of the fetal venous circulation.

Venous Doppler changes appear at a late stage in the process of fetal deterioration. Abnormalities in the umbilical artery and in the central and cerebral arterial fetal circulation can persist for weeks while venous flows remain in the normal range.[92]

What does an abnormal test result mean? A pathologic venous flow (increased pulsatility index for veins (PIV), absent/reverse flow during the a-wave) (Figure 37–3) is indicative of cardiac decompensation and is typical of severe early IUGR (<30–32 weeks). Abnormal venous flows can appear 1 to 2 weeks before the appearance of abnormal fetal heart rate tracings that traditionally prompt fetal delivery.[88,92,137] Longitudinal studies indicate that about 40% of IUGR fetuses who deteriorate in utero have an increased diastolic velocity Doppler index the week before delivery. On the day of delivery, an additional 20% deteriorate further.[89,91] Elevation of venous Doppler indices, either alone, or in combination with umbilical venous pulsations, increases the risk of fetal hypoxia and acidemia.[117,120] Depending on the cutoff used (2 vs. 3 SDs) and the combinations of veins examined, the sensitivity of venous Doppler for the prediction of fetal acidemia ranges from 70% to 90%, and the specificity from 70% to 80%.[136]

The relationship between venous Doppler abnormalities and perinatal outcomes is very important for clinical management. Longitudinal changes in venous Doppler parameters are related to perinatal mortality and morbidity in the form of bronchopulmonary dysplasia (BPD) and severe intraventricular hemorrhage (IVH).[137] Bilardo et al. observed that the prevalence of adverse perinatal outcome in fetuses ($n = 33$) with severe early onset IUGR prior to 30 weeks was 45%, and the perinatal mortality was 36%. The chance of an adverse outcome was increased threefold when the diastolic velocity PI for the veins value was more than 2 SDs at 2 to 7 days before delivery, and 11-fold when the PI for the veins deteriorated to above 3 SDs on the day preceding delivery.

Prediction of stillbirth.

Abnormal venous Doppler parameters are the strongest peripheral Doppler predictors of stillbirth. Even among fetuses with severe arterial Doppler abnormalities (e.g., absent/reversed umbilical artery end-diastolic velocity), the risk of stillbirth is largely confined to those fetuses with abnormal venous Doppler findings. The likelihood of stillbirth increases proportionally with the

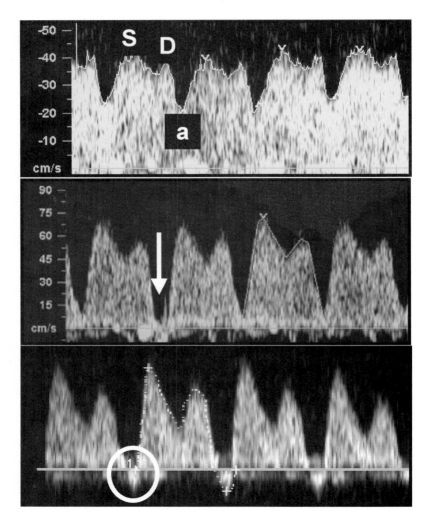

Figure 37-3 Changes in the ductus venosus waveform from positive, to absent. To reverse flow during the a-wave.

degree of venous Doppler abnormality. Venous Doppler findings that are particularly ominous include absence or reversal of the ductus venous a-wave and biphasic/triphasic umbilical venous pulsations. These Doppler findings have 65% sensitivity and 95% specificity for the prediction of stillbirth in a population of preterm severe IUGR fetuses with a 25% stillbirth rate.[138]

Prediction of neonatal mortality.

Neonatal mortality is determined by multiple factors including gestation at delivery and the occurrence and severity of neonatal complications.

An increase in the diastolic velocity Doppler index doubles the mortality rate, although the sensitivity is only 38% in this setting (specificity 98%).[138] Whereas abnormal venous Doppler is associated with a higher rate of postnatal complications, gestational age at delivery has the strongest impact on the overall mortality.[54]

Prediction of neonatal complications.

Gestational age at delivery is the primary determinant of neonatal complications, such as RDS, BPD, and IVH, followed by the degree of IUGR.[54] Advanced fetal circulatory compromise with an abnormal diastolic velocity waveform may have additional impacts, particularly on cardiovascular stability in the neonatal period. Because of the multiple relevant variables, prediction of neonatal outcomes remains difficult. Elevations in compromised fetuses of troponin I, S100B protein levels, and transaminases all provide evidence of ongoing cellular damage in the myocardium, brain, and liver.[139–141] An increased risk of necrotizing enterocolitis in survivors has been attributed to bowel injury secondary to chronic underperfusion.[142]

What does a normal test result mean? The finding of normal diastolic velocity flow at an early gestation means that any placental dysfunction has not yet reached its critical phase. Later in gestation (i.e., >32 weeks), the prevalence of abnormal diastolic velocity flow is lower. Fetal heart rate abnormalities often prompt delivery at this stage before the occurrence of abnormal venous flow.[92,137]

Fetal behavioral responses.

Fetal behavioral responses are related to neurodevelopmental status and the impact of ambient oxygen tension on the central regulation of fetal behaviors. Under normal circumstances, successive fulfillment of behavioral milestones progresses from the initiation of gross body movements and fetal breathing, to coupling of fetal behavior (e.g., heart rate reactivity) and integration of rest–activity cycles into stable behavioral states. These developments are accompanied by a steady decrease in the fetal heart rate baseline (due to rising vagal tone) and increasing short- and long-term variability and variation (reflecting progressive central processing). These milestones are generally completed by 32 weeks when heart rate reactivity by traditional criteria is present in 80% of fetuses. Fetal behavioral responses to placental dysfunction can also be subdivided into early and late. Early changes are due predominantly to delay in the central integration of fetal behaviors and can be characterized by less vigorous fetal movements, delayed acquisition of stable behavioral states, abnormal transition between behavioral states or delayed development of coupling. Detection of these alterations requires sophisticated examination methods. Late changes are readily apparent on ultrasound. They consist of the sequential loss of biophysical variables and are typically due to the impact of declining acid-base balance on central regulatory centers. Fetal breathing ceases with increasing hypoxemia; gross body movements and tone decrease further and are finally lost as acidemia deepens.[143]

■ The Tests

Fetal heart rate continuous recording cardiotocogram (CTG).

Characteristics of the fetal heart rate (FHR) are determined by autonomic control mechanisms superimposed on intrinsic cardiac activity and the modulating effects of oxygen on their central regulatory centers. Successful maturation of these connections is associated with decreasing baseline heart rate, increasing heart rate variability and variation, coupling between episodic accelerations with fetal movement, and the superimposed impact of behavioral states. This level of central integration of fetal heart rate characteristics with fetal behavior is normally accomplished by 28 weeks of gestation.[144]

Visual FHR analysis was traditionally the method of choice creating problems of inter- and intraobserver variability. These problems can be circumvented by computerized analysis of the fetal heart rate (computerized CTG [cCTG]). In addition to the baseline heart rate and the frequency of accelerations and decelerations, the cCTG assesses parameters not amenable to visual analysis, which include short-term, long-term, and mean minute variation, as well as periods of high variation. It remains to be determined how the application of computerized interpretations changes clinical outcomes.

Chronically hypoxic IUGR fetuses are delayed in all aspects of central nervous system (CNS) maturation, which probably relates to altered myelination as well changes in central neurotransmitter availability.[145–149] The delayed development of behavioral milestones and their central integration with fetal heart rate are primary determinants of lower short- and long-term variation (on computerized analysis), and delayed development of heart rate reactivity that is observed in IUGR fetuses.[147,150–153] Despite the maturational delay of some aspects of CNS function, several centrally regulated responses to acid-base status are preserved.

What is the purpose of the tests?

To identify fetal hypoxemia (and/or acidemia).

What is the nature of the tests?

Fetal heart rate is recorded across the maternal abdomen using phono, ultrasound, or electrocardiogram (ECG) techniques. Ultrasound is currently the method of choice. Beat-to-beat intervals are measured and transformed into heart rate and depicted continuously on a paper channel recorder (at 1- to 3-cm/min) together with contraction information using an external tocodynameter.

The following aspects of the FHR tracing are assessed:

- Baseline
- Accelerations (i.e., periodic increases in rate usually associated with fetal movements, exceeding 15 bpm for at least 15 seconds).
- Heart rate variability: This is the bandwidth of the range over a defined period of time, excluding accelerations and decelerations.
- Decelerations: Periodic falls in heart rate, either shallow with reduced variability and following contractions (late decelerations) or variable in onset and return (variable deceleration).

The assessment of FHR tracings must consider gestational age, because FHR variation and the incidence and size of decelerations and accelerations are dependent on it. Moreover, fetal rest–activity cycles develop over time, which affects the FHR pattern.[147]

The FHR tracing is completely flat before 16 weeks.[154] Large heart rate decelerations can occur between 16 and 26 weeks, and decelerations are more numerous than accelerations before 30 weeks. Thereafter, this relationship is reversed, although decelerations following accelerations remain common during normal pregnancy near term.[155,156] During the third trimester, heart rate accelerations increase in number and size, and from about 35 weeks onward, normal fetuses exhibit accelerations above 15 bpm above baseline. However, accelerations of this size are not a consistent phenomenon before this age.[156,157] The use of amplitude above 10 bpm is often used at earlier gestational ages and may be as predictive.[158–161]

The FHR pattern is also affected by a progressive patterning of the heart rate into episodes of low and high heart rate variation. From 27 weeks' gestation onward, these patterns are related to the fetal rest–activity cycles.[157] In the preterm fetus, the median length of a consecutive low and high variation episode is 12.5 minutes.[162,163] After 36 weeks, the median length of a consecutive low- and high-variation episode increases to 80 minutes, whereas the mean length of the low variation episode increases to about 20 minutes (range, 6–40 minutes).[157,164–166] These findings suggest that "nonreactive" heart rate patterns of up to 30 minutes before 36 weeks or 40 minutes near term are normal findings in uncomplicated pregnancies. They reflect quiet sleep and explain why the fetus does not react to external stimuli like shaking of the maternal abdomen.[167]

It is now possible to analyze the antenatal FHR pattern using a computer.[156] This should provide objectivity and reproducibility, considering the inter- and intraobserver variation associated with visual analysis. However, gestational age, time of the day, presence of fetal rest–activity cycles, and duration of recordings should still be taken into account. Between 24 and 40 weeks, there is a curvilinear increase in long-term and short-term FHR variation (median values of the latter increasing from 6.2 to 9.2 milliseconds).[166] The lower limit of the normal range increases until 30 weeks, and remains more or less stable thereafter. Due to the development of fetal rest–activity cycles, the minimal recording time necessary to reliably assess FHR and its variation is at least 30 minutes before 34 weeks and at least 40 minutes thereafter. The lower limits of the normal range are strongly dependent on the recording length. There are wide normal ranges for fetal heart rate and its variation, but the individual fetus shows a certain consistency throughout gestation. Each fetus should be used as its own control for the monitoring of trends, using recordings of standardized duration and appropriate reference ranges.[147] The effects of medication on the FHR pattern must be kept in mind. For example, betamethasone causes a temporary decrease in the FHR variability on days 2 and 3 after the first injection, together with a 50% reduction in fetal body movements and an almost cessation of fetal breathing movements.[168]

What does an abnormal test result mean? Certain abnormalities of the FHR are thought to reflect fetal hypoxemia—a reduction of FHR variation below the normal range and the occurrence of late and or severe variable heart rate decelerations.[160,169,170] There is a direct correlation between FHR variation assessed numerically and pO_2 in the umbilical vein when the sample is obtained at cordocentesis or after cesarean delivery.[151,152] FHR variation usually decreases gradually during the weeks preceding the appearance of late decelerations (and fetal hypoxemia).[187] Longitudinal FHR recordings may, therefore, indicate a gradual deterioration of the fetal condition, even before the onset of hypoxemia. However, a single recording cannot identify the small fetus at risk of developing hypoxemia since the FHR variation is still within the normal range. This indicates that antenatal FHR monitoring is not a useful screening test and should only be applied longitudinally in high-risk populations. The best indication for serial FHR monitoring is the IUGR fetus with abnormal Doppler waveform patterns, in whom hypoxemia is likely.

Hypoxemia does not mean acidemia. The fetal pH is usually normal when first FHR abnormalities first appear.[169,171] Only with a further flattering of the trace and after the appearance of shallow late decelerations ("terminal" FHR trace) does acidemia develop.[172] In IUGR fetuses, the interval between the first abnormal Doppler finding and the onset of FHR abnormalities/hypoxia varies greatly. The interval is shorter in late than in early gestation and shorter in IUGR complicated by preeclampsia.[173–175] It appears that the small fetus in early gestation tolerates reduced placental function for a longer period than the larger IUGR fetus can in later pregnancy-an observation consistent with the higher oxygen requirements. These findings suggest that the deterioration of the placental function in preeclampsia occurs more rapidly than in IUGR fetuses without preeclampsia. The clinical implication of these observations is that once Doppler waveforms become abnormal, FHR monitoring should be carried out more frequently after 30 weeks and in all cases complicated by preeclampsia.

What does a normal test result mean? A normal test result (i.e., "reactive" FHR tracing with two or more accelerations [> 10 bpm and duration > 15 seconds] in a period of less than 30 minutes before 32 weeks or after 36 weeks two or more accelerations [> 15 bpm and duration > 15 seconds] in a period of less than 40 minutes and no decelerations) indicates adequate oxygen for central receptor function at the moment of the FHR recording. It does not mean normal oxygenation. The predictive value of a normal test result depends on the underlying disease process. In instances of acute complications such as partial placental abruption or thrombosis (preeclampsia), oxygenation may be acutely reduced by the worsening of disease shortly after a normal test result.

What is the cost of testing?

An antenatal FHR monitor costs about € 15,000 and can be used for more than 5 years. The major incremental costs are those for personnel. A FHR recording in a high-risk woman will last on average 40 minutes, of which approximately 15 minutes requires the presence of a health care worker to deliver the equipment, establish a satisfying recording, discontinue the recording and interpret the tracing.

Fetal movement.

Fetal movement and tone are the first embryonic activities initiated in the first trimester. Initially, fetal activity is almost constant; eventually, it develops into rest–activity cycles that become integrated into behavioral states. In anatomically normal fetuses, there are three principal reasons for fetal movement to be absent. The most common explanation is the physiologic variation that reflects gestational age and behavioral state. The second reason is maternal administration of centrally active agents such as opiates, magnesium, or diazepam. From the perspective of antenatal surveillance, the third cause, loss of fetal movement due to acidemia is the most important clinically. Fetal movements are generally lost at a mean UA pH of 7.20.[188] It should be borne in mind that an umbilical artery pH should be above 7.32 at term in the non-laboring pregnancy.

Fetal movement is a fundamental biophysical variable perceived by the mother at a gestational age relevant for obstetric intervention (i.e., viability). It has been used for antenatal surveillance in two ways. First, it is part of the five component biophysical profile score. Second, maternal counting of fetal movement (so called "kick counts") forms the simplest form of fetal surveillance as it solely relies on the cooperation and ability of the woman to perceive and record fetal movement.

What is the purpose of the test?

Identify the hypoxemic/acidemic fetus and prevent fetal death.

What is the nature of the test?

Fetal movements may be counted by the pregnant woman, who records the time required to complete ten movements. Alternatively, the number of perceived movements per hour is recorded. The routine recommendation for

women to count fetal movements daily during late pregnancy for the prevention of fetal death has been the subject of several large series.[176,177] Formal, routine movement counting does not prevent antepartum death. In these studies,
most of the fetuses who died antenatally were already dead by the time the
women received medical attention despite the formalized counting policy.
Moreover, there is a high false-positive rate (reduced movements, normal clinical findings), which implies the unnecessary use of considerable resources.

Longitudinal observations of fetal movements in IUGR fetuses by ultrasound
have shown that the frequency of body movements and breathing decline after
FHR abnormalities occur.[143] Body movements decrease gradually, whereas
breathing decreases rather suddenly. The latter change coincides with further
deterioration of the heart rate pattern. The gradual reduction in body movements
may be considered as a sign of fetal adaptation. In these fetuses, FHR variation
decreases gradually until it reaches the lower limit of the normal range, when the
fetuses are likely to be hypoxemic. Thereafter, FHR variation usually remains
constant over a certain period of time, and the frequency of body movements
falls. In other words, it seems likely that the reduction in fetal movements may
contribute to the relative stability of the fetal pO_2 until a further reduction can no
longer contribute. FHR variation declines further; body and breathing movements disappear, and the fetus becomes progressively hypoxemic and acidemic.

What does an abnormal test result mean? Doubling of the time to complete
ten movements or a halving of the number of movements perceived is defined
as an abnormal test result that requires further evaluation[178] From subjective
recordings of fetal body movements kept by pregnant women, it is known that
the movements decline rather suddenly just before fetal death, and that the frequency of movements beforehand is within the normal range.[179,180] This suggests that any dramatic reduction in the quantity of fetal body movements is a
late sign of fetal impairment.

An abnormal test result can fall within physiologic variation or reflect worsening acid-base status. The next step is fetal heart rate recording. As noted above,
there are many false-positive findings with formal movement counting. Reduced
movements during (prolonged) ultrasound recording are more likely to be associated with fetal hypoxemia/acidemia. Alternatively, reduced movements may be
due to medication (betamethasone), congenital malformations (neuromuscular
diseases), or a prolonged episode of "quiet" sleep. Fetal heart rate monitoring and
ultrasound assessment will usually clarify the underlying fetal condition/problem.

What does a normal test result mean? If the mother performs the tests well, a
normal kick count essentially excludes acidemia at the time of the test.

What is the cost of testing?

No direct medical costs are incurred by the test, but the cost of false-positive
tests is likely substantial.

The biophysical profile score.

What is the nature of the test?

The biophysical profile score consists of five components used to quantify fetal behavior by assessing tone, movement, breathing activity, and fetal heart rate reactivity. Amniotic fluid volume assessment is the fifth component. In the second trimester, amniotic fluid production primarily reflects fetal urine production and thus renal perfusion. Through its relationship with vascular status, amniotic fluid volume assessment is the main longitudinal monitoring component of the biophysical profile score (BPS) and accordingly has a higher weight in the overall grading of the score. The BPS is a composite measure applying categorical cutoffs for fetal tone, breathing movement, gross body movement, amniotic fluid volume, and traditional fetal heart rate analysis. The fetal observation period is typically 30 minutes after a 30-minute fetal heart rate tracing. This time interval reflects physiologic variation in fetal behavior. However, the time necessary to complete the test is variable. In rapid eye movement (REM) sleep, all activities are typically observed within 4 minutes, whereas in quiet sleep, this may take up to 26 minutes.[36] If the test is abnormal (score <6) after 30 minutes, the observation is extended to 1 hour. If no other factors can be identified and the test remains abnormal, delivery is recommended.

The association between a reduction in the quantity of movements and (impending) acidemia has been confirmed in studies where occurrence of body and breathing movements was documented sonographically and correlated to blood gas levels and pH at cordocentesis.[181,182] Studies of the BPS have also revealed that changes in the FHR pattern and amniotic fluid volume occur first and that a reduction in movement is a later sign of impairment. The BPS (with three of the five items being related to fetal movements) relates to the UV pH at cordocentesis, but not with the umbilical vein (UV) pO_2, suggesting that movements decrease only with the beginning of acidemia.[181,183] During and after acute hypoxemic events (late FHR decelerations), both body and breathing movements are reduced temporarily,[184] and increase after maternal hyperoxygenation compared to baseline values.[185] These observations again suggest that movements are affected by fetal hypoxemia. The gradual fall in general body movements, as observed with progressive deterioration of the fetal condition, is in line with this hypothesis, but cannot explain the late and rather sudden fall in breathing movements. Experiments in fetal sheep resolve this apparent controversy: breathing activity decreases markedly with acute hypoxemia, but gradually reappears as the hypoxemia becomes chronic.[186]

What does an abnormal test result mean? A BPS of less than 6 suggests fetal acidemia.

Chronic hypoxemia is associated with a decline in global fetal activity.[187] If the severity of hypoxemia increases, fetal breathing, gross body movements, and tone decrease further and are generally lost when acidemia develops. Progressive deterioration of acid-base and vascular status is accompanied by a progressive decline in amniotic fluid volume. Similarly, worsening hypoxemia triggers a decrease in fetal heart rate variation and variability, as well as the onset deceler-ations.[183,188] The decline of the biophysical variables is determined by the central effects of hypoxemia/acidemia independent of the cardiovascular status.[143,189–191] A BPS of less than 6 is associated with a mean pH less than 7.20 (absent labor); the sensitivity of a BPS less than 4 for the prediction of acidemia is 100%.

The five-component BPS has a reliable and reproducible relationship with the fetal pH irrespective of the underlying pathology and gestational age.[181] Because IUGR fetuses preserve their central responses to acid-base status despite their maturational delay, the close relationship between the BPS and arterial pH is maintained in the second half of pregnancy. When the relation-ship between the various testing modalities and fetal acid base status is com-pared, biophysical parameters show a closer relationship with the pH while Doppler parameters have a wider variance (Figure 37–4).

A systematic review of four RCTs concluded there were no differences in the fetal and neonatal outcomes of high-risk pregnancies monitored by BPS testing versus other forms of fetal assessment.[192] The authors conclude that, at the moment, there is not enough evidence to recommend routine use of the BPS as a test of fetal well-being in high-risk pregnancies.

What does a normal test result mean? A BPS of above 6 in the presence of normal amniotic fluid volume excludes hypoxemia and acidemia at the time of testing. However, an abnormal BPS occurs late compared with pathologic Doppler changes in IUGR fetuses. Deterioration of the BPS often occurs rap-idly, making it a poor choice for the prediction of stillbirth unless performed daily.

What is the cost of testing?

The equipment and personnel costs for the BPS include a traditional CTG machine, and a simple grey scale ultrasound machine is sufficient to perform the score. The BPS can be performed by trained nurses and midwives and thus circumvents physician costs. However, testing may be time consuming. Depending on the clinical scenario (nonreactive CTG, abnormal score after 30 minutes), the test may take 90 minutes to reach a conclusion.

■ Conclusions and Recommendations

All antenatal tests of fetal well-being seek to identify fetal hypoxemia. Screen-ing for fetal hypoxemia is a complex issue requiring the integration of infor-mation originating from different assessment modalities.

Antenatal surveillance in IUGR pregnancies due to placental dysfunction must be longitudinal with each fetus as its own control. The assessment fre-quency is tailored to the severity of the condition and includes fetal biometry, amniotic fluid evaluation, Doppler assessment of the fetal arterial and venous

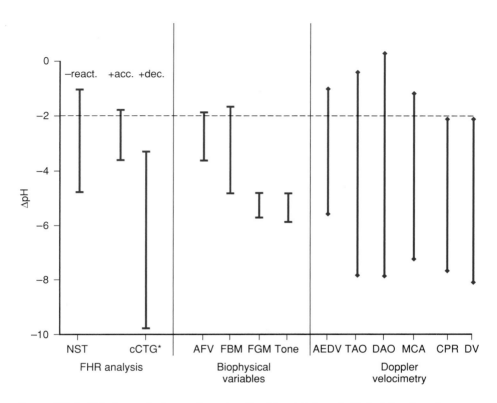

Figure 37-4 This figure displays a diagrammatic representation of pH deviation from the gestational age mean (ΔpH) with abnormal test results in various antenatal tests. These include fetal heart rate (FHR) analysis using traditional nonstress testing (NST; –react = nonreactive) and the computerized cardiotocogram (cCTG; +acc = accelerations present, +dec = obvious decelerations present). Biophysical variables (AFV, amniotic fluid volume; FBM, fetal body movement; FGM, fetal gross movement). The same relationships are expressed for umbilical artery absent end-diastolic velocity (AEDV) and deviation of the arterial or venous Doppler index more than 2 SD from the gestational age mean for the thoracic aorta (TAO), descending aorta (DAO) the middle cerebral artery (MCA), cerebroplacental ratio (CPR) and the ductus venosus (DV). Reproduced with permission from Baschat AA. Integrated fetal testing in growth restriction: combining multivessel Doppler and biophysical parameters. *Ultrasound Obstet Gynecol* 2003;21:1–8.

circulation, FHR monitoring and evaluation of fetal movements and tone. The modalities are complementary.

The two main therapeutic interventions in IUGR pregnancies are the administration of prenatal corticosteroids and delivery. The administration of a completed course of corticosteroids is recommended until 34 weeks' gestation. IUGR fetuses do not derive a maturation benefit from intrauterine stress. Delivery is indicated when the risk of fetal acidemia and/or stillbirth is high (Figure 37–5). Before 30 weeks, delivery is indicated when the ductus venosus Doppler index increases beyond 3 SDs above the mean. Other indicators include the

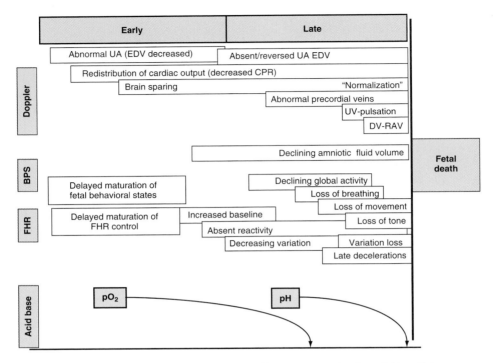

Figure 37-5   This figure summarizes the early and late responses to placental insufficiency. Doppler variables in the placental circulation precede abnormality in the cerebral circulation. Biophysical parameters (BPSs) are still normal at this time and computerized analysis of fetal behavioral patterns is necessary to document a developmental delay. With progression to late responses venous Doppler abnormality in the fetal circulation is characteristic often preceding the sequential loss of fetal dynamic variables and frequently accompanying the decline in amniotic fluid volume. The * in the ductus venosus flow velocity waveform marks reversal of blood flow during atrial systole (a-wave). The decline in biophysical variables shows a reproducible relationship with acid-base status. If adaptation mechanisms fail, stillbirth ensues.

absence of movements, anhydramnios, and fetal heart rate variation below 3.5 milliseconds or repetitive shallow FHR deceleration. After 30 weeks, the clinician may choose to deliver the fetus when umbilical artery velocimetry is severely abnormal or whenever important CTG abnormalities are present. At any gestational age, it is unlikely that clinical decisions can be based on an abnormality of a single monitoring parameter; usually, the vast majority of parameters follow the same deterioration trends.

The single most important variable to critically influence the clinical decision of when to deliver the IUGR fetus is gestational age. An ongoing study of over 300 antenatally identified IUGR fetuses with elevated placental blood flow resistances delivered before 32 weeks suggests the effect of gestational age overshadows all other perinatal variables until 27 weeks, when survival and intact survival in this high-risk cohort first exceed 50% (personal communication Ahmet A. Baschat, September 2005). Intact survival was observed in 80% of fetuses delivered after 29 weeks of gestation, suggesting that this gestational epoch is the time to individualize intervention thresholds. The conclusion of the TRUFFLE study (**Tr**ial of **U**mbilical and **F**etal **Fl**ow in **E**urope) will hopefully clarify whether delivery triggered by arterial Doppler versus computerized fetal heart rate analysis has a measurable impact on outcome. Ongoing efforts are needed to refine our understanding of the relationship between fetal testing variables, intervention, and outcomes. Modification of neonatal management based on prenatally available information of fetal status is an almost unexplored avenue to improve outcome.

■ Summary

1 ■ What Is the Problem that Requires Screening?
Fetal hypoxemia and conditions predisposing to it.

a. *What is the incidence/prevalence of the target condition?*
Placental dysfunction, as a potential cause of fetal hypoxemia, affects about one third of all cases of IUGR and about 3% of all pregnancies.

b. *What are the sequelae of the condition that are of interest in clinical medicine?*
Chronic hypoxemia may cause IUGR, stillbirth, and long-term neurodevelopmental, cardiovascular and endocrine compromise.

2 ■ The Tests
a. *What is the purpose of the tests?*
To detect the presence of fetal hypoxemia or conditions predisposing to fetal hypoxia

b. *What is the nature of the tests?*
There is no single screening test for the detection of fetal hypoxemia. Effective detection requires a combination of tests that focus on fetal adaptive responses to hypoxemia. These include fetal biometry, Doppler velocimetry of maternal and

Continued

■ **Summary—cont'd**

fetal vessels, fetal heart rate testing, fetal kick counts, biophysical profile testing. These tests are intended to detect both hypoxemia and the conditions predisposing fetal hypoxia such as IUGR and placental dysfunction.

c. What are the implications of testing?

1. What does an abnormal test result mean?

An abdominal circumference below the 2.5 percentile (reference ranges based on a mixed group of high- and low-risk pregnancies) or below the tenth percentile (reference ranges based on normal pregnancies only) is the most sensitive biometric parameter to detect IUGR. An abnormal screening test usually triggers the performance of diagnostic tests. Abnormal Doppler velocimetry combining fetal umbilical and middle cerebral arteries plus venous flow determinations are the most sensitive tool for the identification of fetal hypoxia and acidemia. It is the combination of fetal biometry with Doppler that is the best available tool for the identification of the small fetus at risk of fetal hypoxia from placental dysfunction. The complementary use of these two ultrasound imaging modalities is necessary whenever IUGR is suspected.

2. What does a normal test result mean?

A normal test, whether it is fetal heart rate testing, Doppler, or biophysical profile testing suggests the fetus is unlikely to die within 7 days.

d. What is the cost of testing?

Antenatal testing has not been studied from a cost-benefit perspective.

3 ■ Conclusions and Recommendations

The combination of a small abdominal circumference, normal anatomy, low or normal amniotic fluid volume, and abnormal umbilical artery Doppler is strongly suggestive of IUGR due to placental dysfunction. The amniotic fluid volume alone is a poor screening tool for IUGR and acidemia, but could be an important prognostic tool once the diagnosis of IUGR is made. The possibility of aneuploidy, syndromes, and viral infection should always be considered and fetal karyotyping should be offered.

Umbilical artery Doppler is the best first choice method to evaluate the fetal compartment of the placental circulation. Fetal cardiovascular and behavioral deterioration follows a relatively predictable pattern progressing from early to late changes. Direction of surveillance and intervention is inaccurate if based on umbilical artery Doppler alone. Examination of the cerebral and venous circulation is mandatory if umbilical artery Doppler is abnormal and if Doppler is chosen as the primary management tool. For arterial vessels, the Pulsatility Index offers the narrowest reference limits and measurement error. Multiple venous Doppler indices have been described without clear advantage. The monitoring intervals are shortened with progressive cardiovascular compromise. Once delivery becomes imminent, antenatal steroids should be administered if < 34 weeks' gestation. Delivery should be performed when there is strong evidence of fetal acidemia and/or impending stillbirth. Ductus venosus index escalation beyond 3 SDs above the mean or absence or reversal of the a-wave are strong evidence. Corroborating evidence from biophysical and computerized heart rate analysis should be sought whenever possible.

Antenatal FHR monitoring is not a useful screening test and should only be applied longitudinally in high-risk populations. The best indication for serial FHR monitoring is the IUGR fetus with abnormal Doppler waveform patterns, in whom hypoxemia is likely.

Fetal kick counts are a poor screening tool for the prediction of IUGR and fetal acidemia. Late changes in fetal behavior response to placental dysfunction are, however, apparent at ultrasound. Fetal breathing ceases with increasing hypoxemia; gross body movements and tone decrease further and are finally lost as acidemia deepens. There is not enough evidence presently to recommend routine use of the biophysical profile score compared with other discussed modalities as a test of fetal well-being in high-risk pregnancies.

References

1. Kupferminc MJ, Peri H, Zwang E, et al. High prevalence of the prothrombin gene mutation in women with intrauterine growth retardation, abruptio placentae and second trimester loss. *Acta Obstet Gynecol Scand* 2000;79:963–967.
2. Weiner CP. Pathogenesis, evaluation, and potential treatments for severe, early onset growth retardation. *Semin Perinatol* 1989;13:320.
3. Nicolaides KH, Bilardo CM, Soothill P, et al. Absence of end diastolic frequencies in umbilical artery: a sign of fetal hypoxia and acidosis. *BMJ* 1988,209:1026–1027.
4. Bilardo CM, Nicolaides KH, Campbell S. Doppler measurements of fetal and uteroplacental circulations: relationship with umbilical venous blood gases measured at cordocentesis. *Am J Obstet Gynecol* 1990;162:115–120.
5. Nicolaides KH, Soothill PW, Campbell S. Ultrasound guided sampling of umbilical cord and placental blood to assess fetal well-being. *Lancet* 1986:1065–1067.
6. Soothill PW, Nicolaides KH, Rodeck CH, et al. Effects of gestational age on fetal and intervillous blood gas and acid-base values in human pregnancy. *Fetal Ther* 1986;1:168–170.
7. Wilkening RB, Meschia G. comparative physiology of placental oxygen transport. *Placenta* 1992;13:11–15.
8. Soothill PW, Nicolaides KH, Campbell S. Prenatal asphyxia, hyperlacticaemia, hypoglycaemia, and erythroblastosis in growth retarded fetuses. *BMJ* 1987;294:1051–1053.
9. Andres RL, Saade G, Gilstrap LC, et al. Association between umbilical blood gas parameters and neonatal morbidity and death in neonatates with pathological fetal academia. *Am J Obstet Gynecol* 1999;181:867–871.
10. Jones CT, Ritchie JW, Walker D. The effects of hypoxia on glucose turnover in the fetal sheep. *J Dev Physiol* 1983;5:223–235.
11. Nicolini U, Hubinont C, Santolaya J, et al. Maternal-fetal glucose gradient in normal pregnancies and in pregnancies complicated by alloimmunization and fetal growth retardation. *Am J Obstet Gynecol* 1989;161:924–927.
12. Economides DL, Nicolaides KH. Blood glucose and oxygen tension levels in small-for-gestational-age fetuses. *Am J Obstet Gynecol* 1989;160:385–389.
13. Hubinont C, Nicolini U, Fisk NM, et al. Endocrine pancreatic function in growth-retarded fetuses. *Obstet Gynecol* 1991;77:541–544.
14. Van Assche FA, Aerts L, DePrins FA. The fetal endocrine pancreas. *Eur J Obstet Gynecol Reprod Biol* 1984;18:267–272.
15. Cetin I, Marconi AM, Corbetta C, et al. Fetal amino acids in normal pregnancies and in pregnancies complicated by intrauterine growth retardation. *Early Hum Dev* 1992;29:183–186.
16. Cetin I, Corbetta C, Sereni LP, et al. Umbilical amino acid concentrations in normal and growth-retarded fetuses sampled in utero by cordocentesis. *Am J Obstet Gynecol* 1990;162:253–261.
17. Economides DL, Nicolaides KH, Campbell S. Metabolic and endocrine findings in appropriate and small for gestational age fetuses. *J Perinat Med* 1991;19:97–105.
18. Vannucci RC, Vannucci SJ. Glucose metabolism in the developing brain. *Semin Perinatol* 2000;24:107–115.
19. Fisher DJ, Heymann MA, Rudolph AM. Fetal myocardial oxygen and carbohydrate consumption during acutely induced hypoxemia. *Am J Physiol* 1982;242:H657–H661.
20. Spahr R, Probst I, Piper HM. Substrate utilization of adult cardiac myocytes. *Basic Res Cardiol* 1985;80[Suppl 1]:53–56.
21. Pardi G, Cetin I, Marconi AM, Lanfranchi A, Bozzetti P, Ferrazzi E, Buscaglia M. Diagnostic value of blood sampling in fetuses with growth retardation. *N Engl J Med* 1993;328:692–696.
22. Owens JA, Falconer J, Robinsin JS. Effect of restriction of placental growth on fetal uteroplacental metabolism. *J Dev Physiol* 1987;9:225–238.
23. Paolini CL, Marconi AM, Ronzoni S, et al. Placental transport of leucine, phenylalanine, glycine, and proline in intrauterine growth-restricted pregnancies. *J Clin Endocrinol Metab* 2001;86:5427–5432.

24. Wolfe HM, Sokol RJ, Dombrowski MP, et al. Increased neonatal urinary ammonia: a marker for in utero caloric deprivation? *Am J Perinatol* 1989;6:4–7.
25. Bernstein IM, Silver R, Nair KS, et al. Amniotic fluid glycine-valine ratio and neonatal morbidity in fetal growth restriction. *Obstet Gynecol* 1997;90:933–937
26. Roberts A, Nava S, Bocconi L, et al. Liver function tests and glucose and lipid metabolism in growth-restricted fetuses. *Obstet Gynecol* 1999;94:290–294.
27. Battaglia FC. Clinical studies linking fetal velocimetry, blood flow and placental transport in pregnancies complicated by intrauterine growth retardation (IUGR). *Trans Am Clin Climatol Assoc* 2003;114:305–313.
28. Spencer JA, Chang TC, Crook D, et al. Third trimester fetal growth and measures of carbohydrate and lipid metabolism in umbilical venous blood at term. *Arch Dis Child Fetal Neonatal Ed* 1997;76:F21–5.
29. Peeters LLH, Sheldon RH, Jones MD, et al. Blood flow to fetal organs as function of arterial oxygen content. *Am J Obstet Gynecol* 1979;135:637–646.
30. Soothill PW, Ajayi RA, Campbell S, et al. Relationship between fetal acidemia at cordocentesis and subsequent neurodevelopment. *Ultrasound Obstet Gynecol* 1992;2:80–83.
31. Ley D, Wide-Swensson D, Lindroth M, et al. Respiratory distress syndrome in infants with impaired intrauterine growth. *Acta Paediatr* 1997;10:1090–1096.
32. Spinillo A, Capuzzo E, Piazzi G, et al. Significance of low birthweight for gestational age among very preterm infants. *Br J Obstet Gynaecol* 1997;104:668–673.
33. Aucott SW, Donohue PK, Northington FJ. Increased morbidity in severe early intrauterine growth restriction. *J Perinatol* 2004;24:435–440.
34. Ley D, Tideman E, Laurin J, et al. Abnormal fetal aortic velocity waveform and intellectual function at 7 years of age. *Ultrasound Obstet Gynecol* 1996;8:160–165.
35. Barker DJ. Fetal growth and adult disease. *Br J Obstet Gynaecol* 1992;99:275–276.
36. Manning FA. Fetal biophysical profile. *Obstet Gynecol Clin North Am* 1999;26:557–577.
37. Snijders RJM, Sherrod C, Gosden CM, et al. Fetal growth retardation:Associated malformations and chromosome abnormalities. *Am J Obstet Gynecol* 1993;168:547–555.
38. Khoury MJ, Erickson D, Cordero JE, et al. Congenital malformations and intrauterine growth retardation: a population study. *Pediatrics* 1988;82:83–90.
39. Sickler GK, Nyberg DA, Sohaey R, et al. Polyhydramnios and fetal intrauterine growth restriction: Ominous combination. *J Ultrasound Med* 1997;16:609–614.
40. Odegard RA, Vatten LJ, Nilsen ST, et al. Preeclampsia and fetal growth. *Obstet Gynecol* 2000;96: 950–955.
41. Kupferminc MJ, Peri H, Zwang E, et al. High prevalence of the prothrombin gene mutation in women with intrauterine growth retardation, abruptio placentae and second trimester loss. *Acta Obstet Gynecol Scand* 2000;79:963–967.
42. Bukowski R. Fetal growth potential and pregnancy outcome. *Semin Perinatol* 2004;28:51–58.
43. Sabbagha RE. Intrauterine growth retardation, In: Sabbagha RE, ed. *Diagnostic Ultrasound applied to Obstetrics and Gynecology,* 2nd ed. Phildelphia: JB Lippincott, 1987:112–131.
44. Tamura RK, Sabbagha RE. Percentile ranks of sonar fetal abdominal circumference measurements. *Am J Obstet Gynecol* 1980;138:475–479.
45. Baschat AA, Weiner CP. Umbilical artery Doppler screening for detection of the small fetus in need of antepartum surveillance. *Am J Obstet Gynecol* 2000;182:154–158.
46. Divon MY, Chamberlain PF, Sipos L, et al. Identification of the small for gestational age fetus with the use of gestational age-independent indices of fetal growth. *Am J Obstet Gynecol* 1986; 155:1197–1201.
47. Tamura RK, Sabbagha RE, Pan WH, et al. Ultrasonic fetal abdominal circumference: comparison of direct versus calculated measurement. *Obstet Gynecol* 1986;67:833–835.
48. Weiner CP, Robinson D. The sonographic diagnosis of intrauterine growth retardation using the postnatal ponderal index and the crown heel length as standards of diagnosis. *Am J Perinatol* 1989;6:380–383.
49. Hadlock FP, Deter RL, Carpenter RJ, et al. Estimating fetal age: effect of head shape on BPD. *Am J Roentgenol* 1981;137:83–85.

50. Smith PA, Johansson D, Tzannatos C, et al. Prenatal measurement of the fetal cerebellum and cisterna cerebellomedullaris by ultrasound. *Prenat Diagn* 1986;6:133–141.

51. Magann EF, Chauhan SP, Barrilleaux PS, et al. Amniotic fluid index and single deepest pocket: weak indicators of abnormal amniotic volumes. *Obstet Gynecol* 2000;96:737–740.

52. Chamberlain PF, Manning FA, Morrison I, et al. Ultrasound evaluation of amniotic fluid volume, I: the relationship of marginal and decreased amniotic fluid volumes to perinatal outcome. *Am J Obstet Gynecol* 1984;150:245–249.

53. Chauhan SP, Sanderson M, Hendrix NW, et al. Perinatal outcome and amniotic fluid index in the antepartum and intrapartum periods: a meta-analysis. *Am J Obstet Gynecol* 1999;181:1473–1478.

54. McCowan LM, Harding JE, Roberts AB, et al. A pilot randomized controlled trial of two regimens of fetal surveillance for small-for-gestational age fetuses with normal results of umbilical artery Doppler velocimetry. *Am J Obstet Gynecol* 2000;182:81–86.

55. Neilson JP, Alfirevic Z. Doppler ultrasound for fetal assessment in high risk pregnancies (Cochrane review). In: The Cochrane Library, Issue 1,2002. Oxford: Update Software.

56. Westergaard HB, Langhoff-Roos J, Lingman G, et al. A critical appraisal of the use of umbilical artery Doppler ultrasound in high-risk pregnancies: use of meta-analyses in evidence-based obstetrics. *Ultrasound Obstet Gynecol* 2001;17:466–476

57. Ott WJ. Intrauterine growth restriction and Doppler ultrasonography. *J Ultrasound Med* 2000;19:661–665.

58. Strigini FA, De Luca G, Lencioni G, et al. Middle cerebral artery velocimetry: different clinical relevance depending on umbilical velocimetry. *Obstet Gynecol* 1997;90:953–957.

59. Hecher K, Spernol R, Stettner H, et al. Potential for diagnosing imminent risk for appropriate- and small for gestational fetuses by Doppler examination of umbilical and cerebral arterial blood flow. *Ultrasound Obstet Gynecol* 1995;5:247–255.

60. Severi FM, Bocchi C, Visentin A, et al. Uterine and fetal cerebral Doppler predict the outcome of third-trimester small-for-gestational age fetuses with normal umbilical artery Doppler. *Ultrasound Obstet Gynecol* 2002;19:225–228

61. Aplin J. Maternal influences on placental development. *Semin Cell Dev Biol* 2000;11:115–125.

62. Pardi G, Marconi AM, Cetin I. Placental-fetal interrelationship in IUGR fetuses: a review. *Placenta* 2002;23[Suppl A]:S136–S141.

63. Kaufmann P, Scheffen I. Placental development. In: Polin RA Fox WW, eds. *Fetal and Neonatal Physiology*. Philadelphia: WB Saunders, 1998:59–70.

64. Pijnenborg R, Bland JM, Robertson WB, et al. Uteroplacental arterial changes related to interstitial trophoblast migration in early human pregnancy. *Placenta* 1983;4:397–413.

65. Kingdom JC, Burrell SJ, Kaufmann P. Pathology and clinical implications of abnormal umbilical artery Doppler waveforms. *Ultrasound Obstet Gynecol* 1997;9:271–286.

66. Castellucci M, Kosanke G, Verdenelli F, et al. Villous sprouting: fundamental mechanisms of human placental development. *Hum Reprod Update* 2000;6:485–494.

67. Maini CL, Rosati P, Galli G, et al. Non-invasive radioisotopic evaluation of placental blood flow. *Gynecol Obstet Invest* 1985;19:196–206.

68. Molteni RA, Stys SJ, Battaglia FC. Relationship of fetal and placental weight in human beings: fetal/placental weight ratios at various gestational ages and birth weight distributions. *J Reprod Med* 1978;21:327–334.

69. Heinonen S, Taipale P, Saarikoski S. Weights of placentae from small-for-gestational age infants revisited. *Placenta* 2001;22:399–404.

70. Luckhardt M, Leiser R, Kingdom J, et al. Effect of physiologic perfusion-fixation on the morphometrically evaluated dimensions of the term placental cotyledon. *J Soc Gynecol Investig* 1996;3:166–171.

71. White DR, Widdowson EM, Woodard HQ, et al. The composition of body tissues, II: fetus to young adult. *Br J Radiol* 1991;64:149–159.

72. Ziegler EE, O'Donnell AM, Nelson SE, et al. Body composition of the reference fetus. *Growth* 1976;40:329–341.

73. Kingdom J, Huppertz B, Seaward G, et al. Development of the placental villous tree and its consequences for fetal growth. *Eur J Obstet Gynecol Reprod Biol* 2000;92:35–43.

74. Brosens I, Robertson WB, Dixon HG. The physiology response of the vessels of the placental bed to normal pregnancy. *J Pathol Bacteriol* 1967;93:569–579.

75. Brosens I, Dixon HG, Robertson WB. Fetal growth retardation and the arteries of the placental bed. *Br J Obstet Gynaecol* 1977;84:656–663.

76. Meekins JW, Pijnenborg R, Hanssens M, et al. A study of placental bed spiral arteries and trophoblast invasion in normal and severe pre-eclamptic pregnancies. *Br J Obstet Gynaecol* 1994;101:669–674.

77. Khong TY, Mott C. Immunohystologic demonstration of endothelial disruption in acute atherosis in preeclampsia. *Eur J Obstet Gynecol Reprod Biol* 1993;51:193–197

78. Granger JP, Alexander BT, Llinas MT, et al. Pathophysiology of hypertension during preeclampsia linking placental ischemia with endothelial dysfunction. *Hypertension* 2001;38:718–722.

79. Roberts JM, Lain KY. Recent insights into the pathogenesis of pre-eclampsia. *Placenta* 2002;23:359–372.

80. Aardema MW, Oosterhof H, Timmer A, et al. Uterine artery Doppler flow and uteroplacental vascular pathology in normal pregnancies and pregnancies complicated by pre-eclampsia and small for gestational age fetuses. *Placenta* 2001;22:405–411.

81. Ferrazzi E, Bulfamante G, Mezzopane R, et al. Uterine Doppler velocimetry and placental hypoxic-ischaemic lesion in pregnancies with fetal intrauterine growth restriction. *Placenta* 1999;20:389–394.

82. Sebire NJ, Talbert D. The role of intraplacental vascular smooth muscle in the dynamic placenta: a conceptual framework for understanding uteroplacental disease. *Med Hypoth* 2002;58:347–351.

83. Kingdom JC, McQueen J, Connell JM, et al. Fetal angiotensin II levels and vascular (type I) angiotensin receptors in pregnancies complicated by intrauterine growth retardation. *Br J Obstet Gynaecol* 1993;100:476–482.

84. Campbell S, Diaz-Recasens J,Griffin DR, et al. New Doppler technique for assessing uteroplacental blood flow. *Lancet* 1983;26:675–677.

85. Harrington K, Carpenter RG, Goldfrad C, et al. Transvaginal Doppler ultrasound of the uteroplacental circulation in the early prediction of pre-eclampsia and intrauterine growth retardation. *Br J Obstet Gynaecol* 1997;104:674–681.

86. Giles WB, Trudinger BJ, Baird PJ. Fetal umbilical artery flow velocity waveforms and placental resistance: pathological correlation. *Br J Obstet Gynaecol* 1985;92:31–38.

87. Papageorghiou A, Yu CKH, Nicolaides KH. The role of uterine artery Doppler in predicting adverse pregnancy outcome. *Best Pract Res Clin Obstet Gynaecol* 2004;18:383–396.

88. Steel A, Pearce JM, McParland P, et al. Early Doppler ultrasound screening in prediction of hypertensive disorders of pregnancy. *Lancet* 1990;335:1548–1551.

89. Papageorghiou A, Yu CKH, Bindra R, et al. Multicenter screening for pre-eclampsia and fetal growth restriction by transvaginal uterine Doppler artery at 23 weeks of gestation. *Ultrasound Obstet Gynecol* 2001;18:441–449.

90. Martin AM, Bindra R, Curcio P, et al. Screening for pre-eclampsia and fetal growth restriction by uterine artery Doppler at 11-14 weeks of gestation. *Ultrasound Obstet Gynecol* 2001;18:583–586.

91. Ferrazzi E, Bozzo M, Rigano S, et al. Temporal sequence of abnormal Doppler changes in the peripheral and central circulatory systems of the severely growth-restricted fetus. *Ultrasound Obstet Gynecol* 2002;19:140–146.

92. Hecher K, Bilardo CM, Stigter RH, et al. Monitoring of fetuses with intrauterine growth restriction: a longitudinal study. *Ultrasound Obstet Gynecol* 2001;18:564–570.

93. Rigano S, Bozzo M, Ferrazzi E, et al. Early and persistent reduction in umbilical vein blood flow in the growth-restricted fetus: a longitudinal study. *Am J Obstet Gynecol* 2001;185:834–838.

94. Yagel S, Anteby EY, Shen O, et al. Placental blood flow measured by simultaneous multigate spectral Doppler imaging in pregnancies complicated by placental vascular abnormalities. *Ultrasound Obstet Gynecol* 1999;14:262–266.

95. Giles WB, Trudinger BJ, Baird PJ. Fetal umbilical artery flow velocity waveforms and placental resistance: pathological correlation. *Br J Obstet Gynaecol* 1985;92:31–38.

96. Morrow RJ, Adamson SL, Bull SB, et al. Effect of placental embolization on the umbilical artery velocity waveform in fetal sheep. *Am J Obstet Gynecol* 1989;161:1055–1060.

97. Weiner CP. The relationship between the umbilical artery systolic/diastolic ratio and umbilical blood gas measurements in specimens obtained by cordocentesis. *Am J Obstet Gynecol* 1990;162:1198–1202.

98. Bilardo CM, Snijders RM, Campbell S, et al. Doppler study of the fetal circulation during long-term maternal hyperoxygenation for severe early onset intra-uterine growth retardation. *Ultrasound ObstetGynecol* 1991;1:250–257.

99. Al Ghazali W, Chita SK, Chapman MG, et al. Evidence of redistribution of cardiac output in asymmetrical growth retardation. *Br J Obstet Gynaecol* 1987;96:697–704.

100. Reed KL, Anderson CF., Shenker L. Changes in intracardiac Doppler flow velocities in fetuses with absent umbilical artery diastolic flow. *Am J Obstet Gynecol* 1987;157:774–779.

101. Gramellini D, Folli MC, Raboni S, et al. Cerebral-umbilical Doppler ratio as a predictor of adverse perinatal outcome. *Obstet Gynecol* 1992;79:416–420.

102. Wladimiroff JW, Tonge HM, Stewart PA. Doppler ultrasound assessment of cerebral blood flow in the human fetus. *Br J Obstet Gynaecol* 1986;93:471–475.

103. Akalin-Sel T, Nicolaides KH, Peacock J, et al. Doppler dynamics and their complex interrelation with fetal oxygen pressure, carbon dioxide pressure, and pH in growth-retarded fetuses. *Obstet Gynecol* 1994;84:439–444.

104. Arbeille P, Maulik D, Fignon A, et al. Assessment of the fetal PO2 changes by cerebral and umbilical Doppler on lamb fetuses during acute hypoxia. *Ultrasound Med Biol* 1995;21:861–870.

105. Baschat AA. Integrated fetal testing in growth restriction: combining multivessel Doppler and biophysical parameters. *Ultrasound Obstet Gynecol* 2003;21:1–8.

106. Rizzo G, Capponi A, Chaoui R, et al. Blood flow velocity waveforms from peripheral pulmonary arteries in normally grown and growth-retarded fetuses. *Ultrasound Obstet Gynecol* 1996;8:87–92.

107. Gamsu HR, Vyas S, Nicolaides K. Effects of intrauterine growth retardation on postnatal visceral and cerebral blood flow velocity. *Arch Dis Child* 1991;66:1115–1118.

108. Mari G, Abuhamad AZ, Uerpairojkit B, et al. Blood flow velocity waveforms of the abdominal arteries in appropriate- and small-for-gestational-age fetuses. *Ultrasound Obstet Gynecol* 1995;6:15–18.

109. Rhee E, Detti L, Mari G. Superior mesenteric artery flow velocity waveforms in small for gestational age fetuses. *J Matern Fetal Med* 1998;7:120–123.

110. Veille JC, Kanaan C. Duplex Doppler ultrasonographic evaluation of the fetal renal artery in normal and abnormal fetuses. *Am J Obstet Gynecol*. 1989;161:1502–1507.

111. Arduini D, Rizzo G. Fetal renal artery velocity waveforms and amniotic fluid volume in growth-retarded and post-term fetuses. *Obstet Gynecol* 1991;77:370–373.

112. Mari G. Arterial blood flow velocity waveforms of the pelvis and lower extremities in normal and growth-retarded fetuses. *Am J Obstet Gynecol* 1991;165:143–151.

113. Tekay A, Jouppila P. Fetal adrenal artery velocimetry measurements in appropriate-for-gestational age and intrauterine growth-restricted fetuses. *Ultrasound Obstet Gynecol* 2000;16:419–424.

114. Abuhamad AZ, Mari G, Bogdan D, et al. Doppler flow velocimetry of the splenic artery in the human fetus: is it a marker of chronic hypoxia? *Am J Obstet Gynecol* 1995;172:820–825.

115. Karsdorp VH, Dekker GA, Bast A, et al. Maternal and fetal plasma concentrations of endothelin, lipid hydroperoxides, glutathione peroxidase and fibronectin in relation to abnormal umbilical artery velocimetry. *Eur J Obstet Gynecol Reprod Biol* 1998;80:39–44.

116. Harvey-Wilkes KB, Nielsen HC, D'Alton ME. Elevated endothelin levels are associated with increased placental resistance. *Am J Obstet Gynecol* 1996;174:1599–1604.

117. Rizzo G, Montuschi P, Capponi A, et al. Blood levels of vasoactive intestinal polypeptide in normal and growth retarded fetuses: relationship with acid-base and haemodynamic status. *Early Hum Dev* 1995;41:69–77.

118. Saldeen P, Olofsson P, Marsal K. Lack of association between Doppler velocimetry and synthesis of prostacyclin and thromboxane in umbilical cord vessels from growth retarded fetuses. *Acta Obstet Gynecol Scand* 1995;74:103–108.

119. Lyall F, Greer IA, Young A, et al. Nitric oxide concentrations are increased in the feto-placental circulation in intrauterine growth restriction. *Placenta* 1996;17:165–168.

120. Hecher K, Campbell S. Characteristics of fetal venous blood flow under normal circumstances and during fetal disease. *Ultrasound Obstet Gynecol* 1996;7:68–83.

121. Kilavuz O, Vetter K. Is the liver of the fetus the 4th preferential organ for arterial blood supply besides brain, heart, and adrenal glands? *J Perinat Med* 1999;27:103–106.

122. Capponi A, Rizzo G, De Angelis C, et al. Atrial natriuretic peptide levels in fetal blood in relation to inferior vena cava velocity waveforms. *Obstet Gynecol* 1997;89:242–247.

123. Ville Y, Proudler A, Abbas A, et al. Atrial natriuretic factor concentration in normal, growth-retarded, anemic, and hydropic fetuses. *Am J Obstet Gynecol* 1994;171:777–783.

124. Baschat AA, Gembruch U, Reiss I, et al. Demonstration of fetal coronary blood flow by Doppler ultrasound in relation to arterial and venous flow velocity waveforms and perinatal outcome—the "heart-sparing effect." *Ultrasound Obstet Gynecol* 1997;9:162–172.

125. Arduini D, Rizzo G, Romanini C. Changes of pulsatility index from fetal vessels preceding the onset of late decelerations in growth-retarded fetuses. *Obstet Gynecol* 1992;79:605–610.

126. Rizzo G, Arduini D. Fetal cardiac function in intrauterine growth retardation. *Am J Obstet Gynecol* 1991;165:876–882.

127. Rizzo G, Capponi A, Pietropolli A, et al. Fetal cardiac and extracardiac flows preceding intrauterine death. *Ultrasound Obstet Gynecol* 1994;4:139–142.

128. Gosling R.G., King D.H. Ultrasound angiology. In: Marcus AW, Adamson L, eds. *Arteries and Veins*, 2nd ed. Edinburgh: Churchill Livingstone, 1975:61–98.

129. Thompson RS, Trudinger BJ, Cook CM. Doppler ultrasound waveform indices: A/B ratio pulsatility index and Pourcelot ratio. *Br J Obstet Gynaecol* 1988;95:581–588.

130. McGowan LM, Harding JE, Roberts AB, et al. A pilot randomized controlled trial of two regimens of fetal surveillance for small-for-gestational age fetuses with normal results of umbilical artery Doppler velocimetry. *Am J Obstet Gynecol* 2000;182:81–86.

131. Neilson JP, Alfirevic Z. Doppler ultrasound for fetal assessment in high risk pregnancies [Cochrane review]. Cochrane Library, Issue 1, 2002: Oxford: Update Software.

132. Westergaard HB, Langhoff-Roos J, Lingman G, et al. A critical appraisal of the use of umbilical artery Doppler ultrasound in high-risk pregnancies: use of meta-analyses in evidence-based obstetrics. *Ultrasound Obstet Gynecol* 2001;17:466–476.

133. Thornton JG, Lilford R. Do we need randomised trials of antenatal tests of fetal well-being? *Br J Obstet Gynaecol* 1993;100:197–200.

134. Hershkovitz R, Kingdom JC, Geary M, et al. Fetal cerebral blood flow redistribution in late gestation: identification of compromise in small fetuses with normal umbilical artery Doppler. *Ultrasound Obstet Gynecol* 2000;15:209–212.

135. Bahado-Singh RO, Kovanci E, Jeffres A, et al. The Doppler cerebroplacental ratio and perinatal outcome in intrauterine growth restriction. *Am J Obstet Gynecol* 1999;180:750–756.

136. Rizzo G, Capponi A, Talone PE, et al. Doppler indices from inferior vena cava and ductus venosus in predicting pH and oxygen tension in umbilical blood at cordocentesis in growth-retarded fetuses. *Ultrasound Obstet Gynecol* 1996;7:401–410.

137. Bilardo CM, Wolf H, Stigter RH, et al. Relationship between monitoring parameters and perinatal outcome in severe, early intrauterine growth restriction. *Ultrasound Obstet Gynecol* 2004;23:119–125.

138. Baschat AA, Gembruch U, Weiner CP, et al. Qualitative venous Doppler waveform analysis improves prediction of critical perinatal outcomes in premature growth-restricted fetuses. *Ultrasound Obstet Gynecol* 2003;22:240–245.

139. Chaiworapongsa T, Espinoza J, Yoshimatsu J, et al. Subclinical myocardial injury in small-for-gestational-age neonates. *J Matern Fetal Neonatal Med* 2002;11:385–390.

140. Gazzolo D, Marinoni E, di Iorio R, et al. Circulating S100beta protein is increased in intrauterine growth-retarded fetuses. *Pediatr Res* 2002;51:215–219.

141. Roberts A, Nava S, Bocconi L, et al. Liver function tests and glucose and lipid metabolism in growth-restricted fetuses. *Obstet Gynecol* 1999;94:290–294.

142. Hackett GA, Campbell S, Gamsu H, et al. Doppler studies in the growth retarded fetus and prediction of neonatal necrotising enterocolitis, haemorrhage, and neonatal morbidity. *BMJ* 1987;294:13–16.

143. Ribbert LS, Visser GH, Mulder EJ, et al. Changes with time in fetal heart rate variation, movement incidences and haemodynamics in intrauterine growth retarded fetuses: a longitudinal approach to the assessment of fetal well being. *Early Hum Dev* 1993;31:195–208.

144. Manning FA. Fetal biophysical profile. *Obstet Gynecol Clin North Am* 1999;26:557–577.

145. Arduini D, Rizzo G, Romanini C, et al. Computerized analysis of behavioural states in asymmetrical growth retarded fetuses. *J Perinat Med* 1988;16:357–363.

146. Arduini D, Rizzo G, Caforio L, et al. Behavioural state transitions in healthy and growth retarded fetuses. *Early Hum Dev* 1989;19:155–165.

147. Nijhuis IJ, ten Hof J, Nijhuis JG, et al. Temporal organisation of fetal behaviour from 24-weeks gestation onwards in normal and complicated pregnancies. *Dev Psychobiol* 1999;34:257–268.

148. Vindla S, James D, Sahota D. Computerised analysis of unstimulated and stimulated behaviour in fetuses with intrauterine growth restriction. *Eur J Obstet Gynecol Reprod Biol* 1999;83:37–45.

149. Romanini C, Valensise H, Ciotti G, et al. Tryptophan availability and fetal behavioral states. *Fetal Ther* 1989:68–72.

150. Henson G, Dawes GS, Redman CW. Characterization of the reduced heart rate variation in growth-retarded fetuses. *Br J Obstet Gynaecol* 1984;91:751–755.

151. Ribbert LS, Snijders RJ, Nicolaides KH, et al. Relation of fetal blood gases and data from computer-assisted analysis of fetal heart rate patterns in small for gestation fetuses. *Br J Obstet Gynaecol* 1991;98:820–823.

152. Smith JH, Anand KJ, Cotes PM, et al. Antenatal fetal heart rate variation in relation to the respiratory and metabolic status of the compromised human fetus. *Br J Obstet Gynaecol* 1988;95:980–989.

153. Longo LD Packianathan S. Hypoxia-ischemia and the developing brain: hypotheses regarding the pathophysiology of fetal neonatal brain damage. *Br J Obstet Gynaecol* 1997; 104:652–662.

154. Wladimiroff JW. Tachometrie in de vroege zwangerschap;ontwikkeling van de nervus vagus functie. *Nederlands Tijdschrift voor Geneeskunde* 1972;116:1688–1693.

155. Wheeler T, Murrills A. Patterns of fetal heart rate during normal pregnancy. *Br J Obstet Gynaecol* 1978;85:18–27.

156. Dawes GS, Houghton CRS, Redman CWG, et al. Patterns of normal fetal heart rate. *Br J Obstet Gynaecol* 1982;89:276–284.

157. Visser GHA, Dawes GS, Redman CWG. Numerical analysis of the normal human antenatal fetal heart rate. *Br J Obstet Gynaecol* 1981;88:792–802.

158. Nicolaides KH, Sadovsky G, Visser GHA. Heart rate patterns in normoxemic, hypoxemic, and anemic second-trimester fetuses. *Am J Obstet Gynecol* 1989;160:1034–1037.

159. Gagnon R, Campbell K, Hunse C, Patrick J. Patterns of human fetal heart rate accelerations from 26 weeks to term. *Am J Obstet Gynecol* 1987;157:743–749.

160. Visser GHA, Sadovsky G, Nicolaides KH. Antepartum heart rate patterns in small-for-gestational age third trimester fetuses: correlations with blood gases obtained at cordocentesis. *Am J Obstet Gynecol* 1990;162:698–703.

161. Gagnon R, Hunse C, Bocking AD. Fetal heart rate patterns in small-for-gestational age human fetus. *Am J Obstet Gynecol* 1989;161:779–784.

162. Hoppenbrouwers T, Combs D, Ugartechea JC, et al. Fetal heart rates during materal wakefulness and sleep. *Obstet Gynecol* 1981;57:301–309.

163. Visser GHA, Poelmann-Weesjes G, Cohen TMN, et al. Fetal behavior at 30 to 32 weeks of gestation. *Pediatric Res* 1987;22:655–658.

164. Junge HD. Behavioural state and state related heart rate and motor activity patterns in the newborn infant and the fetus antepartum: a comparative study. *J Perinatal Med* 1979;7:85–107.

165. Visser GHA, Goodman JDS, Levine DH, et al. Diurnal and other cyclic variations in human fetal heart rate near term. *Am J Obstet Gynecol* 1982;142:535–544.

166. Nijhuis JG, Prechtl HFR, Martin CB, et al. Are there behavioural states in the human fetus? *Early Hum Dev* 1982;6:177–195.

167. Visser GH, Zeelenberg HJ, de Vries JI, et al. External physical stimulation of the human fetus during episodes of low heart rate variation. *Am J Obstet Gynecol* 1983;145:579–584.

168. Derks JB, Mulder EJ, Visser GH. The effects of maternal betamethasone administration on the fetus. *Br J Obstet Gynaecol* 1995;102:140–146.

169. Bekedam DJ, Visser GHA, Mulder EJH, et al. Heart rate variation and movement incidence in growth-retarded fetuses: the significance of antenatal late heart rate decelerations. *Am J Obstet Gynecol* 1987;157:126–133.

170. Pardi G, Cetin I, Marconi AM, et al. Diagnostic value of blood sampling in fetuses with growth retardation. *N Engl J Med* 1993;328:692–696.

171. Visser GHA, Redman CWG, Huisjes HJ, et al. Nonstressed antepartum heart rate monitoring: implications of decelerations after spontaneous contractions. *Am J Obstet Gynecol* 1980;138: 429–435.

172. Visser GHA,Huisjes HJ. Diagnostic value of the nonstress antepartum cardiotocogram. *Br J Obstet Gynaecol* 1977;84:321–326.

173. Visser GHA. Assessment of fetal well-being in growth retarded fetuses. In: Hanson MA, Spencer JAD, Rodeck CH, eds. *Fetuses and Neonates*, Vol. 3. Oxford: Cambridge University 1995:327–345.

174. Bekedam DJ, Visser GHA, van der Zee AGI, et al. Abnormal velocity waveforms of the umbilical artery in growth retarded fetuses: relationship to antepartum late heart rate decelerations and outcome. *Early Hum Dev* 1990;24:79–90.

175. Arduini d, Rizzo G, Romanini C. The development of abnormal heart rate patterns after absent end-diastolic velocity in umbilical artery. *Am J Obstet Gynecol* 1988;168:43–48.

176. Grant A, Elbourne D, Valentin L, et al. Routine formal fetal movement counting and risk of antepartum late death in normally formed singletons. *Lancet* 1989;345–349.

177. Mangesi L, Hofmeyr GJ. Fetal movement counting for assessment of fetal well-being. The Cochrane Database of Systematic Reviews 2004: CD004909.

178. ACOG practice bulletin. Antepartum fetal surveillance: clinical management guidelines for obstetrician-gynecologists. *Int J Gynaecol Obstet* 2000;68:175–85.

179. Sadovsky E, Yaffe H, Polishuk WZ. Fetal movement monitoring in normal and pathologic pregnancy. *Int J Obstet Gynecol* 1974;12:75–79

180. Pearson JF, Weaver JB. Fetal activity and fetal well-being; an evaluation. *BMJ* 1976;1:1305–1307.

181. Ribbert LS, Snijders RJ, Nicolaides KH, et al. Relationship of fetal biophysical profile and blood gas values at cordocentesis in severely growth-retarded fetuses. *Am J Obstet Gynecol* 1990;163:569–571.

182. Ribbert LSM, Nicolaides KH, Visser GHA. Prediction of fetal acidaemia in intrauterine growth retardation: comparison of quantified fetal activity with biophysical profile score. *Br J Obstet Gynaecol* 1993;100:653–656.

183. Manning FA, Snijders RJM, Harman CR, et al. Fetal biophysical profile score. VI. Correlations with antepartum umbilical venous fetal pH. *Am J Obstet Gynecol* 1993;169:755–763.

184. Bekedam DJ, Visser GHA. Effects of hypoxemic events on breathing, body movements and heart rate variation: a study in growth retarded human fetuses. *Am J Obstet Gynecol* 1985;153:52–56.

185. Bekedam DJ, Mulder EJH, Snijders RJM, et al. The effects of maternal hyperoxia on fetal breathing movements, body movements and heart rate variation in growth retarded fetuses. *Early Hum Dev* 1991;27:223–232.

186. Koos BJ, Kitanaka T, Matsuda K, et al. Fetal breathing adaption to prolonged hypoxaemia in sheep. *J Dev Physiol* 1988;10:161–166.

187. Snijders RJM, Ribbert LSM, Visser GHA, et al. Numeric analysis of heart rate variation in intrauterine growth-retarded fetuses: a longitudinal study. *Am J Obstet Gynecol* 1992;166:22–27.

188. Vintzileos AM, Fleming AD, Scorza WE, et al. Relationship between fetal biophysical activities and umbilical cord blood gas values. *Am J Obstet Gynecol* 1991;165: 707–713.

189. Pillai M, James D. Continuation of normal neurobehavioural development in fetuses with absent umbilical arterial end-diastolic velocities. *Br J Obstet Gynaecol* 1991;98:277–281.

190. Rizzo G, Arduini D, Pennestri F, et al. Fetal behaviour in growth retardation: its relationship to fetal blood flow. *Prenat Diagn* 1987;7:229–238.

191. Arduini D, Rizzo G, Capponi A, et al. Fetal pH value determined by cordocentesis: an independent predictor of the development of antepartum fetal heart rate decelerations in growth retarded fetuses with absent end-diastolic velocity in umbilical artery. *J Perinat Med* 1996;24:601–607.

192. Alfirevic Z, Neilson JP. Biophysical profile for fetal assessment in high risk pregnancies. The Cochrane database of Systematic Reviews 1995, Issue1.Art n.CD000038.

38

Peripartum Coagulopathy

Jamie Star

Jeffrey F. Peipert

■ What Is the Problem that Requires Screening?

Peripartum bleeding abnormalities that may increase the risk of hemorrhage and/or disseminated intravascular coagulation.

What is the incidence/prevalence of the target condition?

Preeclampsia. Preeclampsia complicates 2% to 5% of pregnancies.[1] Depending on the severity of the disease, as well as the presence of HELLP (hemolysis, elevated liver enzymes, low platelet count) syndrome, the risk of coagulopathy is approximately 15%.[2]

Placental abruption. This premature separation of a portion of the placenta from the uterine wall complicates approximately 1% to 2% of all pregnancies.[3] Risk factors include smoking, hypertensive disease, trauma, cocaine use, hydramnios, chorioamnionitis, preterm premature rupture of membranes and history of abruption.[4] Approximately 10% of women with placental abruption also have disseminated intravascular coagulation (DIC), and the prevalence increases with the severity of the abruption such that it is more common in conjunction with complete abruption (i.e., fetal death and/or loss of over 2 L of maternal blood).[3]

Intrauterine fetal death. The coagulopathy associated with an intrauterine fetal death (IUFD) is typically chronic and does not generally occur until 4 to 5 weeks after the demise.[5] Prevalences of up to 25% are reported.[6] The prevalence of DIC when there is a single death in a multiple gestation has been quoted to be as high as 25%, but this appears an overestimate.[7]

Amniotic fluid embolism. This extremely rare but often fatal condition is difficult to diagnose. Reported prevalences ranges from 1/8,000 to 1/80,000 deliveries. The risk of coagulopathy approximates 40%.[8]

Maternal thrombocytopenia. A platelet count of less than $150,000/uL^3$ resulting from any cause complicates 6% to 10% of pregnancies at term. The most common etiologies include preeclampsia (see prior section), gestational thrombocytopenia, and immune thrombocytopenic purpura (ITP) (2–3/1,000 pregnancies).[9] Only preeclampsia is associated with a risk of a clinically significant coagulopathy.

What are the sequelae of the condition that are of interest in clinical medicine?

There are several conditions that predispose a pregnant woman to intrapartum coagulopathy. These include preeclampsia (and/or HELLP syndrome), placental abruption, IUFD, and amniotic fluid embolism, as any of these diagnoses can be associated with DIC and its attendant morbidity and mortality. Certainly, obstetric hemorrhage from other causes, such as uterine atony or placenta previa, may result in DIC due to external consumption of coagulation factors. Additional maternal diseases that increase the bleeding risk include inherited disorders of coagulation (i.e., intrinsic platelet dysfunction, von Willebrand disease, not discussed here) and thrombocytopenia of any cause.

There is normal physiologic shift toward hypercoagulability during pregnancy. With the exception of factors XI and XIII, the soluble coagulation factors increase in concentration. And while fibrinogen increases, plasma fibrinolytic activity decreases. Despite these adaptations, obstetric hemorrhage remains one of the primary causes of maternal mortality. Therefore, the early diagnosis of coagulation disorders and their prompt treatment is critical to the safe practice of obstetrics.

Intrapartum coagulopathy is fortunately an uncommon event. Although hemorrhage is a leading cause of maternal morbidity and mortality, most of it is secondary to postpartum uterine atony.

Preeclampsia creates a high risk of morbidity for both mother and fetus, producing multisystem dysfunction, including the onset of eclampsia or generalized seizures. Maternal death may result from cerebrovascular accident, pulmonary edema, hepatic rupture, renal failure, or complications of severe hypertension and/or DIC. Fetal death can occur in concert with the these problems, often related to severe placental dysfunction.[10]

Placental abruption results in the release of tissue thromboplastin into the maternal circulation, triggering the coagulation cascade.[11] Approximately 10% of patients with an abruption develop clotting abnormalities detectable by laboratory evaluation.[12] In the initial phase of abruption, there is accelerated coagulation, and a decrease in fibrinogen occurs in 5% to 20% of patients followed serially. Fibrinolytic activity results in the formation of fibrin degradation products (FDPs).[13] A separation of more than 50% of the placental surface area is associated with fetal death, and in this setting, the occurrence of a maternal coagulopathy approximates 25% to 30%.[6] Fulminant DIC may develop within 1 to 2 hours after a complete abruption, and rarely persists more than 12 hours after delivery.[3] Milder forms of abruption pose a marked risk to the fetus due to disruption of adequate transfer of nutrients and oxygen.

The coagulopathy associated with a retained IUFD is typically a chronic, compensated DIC. Low-dose heparin has been used with success in case reports. A more acute, uncompensated DIC is seen with an IUFD in the setting of placental abruption.

Amniotic fluid embolism is a rare event characterized by two clinical phases. Approximately 40% of women who survive the initial cardiopulmonary insult develop clotting abnormalities that can present as hemorrhage (uterine atony, incisional bleeding).[8] The exact pathophysiology of DIC in the setting of amniotic fluid embolism is unclear, although amniotic fluid has procoagulant activity.[14]

Bleeding in the adult with ITP is usually mild to moderate and is evidenced by ecchymoses, gingival bleeding, epistaxis, menorrhagia, and/or hematuria.[15] The most serious complication of ITP in nonsurgical patients is intracranial hemorrhage, which occurs in less than 1% of untreated patients. Thrombocytopenia secondary to ITP is unlikely to pose a risk to the fetus (in contrast to alloimmune thrombocytopenia).[16] Gestational thrombocytopenia is not associated with maternal or fetal risks.

■ The Tests

What is the purpose of the tests?

The detection of coagulation abnormalities that place the parturient at increased risk of hemorrhage.

To promptly diagnose the onset of DIC in an attempt to provide expeditious treatment.

What is the nature of the tests?

The laboratory assessment of clotting is approached in stages.

A platelet count is often the initial coagulation screening test in the pregnant woman. Thrombocytopenia accompanies the above disorders of interest, particularly in the setting of preeclampsia and/or HELLP syndrome. Most pregnant women have normal platelet counts (150,000–450,000/uL^3). Decreased counts are typically due to increased consumption rather than decreased synthesis.

The prothrombin time (PT) reflects the integrity of the extrinsic (vitamin K dependent) and common clotting pathways.[17] A normal PT requires a minimum of 100 mg/dL of fibrinogen.[18] The activated partial thromboplastin time (aPTT) evaluates the intrinsic and common pathways, and is most sensitive to a deficiency of factors early in the cascade sequence (i.e., factors XII, XI, IX, and VIII).[19] Both the PT and aPTT may be prolonged if a factor level declines below 25% of normal.[20] This can also occur in the presence of a high concentration of FDPs and/or hypofibrinogenemia.[21] These tests are typically unaffected by normal pregnancy.

A fibrinogen level less than 200 to 250 mg/dL is considered abnormally low in pregnancy.[22]

FDPs are created by the cleavage of fibrin by plasmin. Values above 40 ug/ml is considered abnormal.[23] D-dimer is the primary degradation product of cross-linked fibrin by plasmin, and is measured using monoclonal antibodies, which reduces the chance of a laboratory artifact.[24]

The bleeding time is defined as the time required for bleeding to stop after a standardized puncture of the forearm. It is not a reliable indicator of in vivo platelet function and does not accurately reflect the risk of hemorrhage.[25] It may be used in the assessment of women with von Willebrand disease.

What are the implications of testing?

Preeclampsia. Early studies demonstrated increased fibrin deposition and microvascular thrombosis in the organs of preeclamptic women, establishing the presence of accelerated coagulation.[26] Subsequent research has suggested a component of chronic compensated DIC, with increased fibrinopeptide A, decreased antithrombin III, increased D-dimer, increased FDPs, and increased platelet activation.[10]

What does an abnormal test result mean? Thrombocytopenia is the primary clotting test abnormality in women with preeclampsia, occurring in 15% to 50% of patients.[27] In the absence of thrombocytopenia, other disturbances of common clinical clotting tests (i.e., PT, aPTT) are rare, and additional testing is not indicated. Barron et al suggested that the measurement of lactate dehydrogenase as an adjunct to the platelet count virtually rules out coagulopathy when both tests are normal.[22] Less than 20% of women with severe preeclampsia have a prolonged PT/aPTT. Patients with atypical preeclampsia, the so-called HELLP syndrome, have higher rates of decompensated DIC, which should be investigated.[28]

The options available for analgesia and/or anesthesia in the laboring preeclamptic woman depend largely on the degree of thrombocytopenia. There are no established cutoffs per se, but an individual anesthesiologist may require documentation of a normal PT/aPTT prior to placing an epidural or spinal in the setting of a low platelet count.[29] A platelet count of less than 100,000/uL^3 is generally considered to be a contraindication to regional anesthesia, although counts of 50,000 to 100,000/uL^3 may be deemed acceptable by the responsible anesthesiologist in some circumstances. A bleeding time does not provide additional information regarding risk of hemorrhagic complications.[30]

What does a normal test result mean? A normal platelet count and/or normal coagulation studies essentially rules out the diagnosis of a clinically relevant coagulopathy given the negative predictive values for coagulation tests in this setting are more than 90%.[22]

Placental abruption.
What does an abnormal test result mean? Coagulopathy is uncommon unless there is at least a 50% separation of the placenta, in which case, fetal distress is often evident. A full coagulation workup is recommended in the setting of extensive abruption, up to and including fetal demise. Prolonged clotting times are indicative of DIC, which should prompt product replacement and expeditious delivery.[4] The diagnosis of placental abruption is predominantly clinical, and decisions regarding management are based on evidence of maternal and/or fetal decompensation. Additional studies, such as fibrinogen levels and D-dimer have been used but do not seem to influence management.

What does a normal test result mean? The absence of a coagulopathy does not rule out placental abruption, but may allow for expectant management if both mother and fetus are otherwise stable.

Intrauterine fetal death.
What does an abnormal test result mean? The most consistent clinical laboratory abnormality in the setting of an IUFD is a decreased fibrinogen level,[6] although more sensitive parameters such as fibrinopeptide A and thrombin: antithrombin complex are virtually always abnormal. Evidence of DIC is an indication for product replacement and delivery. Heparin has been used to successfully treat chronic, compensated DIC in a number of case reports.

What does a normal test result mean? The absence of coagulopathy allows for expectant management of an IUFD if desired, which may be critical in circumstances of multiple gestations where there is a remaining live but preterm fetus.

Amniotic fluid embolism.
What does an abnormal test result mean? Acute DIC is common in the first 12 hours following the initial insult of an amniotic fluid embolism.[31] Laboratory findings include thrombocytopenia, hypofibrinogenemia, increased FDPs, and prolonged PT/aPTT, which may occur prior to the onset of clinical bleeding. It is unclear whether the FDP reflects fibrinolysis or fibrinogenolysis or both. Product replacement is indicated.[8]

What does a normal test result mean? The assessment of coagulopathy in the setting of amniotic fluid embolism requires serial evaluation. The absence of laboratory abnormalities during the initial period of diagnosis is reassuring, but does not eliminate the possibility of its later development, particularly in the first 24 hours. Additional testing is dictated by clinical evidence of abnormal clotting.[8]

Maternal thrombocytopenia.
What does an abnormal test result mean? Thrombocytopenia in the gravida with known ITP is expected and is usually mild. Platelet function is normal.

A platelet count may guide the clinician in areas of anesthesia management and transfusion requirements before surgery. Coagulopathy is rare. Although fetal intracranial hemorrhage is a reported risk, its relationship to fetal thrombocytopenia is unclear. Interventions to assess the fetal platelet count are generally not recommended, as there are no data to support alterations in clinical management (i.e., cesarean delivery vs. vaginal).[32]

Spontaneous bleeding secondary to thrombocytopenia is uncommon, provided that platelet function is normal and the platelet count is above 20,000/uL[3].[33] Excessive surgical bleeding is rare when the platelet count is above 50,000/uL[3].[34]

What does a normal test result mean? A normal platelet count suggests there is no increased risk of hemorrhage at delivery.

Acute disseminated intravascular coagulation. DIC is not a disease, but rather the endpoint of many pathways that lead to a disturbance of the coagulation system. Systemic coagulation results in deposition of fibrin in the vasculature. There is enhanced consumption of platelets and coagulation factors, while fibrinolysis creates FDPs, which can further impair fibrin formation and platelet function. It may manifest in a variety of clinical settings, the most common of which in obstetrics are discussed above.[35] Clinical signs range from bleeding from more than two sites to multisystem organ failure. The most likely cause of acute decompensated DIC in obstetrics is hemorrhage. Laboratory evaluation is helpful in determining the degree of coagulopathy, as well as the need for and response to factor replacement. Chronic, compensated DIC is most common in the setting of retained IUFD and may require laboratory testing for diagnosis. Overt hemorrhage is rare.

What does an abnormal test result mean? The prevalences of coagulation abnormalities in the setting of DIC include thrombocytopenia (>90%), prolonged PT (>70%), and prolonged aPTT (50%). The diagnosis is supported by hypofibrinogenemia (50%) and increased FDPs (85%). Schistocytes may be seen on a peripheral smear. Additional tests, such as antithrombin III are highly sensitive for the diagnosis, but are rarely necessary in acute clinical situations.[36]

A bedside clotting assessment (hanging clot) can be helpful in the rapid evaluation of a patient prior to surgery. Approximately 5 mL of whole blood are obtained in a tube free of preservative or anticoagulant. The lack of clot formation in 5 to 10 minutes suggests DIC; the absence of a clot after 10 minutes indicates the fibrinogen is less than 50 mg/dL. Rapid clot breakdown indicates the presence of high levels of FDPs.[37]

What does a normal test result mean? The absence of obvious coagulopathy when DIC is suspected is reassuring. However, serial studies may be necessary depending on the clinical circumstances. Product replacement is generally not indicated when there are no clotting time abnormalities, unless there is ongoing hemorrhage.

Table 38-1	Cost of primary screening tests for intrapartum coagulopathy[1]
Complete blood count (including platelet count)	$33
Prothrombin time	$40
Activated partial thromboplastin time	$52
Fibrinogen	$95
Fibrin degradation products	$109
D-Dimer	$109

[1]These prices reflect the costs incurred by our laboratory and may not represent costs elsewhere.

What is the cost of testing?

The cost of testing is modest (Table 38–1).

■ Conclusions and Recommendations

There are no indications to routinely evaluate the coagulation system of the normal laboring woman. Pregnancies complicated by any disorder that is potentially associated with DIC should be screened accordingly.

■ Summary

1 ■ What Is the Problem that Requires Screening?

Peripartum coagulopathy.

a. What is the incidence of the target condition?

Preeclampsia complicates approximately 2% to 5% of all pregnancies.

Placental abruption complicates approximately 1% to 2% of all pregnancies.

IUFD may be associated with DIC in up to 25% of cases after at least 4 weeks postmortem.

Amniotic fluid embolism is a rare, catastrophic event that has a prevalence of 1/8,000 to 1/80,000 deliveries.

Maternal thrombocytopenia (from any cause) is diagnosed in 6% to 10% of pregnancies. Gestational thrombocytopenia accounts for the majority, and ITP occurs in 2–3/1,000 pregnancies.

b. *What are the sequelae of the condition that are of interest in clinical medicine?*
Each of the above conditions is associated with different morbidities, but maternal hemorrhage may occur in all.

2 ■ The Tests

a. *What is the purpose of the tests?*
To detect the presence of DIC in laboring women and to follow the effects of treatment in patients with the diagnosis.

b. *What is the nature of the tests?*
The primary tests used to assess coagulopathy in the intrapartum period include platelet count, PT, aPTT, fibrinogen, and FDPs.

c. *What are the implications of testing?*
1. What does an abnormal test result mean?
The woman is at risk of or in the midst of developing a significant coagulopathy that requires treatment and may affect decisions regarding delivery.
2. What does a normal test result mean?
The woman is at low risk of developing (or has not yet begun to develop) a clinically important coagulopathy.

d. *What is the cost of testing?*
Modest.

3 ■ Conclusions and Recommendations

There are no indications to routinely evaluate the coagulation system of the healthy laboring woman. Pregnancies complicated by any disorder that is potentially associated with DIC should be screened accordingly.

References

1. Saftlas AF, Olson DR, Franks AL, et al. Epidemiology of preeclampsia eclampsia in the United States, 1979-1986. *Am J Obstet Gynecol* 1990:163:460–465.
2. Sibai BM. Diagnosis, controversies and management of the syndrome of hemolysis, elevated liver enzymes, and low platelet count. *Obstet Gynecol* 2004;103:981–991.

3. Clark SL. Placenta previa and abruption placenta. In: Creasy RK, Resnik R, eds. *Maternal-Fetal Medicine, Principles and Practice*, 4th ed. Philadelphia: WB Saunders, 1999:616–631.

4. Hladky K, Yankowitz J, Hansen WF. Placental abruption. *Obstet Gynecol Survey* 2002;7:299–305.

5. Pitkin RM. Fetal death: diagnosis and management. *Am J Obstet Gynecol* 1987;157:583–589.

6. Pritchard JA. Haematological problems associated with delivery, placental abruption, retained dead fetus and amniotic fluid embolism. *Clin Haematol* 1973;2:563–566.

7. Cleary-Goldman J, D'Alton M. Management of a single fetal demise in a multiple gestation. *Obstet Gynecol Survey* 2004;59:285–298.

8. Clark SL. Amniotic fluid embolism. *Clin Perinatol* 1986;13:801–811.

9. Kam PCA, Thompson SA, Liew ACS. Thrombocytopenia in the parturient. *Anaesthesia* 2004;59:255–264.

10. Norwitz ER, Hsu C-D, Repke JT. Acute complications of preeclampsia. *Clin Obstet Gynecol* 2002;45:308–329.

11. Sher G, Statland BE. Abruptio placentae with coagulopathy: a rational basis for management. *Clin Obstet Gynecol* 1985;28:15–23.

12. Sher G. Pathogenesis and management of uterine inertia complicating abruption placentae with consumption coagulopathy. *Am J Obstet Gynecol* 1966;129:164–170.

13. Bonnar J, McNicol GP, Douglas AS. The behaviour of the coagulation and fibrinolytic mechanisms in abruption placentae. *J Obstet Gynecol Br Commonw* 1969;76:799–805.

14. Phillips LL, Davidson ED. Procoagulant properties of amniotic fluid. *Am J Obstet Gynecol* 1972;113:911–919.

15. Saino S, Kekomaki R, Riikonen R, et al. Maternal thrombocytopenia: a population based study. *Acta Obstet Gynecol Scand* 2000;79:744–749.

16. Payne SD, Resnick R, Moore TR, et al. Maternal characteristics and risk of severe neonatal thrombocytopenia and intracranial hemorrhage in pregnancies complicated by autoimmune thrombocytopenia. *Am J Obstet Gynecol* 1997;177:149–155.

17. Suchman AL, Griner PF. Diagnostic uses of the activated partial thromboplastin time and prothrombin time. *Ann Intern Med* 1986;104:810–816.

18. Bick RL. Disseminated intravascular coagulation and related syndromes: etiology, pathophysiology, diagnosis and management. *Am J Hematol* 1978;5:265–282.

19. Naumann RO, Weinstein L. Disseminated intravascular coagulation—the clinician's dilemma. *Obstet Gynecol Survey* 1985;40:487–492.

20. Burns ER, Goldberg SN, Wenz B. Paradoxic effect of multiple mild coagulation factor deficiencies on the prothrombin time and activated partial thromboplastin time. *Am J Clin Pathol* 1993;100:94–98.

21. Ockelford PA, Carter CJ. Disseminated intravascular coagulation: the application and utility of clinical tests. *Sem Thromb Hemostasis* 1982;8:198–216.

22. Barron WM, Heckerling P, Hibbard JU, et al. Reducing unnecessary coagulation testing in hypertensive disorders of pregnancy. *Obstet Gynecol* 1999;94:364–370.

23. Dixon RE. Disseminated intravascular coagulation: a paradox of thrombosis and hemorrhage. *Obstet Gynecol Survey* 1973;28:385–395.

24. Wakai A, Gleeson A, Winter D. Role of fibrin D-dimer testing in emergency medicine. *Emerg Med J* 2003;20:319–325.

25. Rodgers RPD, Levin J. A critical reappraisal of the bleeding time. *Semin Thromb Hemostasis* 1990;16:1–20.

26. Pritchard JA, Cunningham FG, Mason RA. Coagulation changes in eclampsia: their frequency and pathogenesis. *Am J Obstet Gynecol* 1976;124:855–864.

27. McCrae KR, Samuels P, Schreiber AD. Pregnancy associated thrombocytopenia: pathogenesis and management. *Blood* 1992;80:2697–2714.

28. Perry KG Jr, Martin JN. Abnormal hemostasis and coagulopathy in preeclampsia and eclampsia. *Clin Obstet Gynecol* 1992;35:338–350.

29. Rolbin SH, Abbott D, Musclow E, et al. Epidural anesthesia in pregnant patients with low platelet counts. *Obstet Gynecol* 1988;71:918–920.

30. Douglas MJ. Platelets, the parturient and regional anesthesia. *Int J Obstet Anesth* 2001;10:113–120.

31. Killam A. Amniotic fluid embolism. *Clin Obstet Gynecol* 1985;28:32–36.
32. Laros RK Jr, Kagan R. Route of delivery for patients with ITP. *Am J Obstet Gynecol* 1984;148:901–908.
33. Fellin F, Murphy S. Hematologic problems in the preoperative patient. *Med Clin North Am* 1987;71:477–487.
34. Gill KK, Kelton JG. Management of idiopathic thrombocytopenia purpura in pregnancy. *Sem Hematol* 2000;37:275–283.
35. Levi M. Current understanding of disseminated intravascular coagulation. *Brit J Haematol* 2004;124:567–576.
36. Baglin T. Fortnightly review: DIC, diagnosis and treatment. *BMJ* 1996;312:683–687.
37. Weiner CP. Evaluation of clotting disorders during pregnancy. In: Depp R, Eschenbach DA, Sciarra JJ, eds. *Gynecology and Obstetrics*, Vol. 3. Philadelphia: JB Lippincott, 1993:1–14.

Postpartum Umbilical Cord Blood Testing

Charlene M. Elbert
Ronald G. Strauss

■ What Is the Problem that Requires Screening?

Hemolytic disease of the newborn (HDN); prevention of maternal Rh alloimmunization.

What is the incidence/prevalence of the target condition?

Two percent to 5% of pregnant women exhibit red blood cell (RBC) alloimmunization to antigens other than ABO[1]; a small fraction of their infants develop clinically significant HDN. The prevalence of clinically apparent HDN caused by anti-Rh antibodies approximates 1/1,000. Antibodies to other RBC antigens occur in 3/1,000 livebirths, of which approximately 10% (3/10,000) exhibit clinically significant HDN.[2]

What are the sequelae of the condition that are of significance in clinical medicine?

Rh-negative (i.e., lack D antigen) women who deliver an Rh-positive (i.e., exhibit D antigen) child are at risk of alloimmunization to D. Alloimmunization to Rh (D) is preventable by the maternal administration of anti-D immunoglobulin. Severe RBC alloimmunization, whether secondary to Rh (D) or another RBC alloantibody can cause profound hemolytic anemia with consequent intrauterine fetal death, hydrops fetalis, preterm delivery and, after delivery, hyperbilirubinemia and kernicterus and/or severe anemia requiring RBC transfusions. Although fetal blood obtained from the umbilical cord at the time of birth can be tested for RBC incompatibilities, the results poorly predict the clinical expression of HDN. This is particularly true for HDN secondary to ABO incompatibility, where testing of umbilical cord blood is very poorly predictive of the neonatal course.

■ The Tests

What is the purpose of the tests?

To identify HDN and determine the newborn RBC type and Rh (D) status so as to identify which Rh (D) negative women are at risk of developing alloimmunization.

What is the nature of the tests?

When indicated by clinical history, the blood obtained from the umbilical cord at delivery is tested for ABO grouping, Rh type, direct antiglobulin test (DAT) (also called a direct Coombs test) and RBC antibody screen. Using an umbilical cord sample avoids direct sampling of the neonate. The blood banking tests of interest are the ABO group, Rh (D) type, DAT, and RBC antibody screen. The results of these tests determine whether HDN is a threat—particularly when viewed within the context of the maternal blood group and RBC antibody screen—the clinical setting, the serum bilirubin, the blood hematocrit, and the stained blood smear.

ABO grouping of neonates relies entirely on RBC antigen grouping, eliminating serum grouping for confirmation, because alloantibodies present in umbilical cord blood serum are of maternal, not neonatal origin. Rh typing, including tests for weak D, formerly called D(u), is indicated for infants born to Rh-negative mothers who are not already immunized to the Rh (D) antigen. Accurate Rh testing can be difficult if the RBCs are heavily coated with IgG antibodies (positive direct antiglobulin test)—may give false-negative results—or if samples are contaminated with Wharton jelly—may give false-positive results.[3]

The RBC antibody screen is intended to detect and identify maternal IgG antibodies transported across the placenta and are free in neonatal plasma. The direct antiglobulin test detects *in vivo coating* of umbilical cord blood RBCs by maternal IgG antibody. However, a negative direct antiglobulin test does not guarantee absence of coating antibody, since antiglobulin reagents require approximately 200 molecules of IgG per RBC to give a positive reaction.[4]

A special consideration for the testing of neonates younger than 4 months age is that an initial pretransfusion sample is obtained to determine the ABO group, Rh type, and RBC antibody screen. Repeated testing is then unnecessary for the remainder of the neonate's hospital admission. The serum or plasma of either the neonate or the mother may be used to perform the test for unexpected antibodies. If the initial screen for red cell antibodies is negative, it is unnecessary to crossmatch donor red cells or to request antibody testing for the first 4 months of life during any one hospital admission. If the initial antibody screen demonstrates clinically significant unexpected red cell antibodies, RBC units prepared for transfusion should either not contain the corresponding antigen or be compatible by antiglobulin crossmatch until the antibody is no longer detectable. If a non–group-O neonate (e.g., group A) is to receive non-group-O RBCs (e.g., group A) that are not compatible with the maternal ABO group (e.g., group O), the neonate's serum or plasma should be tested for anti-A or anti-B (in this example, anti-A) by an antiglobulin phase using A_1 or B red cells (in this example, A_1 red cells). If anti-A or anti-B is detected, RBCs lacking the corresponding ABO antigen should be transfused.[5]

What are the implications of testing?

What does an abnormal test result mean? A positive direct antiglobulin test usually indicates the presence of a RBC alloantibody binding to its antigen on the cell surface. The specificity of the antibody is identified by eluting it off the RBC and testing the eluate against a RBC panel. It is usually unnecessary to perform elution studies when the maternal serum contains known clinically significant antibodies. However, this additional information can be of value determining the antibodies responsible for HDN (e.g., multiple maternal alloantibodies and usually difficult instances of ABO hemolytic disease). A positive direct antiglobulin test on the RBCs from infants of women with negative antibody screening tests—using standard group O screening RBCs—suggests either ABO hemolytic disease of the newborn or HDN due to a low-incidence antigen not expressed on the screening cells. An eluate from the umbilical cord blood RBCs is required to confirm the diagnosis. RBC antibody screen using umbilical cord blood plasma or serum serves the same purpose, particularly when reacted with group A_1 or B RBCs. It is preferable to study only those infants who exhibit features of hemolysis, such as anemia and/or indirect hyperbilirubinemia to establish the diagnosis of ABO hemolytic disease of the newborn.

What does a normal test result mean? Rh (D)–negative women who deliver an Rh-positive child with a negative direct antiglobulin test should receive anti-D immunoglobulin 125 to 300 mcg depending on local practices and undergo additional testing (e.g., Rosette, Kleihauer-Betke or flow cytometry studies) to detect a fetomaternal hemorrhage greater than 30 mL. Those women will require additional immunoglobulin. If a hemorrhage of this magnitude or more has occurred, additional anti-D immunoglobulin is necessary.[6,7]

No testing is necessary on the umbilical cord blood of babies born to Rh-positive mothers who have negative antibody screening tests unless there are clinical signs and symptoms of HDN. In that instance, umbilical cord blood studies may aide in the detection and identification of the responsible antibodies.

What is the cost of testing?

Patient charges include reagent costs, labor, and overhead (e.g., space, utilities, insurance, etc.), and often exceed laboratory costs several-fold. It is perhaps better to focus on laboratory costs, not patient charges, as the latter varies greatly among hospitals and does not reflect a true picture because of varying degrees of reimbursement. Actual reagent and supply costs for umbilical cord blood ABO group, Rh (D) type, and direct antiglobulin test are approximately $2.65. Labor costs are $4, based on 12 minutes per test at $20 per hour. Thus, the total laboratory costs are about $6.65.

It is possible to reduce health care costs by limiting umbilical cord blood testing to women with clinically significant maternal RBC antibodies or who are Rh-negative. In the latter, the umbilical cord blood Rh type is used to determine the need for anti-D immunoglobulin administration. But is this cost-effective? Assume 100 Rh (D) negative women who are not immunized to the Rh (D) antigen deliver an infant of unknown Rh (D) type. Statistically, 60 newborns will be Rh-positive and 40 Rh-negative. The pharmacy cost at the University of Iowa for one 300-mcg vial of anti-D immunoglobulin is approximately $80; the cost of administering it (nursing and materials) is another $25. Thus, the total cost of testing the 100 umbilical cord blood samples for their RBC ABO group, Rh-D type, and direct antiglobulin test ($6.65 each) and of treating ($105 each) the 60 women with Rh-positive children is $6,700. In comparison, the cost of simply treating the 100 women with anti-D immunoglobulin is $6300. Unfortunately, the later approach misses the one in 200 to one in 400 women who experience a fetal to maternal transfusion greater than 30 mL whole blood.

■ Conclusions and Recommendations

It is prudent to collect and accurately label an umbilical cord blood sample from all neonates at delivery. This sample can be used to determine the Rh (D) type from all neonates delivered of Rh-negative women who have not been immunized to the Rh (D) antigen. This eliminates the need to sample neonates directly. It is neither wise nor cost-effective to test all umbilical cord blood samples routinely for ABO group, Rh (D) type, DAT, or RBC antibody screen, and the predictive value of test results for HDN is quite poor. Study blood samples only from those infants who exhibit features of HDN to confirm the diagnosis and to identify the antibodies responsible.

Although it is recommended that blood samples be collected from the umbilical cords of all neonates, it is not necessary to test these samples routinely, except when the maternal serum contains clinically significant RBC antibodies or the mother is Rh-negative.[6]

■ Summary

1 ■ What Is the Problem that Requires Screening?

Newborn Rh status, neonatal hemolytic anemia.

a. What is the incidence/prevalence of the target condition?

Two percent to 5% of pregnant women exhibit RBC alloimmunization. The prevalence of clinically apparent hemolytic disease of the newborn for Rh antibodies is about 1/1,000. Antibodies for other RBC antigens occur in 3/1,000 births, of whom approximately 10% (3/10,000) exhibit significant hemolytic disease of the newborn.

b. What are the sequelae of the condition that are of interest in clinical medicine?

Rh-positive women who deliver an Rh-negative child are at risk of alloimmunization to D. Severe RBC alloimmunization, whether secondary to RhD or another alloantibody may cause profound hemolytic anemia ending in intrauterine fetal hydrops, fetal death, preterm delivery and after delivery, hyperbilirubinemia and kernicterus.

2 ■ The Tests

a. What is the purpose of the tests?

To determine the newborn blood type to identify those with HDN and Rh (D)–negative women at risk of developing alloimmunization. Such women should be given anti-D immunoglobulin prophylaxis to prevent the subsequent development of alloimmunization.

b. What is the nature of the tests?

Tests may include ABO grouping, Rh type, direct antiglobulin test, and RBC antibody screen.

c. What are the implications of testing?

1. What does an abnormal test result mean?
   A positive direct antiglobulin test usually indicates the presence of a RBC alloantibody binding to its antigen on the cell

surface. The affected child is at risk of HDN and referred for appropriate evaluation and care.

2. What does normal test result mean?

Rh (D)–negative women who deliver an Rh-positive child with a negative direct antiglobulin test should receive anti-D immunoglobulin 125 to 300 mcg depending on local practices and undergo additional testing to detect a FMH greater than 30 mL. Those women will require additional immunoglobulin.

No testing is necessary on the umbilical cord sample from newborns of Rh-positive mothers who have negative antibody screening tests in the absence of clinical signs and symptoms of hemolytic disease of the newborn.

d. What is the cost of testing?

It is possible to reduce costs by limiting cord blood testing to women with significant maternal RBC antibodies or to those who are Rh negative. In the latter, the cord blood Rh type is used to determine need for anti-D immunoglobulin administration.

3 ■ Conclusions and Recommendations

It is prudent to collect and accurately label an umbilical cord blood sample from all neonates at delivery. It is neither wise nor cost-effective to test all cord blood samples routinely for ABO group, Rh(D) type, direct antiglobulin, or anti-RBC antibody screen. It is better to study blood samples of only those infants who exhibit features of hemolytic disease of the newborn.

References

1. Geifman-Holtzman O, Wojtowycz M, Kosmas E, Artal R. Female alloimmunization with antibodies known to cause hemolytic disease. *Obstet Gynecol* 1997;89:272–275.
2. Moise KJ, Jr. Changing trends in the management of red blood cell alloimmunization in pregnancy. *Arch Path Lab Med* 1994;118:421–428.
3. Brecher, ME, ed. *Technical Manual*, 14th ed. Bethesda, MD: American Association of Blood Banks, 2002: 505–506.
4. Petz LD, Garratty G. *Acquired Immune Hemolytic Anemias*. New York: Churchill-Livingstone, 1980.
5. American Association of Blood Banks. *Standards for Blood Banks and Transfusion Services*, 22nd ed. Bethesda, MD: American Association of Blood Banks, 2003;49–50.

6. Judd WJ, for the Scientific Section Coordinating Committee of the AABB. Practice guidelines for prenatal and perinatal immunohematology, revisited. *Transfusion* 2001;41:1445–1452.

7. Crowther CA, Keirse MJNC. Anti-D administration in pregnancy for preventing rhesus alloimmunisation. *Cochrane Database Syst Rev* 2000; (2): CD000020.

40

When to Screen for Neonatal Hypoglycemia

Diva D. DeLeón

Charles A. Stanley

■ What Is the Problem that Requires Screening?

Hypoglycemia in the newborn period.

What is the incidence/prevalence of the target condition?

Controversy continues on whether the standards for diagnosing and treating hypoglycemia should be different in neonates than in older children and adults.[1–6] Some pediatricians and neonatologists contend that lower limits should be used in neonates based on a statistical definition of normal glucose levels derived from neonates not fed until 8 to 12 hours after delivery. However, the "statistical normal" does not necessarily indicate what is "physiologically normal." We prefer the same standards for diagnosis and treatment of hypoglycemia in neonates as in older children. The concentrations of plasma glucose in the fetus are quite similar to the values maintained in their mothers' blood and to levels found in infants of a few days of age and older. In the absence of convincing evidence to the contrary, it is reasonable to assume that the physiologically optimal requirement for plasma glucose in neonates is the same as that in older children. Based on these considerations, a plasma glucose below 50 mg/dL (2.8 mmol/L) is suggested for the diagnosis of hypoglycemia. This is the same value used in older children and adults and reflects a threshold low enough to include only cases with clearly identifiable disorder.[7] Note that a large proportion of otherwise normal neonates on the first day of life can fall below 50 mg/dL if feedings are delayed for as little as 4 to 6 hours. Such cases do not require investigation and need only simple measures to restore plasma glucose to 70 to 90 mg/dL.

Neonatal hypoglycemia can be classified in three groups according to its duration and etiology:

1. Transient hypoglycemia during the first 24 hours of life is due to immaturity of fasting adaptation systems (gluconeogenesis and ketogenesis) in

otherwise healthy infants who are exposed to excessive fasting on the first postnatal day. Lubchenko and Bard[1] found that 50% of appropriate for gestational age (AGA) term neonates dropped below 50 mg/dL if fasted for 8 hours, 10% dropped below 30 mg/dL, and 2% below 20mg/dL.

2. Prolonged hypoglycemia in at-risk groups (perinatal asphyxia, small for gestational age, large for gestational age, infant of diabetic mother, preterm birth) is usually secondary to hyperinsulinism that eventually resolves but may require 1 to 2 weeks or as long as 2 to 3 months of therapy. Although the prevalence of prolonged hypoglycemia approximates 4.4/1,000 live births, it may be as high as 15.5/1,000 in low-birth-weight infants.[8]

3. Permanent hypoglycemia may result from congenital diseases including genetic disorders of glycogenolysis and gluconeogenesis (glycogen storage diseases), fatty acid oxidation, deficiency of counterregulatory hormones (panhypopituitarism), and congenital hyperinsulinism, which is the most common cause of persistent hypoglycemia. The prevalence of these disorders ranges from 1/8,000 to 1/40,000 live births.

What are the sequelae of the conditions that are of interest in clinical medicine?

Newborns are at high risk of being unable to maintain plasma glucose concentrations during periods of fasting, and neonatal hypoglycemia can cause seizures and permanent brain damage. Neonatal hypoglycemia is especially challenging because of the wide range of potential causes, both transient and permanent, and the outcome may be influenced by the etiology.

Several studies have looked at the long-term sequelae of low plasma glucose levels in symptomatic and asymptomatic neonates.[9–12] Although these studies vary in their definitions of hypoglycemia, neurodevelopmental impairments were documented in up to 50% of children with a history of symptomatic neonatal hypoglycemia. One multicenter study of preterm infants found a correlation between reduced mental and motor developmental scores at 18 months and the number of days with a plasma glucose value below 2.6 mmol/L (47 mg/dL).[9] Children with persistent hypoglycemia had a 3.5-fold greater risk of developmental delay than those without.[9] Long-term follow up of 114 infants with neonatal hypoglycemia due to congenital hyperinsulinism documented that 44% had neurodevelopmental delays.[13] The latter group of infants is at particularly high risk of brain injury because they can not produce ketones as alternative fuels for brain metabolism when glucose levels are low.

To our knowledge, there have not been any randomized trials of the effect of hypoglycemia prevention on neurodevelopmental outcomes. Anecdotally, in severe hypoglycemic disorders that recur in families (e.g., hyperinsulinism) early detection and treatment can prevent damage.

■ The Tests

What is the purpose of the tests?

To identify neonates at risk of recurrent hypoglycemia. Once such infants have been identified, efforts to elucidate the cause should be initiated. Early diagnosis and treatment are considered critical for the prevention of permanent brain damage secondary to hypoglycemia.

What is the nature of the tests?

Screening procedures for neonatal hypoglycemia are designed to allow the rapid detection of low blood glucose levels, to permit rapid corrective measures, and to initiate steps for diagnosis of specific causes in cases where hypoglycemia is a persistent or permanent problem. The measurement of plasma glucose level by the hexokinase method is the gold standard.[14] However, these results are not available quickly enough for timely treatment as they are usually performed in the clinical laboratory. Therefore, point-of-care glucose meters are typically used for the measurement of blood glucose concentration in nursery and neonatal intensive care units.

There are a number of potential artifacts that can interfere with measurement. First, whole-blood glucose concentrations are 10% to 15% lower than plasma glucose levels. Second, bedside meters are less precise than laboratory glucose assays and have an error range of 10% to 15%. Bedside meters are also prone to errors due to outdated strips, or sampling errors, which will result in falsely low or high readings. In light of these issues, point-of-care meters can be used for screening purposes, but any glucose value below 60 mg/dL should be verified by a laboratory measurement. Treatment should not be delayed while waiting for laboratory confirmation.

Routine screening is not recommended for healthy, term infants born following an uncomplicated pregnancy and delivery who have no clinical signs of hypoglycemia and have begun feeding without delay. However, healthy term infants who are being breast-fed poorly are at higher risk of hypoglycemia. Early and frequent feedings with supplementation, if necessary, are recommended until breast milk production is adequate. All infants with clinical signs of hypoglycemia (Table 40–1) should have a blood glucose level measured promptly.

Infants at high risk of hypoglycemia should be screened as soon after birth as possible and any low glucose value should be immediately treated. These include infants at risk due to maternal factors (e.g., diabetes), intrinsic neonatal problems (intrauterine growth restriction, large for gestational age, or perinatal asphyxia) or any suspected endocrine or metabolic disorders (e.g., hepatomegaly, midline defects, micropenis, ambiguous genitalia, etc.) (Table 40–2). It is important that monitoring continues after treatment because these high-risk groups include infants who are also at risk of disorders associated with prolonged and permanent hypoglycemic disorders.

Table 40–1	Clinical signs of hypoglycemia in the neonate

Poor feeding
Cyanosis
Pallor
Tachypnea
Respiratory distress
Apnea
Tachycardia
Hypothermia
Sweating
Irritability
High-pitched cry
Somnolence
Lethargy
Floppiness
Tremors
Seizures
Coma

What are the implications of testing?

What does an abnormal test result mean? An abnormal test means the blood glucose may be too low and therapy should be initiated promptly to restore the plasma glucose to the 70- to 90-mg/dL range. Failure to treat a low glucose

Table 40–2	Etiology of hypoglycemia in neonates

I. Transient Neonatal Hypoglycemia
   A. Developmental immaturity of fasting adaptation (first 12–24 h of life in normal neonates) (mechanism: impaired ketogenesis & gluconeogenesis)
   B. Due to maternal factors
      1. Maternal diabetes (LGA or SGA) (mechanism: hyperinsulinism)
      2. IV glucose administration during labor and delivery (mechanism: hyperinsulinism)
      3. Medications: oral hypoglycemics, terbutaline, propranolol (mechanism: hyperinsulinism)
II. Prolonged Neonatal Hypoglycemia (most, if not all, involve hyperinsulinism)
   A. Intrauterine growth retardation
   B. Birth asphyxia
   C. Maternal toxemia/preeclampsia
   D. Prematurity
   E. Sepsis
   F. Erythroblastosis fetalis, fetal hydrops
   G. Polycythemia
III. Permanent Neonatal Hypoglycemia (caused by congenital Endocrine/Metabolic Disorders)
   A. Hyperinsulinism
   B. Counterregulatory hormone deficiency
      1. Panhypopituitarism
      2. Adrenal Insufficiency
   C. Gluconeogenesis/Glycogenolysis disorders
   D. Fatty Acid Oxidation Disorders

IV, intravenous; LGA, large for gestational age; SGA, small for gestational age.

level can result in permanent brain damage. The postnatal age of the infant and the presence of risk factors should be taken into consideration when interpreting an abnormal blood glucose level (Figure 40–1). These factors help determine the possible etiology and the therapy. The presence of hypoglycemia on the first day of life in the absence of risk factors when appropriate feedings have not been initiated suggests developmental immaturity of fasting adaptation. The neonate must be fed and the blood glucose measurement repeated to ensure it has been corrected. In the presence of risk factors, blood glucose monitoring should continue after correction, and if hypoglycemia persists, appropriate diagnostic evaluation should be started. Hypoglycemia that persists beyond the first 24 hours of life suggests prolonged disorders, such as transient hyperinsulinism induced by perinatal asphyxia, which will resolve eventually; or permanent disorders, like congenital hyperinsulinism, hypopituitarism, or genetic metabolic disorders (Table 40–2). The documentation of a low blood glucose level should initiate not only prompt therapy but also a diagnostic work up in the latter groups to elucidate the cause of hypoglycemia.

What does a normal test result mean? A normal plasma glucose level by a bedside meter is reassuring that the blood glucose is normal at that moment. However, one normal blood glucose level does not exclude a hypoglycemic disorder, and infants with risk factors or symptoms may need further screening.

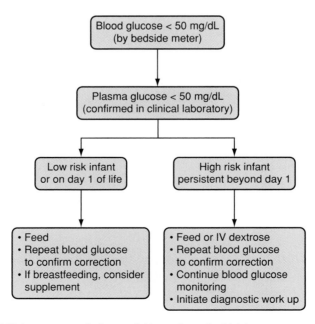

Figure 40-1 Initial management of neonatal hypoglycemia. IV, intravenous.

What is the cost of testing?

The cost of the point-of-care screening varies from $0.50 to $1 per glucose test depending on the instrument used. The cost of a laboratory plasma glucose level is around $40.

Cost-benefit assessments of hypoglycemia screening in various types of high-risk infants have not been performed. For transient hypoglycemia due to developmental delays in fasting adaptation, prevention by early initiation of feeding is probably more efficient than screening. For problems of prolonged hypoglycemia in high-risk newborns (4.4/1000 live births), early detection and treatment of hypoglycemia is likely to be highly cost-effective considering the potential for avoiding severe neurologic handicaps (reported in up to 50%) and the high frequency of hypoglycemia in these infants.

■ Conclusions and Recommendations

Hypoglycemia is a common concern in neonates and when untreated may result in permanent neurodevelopment handicap. Accurate and prompt diagnosis of hypoglycemia in neonates relies on an active surveillance program for clinical signs, identification of risk factors, and the use of an appropriate method to measure glucose levels. Detection of low blood glucose levels should trigger immediate intervention and a diagnostic workup for the underlying cause if indicated by the circumstances.

■ Summary

1 ■ What Is the Problem that Requires Screening?

Neonatal hypoglycemia.

a. What is the incidence/prevalence of the target condition?
4.4/1,000 live births.

b. What are the sequelae of the condition that are of interest in clinical medicine?
Multiple neurodevelopmental deficits, including seizures and permanent brain damage.

2 ■ The Tests

a. *What is the purpose of the tests?*

To identify neonates at risk of recurrent hypoglycemia. Once such infants have been identified, efforts to elucidate the etiology should be initiated.

b. *What is the nature of the tests?*

Blood glucose measurement by bedside glucose meters.

c. *What are the implications of testing?*

1. What does an abnormal test result mean?
   An abnormal test means that the blood glucose is too low and needs prompt treatment; follow-up testing and diagnostic evaluations should be considered in infants with risk factors.
2. What does a normal test result mean?
   A normal plasma glucose level by a bedside meter is reassuring that the blood glucose is normal at that moment; infants with risk factors may need follow-up monitoring.

d. *What is the cost of testing?*

The cost of the point-of-care screening varies from $0.50 to $1 per glucose test depending on the instrument used.

3 ■ Conclusions and Recommendations

Hypoglycemia is common in neonates and when recurrent and untreated may result in permanent neurodevelopment damage. Detection of a low blood glucose level should trigger immediate intervention and a determination of the need for follow-up monitoring. The postnatal age, presence of risk factors for prolonged hypoglycemia (such as small or large for gestational age, birth asphyxia, prematurity) and recurrence of hypoglycemia should be considered in deciding whether a diagnostic workup for the underlying cause is needed.

References

1. Lubchenco LO, Bard H. Incidence of hypoglycemia in newborn infants by birth weight and gestational age. *Pediatrics* 1971;47:831–838.
2. Cornblath M, Hawdon JM, Williams AF, et al. Controversies regarding definition of neonatal hypoglycemia: suggested operational thresholds. *Pediatrics* 2000;105:1141–1145.

3. Koh THHG, Aynsley-Green A. Neonatal hypoglycemia: the controversy regarding definition. *Arch Dis Child* 1988;63:1386–1398.

4. Cornblath M. Neonatal hypoglycemia 30 years later: does it injure the brain? Historical summary and present challenges. *Acta Pediatr Jpn* 1997;39:S7–S11.

5. Srinivasan G, Pildes RS, Cattamanchi G, et al. Clinical and laboratory observations: plasma glucose values in normal neonates: a new look. *J Pediatr* 1986;109:114–117.

6. Heck LJ, Erenberg A. Serum glucose levels in term neonates during the first 48 hours of life. *J Pediatr* 1987;110:119–122.

7. Sperling MA, ed. *Pediatric Endocrinology,* 2nd ed. Philadelphia: Saunders, 2002:796.

8. Gutberlet RL, Cornblath M. Neonatal hypoglycemia, revisited, 1975. *Pediatrics* 1976;58:10–17.

9. Lucas A, Morley R, Cole TJ. Adverse neurodevelopmental outcome of moderate neonatal hypoglycemia. *BMJ* 1988;297:1304–1308.

10. Duvanel CB, Fawer CL, Cotting J. Long-term effects of neonatal hypoglycemia on brain growth and psychomotor developmental in small-for gestational. *J Pediatr* 1999;134:492–496.

11. Koivisto M, Blanco-Sequeiros M, Krause U. Neonatal symptomatic and asymptomatic hypoglycaemia: a follow-up study in 151 children. *Dev Med Child Neurol* 1972;14:603–614.

12. Stenninger E, Flink R, Eriksson B, et al., Long term neurological dysfunction and neonatal hypoglycaemia after diabetic pregnancy. *Arch Dis Child* 1998;79:F174–F179.

13. Meissner T, Wendel U, Burgard P, et al. Long-term follow-up of 114 patients with congenital hyperinsulinism. *Eur J Endocrinol* 2003;149:43–51.

14. Ho HT, Yeung WKY, Young BWY. Evaluation of "point of care" devices in the measurement of low blood glucose in neonatal practice. *Arch Dis Child Fetal Neonatal Ed* 2004;89:F356–F359.

Neonatal Hyperbilirubinemia

Vinod K. Bhutani

Lois H. Johnson

■ What Is the Problem that Requires Screening?

Kernicterus and bilirubin-induced neurologic dysfunction (BIND).

What is the incidence / prevalence of the target condition?

The true contemporary prevalence of kernicterus or BIND is unknown as neither is a reportable condition.[1,2] Further, the natural course of neonatal hyperbilirubinemia is modulated by infant feeding practices (e.g., patterns for breast feeding in the community), early recognition and intervention (early use of phototherapy), and the availability of other bilirubin-reduction strategies.[3-5] Severe hyperbilirubinemia remains the most plausible surrogate indicator for kernicterus,[4] even though the risk of kernicterus at specific total serum bilirubin (TSB) ranges is estimated by clinical consensus rather than evidence-based criteria (Table 41–1). Clinically significant hyperbilirubinemia occurs in from 8% to 11% of infants with approximately 5% being treated with phototherapy and 2.7% requiring readmission for hospital treatment. Total serum bilirubin concentrations increase to 25 mg/dL (250 mg/L; 428 fmol/L) and 30 mg/dL (300 mg/L; 513 fmol/L) in 1:700 and 1 in 10,000 infants, respectively (Table 41–1).

What are the sequelae of the condition that are of interest in clinical medicine?

Kernicterus is a preventable brain injury due to severe, neonatal jaundice with serious and often irreversible posticteric sequelae.[2,6] The hallmark of kernicterus is the icteric (yellow) staining of the basal ganglia (specifically the globus pallidus), which may be demonstrated at autopsy or by echogenicity on neuroimaging. BIND constitutes a wide spectrum of disorders that includes kernicterus in its more severe acute and chronic forms. It results when the total serum bilirubin exceeds the infant's neuroprotective defenses, causing

Table 41-1	Incidence of severe hyperbilirubinemia in term and near-term infants				
Adjective	Total serum bilirubin level	Total serum bilirubin percentile	Incidence		Risk of kernicterus
Significant	>17 mg/dL	>95th centile	8.1 to 10%	1 in 10	Unlikely; subtle effects debated but unproven
Severe	>20 mg/dL	>98th centile	1 to 2%	1 in 70	Unlikely; cases reported.
Extreme	>25 mg/dL	>99.9th centile	0.16%	1 in 700	Of concern, though actual risk unknown
Hazardous	>30 mg/dL	>99.99th centile	0 to 0.032%	1 in 10,000	Increasing likely; unacceptable risk

neuronal injury primarily in the basal ganglia; central and peripheral auditory pathways; hippocampus; diencephalon; subthalamic nuclei; midbrain; pontine and brainstem nuclei for oculomotor function, respiratory, neurohumoral, and electrolyte control; and the cerebellum.[6,7] Approximately 60% of otherwise healthy newborns in the United States develop jaundice associated with increased total serum bilirubin concentration.[1,8] Although most are discharged from their birth hospital by 72 hours of age, the total serum bilirubin does not usually peak until 72 to 120 hours of age. Jaundice usually resolves with a benign outcome by 7 to 10 days of age. Adverse manifestations related to excessive hyperbilirubinemia are as follows:

Acute bilirubin encephalopathy (ABE). Increasing hypertonia, especially of extensor muscles, with retrocolis and opisthotonus, in association with varying degrees of drowsiness, poor feeding, hypotonia, and alternating tone. The early presenting signs and symptoms of ABE are described in terms of mental status, muscle tone, and cry.[1,6] These include feeding difficulties, lethargy with altered awake–sleep pattern, irritability and fussiness, difficult to console, and intermittent arching. Acute-stage mortality is due to respiratory failure and progressive coma or intractable seizures. The rate of clinical progression depends on the rate of bilirubin rise, the duration of hyperbilirubinemia, host susceptibility and the presence of co-morbidities.

Kernicterus, or chronic irreversible bilirubin encephalopathy (CBE). CBE has a variable presentation that includes extrapyramidal movement disorders (dystonia and athetosis), gaze abnormalities (especially upward gaze), auditory disturbances (especially sensorineural hearing loss with central processing disorders and/or auditory neuropathy), and enamel dysplasia of the deciduous teeth.[1,6,7] Cognitive deficits are unusual. Clinically, the minimal to severe range occurs with varying combinations of extrapyramidal disorders and neuromotor abnormalities. Sensorineural hearing loss and visual disability may occur as isolated entities. Neuromotor manifestations of extrapyramidal damage are present in almost all cases. Although unproven, some investigators believe there may be milder and subtler neurologic manifestations of BIND with signs of awkwardness, incoordination, gait abnormalities, fine tremors, and exaggerated extrapyramidal reflexes.[8–11] These subtle signs are difficult to diagnose because of delayed clinical expression and may be the only residual sequelae of ABE.[6,8,12]

■ The Tests

Clinical tests address the need for (a) recognition of early-onset hyperbilirubinemia that is usually due to hemolytic disorders such as alloimmunization, extravascular hemolysis (bruises and hematomas), and intravascular hemolysis (such as neonatal red blood cell or enzyme disorders) and (b) predischarge risk assessment for late-onset hyperbilirubinemia.

What is the purpose of the tests?

Detection of severe hyperbilirubinemia to prevent ABE and CBE, while minimizing the risks of unintended harm such as decreased breast-feeding, undue parental anxiety, and unnecessary treatment.[1,6]

What is the nature of the tests?

Visual assessment of jaundice. All newborns should be routinely monitored for the development of jaundice using established nursery protocols.[6,8] Jaundice is sought whenever the infant's vital signs are measured, but no less than every 8 to 12 hours. It is detected by blanching the skin with digital pressure on the forehead, mid sternum, or knee/ankle to reveal the underlying color of the skin and subcutaneous tissue. Jaundice usually first appears in the face before progressing caudally to the trunk and extremities (Figure 41–1). It can sometimes appear and fade like a suntan. The visual assessment must be done in a well-lit room or, preferably, at a window in daylight. The absence of jaundice does not necessarily mean the absence of hyperbilirubinemia, and estimating the degree of hyperbilirubinemia visually can lead to errors; nor does the absence or severity of jaundice predict subsequent severe hyperbilirubinemia.[3,6,8,13] Before discharge (particularly for those younger than 24 hours), the presence of clinical jaundice must corroborated by a bilirubin measurement (either total serum bilirubin [TSB] or a transcutaneous bilirubin [TcB]).

EXPECTED BILIRUBIN LEVELS FOR
CEPHALO-CAUDAL PROGRESSION

Jaundice progression	Zone	Bilirubin (mg/dL,mean)
None	0	0
Face and neck	1	5
Umbilicus	2	10
Knees	3	15
Ankles	4	20
Toes	5	>20

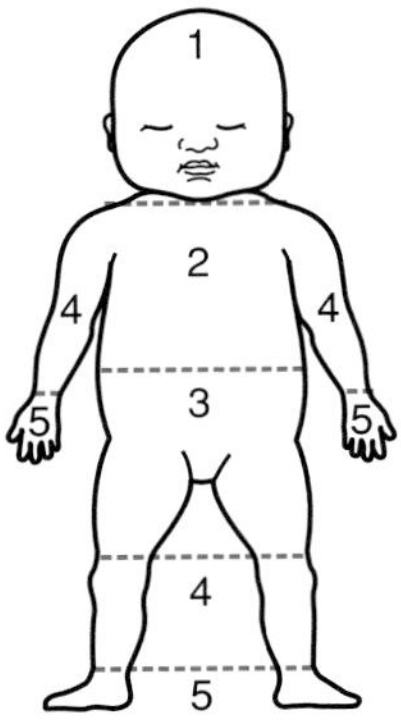

Figure 41-1 Expected bilirubin levels for cephalocaudal progression. From Kramer, LI. Advancement of dermal icterus in the jaundiced newborn. *Am J Dis Child* 1969;118:454–458.

Clinical risk factors. Known clinical risk factors are summarized in Table 41–2.[1,8] Two evidence-based clinical risk factor scoring systems are reported.[14,15] The risk index by Newman et al.[14] is based on exclusive breast-feeding, a sibling history of newborn jaundice, bruising, cephalohematoma, gender, gestational age, maternal race, and age 25 years or older. The score was derived from a nested case-control study and is related to total serum bilirubin above 25 mg/dL (428 fmol/L). Keren et al.[15] developed a clinical risk factor score to identify neonates at risk of a postdischarge total serum bilirubin above the 95th percentile based on birth weight, gestational age less than 38 weeks, oxytocin use during delivery, vacuum extraction, breast-feeding and combination breast and bottle feeding. Neither score has been prospectively validated.

Bilirubin measurement. The American Academy of Pediatrics (AAP) recommends a predischarge assessment that includes a ratio of the total to transcutaneous bilirubin (TSB/TcB) measurement plotted on an hour-specific nomogram of risk zones and /or an assessment of clinical risk factors. The nomogram illustrates the magnitude of hyperbilirubinemia in the context of postnatal age and the percentile level as defined for healthy infants.[5]

TSB and TcB, when plotted on an hour-specific nomogram, are the only clinical tests currently available to predict the risk of severe hyperbilirubinemia (Figure 41–2). When measured in term and near-term newborns concurrent with routine predischarge metabolic screening and plotted on the nomogram in lieu of using a day-specific value, the total serum bilirubin is a powerful screening tool (Figure 41–3) that defines high risk and low risk of postdischarge excessive hyperbilirubinemia. These data allow the identification of high-risk and low-risk populations and has been validated in several prospective studies.[1,16,17]

Table 41–2	**Prenatal, natal and postnatal clinical risk factors reported in the literature**		
Clinical risk factors	**Prenatal**	**Natal**	**Postnatal**
Major	**Race:** East-Asian, Arabic, Chinese, Mediterranean	**Mode of delivery:** forceps, vacuum, birth trauma	**Blood group:** incompatibility
	Mode of Feeding: breast feeding only	**Maternal medication:** oxytocin induction	**Early jaundice** (< 24 hours)
	Sibling treated with phototherapy	**Gestation** at 35 or 36 weeks	**Blood collection:** hematoma, cephal-hematoma, bruising
Minor	**Maternal** hypertension, diabetes mellitus.	**Gestation:** <38 weeks	**Sub-optimal lactation:** infant's inability to breast feed.
	Maternal Age >25 years		**LGA:** large for gestational age
	Family History: sibling with jaundice		**Birth Weight:** more than 3.5kg

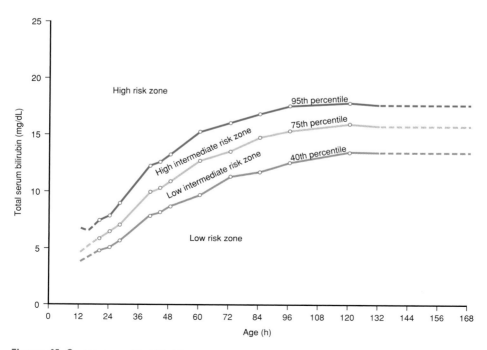

Figure 41-2 Hour-specific bilirubin nomogram.

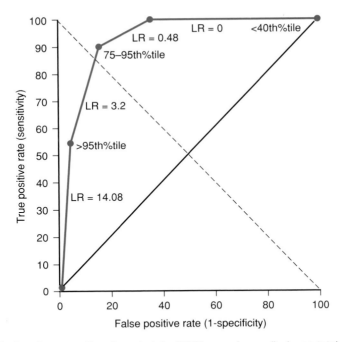

Figure 41-3   Receiver operating characteristic (ROC) curve for predischarge total serum bilirubin level. Adapted from van Pragh R. Diagnosis of kernicterus in the neonatal period. *Pediatrics* 1961;28:870–874. *LR,* Likelihood ratio.

Transcutaneous bilirubin testing. TCB is a noninvasive potential alternative to TSB measurement. Limited data suggest the TcB devices provide a valid estimate of the total serum bilirubinlevel.[17–19] TcB levels may be unreliable during phototherapy or after exposure to sunlight because of skin bleaching by the light. Confounding effects of skin melanin content among different races and manufacturing inconsistency among devices are additional limitations. The BiliChek device (Respironics, Murraysville, PA) seems to have overcome earlier limitations by correcting for skin melanin content.[18] Measurements in newborns using the new TcB devices are within 2 to 3 mg/dL (34–51 μmol/L) of the TSB and useful for total serum bilirubin levels below 15 mg/dL (257 μmol/L).

What are the implications of testing?

Decision analysis in the clinical setting is complicated by variability in bilirubin measurements attributed to laboratory and sampling methodologies, and uncertainty as to which TSB/TcB threshold values can be regarded as safe. By expressing the TSB in terms of risk zone rather than the actual TSB value, the imprecision of TSB measurement is reduced. The low-risk zone is a safe zone for term and healthy neonates.

What does an abnormal test result mean? The hour-specific bilirubin nomogram provides a useful clinical guide for management since the patterns of severity (in milligram per deciliter) at the 95th percentile in a mixed population define the threshold for consideration and the recommendations for intervention.[1] It was developed using data from term and near-term infants free of hemolytic disease or other illnesses requiring neonatal intensive care unit (NICU) admission. The nomogram was not specifically designed for use in preterm infants or infants with co-morbidities requiring intensive neonatal care. These infants are at higher risk than term infants of developing bilirubin toxicity and develop kernicterus at lower bilirubin levels. In term or near-term infants, the nomogram may be helpful in identifying infants who have early hyperbilirubinemia (those in the high-risk zone or with a rapid rate of rise) and those who require further evaluation for a cause of their hyperbilirubinemia. Once it is known an infant has an ABO blood type incompatibility or a glucose 6-phospho-dehydrogenase (G6PD) deficiency, the nomogram may be used to track the progression and resolution of hyperbilirubinemia.

A. **Predischarge management:** A system-based approach in well-baby nurseries with multidisciplinary strategies can address parental education, clinical recognition of jaundice, and predischarge risk assessment as listed in Table 41–3.

B. **Use of hour-specific bilirubin nomogram to guide follow-up:** The primary purpose of the bilirubin nomogram is to provide a simple and accurate method for quantifying the risk a newborn will develop hyperbilirubinemia after discharge from the nursery requiring treatment.[5] Infants in the low-risk zone, particularly those discharged from the hospital before 72 hours of life, and all breast-fed infants should be seen by a health care provider (either in office or home visit) on day 4 or 5 of life to evaluate the nutritional status (hydration, weight loss, breast feeding) and to observe for obvious jaundice. Table 41–4 offers a bilirubin

---

Table 41–3 Strategies for inclusion in a systems approach to screen and manage neonatal hyperbilirubinemia

- Recognize the clinical significance of jaundice at age< 24 hours.
- Recognize the limitations of visual recognition of jaundice.
- Recognize and document clinical jaundice.
- Ensure post-discharge follow-up based on the severity of hyperbilirubinemia.
- Respond to parental concerns of newborn jaundice, poor feeding, lactational difficulties and change in behavior and activity.
- Provide ongoing lactational support to ensure adequacy of intake.
- Recognize the impact of race, ethnicity and family history.
- Diagnose the cause of severe hyperbilirubinemia.
- Institute intervention strategies when bilirubin is rising more rapidly than expected.
- Check serum albumin with TSB levels >95th percentile to gauge susceptibility to neurotoxicity.
- Aggressively and efficiently treat with intensive phototherapy and/or exchange transfusion in a timely manner at recommended thresholds.

Table 41–4	**Post-discharge and follow-up based on pre-discharge total serum bilirubin(mg/dL) level (based on the hour-specific bilirubin nomogram)**			
Pre-discharge total serum bilirubin level at postnatal age (hour-specific)	**Discharge only if total serum bilirubin/ TcB level is**	**TSB/TcB follow-up within**		**Repeat test optional (unless indicated by clinical risk factors)**
		24 hours	**48 hours**	
	< 95th percentile	*> 75th percentile*	*< 75th percentile*	*< 40th percentile*
41–44 hours	<12.3	>10.0	<10.0	<7.9
45–48 hours	<12.7	>10.4	<10.4	<8.2
49–hours	<13.2	>11.0	<11.0	<8.7
57–64 hours	<14.7	>12.2	<12.2	<9.4
65–72 hours	<15.5	>13.0	<13.0	<10.3
>72 hours	<15.5	>14.0	<14.0	<11.0

care map for designating follow-up for a repeated testing based on the predischarge bilirubin risk zone.

C. **Postdischarge follow-up management:** A seamless continuation of care to provide the following services (a) ensuring the arrangement and compliance for an outpatient follow-up appointments; (b) training of personnel to handle outpatient telephone calls for assessment of a symptomatic jaundiced newborn; (c) rapid emergency department/ office intervention plans to transfer a symptomatic neonate to a neonatal intensive care facility; and (d) expeditious and timely intervention with the appropriate and effective bilirubin reduction strategies.[1] It may be necessary to delay discharge until the period of greatest risk has passed (72–96 hours) if the there is an elevated risk of developing severe hyperbilirubinemia and appropriate follow-up cannot be assured (Table 41–5).

What does a normal test result mean? Infants with TSB or TcB values at less than 40th percentile for age are at low risk of hyperbilirubinemia and may be followed less intensively (but according to routine recommendations to allow for efficient targeting of services as well as cost). Importantly, the families can be reassured.

What is the cost of testing?

The actual cost of a TSB measurement when performed with the metabolic screen consists of the laboratory assay and obtaining an additional aliquot of blood. The institutional cost is no more than $1. Additional heel-stick measurements depend on the individual institutional charge. The costs for TcB

Table 41–5   A bilirubin reduction and management approach for term and near-term infants based on the severity of hyperbilirubinemia

Severe hyperbilirubinemia at >72 hours age	Follow rate of total serum bilirubin rise and/or B:A ratio[1]	Interventions
total serum bilirubin level <14 mg/dL total serum bilirubin level >75th percentile	and <0.20 mg/dL/hr	Nutritional support
total serum bilirubin level ≥17 mg/dL total serum bilirubin level >95th percentile	and >0.20 mg/dL/hr	Phototherapy
total serum bilirubin level ≥20 mg/dL total serum bilirubin level >98th percentile	and B:A ratio <7.0	Intensive phototherapy
total serum bilirubin level ≥25 mg/dL total serum bilirubin level >99.9th percentile	and/or B:A ratio ≥7.0 mg/g	Intensive phototherapy and prepare for an exchange transfusion
total serum bilirubin level ≥30 mg/dL total serum bilirubin level >99.99th percentile	and / or B:A ratio ≥7.0 mg/g	Intensive phototherapy and perform an exchange transfusion

[1] B:A ratio is the ratio of total serum bilirubin (mg/dL) value and the concurrent serum albumin (g/dL) value; such that at a total serum bilirubin of 25 mg/dL and a measured serum albumin level of 3.4 g/dL, the B:A ratio is 7.3 mg/g.

measurements are the capital cost of the device (range, $2,000 to $4,000) and the costs of the disposable probes (for calibration and hygiene, about $5 to $7 each). There are the additional costs for TSB measurements related to ensuring accuracy.[1,20,21] To address standardization concerns, the College of American Pathologists (CAP) conducts a neonatal bilirubin (NB) and a chemistry (C) survey every 4 months, providing each participating laboratory an assessment of its bilirubin calibration performance. Before recommending routine bilirubin testing for every newborn, performance standards are essential for both the TSB and TcB devices calibrated to nationally acceptable standards.[22]

■ Conclusions and Recommendations

Acute and chronic BIND can occur in term and preterm infants, but can be effectively prevented by the rapid reduction of the increased bilirubin levels by intensive phototherapy and/or exchange transfusion. However, these interventions leave a very narrow margin of safety for neonates who are at home and not under direct medical supervision during the natural peak of bilirubin (age, 3–5 days). To ensure a safe experience with newborn jaundice and to efficiently prevent excessive hyperbilirubinemia such that BIND (including kernicterus), every infant should be screened systematically for the risk of hyperbilirubinemia by both clinical and total serum hyperbilirubinemia/TcB screening based on the hour-specific bilirubin nomogram.

■ Summary

1 ■ What Is the Problem that Requires Screening?

Hyperbilirubinemia.

a. What is the incidence/prevalence of the target condition?
Clinically significant hyperbilirubinemia occurs in 8% to 11% of newborns.

b. What are the sequelae of the condition that are of interest in clinical medicine?
Bilirubin encephalopathy.

2 ■ The Tests

a. What is the purpose of the tests?

To identify those newborns at increased risk of acute or chronic bilirubin encephalopathy.

b. What is the nature of the tests?

Visual assessment of jaundice, clinical risk factors either singularly or in the form of a score, and the measurement of serum or transcutaneous bilirubin.

c. What are the implications of testing?

1. What does an abnormal test result mean?

   An abnormal test means the neonate has hyperbilirubinemia and is at increased risk of encephalopathy. Affected newborns should be monitored closely and a strategy initiated to reduce bilirubin levels (e.g., phototherapy or exchange transfusion).

2. What does a normal test result mean?

   A normal test means the newborn is unlikely to develop clinically significant hyperbilirubinemia.

d. What is the cost of testing?

The institutional cost of TSB measurement when performed with a metabolic screen is no more than $1.

3 ■ Conclusions and Recommendations

Acute and chronic BIND can occur in term and preterm infants, but can be effectively prevented by the rapid reduction of the increased bilirubin levels by intensive phototherapy and/or exchange transfusion. These interventions leave a very narrow margin of safety for neonates at home and not under direct medical supervision during the natural peak of bilirubin (age, 3–5 days). Every infant should be screened systematically.

References

1. American Academy of Pediatrics. Subcommittee on Hyperbilirubinemia: Maisels MJ, Baltz RD, Bhutani VK, et al. Clinical Practice Guideline: Management of hyperbilirubinemia in the newborn infant—35 weeks of gestation. *Pediatrics* 2004;114:297–316.
2. Bhutani VK, Johnson LH, Maisels MJ, et al. Kernicterus: epidemiological strategies for its prevention through systems-based approaches. *J Perinatol* 2004;24:650–652.

3. Davidson LT, Merritt KK, Weech AA. Hyperbilirubinemia in the newborn. *Am J Dis Child* 1941;61:958–980.
4. Gifford MJ, Gifford K. Normal serum bilirubin levels in the newborn and the effect of breast-feeding. *Pediatrics* 1986;78:837–843.
5. Bhutani VK, Johnson L, Sivieri EM. Predictive ability of a pre-discharge hour-specific serum bilirubin for subsequent significant hyperbilirubinemia in healthy term and near-term newborns. *Pediatrics* 1999;103:6–14.
6. Johnson L, Brown AK, Bhutani VK. System-based approach to management of neonatal jaundice and prevention of kernicterus. *J Pediatr* 2002;93:488–449.
7. van Pragh R. Diagnosis of kernicterus in the neonatal period. *Pediatrics* 1961;28:870–874.
8. Johnson L, Bhutani VK. Guidelines for management of the jaundiced term and near-term infant. *Clin Perinatol* 1998;25:555–574.
9. Soorani-Lunsing I, Woltil A, Hadders-Algra M. Are moderate degrees of hyperbilirubinemia in healthy term neonates really safe for the brain? *Pediatr Res* 2001;50:701–705.
10. Hintz S, Stevenson DK. Just when you thought it was safe. *Pediatr Res* 2001;50:674–676.
11. Bhutani VK. Neonatal hyperbilirubinemia and the potential risk of subtle neurological dysfunction. *Pediatr Res* 2001:50:679.
12. Johnson L. The hyperbilirubinemic term infant: When to worry, when to treat. *N Y State J Med* 2001;11:483–488.
13. Moyer VA, Ahn C, Sneed B. Accuracy of clinical judgement in neonatal jaundice. *Arch Pediatr Adolesc Med* 2000;154:391–394.
15. Keren R, Bhutani VK, Luan XQ, et al. Identifying newborns at risk of severe hyperbilirubinemia: a comparison of two recommended approaches, Pediatric Research. (Abstracts from Pediatric Academic Societies' Annual Meeting, San Francisco, CA, 2004.)
16. Stevenson DK, Fanaroff AA, Maisels MJ, et al. Prediction of hyperbilirubinemia in term and near-term newborn infants. *Pediatrics* 2001;108:31–39.
17. Ip S, Glicken S, Kulig J, et al. Management of Neonatal Hyperbilirubinemia. Rockville, MD: U.S. Department of Health and Human Services, Agency for Healthcare Research and Quality. 03, E011. AHRQ Publication, 2003.
18. Bhutani VK, Gourley G, Kreamer BL, et al. Non-invasive measurement of total serum bilirubin in a multi-racial pre-discharge newborn population to assess the risk of severe hyperbilirubinemia. *Pediatrics* 2000;106:e17.
19. Maisels MJ, Ostrea EM Jr, Touch S, et al. Evaluation of a new transcutaneous bilirubinometer. *Pediatrics* 2004;113:1628–1635.
20. Vreman HJ, Verter J, Stevenson DK Interlaboratory variability of bilirubin measurements. *Clin Chem* 1996;42:869–873.
21. Bhutani VK, Johnson LH. Urgent clinical need for accurate and precise bilirubin measurements in the United States to prevent kernicterus. *Clin Chem* 2004;50:477–480.
22. Ip S, Glicken S, Kulig J, Obrien R, Sege R, Lau J. Management of neonatal hyperbilirubinemia—U.S. Department of Health and Human Services, Rockville, MD, Aging for Healthcare Research and Quality 03, E011, 2003. AHRQ Publication.

Screening for Neonatal Genetic Disorders

Monique Williams

Neonatal screening for genetic disorders seeks to identify inheritable diseases that are asymptomatic at birth. The investigation may be clinical or laboratory based. When the child belongs to a group at high risk of a particular disease, such as Tay Sachs disease in the Ashkenazi Jewish population, investigations may go much further. Genetic counseling may to a great extent influence family life.

The application of tandem mass spectrometry to neonatal screening has led to the detection of both treatable and untreatable diseases. Parents will need to be informed about these disorders, of which the outcome is not always known, especially in diseases with different clinical spectra. Do parents really want to know about a disease that will present later in life if there is no therapeutic option? In some situations, knowing about the disease in advance may prepare parents for the future, though detection of the disease does not always automatically mean it will be symptomatic.[1]

Screening includes testing, providing information to the tested individual or obtaining informed consent from the tested individuals or their lawful caretakers, and providing an explanation of the test results.

The consequences of neonatal genetic screening will affect future generations. For example, female phenylketonuria patients may adversely affect their offspring if their phenylalanine levels are not strictly controlled before and during pregnancy. The development of new treatments, such as enzyme replacement therapy for lysosomal storage diseases, will make it necessary to detect the disease as soon as possible to prevent the onset of irreversible pathologies[2]

PHENYLKETONURIA

■ What Is the Problem that Requires Screening?

Mental retardation secondary to phenylketonuria (PKU).

What is the incidence/prevalence of the target condition?

The initial frequency of PKU (1/25,000 births) was based on the number of affected individuals in institutions for the mentally retarded. After newborn screening began in 1963, the prevalence was found to be much higher and vary considerably among populations: 1/2,400 in the Middle East to 1/4,000–6,000 births in Ireland; 1/6,000 in Scotland; 1/8,000 to 1/10,000 in former West Germany; and 1/16,000 Italy. Populations differ with respect to intermarriages between families and for example the frequency of consanguinity. The lowest prevalence is found in the Asian race; China and Japan, 1/60,000, in the Jewish population, it ranges from 1/6,000 among Yemenite Jews to 1/60,000 among Ashkenazi Jews.[3] Non–PKU-mediated hyperphenylalaninemia was previously known as benign hyperphenylalaninemia: panethnic, 1/65,000 (average).[4,5]

What are the sequelae of the condition that are of interest in clinical medicine?

PKU is an autosomal recessive metabolic disorder whose controlling gene is located on chromosome 12 q22-q24. The disease was first described by Folling in 1934.[6] A deficiency in phenylalanine hydroxylase results in poor conversion of phenylalanine (phe) into tyrosine (tyr).[7] High perinatal levels of phe impair the development of the central nervous system.

The result of untreated PKU is severe mental retardation (microcephaly) in half the patients (IQ < 35). Only 5 % of patients have an IQ of 86 or higher. Epilepsy occurs in 25%.[8] Other consequences described include abnormalities of the skin, teeth, and eyes, postnatal growth, and problems in behavior.[9] A phenylalanine-restricted diet dramatically improves clinical outcome and is the basis of treatment for PKU.[10]

■ The Tests

Newborn PKU screening in the United States is performed using either the semiquantitative Guthrie inhibition assay or the quantitative McCaman–Robins Fluorometric test.[11,12] In these tests, phenylalanine is measured in dried capillary drawn blood. However, these tests will probably be replaced worldwide in the near future with tandem mass spectrometry (TMS) screening, when it will then be possible to screen for 15 to 20 other genetically inherited metabolic disorders simultaneously.

It is only after separation from the umbilical cord that phenylalanine levels rise. Blood specimens are taken in the United States after 24 hours of age. If the test is positive, it should be repeated as soon as possible. In Europe samples are drawn at a later age to prevent impairment of test sensitivity. False-negative tests can occur with semiquantitative for hyperphenylalaninemia.[13]

The normal blood phenylalanine level is 40 to 60 µM/L. Carriers of the disease show slightly higher levels of 100 to 200 µM/L.

What are the implications of testing?

What does an abnormal test result mean? A test is positive if the level is greater than 240 µM/L (hyperphenylalanemia). Hyperphenylalaninemia can result from mutations at the locus encoding the enzyme PAH, at the loci for at least two enzymes in the pathway for the synthesis of tetrahydrobiopterin (BH4), the cofactor for the hydroxylation reaction, and at the locus for dihydropteridine reductase, the enzyme that regenerates BH4 from the oxidized product of the hydroxylation reaction. Mutations of the *PAH* gene described include missense mutations, deletions, and splice site mutations.

The serum phenylalanine level is repeated and the effect of BH4 oral supplementation on the level of phenylalanine assessed. Depending on the test results, the affected child is put on a low-protein diet to lower their intake of phenylalanine. The intake of carbohydrates and lipids is adjusted to a normal caloric intake for a newborn. Amino acid supplements are introduced as soon as possible. In case of hyperphenylalanemia due to BH4 deficiency, the patient requires only BH4.

False-positive tests are seen in patients with liver disease. Children with galactosemia, which results in liver failure, may have higher phenylalanine levels producing a false-positive test. For example, in The Netherlands, where neonatal screening for PKU is performed on the fourth day of life, about one to two patients with galactosemia are detected in this fashion annually.

What does a normal test result mean? A normal test result means either the newborn does not have PKU, or the test is false negative. In breast-fed infants, the levels are about half of those obtained from infants fed commercial formulas. This may lead to false-negative results especially if the blood samples are obtained during the first 24 to 48 hours of life. In patients with developmental delay, blood amino acid analysis should be performed in search of abnormalities of amino acid metabolism.

What is the cost of testing?

Historically, program costs of $1 to $2 for specimen handling, administration, and overhead were ascribed to PKU. Currently, state costs range from no fee to $50 for an all-inclusive program including follow-up confirmatory testing. These costs do not include the total system's cost for second tests and tests confirming the previous test. Education, patient and physician notification and contact, follow-up of affected patients, and the cost of special dietary supplements are also not likely included. Also excluded are the costs of the false-positive results (1%–3%). These include not only economic but also psychological costs. All abnormal test results result in diagnostic and sometimes therapeutic interventions with their associated financial implications, whether related to parental anxiety or iatrogenic side effects.

The costs for newborn screening are variable and are generally cited as initial fees for neonatal testing in a state (United States) or regionalized laboratory[4,5] and vary between $27 and $59.50 in the United States and from $6 in New Zealand to $25 in the Czech Republic.[14] Studies of cost-effectiveness of screening for PKU are not of a recent date,[15] but costs of caring for an institutionalized mentally retarded individual with a life expectancy of about 50 years would approximate $1,500,000 (United States).[16] The costs of a life-long diet without phenylalanine and supplemental amino acids are not always calculated in the cost-effectiveness of screening. It is likely with the introduction of TMS, which brings the possibility of detecting more metabolic disorders that the cost benefit of neonatal screening will become more effective.[17]

■ Conclusions and Recommendations

PKU screening is cost-effective and beneficial when conducted alone or as part of an organized neonatal screening program. Though new methods of screening (TMS) may have greater costs, it can be overcome by the detection of new diseases simultaneously such as medium chain acyl CoA dehydrogenase (MCAD) deficiency. In countries such as China where newborn screening was introduced in the not-too-distant past, and only covers 10% of the total population, the goal remains to expand coverage with gradual incorporation of new screening techniques. Although neonatal screening for disease is part of everyday life in most developed countries, it is still not policy worldwide. Individual country finances and medical organization play an important role in determining the feasibility of neonatal screening programs.

HYPOTHYROIDISM

■ What Is the Problem that Requires Screening?

Congenital hypothyroidism (CH).

What is the incidence/prevalence of the target condition?

Prevalence of congenital hypothyroidism in the United States determined from population-based screening ranges from 1/3,600 to 1/5,000. In Central Europe, the prevalence reported by screening programs approximates 1/3,000. In Sweden, prevalence rates of 1/6,600 to 1/7,300 are reported on the basis of clinical diagnosis. In Japan, prevalence is 1/5,700. Thus, there is racial and ethnic variability in the prevalence of congenital hypothyroidism. Hypothyroidism occurs considerably less often in black populations (1/17,000 in Georgia and 1/10,000 in Texas). It is more frequent in Hispanic populations: 1/2,700.[18,19]

What are the sequelae of the condition that are of interest in clinical medicine?

Hypothyroidism results from the inadequate production of thyroid hormone. This may result from one of several conditions including agenesis or ectopic thyroid gland, genetic disorders of thyroid hormone production, endemic cretinism, hypopituitarism, and maternal blocking antibodies. The most common are nongenetic causes. Untreated patients develop mental retardation and variable growth failure, deafness, and neurologic abnormalities. Apart from these symptoms, abnormalities due to a low metabolic state can be observed.[19–21]

■ The Tests

What is the purpose of the tests?

The purpose of the test is to identify newborns with CH, whether of primary, secondary, or tertiary causes. Once detected, treatment can be initiated early, often within the first week after birth, so as to minimize the risk of neurodevelopmental compromise.

What is the nature of the tests?

Dussault et al.[22] developed the first screening test for congenital hypothyroidism in the early 1970s. Although it followed PKU as a screening test, more newborns are screened today for CH than for PKU. Treatment with T_4 has improved outcome dramatically, although most patients show some impairment when neuropsychological test are given. This likely reflects inadequate hormone availability in utero.

Two types of tests are currently used: radioimmunoassay for T_4, thyroid-stimulating hormone (TSH), or both. In North America, TSH is measured only when the T_4 values are in the lowest 5% to 10%. In Europe and Japan, screening is based primarily on TSH. Simultaneous screening by measuring both T_4 and TSH allows the detection of patients with either secondary or tertiary CH. The T_4-screening approach also identifies infants with T_4-binding globulin deficiency (1/5,000 to 1/10,000) or hypothalamic–pituitary hypothyroidism (1/50,000). Iodine deficiency and the efficacy of treatment can be screened/determined using TSH analysis.[23]

Specimens collected during the first 24 to 48 hours of life may lead to an erroneous conclusion because of the normal spike in TSH and T_4 following delivery. Testing a second sample for T_4 identifies an additional 6% to 12% of cases.

What are the implications of testing?

What does an abnormal test result mean? An abnormal test is suggestive of CH. Infants with a low T_4 level and TSH concentration above 40 mU/L are considered to have primary hypothyroidism. Though treatment should start immediately, confirmatory serum tests (T_4 and TSH) are necessary to verify the hypothyroidism. In newborns with only a slightly elevated screening TSH (>20 mU/L but <40 mU/L), another filter-paper specimen should be obtained for repeat screening. To determine whether there is secondary or tertiary hypothyroidism, the response to TSH-releasing hormone may be determined. Radioisotope scanning is usually necessary to identify the cause of the hypothyroidism. T_4 testing alone has low specificity, with a false-positive rate as high as 0.3%. T_4 testing followed by TSH testing, and when indicated, $T_4$4-binding globulin, reverse T_3, or free T_4, produces high specificity. Recall rates vary from 0.04% to 0.5%.

What does a normal test result mean? A normal test indicates the neonate is unlikely to have CH. The normal range of T_4 values and the T_4 percentile cutoff level for TSH testing are usually established by the individual screening programs. The cutoff for the TSH assay is typically the tenth percentile. Thus, about 10% of CH infants will be missed if not screened a second time. These infants show a low TSH value and a delayed TSH increment, but a normal T_4 value. These infants can only be detected through clinical suspicion.[24-26] The false-negative rate reflects the cutoff and screening methods used, and the age of the infant. Approximately 10% of cases are detected only by a second screening at 2 to 6 weeks of age. The false-negative rate of the population screened is about 1.1% after two tests. Primary TSH screening does not detect secondary and tertiary hypothyroidism.

What is the cost of testing?

Most U.S. states mandate routine neonatal screening for hypothyroidism. At a screening cost of $5 per child, (covering TSH, T_4, and all processing and notification costs), the average cost of detecting subclinical hypothyroidism is $5,000 per affected child.[27] Taking into account the costs of institutionalization and special schooling for an undetected child, the cost: benefit ratio approximates 1:8.9.[28] The second test at an age of 4 to 6 weeks is also cost-effective, with a cost of about $31,881 per child detected.[29]

■ Conclusions and Recommendations

Although newborn screening for hypothyroidism has greatly improved the outcome of affected infants for the better, many have a lag in neurodevelopmental compared with their siblings. This could be caused by a number of reasons such as inadequate hormone availability in utero, late onset of the disease, inadequate dosage of substitute medication, or defects of transcription factors not only leading to hypothyroidism but also to defective central nervous system development. The latter could in the future be detected earlier by genetic screening.[30]

CONGENITAL ADRENAL HYPERPLASIA

■ What Is the Problem that Requires Screening?

Congenital adrenal hyperplasia (CAH) is an autosomal recessive disorder where a lack of cortisol and or aldosterone secondary to a deficiency of 21-hydroxylase or 11-hydroxylase deficiency results in an over production of adrenal corticotrophin hormone (ACTH) and the overproduction of androgenic steroids. There are two clinical presentations: salt losing and virilization.[31,32]

What is the incidence/prevalence of the target condition?

The overall prevalence of CAH is 1:12,000–15,000, most of which is salt wasting. The prevalence is 1/18,850 for salt wasting and 1/57,543 for the virilizing form. It is most common among Yupik Eskimos (1/282), followed by the inhabitants of the island of La Reunion, France (1/2,141). The prevalence in Italy approximates 1/5,500–10,000. Case detection and thus prevalence has increased with the introduction of neonatal screening.[33]

What are the sequelae of the condition that are of interest in clinical medicine?

The increased androgen production causes the somatic and sexual precocity seen in these patients. High fetal adrenal androgens may masculinize the external genitalia of the female resulting in a male sex assignment. In one study by Thilen et al.,[34] 15 girls of 38 with ambiguous genitalia were assigned the wrong sex for the first 40 days of there life. In three fourths of affected males, a salt-losing syndrome is the initial clinical finding. Salt losing and cortisol deficiency may lead to early neonatal death. Treatment suppresses the abnormal steroidal pattern, and avoids the consequences of excess virilization, short stature (due to increased androgen production), and cortisol deficiency. Treatment with glucocorticosteroids serves the dual purpose of replacing cortisol and suppressing excessive corticotrophin production. Salt losing patients with elevated plasma renin activity should receive mineralocorticoid therapy with their hydrocortisone and may need supplemental salt intake.

■ The Tests

What is the purpose of the tests?

Possible benefits of neonatal screening are: the avoidance of a serious salt-loss crisis; prevention of death due to adrenal crises in the neonatal period; earlier diagnosis and correct gender assignment in virilized girls; decreased virilization, growth acceleration and rates of premature pubarche; and reduced negative consequences for psychosocial development and final height. Although screening occurs within the first week of life, it is still not possible to prevent all deaths in the days immediately after birth.

What is the nature of the tests?

Screening test. Screening for a 21-hydroxylase deficiency is performed on dried blood spots using an enzyme immunoassay or radioimmunoassay for measurement of 17-hydroxy-progesterone (17-OHP). The 17-OHP is elevated at birth, although the levels obtained during the first 24 hours of age may be physiologically high. Preterm infants may also have false-positive test results. Screening in the first 48 hours may increase the false-positive rate, but further study is needed. Screening at 1 to 2 weeks of age detects some additional cases of simple virilizing CAH and increased numbers of the nonclassic form of 21-hydroxylase deficiency.[35,36]

What are the implications of testing?

What does an abnormal test result mean? An abnormal test means the child likely has CAH and treatment should be instituted. Ninety-five percent of newborns with a 21-hydroxylase deficiency will be detected using a cutoff value of 65 ng/mL. The percentage of false-positive tests ranges from 0.2% to 0.5%, depending on the cutoff level selected.

What does a normal test result mean? A normal test result virtually eliminates the possibility the child has CAH. The number of false-negative tests is low-about 3% of neonates with salt losing may be missed if screened before 24 hours of age.

What is the cost of testing?

Based on Swedish data, the screening program costs about £1 ($2.70 US) per neonate screened (including reagent fluid). This gives a total cost of £700,000 per year and a cost per adverse event avoided of about £20,000. It is unclear whether this includes the prevention of death or brain damage due to serious illness in the newborn period.[37,38] A second test will also be able to detect the virilizing type of the disease. However, this second test is not as cost-effective as the first test.[39]

■ Conclusions and Recommendations

Further quantification of the false-negative and false-positive rates and follow up to determine the extent the clinical outcome has improved by early diagnosis and treatment is greatly needed. The importance of a quick response time is essential to increasing the efficacy of the screening program. Screening for a 21-hydroxylase deficiency has not been universally adopted in great part because of the high false positive rate, mostly in preterm infants. The problems with screening preterm infants can be overcome by giving additional information (birth weight and gestational age) of the child to be screened.[40] Although prevention of neonatal death from acute adrenal insufficiency can also be achieved by increasing clinical awareness, biochemical screening still allows for earlier treatment.[41]

MEDIUM-CHAIN ACYL-COA DEHYDROGENASE DEFICIENCY

■ What Is the Problem that Requires Screening?

Medium-chain acyl-CoA dehydrogenase deficiency (MCAD) results from a defect in mitochondrial fatty acid oxidation. It is an autosomal recessive disorder caused by a variety of mutations in the single *MCAD* gene on chromosome 1. Most clinical cases are caused by an A985G transition in exon 11.[42]

What is the incidence/prevalence of the target condition?

The reported prevalence of MCAD deficiency in some parts of the United Kingdom is about 1/10,000.[43] It affects mainly whites of Northern European origin. In the United States (Wisconsin), the prevalence in one screening study was 4.5/100,000.[44] Before this study, the prevalence was thought to be about 2.5/100,000.

What are the sequelae of the condition that are of interest in clinical medicine?

The disorder presents with hypoglycemia and encephalopathy after an intercurrent illness, such as vomiting or after childhood immunization. Sometimes the mental state is changed and hepatic failure follows. These symptoms are known as Reye-like features. There is a high risk of death (about 25 %) or permanent neurologic sequelae[with] the attacks.[45,46] In one prospective study from the United States (Pennsylvania), many mutations other than the A985G were found, but that the typical clinical presentations were related to the A985G mutations.[47] Two prospective studies found that 25% of affected children were asymptomatic at testing,[48,49] reflecting different mutations.

■ The Tests

What is the purpose of the tests?

The purpose of the test is to detect neonates with MCAD deficiency to prevent sequelae resulting from the inability to metabolize medium chain fatty acids.

What is the nature of the tests?

The abnormal acylcarnitines present in a dried blood spot are detected by tandem mass spectrometry. The profile of acylcarnitines is unique and specific for MCAD deficiency.[50]

What are the implications of testing?

What does an abnormal test result mean? An abnormal test means the neonate likely has MCAD deficiency, and diet therapy should be instituted. Repeat tests are performed when increased C6, C8, and C10:1 acylcarnitines are detected in the blood spots. Different laboratories have different cutoff levels. In Sydney, for example, screened infants with a blood octanoylcarnitine level of 1 μmol/L are further analyzed. Patients with the classical mutation have higher levels of octanoylcarnitine than with other mutations or only one common mutation.[51] Additional testing for demonstrating enzyme deficiency or by DNA testing for known mutations will confirm the diagnosis. In Wisconsin, testing confirmed the diagnosis in seven of nine affected infants from a pool of 155,000 screened infants, yielding a test specificity of 99.9%.[52]

The significant heterogeneity in the phenotype, even within families, and the detection of a much higher frequency of abnormal acylcarnitines after neonatal screening (4–5/100,000) than anticipated suggest there are phenotypes that never present clinical symptoms.[52,53] Carriers show a normal acylcarnitine profile.[54]

What does a normal test result mean? A normal test means the newborn is not an MCAD-deficient patient. Carriers of a MCAD deficiency gene have a normal test. Theoretically, individuals with unknown mutations with decreased enzyme activity but no clinical symptoms could be missed, but without clinical implication.

What is the cost of testing?

The cost of testing of screening alone is about $3.99 per sample. Taking into account the costs saved preventing neurologic impairment or a fatal outcome, screening is cost-effective ratio with a cost of $41,862 per quality adjusted life-year[52]

■ Conclusions and Recommendations

The high morbidity and mortality of the disease coupled with the efficacy of early treatment justifies screening for MCAD deficiency.[55] But the lack of knowledge of the clinical symptoms and outcome in patients with a mutation other than the classical A985G mutation may lead to unnecessary intervention in some people who would never have clinical symptoms.

CYSTIC FIBROSIS

■ What Is the Problem that Requires Screening?

Cystic fibrosis (CF) is autosomal recessively inherited disorder caused by one of many different mutations in the CF gene. The result is a disorder of exocrine glands, characterized by thickened secretions leading to multisystem dysfunction and failure (see related information in Chapter 9).

What is the incidence/prevalence of the target condition?

The prevalence of CF in Caucasian ranges between 1/2,000–4000 in the United States and European-derived populations. A higher prevalence is found in Celts from Brittany, Afrikaners from southwest Africa, and in French Canadians from the Saugueny-Lac St. Jean region in Canada. Genetic drift and founder effect account for the much higher prevalence in these populations (frequency of 1/377, 1/622, and 1/895, respectively). The carrier frequency of the mutation in the gene encoding for the cystic fibrosis transmembrane conductance regulator (CFTR) is 1/22–28. More than 800 mutations have been identified.[56] In the United States, some 30,000 persons are affected.[57,58]

What are the sequelae of the condition that are of interest in clinical medicine?

CF is the most common lethal disease in whites, having an overall median survival of just 32.3 years.[59] The disease affects multiple organ systems. The main problems are: pulmonary mucus plugging, infection (particularly with *Pseudomonas aeruginosa*), and inflammation leading to structural injury; bronchiectasis, and bronchiolectasis. The development of bronchiectatic cysts and abscesses is prominent. Pulmonary hypertension develops as a consequence.

The pancreas is another organ affected. Exocrine pancreatic insufficiency is present in more than 80% and highly correlated with genotype. Patients homozygous for ΔF508 mutation have pancreatic insufficiency. Pancreatic insufficiency leads to fat and protein malabsorption (also deficient absorption of fat-soluble vitamins), and thus to an abnormal stool (steatorrhea) with failure to thrive. Meconium ileus can sometimes be identified antenatally as a symptom of gastrointestinal CF. The risk of CF in these case ranges from 1.3% to 13.3% depending on the sonographic findings.[60] The higher energy demand required for respiration and the frequent pulmonary infections further contribute to malnutrition and growth failure. Pancreatic disease can lead to recurrent pancreatitis and diabetes mellitus. Other manifestations of the disease include hepatobiliary disease, infertility, and osteoporosis.[61]

■ The Tests

Carrier screening is only possible by DNA screening for the mutation. General-population screening is not yet recommended. In the United States, screening is offered to individuals with a family history of CF, reproductive partners of people who have CF, and couples in whom one or both members are white and who are planning a pregnancy or seeking prenatal care.[62]

In the United Kingdom, there are currently seven local CF screening programs.[63] In France, pediatricians have requested a neonatal screening program for CF be set up. L'association Française pour le depistage et la prévention des handicaps de l 'enfant (AFDPHE) defined the terms of implementation and rules to be followed with respect to patient care.[64] The national insurance and the Directorate General of Health (DGS) assisted setting this program up and will evaluate the results.[63,65]

What is the purpose of the tests?

The purpose of the test is to detect CF patients. A cure for the disease is not available and treatment remains symptomatic. Gene therapy may be a future option. Screening reduces parental stress.[66] There is some circumstantial evidence[67] of long-term benefit when patients are detected via neonatal screening.[68]

What is the nature of the tests?

Blood spot immunoreactive trypsinogen (IRT). Complementary mutation analysis of the *CFTR* gene is performed when high IRT values are found.[69] When no mutation is found, the IRT test is performed again on day 21, and if still positive, a sweat test is performed. Because additional genetic testing is involved, the parents or legal guardians must authorize the test. The cutoff value for the IRT test is 60 g/L on day 3 of testing (results in 0.5 % of positive IRT tests). IRT test performance is evaluated regularly to the appropriateness of the test kit, and the threshold adjusted when necessary. Depending on the population, genetic testing identifies only up to 80% to 85% of mutations known to date because the test panels include only those with the greatest prevalence. Cutoff levels vary among screening programs.

What are the implications of testing?

What does an abnormal test result mean? An abnormal IRT value necessitates further investigation. In about 10% of abnormal IRT tests, genetic testing will reveal either one or two mutated genes. In the instance of homozygous or compound heterozygous children, the severity and clinical manifestations of the disease reflect the mutation found. Affected and carrier neonates should be referred for clinical assessments. Up to 10% of presumed carrier infants will be affected.[70] Parents of carrier infants should be referred for counseling.

What does a normal test result mean? A normal IRT means the child is likely normal, as an IRT has a sensitivity of 94%.[71] Those that are affected are usually modest. A false-negative test would mean the child screened carries either an unknown mutation or one not on the panel. In this instance, the clinical picture is likely to be mild for homozygous patients. The cutoff values chosen for the screening test will have to be further evaluated in the coming years.

What is the cost of testing?

Earlier treatment allowed by neonatal screening changes neither the therapy nor the outcome. Thus, the cost of delivery is central to any argument for neonatal CF screening. Lee et al.[72] compared the cost of neonatal screening to the normal costs for the CF detection in Wisconsin. The number of sweat tests was reduced by the introduction of the screening program. The annual cost of screening for CF per child is $4.58, whereas the traditional detection costs approximate $4.97, and without the need to perform the sweat test, costs are even lower.[72] Thus, newborn screening for CF is cost-effective compared to the traditional approach.

■ Conclusions and Recommendations

CF screening was the first disease screened for using genomic material, which has changed neonatal screening. Because there is no therapy for CF other than palliative care, it bypasses many of the criteria for a screening test suggested by Wilson and Jungner in 1968.[73] False-positive tests can create unnecessary anxiety, as despite several trials with gene therapy, there is still no treatment for CF. Approximately 1% of the screened neonates will have a positive IRT test, of whom 10% will either be affected (homozygous or compound heterozygous) or a carrier. These infants should be referred for further clinical assessment and genetic counseling. Infants with a normal IRT result are very unlikely to be affected given the high sensitivity and the low prevalence of the disease. Nonetheless, there are screen negative infants that may be carriers or homozygous with mild disease.

CONGENITAL HIP DYSPLASIA OR DEVELOPMENTAL DYSPLASIA OF THE HIP

■ What Is the Problem that Requires Screening?

Risk factors for congenital hip dysplasia (CHD) or developmental dysplasia of the hip (DDH) include a positive family history (20% have a positive family history), female sex, foot abnormalities, breech presentation, oligohydramnios and primiparity.[74–76] The presentation spectrum of DDH is wide. It includes neonatal instability, limping in the toddler, painful dysplasia in youth and osteoarthritis in the adult and can develop without treatment that limits limb abduction.[77] The prognosis improves with the early detection of the disorder; thus early diagnosis is the cornerstone of management.[77]

What is the incidence/prevalence of the target condition?

The prevalence of hip dislocation in unscreened populations is estimated at 1–2/1,000 children of European origin.[78,79] It is rare in African blacks.[80,81] It is also more common in populations that practice swaddling or use infant cradle boards.[82,83]

The prevalence of DDH in Croatian infants screened in the fourth month of age is 3.3 %, though the clinical prevalence was only 1.7 %.[84] The prevalence of DDH can also vary with the time of detection since dislocatable hips may spontaneously normalize.[85]

What are the sequelae of the condition that are of interest in clinical medicine?

The natural history of developmental dysplasia of the hip is not completely understood,[86] but an abnormal gait, pain and osteoarthritis are each thought to be consequences of untreated DDH. Ultrasound at birth identified DDH that was not clinically detectable at two months of age in 80%.[87] These observations were confirmed in a study where 90% normalized spontaneously.[85] In these studies, neonates with normal hip ultrasound investigations did not develop DDH during the examination period.

Surgical intervention may still be necessary even when DDH is detected early. A small number of children (not more than 1/5,000) appear to have a poor outcome and require surgical correction of the abnormality.[85] The prevalence rate for first operations in a screened German population was 0.26/1,000 live births.[88]

■ The Tests

What is the purpose of the tests?

The early detection of developmental hip dysplasia coupled with the treatment of hip instability reduces the need for surgical intervention and prevents the sequelae of the undetected DDH such as unstable gait, pain, and osteoarthritis.

What is the nature of the tests?

Clinical examination consists of the standardized Ortolani and Barlow maneuvers.[87,89] Ultrasound screening of newborn hips is performed either as the initial screen for congenital hip dysplasia, or after a clinical abnormal finding.

What are the implications of testing?

What does an abnormal test result mean? An abnormal clinical test leads to an ultrasound of the hips. An abnormal ultrasound test means that the hip is abnormal but does not imply that intervention is mandatory as a considerable percentage resolves over time.[85,87]

What does a normal test result mean? A normal ultrasound means that the hip is normal and no further dislocations of the hip will develop in the future.

What is the cost of testing?

A postnatal clinical examination is part of the normal care for the newborn. Thus, it is difficult to separate out the cost of the clinical hip examination. The cost of a neonatal hip ultrasound varies from £50 to from $75 US. Elbourne et al.[90] studied the clinical and economic results of a multi-center randomized trial and compared the cost of clinical screening only and screening with ultrasound examinations. They concluded that infants in the ultrasonography group incurred markedly higher ultrasound costs over the first 2 years (£42) compared with the clinical examination only (£23). The combination of clinical and ultrasound screening prevents abduction splinting and does not lead to an increase in either abnormal hip development, or more surgical interventions by 2 years of age.

Brown et al.[91] looked at the additional cost of ultrasound when restricted to infants with risk factors. The estimated total cost per 100,000 live births was approximately £4 million for universal ultrasound, £3 million for selective ultrasound, £1 million for clinical screening alone, and £0.4 million for no screening. The efficiency of selective ultrasound and clinical screening is poorly differentiated, and depends on the selection criteria for ultrasound as well as the expertise of clinical examiners. If training costs less than £20 per child screened, clinical screening alone would be more efficient than selective ultrasound. Policy choice depends on values attached to the different outcomes, willingness to pay to achieve these and the total budget available.[91]

■ Conclusions and Recommendations

The Medical Research Council on Congenital Dislocation of the Hip in 1998 concluded that screening by clinical examination of the hip had not reduced the prevalence of late presentation of DDH requiring surgical therapy, and as a result, a formal evaluation of current and alternative policies such as primary ultrasound imaging was necessary.[92] Since then, a number of nondefinitive studies have concluded that either primary or additional ultrasound could be useful. Puhan et al.[93] conducted a meta-analysis of 49 observational studies. The prevalence of DDH ranged from 0.5% to 30% depending largely on definition. Less than 0.1% of patients with DDH were missed by ultrasound regardless of the scan technique used. About 80% to 90% of newborns with abnormal ultrasounds initially did not develop DDH. Only six studies with 23,108 newborns reported complications, and of those newborns there was only one infant with an avascular necrosis of the femoral head. However, reports were often incomplete and clinical follow-up of newborns with normal findings not routinely carried out. Thus, clinical outcome data as well as appropriate controls were missing. These authors concluded that there was still insufficient study, and while there was evidence in favor of ultrasound screening, there remained a great need for randomized controlled trials comparing the effectiveness of different screening regimens.

HEMOGLOBINOPATHY

■ What Is the Problem that Requires Screening?

Hemoglobinopathy.

What is the incidence/prevalence of the target condition?

There is a high prevalence of sickle hemoglobinopathies in African and African Americans. Sickle cell disease (SCD) is the most common form of sickle cell anemia with a prevalence rate of 1/400 African Americans.[94] One of 333 black newborns in the United States is affected. In northwest London, the prevalence of SCD is 1/1,915 births.[95] There will be in the year 2000 more than 10,000 patients with SCD in the United Kingdom. In addition, there are about 600 patients with a-thalassemia major in the United Kingdom.[96]

What are the sequelae of the condition that are of interest in clinical medicine?

There is abnormal hemoglobin in sickle cell disease causing the RBC to assume a dysmorphic shape is more rigid and thus less pliable than the normal erythrocyte.[97] Sickle cell anemia is the homozygous disease form (HbSS), whereas compound heterozygous disease forms include HbSC. α-thalassemia major is detected by the same tests[98] (see Chapter 16 for related information). The clinical manifestations reflect decreased oxygen transport and exchange. The abnormal cell form is easily destroyed resulting in hemolytic anemia. The trapped erythrocytes cause bone infarction and subsequent pain crises. The accumulation of erythrocytes in the spleen causes dysfunction associated with an increased susceptibility to bacterial infection, especially *Streptococcus pneumoniae*.[99,100] Morbidity and mortality has been reduced markedly with the use of antibiotic prophylaxis.[99]

Patients with α-thalassemia are transfusion dependent and require regular red blood cell transfusions.

■ The Tests

What is the purpose of the tests?

The purpose of the sickle cell detection test is to identify affected patients at a young age so as to begin treatment early and prevent mortality and morbidity.

What is the nature of the tests?

Hemoglobinopathies may be screened for using either isoelectric focusing or high-performance liquid chromatography (HPLC). The former test is more convenient when large number of tests should be processed. The latter is easier to interpret.[101]

What does an abnormal test result mean? These tests have very low false positive test rates. An abnormal test means the patient has an abnormal form of hemoglobin.[102] However, abnormal tests must be confirmed, as some abnormal hemoglobins are not easily distinguished from HbS. In these cases, a DNA test will identify the variant Hb form (Hb G Madagaskar).[98] Sickle cell anemia is the homozygous disease form (HbSS), while compound heterozygous disease forms include HbSC. α-thalassemia major is detected by the same tests[103] (see Chapter 16 for related information).

What does a normal test result mean? A normal test does not exclude the possibility of some other rare hemoglobin forms, rare sickling variants, persistent fetal hemoglobinemia, or α-thalassemia trait.[98] These forms are, however, very rare. Almeida et al.[95] screened a neonatal population of 414,801, with 19% non-white individuals. They were unable to obtain a definitive result in only 0.26 % of the population tested. In most individuals ($n = 901$), this was due to a prior blood transfusion.

What is the cost of testing?

The results suggest that screening services should aim to cover populations that generate a workload of over 25,000 births per year, and preferably over 40,000. IEF and HPLC are very similar in terms of average cost per test.[96] In one 1991 study, the cost-effectiveness of antibiotic treatment was compared in two populations, one detected by neonatal screening and the other group treated with antibiotics only after appearance of symptoms.[104] Screening and treating patients in a high-risk population (black infants) only cost $ 3,100 per life saved compared with $1.4 million per life saved in a population with a high prevalence of HbS in a nonblack population. Screening low-prevalence populations would cost $450 billion per life saved. Cost-effectiveness reflects the first 3 years of life.

■ Conclusions and Recommendations

When the number of carriers in the screened population is 16/1,000 and 0.5/1,000 screened have sickle cell disease, there is no significant difference in the detection component cost between universal and targeted programs. Below this prevalence, a targeted program is likely to be less expensive but will miss cases.[96,104]

HEARING IMPAIRMENT

■ What Is The Problem That Requires Screening?

Hearing impairment.

What is the incidence/prevalence of the target condition?

The overall rate of congenital hearing loss in one U.S. screening study was 2–3/1,000 newborns; of these, 75 % suffered bilateral hearing loss.

Severity of hearing impairment is mild to moderate in 78%, and severe to profound in 22%.[105] Approximately 2% to 4% of infants who leave neonatal intensive care units are hearing impaired.[106–108]

In 1999, the United States began to provide funds to states for the development of hearing screening programs.[109] Presently, 37 states have mandatory screening programs for newborn hearing, as have many of the larger hospitals with many births and a newborn intensive care unit. Some hospitals currently screen only "high-risk" infants, such as those with a family history of congenital deafness, congenital infection (such as measles, cytomegalovirus), infants with craniofacial abnormalities, infants under 1,500 g, infants with extremely high bilirubin levels, infants who have received medications that may be toxic to the otic nerves, infants with bacterial meningitis, and infants who have had prolonged and assisted ventilation.[110]

What are the sequelae of the condition that are of interest in clinical medicine?

Hearing impairment leads to delayed speech development, and impairment of social and emotional development.[111]

■ The Tests

What is the purpose of the tests?

To detect a hearing impairment.

An intervention program is started immediately after hearing impairment has been detected to aid the development of language skills and preserve social and emotional development. With early amplification and appropriate therapy, hearing-impaired children are capable of achieving normal speech–language developmental milestones. Yoshinaga-Itano and coworkers[112] demonstrated in a cohort of affected newborns identified through newborn screening near-normal language development, significantly exceeding the language development of comparable children not identified until after 6 months of age.

What is the nature of the tests?

Otoacoustic emissions. One of the tests is called otoacoustic emissions or OAEs. For this test, a miniature earphone and microphone are placed in the ear, sounds played, and the response measured. An echo is reflected back into the ear canal if a neonate hears normally, which is picked up by the microphone. No echo is detected on OAE testing if the infant has a hearing impairment.[113]

Auditory brainstem response The second test is called auditory brainstem response or ABR. This test actually measures the brain responding to sound. Band-aid–like electrodes are placed on the neonate's head to detect brain waves and sounds played to the neonate's ears.[113]

What does an abnormal test result mean? Two test regimens are used to screen newborns for hearing loss. The sensitivity and specificity of the automated ABR test are reported to be 100% and 98 %, respectively.[114] The sensitivity and specificity of the OAEs are reportedly 100% and 82%, respectively.[115] Reported sensitivities may differ with the populations screened. An abnormal test means there is a hearing impairment of some etiology because the current tests have a high sensitivity. Further testing may be required to determine the etiology.

What does a normal test result mean? A normal test shows indicates there is no significant hearing impairment at the moment of screening, but it is does not guarantee the child will not develop a hearing impairment in the future.

What is the cost of testing?

Screening for congenital hearing impairment is a significant undertaking. The true cost for each infant screened is estimated to be $25 per infant, including labor costs, disposable supplies, and amortized capital equipment costs. (To date, the costs in Colorado of screening range from $18.30 per infant when performed by supervised volunteers, to $25.60 per infant when performed by a paid technician, and to $33.30 per infant when performed by an audiologist. Refined echnology with improved speed of testing has decreased these 1997 estimates.) The cost per case of congenital hearing impairment detected approximates $9,600. This model for cost predictions and subsequent intervention savings shows that recovery of all screening costs will occur after only 10 years of universal screening.[116]

■ Conclusions and Recommendations

Neonatal hearing screening has become widespread, with the benefit of speech and language development comparable to that of hearing children. It is likely the beneficial aspects of screening for hearing impairment will continue its adoption by more countries.

■ Summary

1 ■ What Is the Problem that Requires Screening?
Neonatal genetic disorders.

a. What is the incidence/prevalence of the target condition?
Variously ranges from 1/400 to 1/60,000 depending on the disorder and the geographic location.

b. What are the sequelae of the condition that are of interest in clinical medicine?
Premature death and lifelong suffering.

2 ■ The Tests

a. What is the purpose of the tests?
To detect affected individuals and in some disorders, the carriers.

b. What is the nature of the tests?
The measurement of metabolites, enzyme activity, detection of mutated genes, and the clinical examination/sonography of the affected joint.

c. What are the implications of testing?

1. What does an abnormal test result mean?
   The neonate is likely to be affected by the disorder in question.
2. What does a normal test result mean?
   All tests have a high sensitivity. A normal result typically excludes the likelihood of an affected neonate.

d. What is the cost of testing?

Many screens are part of a neonatal panel. All of these are cost beneficial. Other screens are cost beneficial under certain circumstances.

3 ■ Conclusions and Recommendations

All screening tests for disorders covered in this chapter have high sensitivity. Early intervention has the potential to change long-term outcome.

References

1. Weisbren SE, Albers SA, Amato S, et al. Effect of expanded newborn screening for biochemical genetic disorders on child outcomes and parental stress. *JAMA* 2003;290:2564–2572.
2. Meikle PJ, Hopwood JJ. Lysosomal storage disorders: emerging therapeutic options require early diagnosis. *Eur J Ped.* 2003;162[Suppl l]:S34–S37.
3. De la Cruz F, Koch R. Genetic implications for newborn screening for phenylketonuria. In: Evans MI, ed. *Clinics in Perinatology. Metabolic and Genetic Screening.* 2001;28:419–425.
4. American Academy of Pediatrics, Committee on Genetics. Newborn screening fact sheets. *Pediatrics* 1989;83:449–464.
5. American Academy of Pediatrics, Committee on Genetics. Issues in newborn screening. *Pediatrics* 1992;89:345–349.
6. Folling A. Phenylpyruvic acid as a metabolic anomaly in connection with imbecility. *Z Physiol Chem* 1934;227:169.
7. Jervis GA. Studies on phenylpyruvic oligophrenis: position of metabolic error. *J Biol Chem* 1947;169:651.
8. Pitt DB, Danks DM. The natural history of untreated phenylketonuria. *J Pediatr Child Health* 1991;27:189–190.
9. Sciver CR, Kaufman S, Woo SLC. The hyperphenylalaninemias. In: Scriver CR, Beaudet AL, Sly WS, et al., eds. *The Metabolic Basis of Inherited Disease.* New York: McGraw-Hill, 1989:495.
10. Bickel H, Gerrard JW, Hickmans EM. Influence of phenylalanine on phenylketonuria. *Lancet* 1953;2:812–813.
11. Guthrie R. Blood screening for phenylketonuria. *JAMA* 1961;178:863.
12. McCaman MW, Robins E. Fluorimetric method for the determination of phenylalanine in serum. *J Lab Clin Med* 1965;59:885.

13. Smith I, Cook B, Beasley M. Review of neonatal screening programme for phenylketonuria. *BMJ* 1991;303:333–335.

14. Genetic Science Learning Center, University of Utah, Section 8: Cost Considerations, pp40-43, Salt Lake City, 2001.

15. National Institute of Health Consensus Statement. Phenylketonuria: screening and management. October 16-18, 2000;17:31–37.

16. South California Department of Health and Environmental Control. Newborn Screening Section. Phenylketonuria.

17. Pandor A, Eastham J, Beverley C, et al. Clinical effectiveness and cost-effectiveness of neonatal screening for inborn errors of metabolism using tandem mass spectrometry: a systematic review. *Health Technol Assess* 2004;8:1–121.

18. American Academy of Pediatrics, Section on Endocrinology and Committee on Genetics, and American Thyroid Association Committee on Public Health. Newborn screening for congenital hypothyroidism: recommended guidelines. *Pediatrics* 1993;91:1203-1209.

19. LaFranchi S, Disorders of the thyroid gland. In: Behrman RE, Kliegman PM, Nelson WE, et al., eds. *Nelson Textbook of Pediatrics*, 17th ed., WB Saunders: Philadelphia, 2004.

20. Rovet JF, Ehrlich RM, Sorbara DL. Neurodevelopment in infants and preschool children with congenital hypothyroidism: etiological and treatment factors affecting outcome. *J Pediatr Psychol* 1992;17:187–213.

21. Tillotson S, Fuggle PW, Smith I, et al. Relation between biochemical severity and intelligence in early treated congenital hypothyroidism: a threshold effect. *BMJ* 1994;309:440–445.

22. Dussault JH Laberge C. dosage de la T4 (T4) par methode radio-immunologique dans l' eluat de sang seche : nouvelle methode de depistage de l'hypothytoidie neonatale ? *Union Med Can* 1973;10:2062–2064.

23. Zamboni G, Zaffanello M, Rigon F, et al. Diagnostic effectiveness of simultaneous thyroxine and thyroid stimulating hormone screening measurements: thirteen years experience in the Northeast Italian Screening Programme. *J Med Screen* 2004;11:18–20.

24. American Academy of Pediatrics, Section on Endocrinology and Committee on Genetics, and American Thyroid Association Committee on Public Health. Newborn screening for congenital hypothyroidism: recommended guidelines. *Pediatrics* 1993;91:1203–1209.

25. National Committee for Clinical Laboratory Standards. Blood Collection on Filter Paper for Neonatal Screening Programs: Approved Standard. Villanova, PA: National Committee for Clinical Laboratory Standards; NCCLS Publication LA4-A2, 1992.

26. Delange F. Neonatal screening for congenital hypothyroidism: Results and perspectives. *Horm Res* 1997;48:51–61.

27. Dr Marvin Mitchell, of the State Laboratory Institute and University of Massachusetts Medical School

28. Layde PM, Von Allmen SD, Oakley GP Jr. Congenital hypothyroidism control programs: a cost-benefit analysis. *JAMA* 1997;241:2290–2292.

29. LaFranchi SH, Hanna CE, Krainz PL, et al. Screening for congenital hypothyroidism with specimen collection at two time periods: results of the Northwest Regional Screening Program. *Pediatrics* 1985;76:734–740.

30. Gruters A, Jenner, A, Krude H. Long term consequences of congenital hypothyroidism in the era of screening programs. *Best Pract Res Clin Endocrinol Metab* 2002;16:369–382.

31. White PC, Speiser PW. Congenital adrenal hyperplasia due to 21-hydroxylase deficiency. *Endocr Rev* 2000;21:245–291.

32. Cacciari E, Balsamo A, Cassio A, et al. Neonatal screening for congenital adrenal hyperplasia. *Arch Dis Child* 1993;58:803–806.

33. Pang S, Wallace MA, Hofman L, et al. Worldwide experience in newborn screening for classical congenital adrenal hyperplasia due to 21-hydroxylase deficiency. *Pediatrics* 1988;81:866–874.

34. Thilen A, Larsson A. Congenital adrenal hyperplasia in Sweden 1969-1986. Prevalence, symptoms and age at diagnosis. *Acta Paediatr Scand* 1990;79:168–175.

35. Wallace AM, Beastall GH, Cook B, et al. Neonatal screening for congenital adrenal hyperplasia: a program based on a novel direct radioimmunoassay for 17-hydroxyprogesterone in blood spots. *J Endocrinol* 1986;108:299–308.

36. Thompson R, Seargeant L, Winter JSD. Screening for congenital adrenal hyperplasia: distribution of 17 alpha-hydroxyprogesterone concentrations in neonatal blood spot specimens. *J Pediatr* 1989;114:400–404.

37. Thil'en A, Nordenstrom A, Hagenfeldt L, et al. Benefits of neonatal screening for congenital adrenal hyperplasia (21-hydroxylase deficiency) in Sweden. *Pediatrics* 1998;101:E11.

38. Brosnan CA, Brosnan PG, Swint JM, et al. Analyzing the cost of neonatal screening for congenital adrenal hyperplasia. *Pediatrics* 2001;107:1238.

39. Brosnan CA, Brosnan P, Therrell BL, et al. A comparative cost analysis of newborn screening for classic congenital adrenal hyperplasia in Texas. *Public Health Rep* 1998;113:170–178.

40. Olgemoller B, Roscher AA, Liebl B, et al. Screening for congenital adrenal hyperplasia: adjustment of 17-hydroxyprogesterone cut-off values to both age and birth weight markedly improves the predictive value. *J Clin Endocrinol Metab* 2003;88:5790–5794.

41. Van Vliet G, Czernichow P. Screening for neonatal endocrinopathies: rationale, methods and results. *Semin Neonatol* 2004;9:75–85.

42. Roe CR, Ding J. Mitochondrial fatty acid oxidation disorders. In: Scriver CR, Beaudet AL, Sly WS, et al., eds. *The Metabolic and Molecular Bases of Inherited Disease*, 8th ed. McGraw-Hill: New York, 2001, P. 2313.

43. Seddon HR, Green A, Gray RGF, et al. Regional variations in medium-chain acyl-CoA dehydrogenase deficiency [letter]. *Lancet* 1995;345:135–136.

44. Insinga RP, Laessig RH, Hoffmann GL. Newborn screening with mass spectrometry: Examining its cost-effectiveness in the Wisconsin Newborn Screening Panel. *J Pediatr* 2002;141: 524–531.

45. Iafolla AK, Thompson RJ, Roe CR. Medium-chain acyl-CoA dehydrogenase deficiency: clinical course in 120 affected children. *J Pediatr* 1994;124:409–415.

46. Wilcken B, Hammond J, Silink M. Mortality and morbidity in medium chain acyl coenzyme A dehydrogenase deficiency. *Arch Dis Child* 1994;70:410–412.

47. Ziadeh R, Hoffman EP, Finegold DN, et al. Medium chain acyl-CoA dehydrogenase deficiency in Pennsylvania: neonatal screening shows high incidence and unexpected mutation frequencies. *Pediatr Res* 1995;37:675–678.

48. Pollit RJ, Leonard JV. Prospective surveillance study of medium chain acyl-CoA dehydrogenase deficiency in the UK. *Arch Dis Child* 1998;79:116–119.

49. Zschocke J, Schulze A, Lindner M, et al. Molecular and functional characterization of mild MCAD deficiency. *Human Genet* 2001;108:404–408.

50. Millington DS, Kodo N, Norwood DL, et al. Tandem mass spectrometry: a new method for acylcarnitine profiling with potential for neonatal screening for in born errors of metabolism. *J Inherit Metab Dis* 1990;13:321–324.

51. Carpenter K, Wiley V, Sim KG, et al. Evaluation of newborn screening for medium chain acyl-CoA dehydrogenase deficiency in 275 000 babies. *Arch Dis Child Fetal Neonatal Ed* 2001;85:105–109.

52. Insinga RP, Laessig RH, Hoffmann GL. Newborn screening with tandem mass spectrometry: examining cost effectiveness in the Wisconsin Newborn Screening panel. *J Pediatr* 2002;141:524–531.

53. Zytkovitz TH, Fitzgerald EF, Marsden D, et al. Tandem mass spectrometric analysis for amino acid, organic and fatty acid disorders in newborn dried blood spots: a two year summery from the New England Newborn Screening Program. *Clin Chem* 2001;47:1945–1955.

54. Roe CR, Ding J. Mitochondrial fatty acid oxidation disorders. In: Scriver CR, Beaudet AL, Sly WS, et al., eds. *The Metabolic and Molecular Bases of Inherited Disease*, 8th ed. McGraw-Hill: New York, 2001, p. 2313–2315.

55. Pourfarzam M, Morris A, Appleton M, et al. Neonatal screening for medium-chain acyl-CoA dehydrogenase deficiency. *Lancet* 2001;358:1063–1064.

56. Riordan JR, Rommens, JM, Buchanan D. et al. Identification of the cystic fibrosis gene : Cloning and characterization of complementary DNA. *Science* 1989;245:1066–1073.

57. Quinton P. Physiological basis of cystic fibrosis: a historical perspective. *Physiol Rev* 1999;79:S3–S22.

58. Welsh MJ, Ramsey BW. Research on cystic fibrosis: a journey from the heart house. *Am J Resp Crit Care Med* 1998;157:148–154.

59. Cystic Fibrosis Foundation: Patient Registry 1998 Annual Data Report. Bethesda, MD: Cystic Fibrosis Foundation, 1999.

60. Muller F, Dommergues M, Simon-Buoy B. et al. Cystic fibrosis screening : A fetus with hyperechogenic bowel may be an index. *J Med Gen* 1998;35:657–660.

61. Welsh MJ, Ramsey BW, Accurso F, et al. Cystic fibrosis. In: Scriver, Beaudet, Valle, et al., eds. *The Metabolic and Molecular Bases of Inherited Disease*, 8th ed. McGraw-Hill: New York, 2001:1521–1588.

62. National Institutes of Health: National Institutes of Health Consensus Development Conference Statement on genetic testing for cystic fibrosis: Genetic testing for cystic fibrosis. *Arch Intern Med* 1999;159:1529–1539.

63. Pollit, RJ. Newborn screening for cystic fibrosis: science, legislation, and human values. *J Inherit Met Dis* 2003;26:729–744.

64. Turck D, Clement A, Reinert P, et al., AFDPHE study group. Criteria for CF centers. Neonatal screening for cystic fibrosis: France rises to the challenge. *J Inherit Met Dis* 2003;26:729–744.

65. Farriaux JP, Vidailhet M, Briard ML, et al. Neonatal screening for cystic fibrosis: France rises to the challenge. *J Inherit Met Dis* 2003;26:729–744.

66. Merelle ME, Huisman J, Alderen-ven der Vecht A, et al. Early versus late diagnosis: psychological impact on parents. *Pediatrics* 2003;111:346–350.

67. Mastella G, Zanulla L, Castellani C, et al. Neonatal screening for cystic fibrosis: long term clinical balance. *Pancreatology* 2001;15:531–537.

68. Murray J, Cuckle H, Taylor G, et al. Screening for cystic fibrosis. *Health Technol Assess* 1999;3:i–iv, 1–104.

69. Corbetta C, Seia M, Basotti A, et al. Screening for cystic fibrosis in newborn Infants: Results of a pilot programme based on a two tier protocol (IRT/DNA/IRT) in the Italian population. *J Med Screen* 2002;9:60–63.

70. Ranieri E, Lewis BD, Gerace RL, et al. Neonatal screening for cystic fibrosis using immunoreactive trypsinogen and direct gene analysis: four years' experience. *BMJ* 1994;308:1469–1472.

71. Corbetta C, Seia M, Bassotti A, et al. Screening for cystic fibrosis in newborn infants: results of a programme based on two tier protocol (IRT/DNA/IRT) in the Italian population. *J Med Screen* 2002;9:60–63.

72. Lee DS, Rosenberg MA, Peterson A, et al. Analysis of the costs of diagnosing cystic fibrosis with a newborn screening program. *J Pediatr* 2003;142:617–623.

73. Wilson JMG, Jungner G. *Principles and Practice of Screening for Disease: Public Health Papers, No. 34.* Geneva: World Health Organization, 1968.

74. Holen KJ, Terjesen T, Tegnander A, et al. Ultrasound screening for hip dysplasia in newborns. *J Pediatr Orthop* 1994;14:667–673.

75. Chan A, McCaul KA, Cundy PJ, et al. Perinatal risk factors for the developmental dysplasia of the hip. *Arch Dis Child Fetal Neonatal Ed* 1997;76:94–100.

76. Clark NM. Role of ultrasound in congenital hip dysplasia. *Arch Dis Child* 1994;70:362–363.

77. Jones D. Neonatal detection of developmental dysplasia of the hip. *J Bone Joint Surg Br* 1998;80:943–945.

78. Asher MA. Screening for congenital dislocation of the hip, scoliosis and other abnormalities affecting the neuromuscular system. *Pediatr Clin North Am* 1986;33:1335–1353.

79. Bennet GC. Screening for congenital dislocation of the hip [editorial]. *J Bone Joint Surg Br* 1992;74:643–644.

80. Aronsson DD, Goldberg MJ, Kling TF Jr, et al. Developmental dysplasia of the hip. *Pediatrics* 1994, 94:201–208 [Published erratum in *Pediatrics* 1994;94:470].

81. Skriving AP, Scadden WJ. The African neonatal hip and its immunity from congenital dislocation. *J Bone Joint Surg Br* 1979;61:339–341.

82. Kutlu A, Memik R, Mutlu M, et al. Congenital dislocation of the hip and its relation to swaddling used in Turkey. *J Pediatr Orthop* 1992;12:598–602.

83. Churgay CA, Caruthers BS. Diagnosis and treatment of congenital dislocation of the hip. *Am Fam Phys* 1992;45:1217–1228.

84. Krolo I, Viskovic K, Kozic S, et al. The advancement in the early diagnosis of developmental hip dysplasia in infants: the role of ultrasound screening. *Coll Anthropol* 2003;27:27–34.

85. Marks DS, Clegg J, Al-Chalabi AN. Routine ultrasound screening for neonatal hip instability: can it abolish late presenting congenital dislocation of the hip? *J Bone Joint Surg Br* 1994;76: 534–538.

86. Bennet GC. Screening for congenital dislocation of the hip (editorial). *J Bone Joint Surg Br* 1992;74:643–644.

87. Barlow TG. Early diagnosis and treatment of congenital dislocation of the hip. *J Bone Joint Surg Br* 1962;44:292–301.

88. Von Kries R, Ihne N, Oberle D, et al. Effect of ultrasound screening on the first rate operative procedures for developmental hip dysplasia in Germany. *Lancet* 2003;6:1883–1887.

89. Ortholani M. Early diagnosis and therapy of congenital hip luxation. *Kinderarztl Prax* 1951;19: 404–407.

90. Elbourne D, Dezateux C, Arthur R, et al., and the UK Collaborative Hip Trial Group. Ultrasonography in the diagnosis and management of developmental hip dysplasia (UK Hip Trial): clinical and economic results of a multicentre randomised controlled trial. *Lancet* 2002;360:2009–2017.

91. Brown J, Dezateux C, Karnon J, et al. Efficiency of alternative policy options for screening for developmental dysplasia of the hip in the United Kingdom. *Arch Dis Child* 2003;88: 760–766.

92. Godward S, Dezateux C. Surgery for congenital dislocation of the hip in the UK as a measure of outcome of screening. *Lancet* 1998;351:1149–1152.

93. Puhan MA, Woolacott N, Kleijnen J, et al. Observational studies on ultrasound screening for the developmental dysplasia of the hip in newborns-a systematic review. *Ultraschall Med* 2003;24:377–382.

94. Larsson A, Therrel BL. Newborn screening: the role of the obstetrician. *Clin Obstet Gynecol* 2002;45:697–710.

95. Almeida AM, Henthorn JS, Davies SC. Neonatal screening for haemoglobinopathies: the result of a 10 year programme in an English Health Region. *Br J Haematol* 2001;112:32–35.

96. Davies SC, Cronin E, Gill M, et al. Screening for sickle cell disease and thalassemia: a systematic review with supplementary research. *Health Technol Assess* 2000;4:1–99.

97. Larsson A, Therrel BL. Newborn screening: the role of the obstetrician. *Clin Obstet Gynecol* 2002;45:697–710.

98. Henthorn JS, Almeida AM, Davies SC. Neonatal screening for sickle cell disorders. *Br J Haematol* 2004;124:259–263.

99. Pass KA, Harris K. Update: newborn screening for sickle cell disease—California, Illinois and New York. *MMWR Recomm Rep* 2000;49:729–731.

100. Pass KA, Lane PA, Fernhoff PM, et al. US newborn screening system guidelines, II: follow-up of children, diagnosis, management and evaluation. Statement of the council of Regional Networks for Genetic Services (CORN). *J Pediatr* 2000;137:S1–46.

101. Campbell M, Henthorn, JS, Davies SC Evaluation of cation-exchange HPLC compared with isoelectric focusing for neonatal hemoglobinopathy screening. *Clin Chem* 1999;45:969–975.

102. Papadea C, Eckman JR, Kuehnert RS, et al. Comparison of liquid and dried blood for neonatal hemoglobinopathy screening: laboratory and programmatic issues. *Pediatrics* 1994;93: 427–432.

103. Henthorn JS, Almeida AM, Davies SC. Neonatal screening for sickle cell disorders. *Br J Haematol* 2004;124:259–263.

104. Tsevat J, Wong JB, Pauker SG, et al. Neonatal screening for sickle cell disease: a cost-effective analysis. *J Pediatr* 1991;118:546–554.

105. Texas Department of Health. *State Health Data,* Austin TX, 1995

106. Cevette MJ. Auditory brainstem response testing in the intensive care unit. *Semin Hear* 1984;5:57–68.

107. Galambos R, Wilson MJ, Silva PD. Identifying hearing loss in the intensive care nursery: A 20 year summary. *J Am Acad Audiol* 1994;5:151–162.

108. Task Force on Newborn and Infant Hearing. Newborn and infant hearing loss: detection and Intervention. *Pediatrics* 1999;103:527–530.

109. Position Statement: Principles and guidelines for early detection and intervention programs from the AAP Joint Committee on Infant Hearing. *Pediatrics* 2000;106:798–817.
110. Downs MP. Auditory screening. *Otolaryngol Clin North Am* 1978;11:611–629.
111. Yoshinaga-Itano C, Sedey AL, Coulter DK, et al. Language of early-and-later identified children with hearing loss. *Pediatrics* 1998;5:161–171.
112. Yoshinaga-Itano C. Efficacy of early identification and early intervention. *Semin Hear* 1995;16:115–123.
113. De Michele AM, Ruth RA. Newborn hearing screening. Available at www.emedicine.com, 2004.
114. Jacobson JT, Jacobsen CA, Spahr RC. Automated and conventional ABR screening techniques in high risk infants. *J Am Acad Audiol* 1990;1:187–195.
115. White KR. Universal newborn hearing screening using transient evoked Otoacoustic emissions: past, present, and future. *Semin Hear* 1996;17:171–183.
116. Mehl AL, Thomson V. Newborn hearing screening: the great omission. *Pediatrics* 1998;101:e4.

The Annual Bimanual Examination

Susan R. Johnson

Ann Laros

■ What Is the Problem that Requires Screening?

Gynecologic malignancy.

What is the incidence/prevalence of the target condition?

The average lifetime risk of ovarian cancer for women in the United States is 1/70, or about 1.7%.[1] The 2000 SEER (Surveillance, Epidemiology, and End Results) data for ovarian cancer in the United States showed an age-adjusted overall rate of 15.8 (15.5–16.0) cases per 100,000 women, with a higher rate for white women (16.4 cases/100,000) and a lower rate for black women (10.5 cases/100,000). This rate translates into about 25,000 new cases per year in the United States.[2] Rates are low before age 50, and then rise until a peak rate of about 40 to 60 cases per year (depending on race) in the seventh decade. There is some evidence that the incidence has declined since 1990, at least among white women.[3]

Women at greatest risk are those in families with a genetically transmitted cancer syndrome, in particular *BRCA1* and *BRCA2* mutations (see related information in Chapter 47). Women with two or more first-degree relatives with ovarian cancer have a lifetime risk as high as 50%, and women with a single first-degree relative with ovarian cancer may have a 5% risk, which is approximately three times the average risk. Based on this epidemiologic picture, screening strategies have been studied for women older than 50 years and on women of any age whose high risk is based on their genetic profile.

What are the sequelae of the condition that are of interest in clinical medicine?

Ovarian cancer is the fifth leading cause of death among American women after lung, colon, breast, and pancreatic cancers.[3] The mortality rate for ovarian cancer has changed little over the past 40 years, although there was a slight, but statistically significant decline between 1992 and 2001.[4] The overall 5-year survival rate is about 50%, somewhat improved from about 40% in the early 1970s. Survival is associated with the stage of the disease at diagnosis, and unfortunately, most cases are diagnosed at an advanced stage. Indicating the potential importance of early detection, localized disease has a reported 5-year survival rate approximating 90%[5,6] Other malignancies that may be discovered at the time of the examination include vulvar and vaginal.

■ The Tests

What is the purpose of the tests?

To identify women with early-stage ovarian cancer by the detection of a pelvic mass.

What is the nature of the tests?

The bimanual examination is usually performed as a routine component of a complete gynecologic screening examination to assess the pelvic structures. This examination is clearly useful in the evaluation of women who present with symptoms such as pelvic or abdominal pain, dyspareunia, abnormal bleeding, or a feeling of lower abdominal fullness. In the presence of such symptoms, the finding of an enlarged or irregularly shaped uterus, pelvic mass, or tenderness has a high positive predictive value. In the absence of symptoms, on the other hand, these findings are most likely to represent conditions, such as a uterine leiomyomas, benign adnexal mass, or endometriosis, for which routine screening is probably not cost-effective.[7,8]

The identification of malignant masses in the presymptomatic state, particularly cancer of the ovary, is potentially of more value. We recognize that on very rare occasions other asymptomatic gynecologic malignancies, such as uterine sarcoma or fallopian tube carcinoma will also be detected, but these conditions are extremely rare and not candidates for routine screening.

The bimanual examination is part of the physical examination. The examiner places one or two fingers in the vagina, and the opposite hand on the abdomen, allowing palpation of the uterine cervix and corpus and the adnexal structures. The examiner can then assess the location, size, consistency, and mobility of an abnormal mass.

The size of the normal ovary in a premenopausal woman approximates $3.5 \times 2 \times 1.5$ cm; in the postmenopausal woman it is 2×0.5 cm or less, which is not palpable by bimanual examination. In the premenopausal woman, asymptomatic masses of 5 cm or larger are considered abnormal, and require follow-up. The finding of a palpable ovary, or a pelvic mass, of any size in a postmenopausal woman mandates further evaluation.

The bimanual examination is difficult to standardize, and many factors affect accuracy and reproducibility. These include the experience of the examiner, and the habitus and cooperation of the woman.[9] Jacobs et al.[10] suggested that a positive predictive value of at least 10% is required for either a single test or combination of tests to provide cost-effective screening for ovarian cancer. Assuming 40 women per 100,000 screened have ovarian cancer, it would require a sensitivity of 60% and a specificity of 99.6% for screening to be cost-effective. Test performance characteristics have not been well studied for the bimanual examination, but the data available suggest that neither sensitivity nor specificity is adequate for screening purposes.

A study of the ability of internal medicine resident physicians to identify pelvic masses on a synthetic pelvic trainer model noted a sensitivity of 67% for 3- to 6-cm masses with 100% specificity.[11] Table 43-1 summarizes studies in which the investigators report the agreement between preoperative examination and surgical findings.[9,12–16] Sensitivity ranges from 21% to 90%, and specificity from 79% to 94%. The positive predictive value is not meaningful in these samples, because the women in the study were generally selected either because of a known mass or a high suspicion of a mass. Frederick et al.[13] included a large number of women with uterine leiomyomata, and so the same level of sensitivity may not be seen for ovarian masses alone. The very high sensitivity reported by Rulin et al.[15] may reflect the high number of very large masses (up to 10 cm in diameter.) In contrast, Popp et al.[14] observed that almost half of the masses smaller than 5 cm were missed at pelvic examination, which is particularly relevant since prognosis is improved with the identification of early ovarian tumors. Padilla et al.[9] found a difference in sensitivity depending on the side of the pelvis being examined, and no difference in the accuracy among practicing gynecologists and medical students; residents in obstetrics and gynecology were the most accurate!

Table 43-1	**Studies of preoperative pelvic examination findings compared with surgical findings**

Study	No. patients	Sensitivity, %	Specificity, %
Rulin and Preston, 1987	150	90[1]	—
Andolf and Jorgenson, 1988	194	67	94
Frederick et al., 1991	133	65.7	92.5
Popp, 1993	157	56[2]	—
Padilla, 2000	140	21,[3] 33[4]	79,[3] 88[4]

[1] For adnexal masses less than 10 cm in diameter.
[2] For adnexal masses less than 5 cm in diameter.
[3] For right-sided adnexal masses.
[4] For left-sided adnexal masses.
From Rulin MC, Preston AL. Adnexal masses in postmenopausal women. *Obstet Gynecol* 1987;70:578–581; Andolf E, Jorgensen C. A prospective comparison of clinical ultrasound and operative examination of the female pelvis. *J Ultrasound Med* 1988;7:617–620; Frederick JL, Paulson RJ, Sauer MV. Routine use of vaginal ultrasonography in the preoperative evaluation of gynecologic patients: an adjunct to resident education. *J Reprod Med* 1991;36:779–782; Popp LW, Gaetje R, Stoyanov M. Accuracy of bimanual palpation versus vaginosonography in determination of the measurements of pelvic tumors. *Arch Gynecol Obstet* 1993;252:197–202; and Padilla LA, Radosevich DM, Milad MP. Accuracy of the pelvic examination in detecting adnexal masses. *Obstet Gynecol* 2000;96,4 593–598.

Schutter et al.[16] compared presurgical pelvic examination, ultrasound and cancer antigen 125 (CA-125) (see Chapter 52) in women with a known mass to determine which test, or combination of tests, was most helpful in distinguishing benign and malignant tumors. Pelvic examination was as sensitive for the identification of malignancy as the other two modalities (approximately 75% accurate), and the best predictor of "no malignancy" was when findings of all three tests were negative. However, this study was not designed to assess the sensitivity or specificity of these modalities in a screening setting. Two studies have examined the independent role of pelvic examination in a general population screening setting.[7,10] Jacobs et al.[10] screened 1,010 postmenopausal women using bimanual examination, pelvic ultrasonography, and CA-125 testing. Bimanual examination alone had a specificity of 97.3%, but the sensitivity could not be assessed because only one cancer was found in the study. Similarly, Grover et al.[7] noted a high specificity (99.9%), but was unable to assess sensitivity because no cancers were found in the sample of 2,623 women. Piver and Barlow[17] found that only 15% of 100 consecutive patients with ovarian cancer were initially identified by a routine pelvic examination.

What are the implications of testing?

What does an abnormal test result mean? The differential diagnosis of an adnexal mass varies with the age and menopausal status of the patient. Many benign conditions cause enlargement of the ovaries in premenopausal women and the risk of ovarian cancer is low. However, a cystic mass larger than 5 cm that persists after one or two menstrual cycles or a mass that has worrisome characteristics (i.e., solid, bilateral, nodular, or very large) should be investigated immediately.[18]

The historical practice has been to recommend immediate surgical evaluation for any palpable mass found in a postmenopausal woman.[19] However, a more conservative approach is now suggested for masses smaller than 5 cm in diameter that appear sonographically as simple cysts. Small simple cysts of the ovary are commonly found in postmenopausal women during transvaginal ultrasound examination, and current evidence supports careful observation of these cysts with serial ultrasound and tumor marker measurement rather than immediate surgery.[20–22]

What does a normal test result mean? Although a normal examination does not exclude the presence of disease, the pelvic examination does have a reasonable level of specificity (Table 43–1). Women who have a normal examination and are asymptomatic should be reexamined at the time of their next gynecologic appointment.

What is the cost of testing?

The bimanual examination adds little direct cost to the health care system when performed at the time of a recommended Pap smear or sexually transmitted diseases testing. The examination typically takes less than a minute of provider time, and the provider fee is generally included as part of the consultation fee. The cost of evaluation of abnormal findings, however, can be high. Follow up with transvaginal ultrasound and a CA-125 level may cost hundreds of dollars, although this is much less than the several thousand dollars required for surgical evaluation.

■ Conclusions and Recommendations

An annual bimanual examination is not sufficient as a screening test for ovarian cancer. Because it is inexpensive, minimally invasive, and a small percentage of asymptomatic ovarian cancers will be identified, performance of a bimanual examination is reasonable if a pelvic examination is being done for other reasons.

■ Summary

1 ■ What Is the Problem that Requires Screening?

Gynecologic malignancy.

  a. What is the incidence/prevalence of the target condition?
  The lifetime risk of ovarian cancer in the United States is 1/70. Rates are late before age 50, and rise thereafter with peaks in the seventh decade.

  b. What are the sequelae of the condition that are of interest in clinical medicine?
  Ovarian cancer is the fifth leading cause of death in American women. The 5-year survival rate approximates 50% and reflects the stage of disease at diagnosis. Other cancers that may be noted at the time include vulva and vaginal.

2 ■ The Tests

  a. What is the purpose of the tests?
  To identify women with early-stage gynecologic cancer, primarily ovarian.

Continued

■ Summary—cont'd

b. ***What is the nature of the tests?***
Bimanual examination of the pelvic organs.

c. ***What are the implications of testing?***
1. What does an abnormal test result mean?
An abnormal test means further evaluation, which may include ultrasound, biochemical testing where indicated, and subsequent surgery. Small simple cysts (<5 cm) of the ovary are commonly found in the ovaries of post-menopausal women during transvaginal ultrasound examination. Evidence supports serial observation of these cysts and tumor marker measurements rather than immediate surgery.
2. What does a normal test result mean?
Although a normal examination does not exclude the presence of disease, the pelvic examination does have a reasonable level of specificity

d. ***What is the cost of testing?***
The bimanual examination adds little direct cost to the health care system when performed at the time of a recommended Pap smear or sexually transmitted diseases testing.

3 ■ Conclusions and Recommendations

An annual bimanual examination is not sufficient as a screening test for ovarian cancer. However, because it is inexpensive and minimally invasive and a small percentage of asymptomatic ovarian cancers will be identified, a bimanual examination should be performed if a pelvic examination is being performed for other reasons.

References

1. Ries LAG, Eisner MP, Kosary CL, et al. SEER cancer statistics review, 1973–1997. (NIH Pub. No. 00-2789). Bethesda, MD: National Cancer Institute, 2000.
2. U.S. Cancer Statistics Working Group.. United States Cancer Statistics: 2000 Incidence. Atlanta, GA: Department of Health and Human Services, Centers for Disease Control and Prevention and National Cancer Institute, 2003.

3. Goodman MT, Howe HL. Descriptive epidemiology of ovarian cancer in the United States, 1992-1997. *Cancer* 2003;97[10 Suppl]:2615–2630.

4. Jemal A, Clegg LX, Ward E, et al. Annual report to the nation on the status of cancer, 1975-2001, with a special feature regarding survival. *Cancer* 2004;101:3–27.

5. Dembo AJ, Davy M, Stenwig AE, et al. Prognostic factors in patients with stage I epithelial ovarian cancer. *Obstet Gynecol* 1990;75,2 263–273.

6. Young RC, Walton LA, Ellenberg SS, et al. Adjuvant therapy in stage I and stage II epithelial ovarian cancer. Results of two prospective randomized trials [see comment]. *N Engl J Med* 1990;322:1021–1027.

7. Grover SR, Quinn MA. Is there any value in bimanual pelvic examination as a screening test [see comment]. *Med J Austral* 1995;162:408–410.

8. Oboler SK, LaForce FM. The periodic physical examination in asymptomatic adults. *Ann Intern Med* 1989;110:214–226.

9. Padilla LA, Radosevich DM, Milad MP. Accuracy of the pelvic examination in detecting adnexal masses. *Obstet Gynecol* 2000;96,4 593–598.

10. Jacobs I, Stabile I, Bridges J, et al. Multimodal approach to screening for ovarian cancer. *Lancet* 1988;1:268–271.

11. Ferris AK, Schapira MM, Young MJ. Accuracy of pelvic examination. *Ann Intern Med* 1991;114:522.

12. Andolf E, Jorgensen C. A prospective comparison of clinical ultrasound and operative examination of the female pelvis. *J Ultrasound Med* 1988;7:617–620.

13. Frederick JL, Paulson RJ, Sauer MV. Routine use of vaginal ultrasonography in the preoperative evaluation of gynecologic patients: an adjunct to resident education. *J Reprod Med* 1991;36:779–782.

14. Popp LW, Gaetje R, Stoyanov M. Accuracy of bimanual palpation versus vaginosonography in determination of the measurements of pelvic tumors. *Arch Gynecol Obstet* 1993;252:197–202.

15. Rulin MC, Preston AL. Adnexal masses in postmenopausal women. *Obstet Gynecol* 1987;70:578–581.

16. Schutter EM, Kenemans P, Sohn C, et al. Diagnostic value of pelvic examination, ultrasound, and serum CA 125 in postmenopausal women with a pelvic mass. An international multicenter study. *Cancer* 1994;74:1398–1406.

17. Piver MS, Barlow JJ. Preoperative and intraoperative evaluation in ovarian malignancy. *Obstet Gynecol* 1996;48:312–315.

18. Spanos WJ. Preoperative hormonal therapy of cystic adnexal masses. *Am J Obstet Gynecol* 1973;116:551–556.

19. Barber HR, Graber EA. The PMPO syndrome (postmenopausal palpable ovary syndrome). *Obstet Gynecol* 1971;38:921–923.

20. Ekerhovd E, Wienerroith H, Staudach A, et al. Preoperative assessment of unilocular adnexal cysts by transvaginal ultrasonography: a comparison between ultrasonographic morphologic imaging and histopathologic diagnosis. *Am J Obstet Gynecol* 2001;184:48–54.

21. Nardo LG, Kroon ND, Reginald PW. Persistent unilocular ovarian cysts in a general population of postmenopausal women: is there a place for expectant management? *Obstet Gynecol* 2003;102:589–593.

22. Oyelese Y, Kueck AS, Barter JF, et al. Asymptomatic postmenopausal simple ovarian cyst. *Obstet Gynecol Surv* 2002;57:803–809.

Dyslipidemia

Eric J. G. Sijbrands
Janneke G. Langendonk

■ What Is the Problem that Requires Screening?

Dyslipidemia.

What is the incidence/prevalence of the target condition?

Approximately 25% of the adult population in the United States has hyperlipidemia, mostly secondary to environmental factors such as poor diet, inadequate exercise, and the metabolic syndrome. Other secondary causes of hypercholesterolemia include renal and liver diseases, corticosteroid use, nephrotic syndrome, and hypothyroidism (Table 44–1). One study suggests that 20% of women older than 40 years with hypercholesterolemia are hypothyroid.[1]

Familial hypercholesterolemia (FH) is the most common primary inheritable dyslipidemia with a prevalence of 1/400–500 in Western countries. This autosomal dominant disorder is caused by a mutation in the gene for the low-density lipoprotein (LDL) receptor. Over 700 sequence variations in the LDL receptor have been identified to date.[2,3] Homozygosity for the gene mutation occurs in 1/1,000,000, whereas compound heterozygosity occurs in 1/200,000.

The estimated prevalence of dysbetalipoproteinemia approximates 1/5,000. The estimated prevalence of severe hypertriglyceridemia caused either by lipoprotein lipase or apolipoprotein C2 deficiency is 1/1,000,000.[4]

What are the sequelae of the condition that are of interest in clinical medicine?

Cardiovascular disease (CVD) is the leading cause of death in the Western world. More than 140,000 papers have been published on cholesterol since elucidation of the receptor-mediated cholesterol pathway by Brown and Goldstein. Many risk factors for CVD are now recognized, and hypercholesterolemia enhances their effect (Figure 44–1).[5]

Table 44–1 **Secondary causes of dyslipidemia**	
Hypercholesterolemia	Hypothyroidism
	Nephrotic syndrome
	Obstructive liver disease (Lipoprotein X)
	Anorexia nervosa
	Pregnancy
	Drugs (prostagens, cyclosporine, thiazide diuretics)
Hypertriglyceridemia	Obesity
	Diabetes mellitus
	Chronic renal insufficiency
	Hypothyroidism
	Alcohol
	Sepsis
	Monoclonal gammopathies
	Drugs such as corticosteroids, antiretrovirals, estrogens and tamoxifen, retinoids, and beta-blockers in high dosages
	Glycogen storage disease
	Pregnancy

FH follows autosomal dominant inheritance, with clinical heterogeneity and variable penetrance; the phenotype differs between patients, families and specific mutations in the LDL receptor gene on chromosome 19 (Figure 44–2).[6] Cholesterol values are usually above 8 mmol/L (309 mg/dL). The excess mortality rate for the untreated disorder varies considerably even among carriers of an identical mutation.[7] Heterozygous FH is characterized by isolated hypercholesterolemia, premature corneal arcus, tendon xanthomas, premature xanthe-

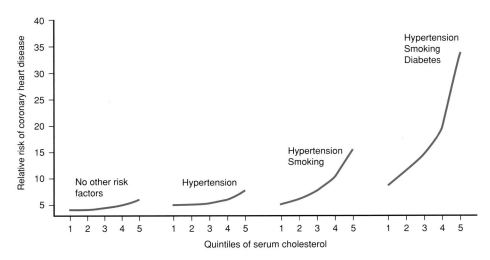

Figure 44–1   Interaction between hypertension, smoking, diabetes mellitus, and hypercholesterolemia, according to the data from the Framingham Heart Study. From Castelli WP. Lipids, risk factors, and ischaemia disease. Atherosclerosis 1996;124:51–59.

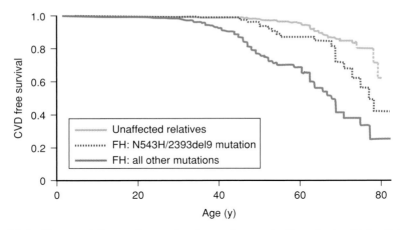

Figure 44-2 The cumulative cardiovascular disease-free survival in patients with familial hypercholesterolemia. Carriers have an eight times higher chance of coronary vascular disease compared to their family members without the mutation. From Umans-Eckenhausen MAW, Sijbrands EJG, Kastelein JJP, Defesche JC. LDL-receptor gene mutations and cardiovascular risk in a large genetic cascade screening population. *Circulation* 2002;106:3031-6.

lasmata, and premature cardiovascular disease. The lifetime risk of CVD for affected individuals is eight times that of normocholesterolemic rates. More than half of untreated male patients with FH have their first coronary event before the age of 50 years. The corresponding age for women is 60 years.[8]

Homozygosity is rare and typically associated with consanguinity. It is characterized by extremely high LDL cholesterol levels (>15 mmol/L). Fatal myocardial infarction has been reported in a homozygous fetus. The lifetime prognosis has improved significantly since the advent of statin therapy and LDL apheresis. Compound heterozygosity is more common, and cholesterol levels and the disease burden range widely.

■ The Tests

What is the purpose of the tests?

The detection of dyslipidemia.

What is the nature of the tests?

Screening for dyslipidemia is accomplished by measuring a fasting lipid profile. Cholesterol and triglycerides are measured with standard biochemical automated methods. High-density lipoprotein (HDL) is measured either directly or after precipitation. LDL cholesterol can also be measured directly or, more commonly, estimated with a formula described by Friedewald et al.[9]

LDL cholesterol = total cholesterol – HDL cholesterol – triglycerides ÷ 5
if all concentration are in mg/dL.
(LDL cholesterol = total cholesterol – HDL cholesterol – triglycerides ÷ 2.2
if all concentrations are in mmol/L.)

The Friedewald formula cannot be used in patients with hypertriglyceridemia.

Molecular testing of the total coding sequence of the LDL receptor gene and the apolipoprotein B gene is performed in the first family member when FH is suspected. Subsequent family members will only need to be tested for the specific mutation.

What are the implications of testing?

What does an abnormal test result mean? An abnormal lipid profile identifies a primary or secondary dyslipidemia that contributes to an increased risk of cardiovascular disease. Reducing the cholesterol to normal levels generates a proportionate reduction in the risk of CVD.

The present-day classification of dyslipidemias is based on the most characteristic abnormality of the lipid profile: hypercholesterolemia, hypertriglyceridemia, combined hyperlipidemia, and isolated low HDL. Severe elevations suggest a primary dyslipidemia (see Table 44–2).[10] Within these groups, the diagnosis of subtypes is based on the most probable underlying molecular defect.

Secondary dyslipidemia can be treated with lifestyle intervention or specific treatment for the underlying illness. Should the intervention be insufficient to lower the lipids so that the 10-year cardiovascular risk is increased, statin agents may be started. The Framingham Heart Study developed a coronary-prediction algorithm that provides estimates of total CHD risk over the course of 10 years. Separate score sheets are used for men and women. The factors used to estimate risk include age, blood cholesterol (or LDL cholesterol), HDL cholesterol, blood pressure, cigarette smoking, and diabetes mellitus. There is free access to the study's findings is available at www.nhlbi.nih.gov/about/framingham/riskabs.htm. Statin treatment for women is rarely indicated except for a primary hereditary dyslipidemia or when there are several independent risk factors.

Statins are highly effective in lowering plasma LDL cholesterol and triglycerides. Clinical endpoint statin trials have demonstrated safety and effectiveness for primary and secondary prevention of CVD.[11–14]

Familial hypercholesterolemia. The criteria for FH include the following:

1. Cholesterol > 8 mmol/L (309 mg/mL) after excluding secondary causes.
2. Symptoms including xanthelasmata in childhood, arcus lipoides cornea before 40 years of age, and tendon xanthomas.

Table 44-2 **ATP III Classification of cholesterol and triglycerides in mg/dl (mmol/l)[1]**

Total Cholesterol		LDL Cholesterol		Triglycerides		HDL Cholesterol	
< 200	(< 5.17)	Desirable	<100	(< 2.59)	Optimal	< 150	(< 1.69)	Normal	> 60	(> 1.55)	Desirable
200–239	(5.17-6.18)	Borderline High	100–129	(2.59-3.34)	Near/Above Optimal	150–199	(1.69-2.25)	Borderline-High	< 40	(< 1.03)	Low
> 240	(> 6.21)	High	130–159	(3.35-4.11)	Borderline High	200–499	(2.26-5.63)	High			
			160–189	(4.12-4.89)	High	> 500	(> 5.65)	Very high			
			>190	(> 4.91)	Very high						

HDL, high-density lipoprotein; LDL, low-density lipoprotein.

[1]These values can be used with tests taken after the implementation of lifestyle intervention (most laboratories have their own normal values depending on the methods and the population).

Expert Panel on detection, evaluation, and treatment of high blood cholesterol in adults (Adult Treatment Panel III). *Third report of the National Cholesterol Education Program (NCEP)*. NIH Publication No. 02-5215. Bethesda: National Institutes of Health, 2002.

3. Family history of premature CVD in first-degree relatives (men younger than 55 years and women younger than 60 years with angina pectoris, myocardial infarction, coronary bypass surgery, percutaneous transluminal coronary angioplasty (PTCA), CVA, or peripheral vascular disease).
4. Proven LDL receptor (or apolipoprotein B) mutation tested with molecular diagnostics.

The presence of criterion 4 or criteria 1 and 2 allows a definite diagnosis of FH. Individuals with criteria 1 and 3 probably have FH. The differential diagnosis of FH includes familial defective apolipoprotein B, autosomal recessive hypercholesterolemia, sitosterolemia, and cerebrotendinous xanthomatosis. Approximately 5% of apparently unrelated patients with hypercholesterolemia (total cholesterol > 7.5 mmol/L) have mutations in the apolipoprotein B gene. Compared to carriers of LDL receptor mutations, they have lower LDL cholesterol levels and a smaller increase in their risk of CVD. The remaining disorders are very rare.

Primary and secondary prevention trials with statins have not been conducted specifically in FH patients. The treatment of FH with statin agents is considered to be causal therapy of an inborn error of metabolism. Therefore, the risk reduction is expected to be larger than that observed in the aforementioned trials.

Familial combined hypercholesterolemia. Familial combined hypercholesterolemia is characterized by increased LDL and very-low-density lipoprotein (VLDL), resulting in increased levels of cholesterol and triglycerides and an increased risk of cardiovascular disease. A molecular diagnosis is not yet available because of the considerable genetic heterogeneity. If discovered during pregnancy or while breast-feeding, the lipid profile should be repeated after weaning to confirm the presence of disease.

Dysbetalipoproteinemia. Dysbetalipoproteinemia is characterized by high levels of triglyceride-rich remnant particles due to homozygosity for apolipoprotein E2. This results in a lipid profile with equally increased levels of cholesterol and triglycerides. This phenotype is expressed mainly in the presence of hyperinsulinemia and variations in other genes that are involved in the clearance of lipoproteins.[15] These patients should be referred to a lipid clinic for treatment. Dietary intervention improves the lipid profile of most patients. Nonetheless, deterioration of the lipid profile during pregnancy can lead to severe hypertriglyceridemia and an increased risk of gestational pancreatitis.

Increased lipoprotein. Increased lipoprotein A[Lp(a)] Lp(a) is an untreatable independent risk factor for cardiovascular disease. High concentrations of Lp(a) in pregnancy may induce or contribute to the development of preeclampsia by promoting endothelial dysfunction. Lp(a) levels, however, have no value for the prediction of preeclampsia.

Hypertriglyceridemia. Hypertriglyceridemia is typically secondary to other disorders. Lifestyle factors such as excessive alcohol consumption, overweight, physical inactivity, and high carbohydrate diet (> 60% total calories) contribute to hypertriglyceridemia. Medical disorders associated with hypertriglyceridemia include type 2 diabetes mellitus, chronic renal failure, nephrotic syndrome, and systemic lupus erythematosus. Antiretroviral medications, corticosteroids, estrogens and tamoxifen, retinoids, and beta-blockers in high dosages also may cause or worsen hypertriglyceridemia.[16] Hypertriglyceridemia may be the main finding in patients with familial combined hyperlipidemia and familial dysbetal-ipoproteinemia. The diagnosis of primary (inherited) hypertriglyceridemia or familial hypertriglyceridemia is reserved for patients with triglycerides in the range of 4 to 10 mmol/L (354–887 mg/dL; mild hypertriglyceridemia) and above 10 mmol/L (887 mg/dL; severe hypertriglyceridemia). The molecular defect underlying mild hypertriglyceridemia is unknown.

High triglyceride levels and decreased HDL cholesterol levels are interrelated, but they nonetheless remain independent risk factors for CVD. Mild hypertriglyceridemia is prevalent and can often be treated by refraining from alcohol and adhering to a reduced fat and carbohydrate diet. Statin and fibrate agents may be considered to improve the lipid profile if needed.

After excluding secondary causes of severe hypertriglyceridemia, a rare lipoprotein lipase or apolipoprotein C2 deficiency can be considered. Patients with severe hypertriglyceridemia should be referred to a specialized clinic where DNA testing and appropriate care are available. The patients with lipoprotein lipase deficiency typically presents with acute pancreatitis, hepatosplenomegaly, and eruptive xanthomas. They are advised to follow a diet containing less than 10% fat, mostly from a special oil consisting of medium-chain triglyceride (MCT). Unfortunately, patient compliance with this dietary intervention is low, and patients with lipoprotein lipase deficiency do not respond to fibrate and/or statin agents.

Hypertriglyceridemia treatment during pregnancy and breast-feeding. The peak levels of hypertriglyceridemia during pregnancy occur in the third trimester.[17,18] Women with hypertriglyceridemia are prone to gestational pancreatitis, a condition carrying substantial maternal and fetal risk.[19] Dietary intervention remains the cornerstone of the treatment.[20] It is especially important to refrain from alcohol consumption. When severe hypertriglyceridemia persists, an MCT diet should be considered. Fibrates and nicotinic acids are considered to be contraindicated during pregnancy and breast-feeding, although there is little information about their effects on human gestation available.[21] Maternal fenofibrate treatment of pregnant rats increases maternal and fetal plasma triglyceride concentrations,[22] and embryotoxicity has occurred at toxic doses. The current medical advice to women planning pregnancy is to discontinue fibrates and nicotinic acids 3 months before conception. Aggressive dietary therapy and intermittent intravenous feeding have been shown to be effective in reducing triglycerides should they exceed an arbitrarily selected threshold of 28 mmol/L (2,480 mg/dL). The efficacy of intermittent intravenous feeding can be explained by the observation that low-fat (high carbohydrate) isocaloric diets elevate serum triglyceride levels by the oral, but not the intravenous, route in normal individuals.[23]

The treatment options for women with hypertriglyceridemia who develop gestational pancreatitis include dietary control and lipoprotein apheresis during the acute phase. Heparin has been reported to effectively decrease triglyceride levels in a patient with severe hypertriglyceridemia-associated gestational pancreatitis. Heparin liberates the endothelial-bound lipoprotein lipase into the plasma.[24] However, the reduction of the triglycerides by heparin is only temporary, and long-term use may paradoxically increase the triglyceride level as a result of lipoprotein lipase depletion. Some authors suggest that the routine determination of fasting plasma cholesterol and triglyceride levels, or a visual examination of the fasting plasma for triglyceride-induced opacity or "milky" appearance, be performed during early pregnancy to identify at-risk women.[19]

Implications of familial hypercholesterolemia before conception. Each child of a parent heterozygous for FH has a 50% risk of being affected. However, prenatal screening is not indicated because treatment of heterozygous neonates is unnecessary. Genetic counseling is advised when both future parent have familial hypercholesterolemia; referral to a lipid clinic for an accurate diagnosis and treatment may be necessary. Prenatal molecular diagnosis via chorionic villus sampling or amniocentesis is possible but seldom performed because medical therapy is effective. The risk of fetal death is increased among homozygous progeny. The lipid profile of the rare newborns born to two parents with FH should be tested in a specialized pediatric clinic and treatment begun immediately if homozygosity is suggested. All children of a homozygous parent are heterozygous for FH. The risk of a fetal death when the mother is homozygous is unknown with present-day treatment. Ideally, homozygous women should undergo electrocardiographic exercise testing before conception and refrain from pharmaceutical treatment temporarily, at least during the first trimester. Alternative therapy during the interval off medical therapy includes weekly selective LDL apheresis.

Implications of hypercholesterolemia during pregnancy. Gestation is associated with increased levels of blood lipids, especially triglycerides. The dyslipidemia is more pronounced in patients with preeclampsia. Compared with controls, preeclamptic women have increased LDL cholesterol, Lp(a), and triglycerides, and decreased levels of HDL cholesterol. Moreover, the mean particle size of LDL is reduced. This atherogenic lipid profile may contribute to the endothelial dysfunction typical of preeclampsia. However, preeclampsia has not been described among women with inherited hypercholesterolemia and known endothelial dysfunction beginning at very young age.

Diet and other lifestyle interventions can be safely continued during pregnancy. Although animal studies suggest that statin agents are teratogenic when given at toxic dosages, the available human data have been generally reassuring.[25] However, an analysis of the U.S. Food and Drug Administration (FDA) surveillance database suggests a possible increase in congenital central nervous system and limb abnormalities with exposure to lipophilic statins during the first trimester.[26] Although statins are relatively contraindicated during pregnancy, follow up of the hypercholesterolemia is necessary. Untreated hypercholesterolemia may further deteriorate due to the hormonal changes of pregnancy. Cholestyramine may be given if the LDL cholesterol has risen in the first trimester above 15 mmol/L (570 mg/dL). Bile acid sequestrants such as cholestyramine are not absorbed from the intestine, though it may induce or exacerbate hyperemesis in early pregnancy. Resumption of statin treatment should be considered if the LDL levels become unacceptably high and the patient cannot tolerate cholestyramine.

There are only a few reports of pregnancies in FH homozygote women. These reports indicate successful outcomes after LDL apheresis,[27–30] even when the patient has overt coronary artery disease.

Primary dyslipidemia in gynecology. Patients with severe hereditary dyslipidemia are at increased risk of CVD despite a young age. In addition, perioperative myocardial ischemia, severe atherosclerosis of peripheral arteries and cholesterol emboli can also complicate surgery. Preoperative tests such as coronary angiography, perioperative monitoring and preoperative medical therapy should be considered depending on the estimated absolute risk of cardiovascular disease. In patients with primary dyslipidemia on medical treatment, strict birth control procedures are indicated. Oral contraceptives are acceptable despite the potential for mild deterioration of lipids.

What does a normal test result mean? The individual is unlikely to have a primary or secondary dyslipidemia.

What is the cost of testing?

A lipid profile and a minimal set of measurements to exclude secondary causes cost only a few dollars. DNA sequencing in the first patient costs about $600. When the family DNA mutation is known, the cost is less than $50.

Molecular testing is an effective and a more sensitive way to screen for FH among family members. Using a clinical diagnosis of FH for family screening that is solely based upon LDL cholesterol, values above the 95th percentile produces a 43% false-positive diagnosis rate among the family members.[31]

Systematic genetic screening of family members of persons diagnosed with FH is cost-effective. New cases diagnosed by the screening program gained 3.3

years of life each. Twenty-six myocardial infarctions will be avoided for every 100 persons treated with statins between the ages of 18 and 60 years. Several analysis reveal that the cost per life-year gained approximates $8,700.[32-34] One randomized screening study of 16-year-olds for FH resulted in 470 new diagnoses, and over 10 subsequent years averted an estimated 12 deaths. In contrast, screening first-degree relatives of known FH cases resulted in 13,248 new diagnoses and 560 averted deaths over 10 years. The price of statins is the main determinant of the costs. However, since most of the successful and effective statins have gone or will soon go off patent, the cost-effectiveness should improve further.

■ Conclusions and Recommendations

The identification of primary dyslipidemias is important for several reasons. Patients with either hypercholesterolemia or hypertriglyceridemia need further testing to diagnose secondary causes. When a primary dyslipidemia is suspected, the patient should be referred to a specialized clinic for treatment with diet, statin and/or fibrate agents. Family members should be examined as well when a primary dyslipidemia, such as FH, is diagnosed.

Patients with FH should discontinue statin treatment before conception. Untreated and pregnant heterozygotes can have lipid profiles that mimic the homozygous phenotype and this creates a severe CVD risk. When both parents have FH, prenatal or neonatal diagnosis is important to facilitate timely treatment of the rare homozygous children.

Severe hypertriglyceridemia is associated with acute gestational pancreatitis. When the dyslipidemia worsens during pregnancy despite lifestyle interventions, referral to a lipid clinic is recommended for additional treatment during pregnancy (pharmaceutical, apheresis, heparin infusion, etc.).

■ Summary

1 ■ What Is the Problem that Requires Screening?
Dyslipidemia and subsequent cardiovascular disease.
a. What is the prevalence of the target condition?
Pregnancy is associated with more pronounced dyslipidemia. Approximately 25% of the adult population in the United

Continued

■ **Summary—cont'd**

States has dyslipidemia, mostly secondary to environmental factors such as poor diet, inadequate exercise, diabetes, and the metabolic syndrome. Familial hypercholesterolemia is the most common primary dyslipidemia with a prevalence of 1/400–500 in Western countries. This autosomal dominant disorder is caused by a mutation in the gene for the LDL receptor. Over 700 sequence variations in the LDL receptor have been identified to date.

b. *What are the sequelae of the condition that are of interest in clinical medicine?*
A number of clinical disorders are associated with secondary dyslipidemia that contributes to an increased risk of cardiovascular disease. In this context, the most frequently encountered form of secondary dyslipidemias occurs in association with the metabolic syndrome, diabetes mellitus type 2, and hypothyroidism. Dyslipidemia may be aggravated by excessive alcohol consumption, overweight, and physical inactivity. Premature cardiovascular disease, xanthomas of the tendons, and xanthelasmata constitute the major manifestations of familial hypercholesterolemia.

2 ■ **The Tests**

a. *What is the purpose of the tests?*
To identify persons at increased risk of cardiovascular disease.

b. *What is the nature of the tests?*
Plasma lipid profile.

c. *What are the implications of testing?*
1. What does an abnormal test result mean?
An abnormal lipid profile identifies a primary or secondary dyslipidemia. Further diagnostic tests for identifying secondary causes and implementation of lifestyle interventions are needed. In severe cases, referral to a specialized clinic is strongly advised.
2. What does a normal test result mean?
A normal test result indicates that hereditary dyslipidemia is unlikely.

d. What is the cost of testing?

A lipid profile and a minimal set of measurements costs only a few dollars.

3 ■ Conclusions and Recommendations

Individuals with a history of dyslipidemia and/or a family history of premature cardiovascular disease, pancreatitis, or hypercholesterolemia or a milky-appearing plasma on visual inspection, should undergo a routine determination of plasma cholesterol and triglycerides. In cases of dyslipidemia the patient should be referred to a specialized clinic.

References

1. Series JJ, Biggart EM, O'Reilly DS, Shepherd J. Thyroid dysfunction and hypercholesterolemia in the general population of Glasgow, Scotland. *Clin Chim Acta* 1988;172:217–221.
2. Heath KE, Gahan M, Whittall RA, et al. Low-density lipoprotein receptor gene (LDLR) world-wide website in familial hypercholesterolaemia: update, new features and mutation analysis. *Atherosclerosis* 2001;154:243–246.
3. Villeger L, Abifadel M, Allard D, et al. The UMD-LDLR database: additions to the software and 490 new entries to the database. *Hum Mutat* 2002;20:81–87.
4. Evans V, Kastelein JJ. Lipoprotein lipase deficiency: rare or common? *Cardiovasc Drugs Ther* 2002;16:283–287.
5. Castelli WP. Lipids, risk factors and ischaemic disease. *Atherosclerosis* 1996;124:S1-S9.
6. Umans-Eckenhausen MAW, Sijbrands EJG, Kastelein JJP, Defesche JC. LDL-receptor gene mutations and   cardiovascular risk in a large genetic cascade screening population. *Circulation* 2002;106:3031–3036.
7. Sijbrands EJG, Westendorp RGJ, Defesche JC, de Meijer PHEM, Smelt AHM, Kastelein JJP. Mortality over two centuries in a large pedigree with familial hypercholesterolaemia. *BMJ* 2001;322:1019–1023.
8. Mabuchi H, Koizumi J, Shimizu M, et al. Development of coronary heart disease in familial hypercholesterolemia. *Circulation* 1989;79:225–232.
9. Friedewald WT, Levy RI, Fredrickson DS. Estimation of the concentration of low-density lipoprotein cholesterol in plasma, without use of the preparative ultracentrifuge. *Clin Chem* 1972;18:499–502.
10. Expert Panel on detection, evaluation, and treatment of high blood cholesterol in adults (Adult Treatment Panel III). *Third report of the National Cholesterol Education Program (NCEP)*. NIH Publication No. 02-5215. Bethesda: National Institutes of Health, 2002.
11. Sacks FM, Pfeffer MA, Moye LA, et al. The effect of pravastatin on coronary events after myocardial infarction in patients with average cholesterol levels. Cholesterol and Recurrent Events Trial investigators. *N Engl J Med* 1996;3;1001–1009.
12. Shepherd J, Cobbe SM, Ford I, et al. Prevention of coronary heart disease with pravastatin in men with hypercholesterolemia. West of Scotland Coronary Prevention Study Group. *N Engl J Med* 1995;333:1301–1307.

13. Randomised trial of cholesterol lowering in 4444 patients with coronary heart disease: the Scandinavian Simvastatin Survival Study (4S). *Lancet* 1994;344:1383–1389.

14. Prevention of cardiovascular events and death with pravastatin in patients with coronary heart disease and a broad range of initial cholesterol levels: the Long-Term Intervention with Pravastatin in Ischaemic Disease (LIPID) Study Group. *N Engl J Med* 1998;5:1349–1357.

15. Sijbrands EJ, Hoffer MJ, Meinders AE, et al. Severe hyperlipidemia in apolipoprotein E2 homozygotes due to a combined effect of hyperinsulinemia and an SstI polymorphism. *Arterioscler Thromb Vasc Biol* 1999;19:2722–2729.

16. Glueck CJ, Lang J, Hamer T, et al. Severe hypertriglyceridemia and pancreatitis when estrogen replacement therapy is given to hypertriglyceridemic women. *J Lab Clin Med* 1994;123:59–64.

17. Herrera E, Gomez-Coronado D, Lasuncion MA. Lipid metabolism in pregnancy. *Biol Neonate* 1987;51:70–77.

18. Herrera E, Lasuncion MA, Gomez-Coronado D, et al. Role of lipoprotein lipase activity on lipoprotein metabolism and the fate of circulating triglycerides in pregnancy. *Am J Obstet Gynecol* 1988;158:1575–1583.

19. Glueck CJ, Christopher C, Mishkel MA, et al. Pancreatitis, familial hypertriglyceridemia, and pregnancy. *Am J Obstet Gynecol* 1980;136:755–761.

20. Sanderson SL, Iverius PH, Wilson DE. Successful hyperlipemic pregnancy. *JAMA* 1991;265:1858–1860.

21. Weiner CP, Buhimschi C. *Drugs for Pregnant and Lactating Women.* Philadelphia: Churchill Livingston, 2004.

22. Soria A, Bocos C, Herrera E. Opposite metabolic response to fenofibrate treatment in pregnant and virgin rats. *J Lipid Res* 2002;43:74–81.

23. DenBesten L, Reyna RH, Connor WE, Stegink LD. The different effects on the serum lipids and fecal steroids of high carbohydrate diets given orally or intravenously. *J Clin Invest* 1973;52:1384-1393.

24. Loo CC, Tan JY. Decreasing the plasma triglyceride level in hypertriglyceridemia-induced pancreatitis in pregnancy: a case report. *Am J Obstet Gynecol* 2002;187:241–242.

25. Hosokawa A, Bar-Oz B, Ito S. Use of lipid-lowering agents (statins) during pregnancy. *Can Fam Physician* 2003;49:747–749.

26. Edison RJ, Muenke M. Central nervous system and limb anomalies in case reports of first trimester statin exposure. *N Engl J Med* 2004;350:1579–1582.

27. Naoumova RP, Thompson GR, Soutar AK. Current management of severe homozygous hypercholesterolaemias. *Curr Opin Lipidol* 2004;15:413–422.

28. Makino H, Harada-Shiba M. Long-term effect of low-density lipoprotein apheresis in patients with homozygous familial hypercholesterolemia. *Ther Apher Dial* 2003;7:397–401.

29. Klingel R, Gohlen B, Schwarting A, et al. Differential indication of lipoprotein apheresis during pregnancy. *Ther Apher Dial* 2003;7:359–364.

30. Kroon AA, Swinkels DW, van Dongen PW, et al. Pregnancy in a patient with homozygous familial hypercholesterolemia treated with long-term low-density lipoprotein apheresis. *Metabolism* 1994;43:1164–1170.

31. Umans-Eckenhausen MA, Defesche JC, Sijbrands EJ, et al. Review of first 5 years of screening for familial hypercholesterolaemia in The Netherlands. *Lancet* 2001;357:165–168.

32. Wonderling D, Umans-Eckenhausen MA, Marks D, et al. Cost-effectiveness analysis of the genetic screening program for familial hypercholesterolemia in The Netherlands. *Semin Vasc Med* 2004;4:97–104.

33. Marks D, Thorogood M, Neil HA, et al. Comparing costs and benefits over a 10 year period of strategies for familial hypercholesterolaemia screening. *J Public Health Med* 2003;25:47–52.

34. Marks D, Wonderling D, Thorogood M, et al. Cost effectiveness analysis of different approaches of screening for familial hypercholesterolaemia. *BMJ* 2002;324:1303.

45

Diabetes Mellitus

Hajo I. J. Wildschut

■ What Is the Problem that Requires Screening?

Diabetes mellitus, types 1 and 2.

What is the incidence/prevalence of the target condition?

The prevalence of diabetes is difficult to determine as criteria have been promulgated. In the United States, there is evidence of a substantial increase in the prevalence of diabetes among adults of both sexes.[1,2] The estimated lifetime risk in the United States of developing diabetes for individuals born in 2000 is 33% for males and 39% for females.[3] Females have higher residual lifetime risks at all ages. The highest estimated lifetime risk of diabetes is among Hispanic groups.

Approximately three fourths of all newly diagnosed cases of type 1 diabetes occur in individuals younger than 18 years.[4] The highest prevalences of type 1 diabetes are found in Scandinavia and Northern Europe, whereas the lowest are found in China.

Type 2 diabetes is a heterogeneous disease typically affecting those older than 40 years and obese individuals. However, the prevalence of type 2 diabetes in children and adolescents has increased dramatically over the last decade, especially among ethnic minority groups.[5] Type 2 diabetes accounts for 90% to 95% of all cases of diabetes.[6] The estimated global prevalence of diabetes in adults older than 20 years is 5%, with prevalences being higher in developed than in developing countries.

What are the sequelae of the condition that are of interest in clinical medicine?

Type 1 diabetes is due to a deficiency in insulin secretion secondary to pancreatic islet cell B cell destruction typically by an autoimmune process. Circulating islet cell antibodies are detected in as many as 85% of patients tested during the first weeks after diagnosis.[8] The observation of a high concordance in monozygotic twins favor an important genetic influence.[9,10] Type 1 diabetes may also be caused by extrinsic events that cause B cell damage, such as mumps, Coxsackie B4 virus, toxic chemical agents and destructive cytotoxins. Type 1 diabetes usually develops in school-aged children and is characterized by polyuria, polydipsia, and weight loss. The initial clinical presentation may be altered consciousness or frank coma secondary to acute metabolic decompensation with ketoacidemia and ketonuria. Insulin is required for all patients with type 1 diabetes.

Type 2 diabetes results from either tissue insensitivity to insulin, aberrant insulin release, inadequate insulin release or a combination thereof.[8] Type 2 diabetes has been attributed to several interrelating factors such as ethnicity, age, sedentary lifestyle, and abdominal–visceral obesity. The cause is unknown in most cases of type 2 diabetes in nonobese patients. Unfortunately, type 2 diabetes frequently remains undiagnosed until complications appear. About one third of all diabetic patients are unrecognized.[4] The characteristic clinical signs and symptoms of type 2 diabetes begin more gradually than type 1. Monilial vaginitis may be the initial manifestation of type 2 diabetes in women. The diagnosis is frequently made after an asymptomatic individual is found to have elevated plasma glucose on routine laboratory examination. Depending on the population studied and the investigators' assumptions, the time from the onset of preclinical diabetes to clinically manifest disease is 5 to 12 years.[11]

Hypertension (blood pressure 140/90 mm Hg) is a common comorbidity of diabetes, ultimately affecting the majority of individuals with diabetes. In type 1 disease, hypertension is often the result of an underlying nephropathy, whereas in type 2 diabetes, hypertension may present as part of the metabolic syndrome (i.e., obesity, hyperglycemia, dyslipidemia) that is associated with high rates of cerebrovascular disease.[4] Type 2 diabetes seldom causes ketoacidosis and coma. Long-term complications of diabetes involve eyes, kidneys, nerves, and blood vessels. The life expectancy patients with type 2 diabetes is shortened by as much as 15 years, with up to 75% dying of macrovascular complications.[12] Prediabetes is considered a risk factor for future overt diabetes and cardiovascular disease.[4]

■ The Tests

What is the purpose of the tests?

To identify asymptomatic individuals who are likely to have diabetes mellitus.

What is the nature of the tests?

Fasting plasma glucose. Fasting is defined as no consumption of food or beverages other than water for at least 8 hours before testing.[6] Laboratory testing of plasma glucose concentration is performed on venous samples with enzymatic assay techniques (typically glucose oxidase). Capillary blood glucose testing using reflectance blood glucose meter is not suitable for screening, because of the relative imprecision.[6] The same is true for urinary glucose measurements.[11]

Reference test. In 1999, the World Health Organization (WHO) set new criteria classifying individuals as either having normal or impaired glucose tolerance after a 75-g oral glucose tolerance test (GTT) following an overnight fast.[11] Based on a fasting glucose and a 2-hour blood glucose measurement, the WHO distinguishes three diagnostic categories: (a) normal, fasting glucose less than 7.0 mmol/L (126 mg/dL) and a 2-hour glucose less than 7.8 mmol/L (140 mg/dL); (b) prediabetes: fasting glucose less than 7.0 mmol/L (126 mg/dL) and a 2-hour glucose 7.8 to 11.0 mmol/L (140–199 mg/dL); and (c) diabetes: fasting glucose 7.0 mmol/L (126 mg/dL) or a 2-hour glucose 11.1 mmol/L (200 mg/dL).[13]

In 1997, an expert committee of the American Diabetes Association (ADA) recommended that oral glucose tolerance testing not be routinely performed in clinical practice or for epidemiologic studies. Rather, they recommended a fasting glucose above 7.0 mmol/L (126 mg/dL) be used to classify individuals as having diabetes.[4,14] The ADA fasting criteria defined diabetes as a fasting glucose above 7.0 mmol/L (126 mg/dL) and impaired fasting glucose tolerance (prediabetes) as a fasting glucose between 5.6 mmol/L (100 mg/dL) and 6.9 mmol/L (125 mg/dL).[4,14] The sensitivity of the ADA criteria to diagnose diabetes compared to the WHO definitions is poor at 48% (95% confidence interval [CI], 36%–61%).[15] It is not known which definition, if either, is a superior predictor of diabetic sequelae. Additional testing by glycosylated hemoglobin increases sensitivity of the ADA definition using the WHO as a gold standard (see section on Hemoglobin A1c). An oral GTT may be required in the diagnostic evaluation of the individual with impaired fasting glucose or when diabetes is still suspected despite a normal fasting plasma glucose.[4]

Random plasma glucose. Plasma glucose testing may also be performed on subjects who have eaten or drunk shortly before testing. Such tests are referred to as random or casual plasma glucose measurements. A random plasma glucose above 11.1 mmol/L (200 mg/dL) with clinical symptoms of diabetes is considered diagnostic of the disease.[4] A confirmatory fasting plasma glucose or oral GTT should be carried out only when the clinical condition of the patient allows.

Hemoglobin A1. The major form of glycosylated hemoglobin is termed "hemoglobin A_{1c}" (HbA1c), which normally comprises 4% to 6% of the total hemoglobin. HbA1c is abnormally high in diabetic subjects with chronic hyperglycemia, and reflects the overall glycemic state during the preceding 8 to 12 weeks. HbA1c is measured using low-pressure cation exchange chromatography.[16] Using a receiver operator characteristic curve, the optimum combined cutpoint using fasting plasma glucose and HbA1c to diagnose diabetes is a fasting plasma glucose of 5.7 mmol/L and an HbA1c of 5.9%.[15] These cutpoints have a sensitivity and specificity of 72% and 95%, respectively, using the WHO standard. Marked ethnic variation in the sensitivity and specificity of this approach is reported: 47% and 98% among Europeans, 79% and 96% among Chinese, and 85% and 91% among South Asians, respectively.[15] HbA1c is a valuable tool for monitoring glycemia, but is currently not recommended by the ADA as a screening tool for diabetes.[4]

What are the implications of testing?

What does an abnormal test result mean? A fasting plasma glucose above 7.0 mmol/L (126 mg/dL) is an indication for retesting, which should be performed on a different day to confirm the diagnosis. If the fasting plasma glucose is below 7.0 mm/l (126 mg/dL) but there is high suspicion of diabetes mellitus, an oral GTT could be performed. Alternatively, the combination of fasting plasma glucose level and HbA1c may be used to confirm diabetes.[15]

Glycemic control is fundamental in the management of diabetes.[4] Achieving euglycemia attenuates many of the complications in patients with both type 1 and type 2 diabetes.[4,15] In patients with type 1 diabetes, treatment with insulin is required to achieve euglycemia. The management of patients with newly diagnosed type 2 diabetes includes a complete medical evaluation and integrated care focussing on diet, lifestyle, counseling for the timely identification and treatment of future diabetic complications, and oral drug therapy or insulin, where indicated.[4,17] Weight reduction in obese subjects may "cure" their diabetes mellitus. HbA1c should be measured at regular intervals, as the risk of complications in diabetic patients is directly related to glycemic control. The management plan should seek preprandial plasma glucose measurements between 5.0 mmol/L (90 mg/dL) and 7.2 mmol/L (130 mg/dL), 2-hour postprandial plasma glucose measurements below 10.0 mmol/L (180 mg/dL) and an HbA1c target of below 7%.[4] Quality indicators for optimal care include the periodic measurement of blood pressure, cholesterol, and microalbuminuria; regular examination of feet; retinal screening; and influenza vaccination.[17] Adults diagnosed with prediabetes may be advised to reduce weight and increase physical activity in order to reduce the rate of progression to frank diabetes.[4]

What does a normal test result mean? The chance of an asymptomatic individual without any risk factors having or developing diabetes is relatively low. It is recommended that screening be repeated at 3-year intervals beginning at age 45, particularly in those who are overweight and have additional risk factors (Table 45–1). The rationale for this interval is that testing will be repeated before a substantial time elapses in which the individual with a (false) negative screening test result is unlikely to develop any serious diabetic complications.[6]

Table 45–1	**Risk Factors for diabetes type 2**

Sedentary life style
Obesity
Hypertension
Dyslipidemia
First-degree relative with diabetes
Member of a high-risk ethnic population
Delivered of an infant with macrosomia
Have been diagnosed with gestational diabetes
Polycystic ovarian syndrome
History of vascular disease
On previous testing, impaired glucose tolerance or impaired fasting glucose

Copyright © 2004 American Diabetes Association. From *Diabetes Care* 2004;27[Suppl 1]:S15–35. Reprinted with permission from The American Diabetes Association.

What is the cost of testing?

Costs of screening and early treatment of those identified as having diabetes are generally higher when compared with the current practice of standard diagnosis. Early diagnosis and treatment of type 2 through opportunistic screening (i.e., case finding during routine contact with the medical care system) is considered cost-effective, in particular when patients at increased risk of microvascular complications are targeted (Table 45–1).[12,18,19] One study from the Centers for Disease Control and Prevention (CDC) identified the costs per case detected in 1998 through opportunistic screening as $1,200, which included the costs incurred for a fasting plasma glucose screening test, an oral GTT test for those with a positive screen test, and physician time for test interpretation.[11,18] The average annual costs for treatment of newly diagnosed patients was $1,007.[11] Overall, the lifetime cost of diabetes treatment was $3,400 higher with screening than treatment following standard diagnosis.[11] Compared with other specific interventions for diabetes (e.g., intensive glycemic control, blood pressure and lipid management) the overall costs for opportunistic screening for diabetes are higher.[11]

■ Conclusions and Recommendations

Diabetes is a chronic illness that requires continuing medical care and patient self-management education to prevent acute complications and to reduce the likelihood of long-term complications.[4]

Almost all patients with type 1 diabetes present with acute symptoms of severe hyperglycemia. Hence, screening asymptomatic individuals for type 1 diabetes is not useful. Clinical studies are being conducted to test various methods of preventing type 1 diabetes in high-risk individuals, such as siblings of individuals with type 1 diabetes.

Type 2 diabetes frequently remains undiagnosed until complications mani-fest. In fact, approximately one third of all patients with diabetes go undiag-nosed.[4] To detect preclinical type 2 diabetes, the ADA recommends a two-stepped approach based on risk status, the measurement of fasting plasma glucose and if indicated, further testing by using HbA1c instead of an oral GTT as recommended by the WHO. The ADA acknowledges their approach will lead to slightly lower estimates of prevalence of abnormal glycemic status com-pared to the WHO criteria.[14,20] However, such two-stage screening test strategy may allow a more efficient use of resources.[11]

Although it is well established that treating overt diabetes diagnosed through standard clinical practice is effective in decreasing diabetic microvas-cular complications,[12] it is unknown whether the additional years of treatment provided to individuals with asymptomatic (preclinical) diabetes diagnosed through screening will result in any clinically relevant improvement in dia-betes-related outcomes.[6,12] Furthermore, screening for diabetes may be poorly targeted (i.e., fail to reach the groups most at risk) and inappropriately test those at low risk (the worried well) or even those already diagnosed with diabetes.[4]

As a stand-alone test, the oral GTT is not recommended for screening because of its poor reproducibility, low acceptability and high costs. Oppor-tunistic screening using biochemical tests among individuals identified as high risk of developing diabetes (Table 45–1) performs best, in terms of a lifetime reduction of microvascular disease and cost-effectiveness.[6,11,19,20] Risk assess-ment questionnaires have generally performed poorly as stand-alone tests.[11]

Population-based and selective screening programs in community settings (outreach programs, health fairs, or shopping malls) have demonstrated uni-formly low yield and poor follow up.[11] Until definitive studies of the effective-ness of screening for type 2 diabetes are available, community screening for diabetes type 2 is not recommended.

■ Summary

1 ■ What Is the Problem that Requires Screening?

Diabetes mellitus, type 1 and type 2.

a. What is the incidence/prevalence of the target condition?

The prevalences of types 1 and 2 are not known exactly as it depends upon the diagnostic criteria, geographic location, and demographic profile. Type 2 diabetes accounts for 90% to 95% of all cases of diabetes. Worldwide, an estimated one in 20 adults older than 20 years has diabetes. The prevalence of diabetes is higher in developed countries than in developing countries.

b. **What are the sequelae of the condition that are of interest in clinical medicine?**

Diabetes is a common disease strongly associated with long- and short-term morbidity, including retinopathy, nephropathy, neuropathy, microvascular disease, cardiovascular disease, and death. Type 2 diabetes is often associated with obesity, hyperlipidemia, atherosclerotic vascular disease, and hypertension. There is ample evidence that adequate glycemic control of patients with diabetes has a favorable effect in terms of reducing the complications of diabetes. About one third of the patients with type 2 diabetes are asymptomatic. Diabetes can be diagnosed in asymptomatic individuals using either the WHO or ADA criteria for abnormal plasma glucose threshold values. It is unknown whether the additional years of treatment provided to individuals with asymptomatic (preclinical) diabetes detected through screening will result in any clinically relevant improvement in diabetes related outcomes. Prediabetes is a risk factor for future diabetes and cardiovascular disease.

2 ■ The Tests

a. **What is the purpose of the tests?**

To identify asymptomatic individuals who are likely to have diabetes mellitus.

b. **What is the nature of the tests?**

Screening tests: Fasting plasma glucose and glycosylated hemoglobin (HbA1c).

Standard reference tests: Oral glucose tolerance test (GTT). Based on fasting glucose and a 2-hour blood glucose measurements following a 75-g glucose load, three diagnostic categories are considered: (a) normal: fasting glucose below 7.0 mmol/L (126 mg/dL) and a 2-hour glucose below 7.8 mmol/L (140 mg/dL); (b) prediabetes: fasting glucose below 7.0 mmol/L (126 mg/dL) and a 2-hour glucose 7.8 to 11.0 mmol/L (140–199 mg/dL); and (c) diabetes: a fasting glucose above 7.0 mmol/L (126 mg/dL) or a 2-hour glucose 11.1 mmol/L (200 mg/dL)

Continued

■ **Summary—cont'd**

c. *What are the implications of testing?*
  1. What does an abnormal test result mean?
     A fasting plasma glucose above 7.0 mmol/L (126 mg/dL) is an indication for retesting, which should be performed on a different day to confirm the diagnosis. If the fasting plasma glucose is below 7.0 mmol/L (126 mg/dL) and there is high suspicion of diabetes, an oral GTT could be performed. Alternatively, the combination of fasting plasma glucose level and HbA1c could be used to confirm diabetes. Once the diagnosis of diabetes is established, the patient should receive adequate treatment in order to achieve acceptable plasma glucose values and an HbA1c below 7%. A management plan should encompass quality indicators for optimal care. Adults diagnosed with prediabetes may be advised to reduce weight and increase physical activity.
  2. What does a normal test result mean?
     The chance of an asymptomatic individual without any risk factors having or developing diabetes is relatively low.

d. *What is the cost of testing?*
   Costs of screening and early treatment are generally higher when compared with current clinical practice of diagnosis and subsequent treatment. Opportunistic screening (i.e., case finding during routine contact with the medical care system) may be considered cost-effective, in particular when targeted at patients at increased risk of microvascular complications (Table 45–1).

3 ■ **Conclusions and Recommendations**

Screening of asymptomatic individuals for type 1 diabetes is not recommended as the onset of disease is usually not manifested by an identifiable preclinical phase that permits effective preventive measures.

The effectiveness of screening for type 2 diabetes has not been directly demonstrated. However, there is indirect evidence of potential benefits of opportunistic screening for diabetes individuals at high risk as this results in improved glycemic control and a lifetime reduction of microvascular disease.[6,11] Population-based and selective screening programs in community settings have uniformly demonstrated low yield and poor follow up.[11] Such screening programs cannot be recommended.

References

1. Engelgau MM, Geiss LS, Saaddine JB, et al. The evolving diabetes burden in the United States. *Ann Intern Med* 2004;140:945–950.
2. Mokdad AH, Ford ES, Bowman BA, et al. Prevalence of obesity, diabetes, and obesity-related health risk factors, 2001. *JAMA* 2003;289:76–79.
3. Narayan KM, Boyle JP, Thompson TJ, et al. Lifetime risk for diabetes mellitus in the United States. *JAMA* 2003; 290:1884–1890.
4. American Diabetes Association. Standards of medical care in diabetes. *Diabetes Care* 2004;27[Suppl 1]:S15–35.
5. Fagot-Campagna A, Pettitt DJ, Engelgau MM, et al. Type 2 diabetes among North American children and adolescents: an epidemiologic review and a public health perspective. *J Pediatr* 2000;136:664–672
6. American Diabetes Association. Screening for type 2 diabetes. *Diabetes Care* 2004;27[Suppl 1]:S11–14.
7. King H, Aubert RE, Herman WH. Global burden of diabetes, 1995-2025: prevalence, numerical estimates, and projections. *Diabetes Care* 1998;21:1414–1431.
8. Masharani, U. Diabetes mellitus and hypoglycemia. In: Tierney Jr LM, McPhee SJ, Papdakis MA, eds. *Current Medical Diagnosis and Treatment.* New York: Lange Medical Books/McGraw-Hill, 2004:1146–1190.
9. Redondo MJ, Yu L, Hawa M, et al. Heterogeneity of type I diabetes: analysis of monozygotic twins in Great Britain and the United States. *Diabetologia* 2001;44:354–362.
10. Hyttinen V, Kaprio J, Kinnunen L, et al. Genetic liability of type 1 diabetes and the onset age among 22,650 young Finnish twin pairs: a nationwide follow-up study. *Diabetes* 2003;52:1052–1055.
11. Engelgau MM, Narayan KM, Herman WH. Screening for type 2 diabetes. *Diabetes Care* 2000;23:1563–1580.
12. Davies MJ, Tringham JR, Troughton J, et al. Prevention of Type 2 diabetes mellitus. A review of the evidence and its application in a UK setting. *Diabet Med* 2004;21:403–414.
13. World Health Organization. *Definition, Diagnosis and Classification of Diabetes Mellitus and its Complications.* Geneva: World Health Organization, 1999.
14. The Expert Committee on the Diagnosis and Classification of Diabetes Mellitus. Report of the Expert Committee on the Diagnosis and Classification of Diabetes Mellitus. *Diabetes Care* 1997;20:1183–1197.
15. Anand SS, Razak F, Vuksan V, et al. Diagnostic strategies to detect glucose intolerance in a multiethnic population. *Diabetes Care* 2003;26:290–296.
16. Little RR, Rohlfing CL, Wiedmeyer H-M, et al., for the NGSP Steering Committee. The national glycohemoglobin standardization program: a five-year progress report. *Clin Chem* 2001;47:1985–1992.
17. Hippisley-Cox J, Pringle M. Prevalence, care, and outcomes for patients with diet-controlled diabetes in general practice: cross sectional survey. *Lancet* 2004;364:423–428.
18. No authors listed. The cost-effectiveness of screening for type 2 diabetes. CDC Diabetes Cost-Effectiveness Study Group, Centers for Disease Control and Prevention. *JAMA* 1998; 25;280:1757–1763.
19. Hoerger TJ, Harris R, Hicks KA, et al. Screening for type 2 diabetes mellitus: a cost-effectiveness analysis. *Ann Intern Med* 2004;140:689–699.
20. Colagiuri S, Hussain Z, Zimmet P, et al. Screening for type 2 diabetes and impaired glucose metabolism: the Australian experience. *Diabetes Care* 2004;27:367–371.

46

Screening Tests for Contraceptive Users

Donna M. LaFontaine

Jeffrey F. Peipert

The number of contraceptive methods available to women has increased dramatically over the past few decades especially in Europe and the United States. The woman's choice of a contraceptive method may depend on many factors including efficacy, safety, convenience, cost, noncontraceptive benefits, and personal considerations.[1] In addition, many women will use more than one method during the course of their reproductive lives.

More than 90% of women who are at risk of unintended pregnancy (women who are sexually active, able to become pregnant, and neither pregnant nor trying to become pregnant) are using a contraceptive method.[2] Oral contraceptive pills remain the most popular form of reversible contraception, although there has been a slight decline in pill use with the availability of new hormonal delivery systems. In general terms, current contraceptive methods pose few health risks (pregnancy and pregnancy termination are more dangerous), but their associations with serious medical conditions raise questions as to whether specific screening strategies are indicated. Therefore, two widely used and extensively studied forms of contraception are focused on here: oral contraceptive pills in the first section, and the intrauterine device in the second section. Information is still being accumulated on the newer contraceptive choices.

ORAL CONTRACEPTIVES

■ What Is the Problem that Requires Screening?

Major medical complications reported to be associated with oral contraceptive (OC) usage include myocardial infarction, venous thromboembolic events, such as deep-vein thrombosis or pulmonary embolism, stroke, hypertension, changes in carbohydrate and lipid metabolism, and certain malignancies including breast and cervical cancers.[3,4]

What is the incidence/prevalence of the target condition?

Myocardial infarction. Studies as early as 1963 linked the original higher dose estrogen preparations with an increased risk of myocardial infarction. Recent studies have shown conflicting results. Two studies from 1997 reported a two- to fivefold increase in the overall relative risk of myocardial infarction in current OC users.[5,6] In contrast, a pooled analysis from two case-control studies showed current OC users do not have an increased relative risk of myocardial infarction compared to nonusers.[7] The Myocardial Infarction and Oral Contraceptives Study reported a statistically nonsignificant increase in the relative risk among OC users of 1.4.[8] The studies that reported an increased risk of myocardial infarction did not account for the high prevalence of cigarette smoking and hypertension in the studied populations, factors that themselves increase the risk of myocardial infarction. For OC users overall, heavy smokers (defined by more than 15 cigarettes per day) are at higher risk of myocardial infarction than light smokers;[9,10] more specifically, the World Health Organization (WHO) concluded that the use of OCs among women older than 35 years who smoke is associated with a substantial excess risk of myocardial infarction (incidence rate about 400/100,000 women-years).[7,11] The incidence rate of myocardial infarction among young nonsmoking women (younger than 35 years) is rare (0.8/100,000 women per year), whereas the incidence rate among young smoking women is relatively low (4/100,000 women per year).[7]

Venous thromboembolism. An increased prevalence of venous thromboembolism has been associated with the use of both high- and low-dose estrogen preparations. It is debated whether the progestin component of an OC has an effect on that risk. Some studies report an increase in the risk of venous thromboembolism with third-generation progestins (i.e., desogestrel or gestodene) compared with the second-generation progestins (i.e., levonorgestrel).[12–14] The risk of venous thromboembolism for women using OCs containing third-generation progestins is quoted as 1.5- to 2.7-fold greater than the risk of the second-generation OCs.[15] The estimated annual occurrence of nonfatal venous thromboembolism is 16/100,000 in otherwise healthy women using second-generation OCs and 29/100,000 healthy women using third-generation OCs.[15] The probability of death due to venous thromboembolism for women using third-generation products is about 20 per million users per year, whereas for women using second-generation products it is about 14 per million users per year, and for nonusers it is five per million per year.[13] Although some have argued the studies that demonstrate these increases are biased, most experts now agree the increase in thromboembolism risk is small, but real and of clinical relevance.[16,17]

In the 1990s, the factor V Leiden mutation was identified, introducing a new risk consideration in OC users. Approximately 5% of American and European white women carry the factor V Leiden mutation, whereas the prevalence is much lower in nonwhite ethnic populations.[18] (see also Chapter 26).

One case-control study found that carriers of the factor V Leiden mutation have an eightfold increase in the risk of deep venous thrombosis compared with noncarrier controls.[19] When compared with women who did not use OCs and were not carriers of the mutation there was a 35-fold increase in risk of thrombosis for carriers who used OCs.[20]

Ischemic stroke. Similar to myocardial infarction, older studies of women using higher-dose estrogen pills showed a clear increase in the risk of ischemic stroke. More recent studies with the low-dose preparations report no increased risk of ischemic stroke in OC users in the United States[20] and Europe.[21] The small but statistically significant increased risk of ischemic stroke among low-dose OC users in developing countries is ascribed to other risk factors among the studied populations.[22] A meta-analysis of 16 epidemiologic studies concluded it would require 24,000 normotensive, nonsmoking low-dose OC users to account for an increase of one ischemic stroke/year over the baseline risk.[21] The estimated incidences of ischemic stroke and hemorrhagic stroke among women aged 18 to 44 years are very low (i.e., 4.3 and 6.4 per 100,000 women-years, respectively).[22]

Hypertension. Early studies reported an increased prevalence of hypertension (5%) in high-dose OC users. A large cohort study of 68,297 healthy female nurses aged 25 to 42 with no cardiovascular risk factors showed that, after adjustment for age, weight, smoking, family history of hypertension, parity, and ethnicity, the relative risk of hypertension compared with women who never used OCs was 1.8 for current users and 1.2 for "ever users".[23] From this study it was concluded that current users of OCs have a moderately increased risk of hypertension. Among the study group, the incidence of hypertension was 42 per 10 0000 woman-years.[24] The recognition of hypertension in women using OCs may be important in determining an increase in risk of cardiovascular diseases.

Metabolic changes. Higher-dose OCs were associated with abnormal oral glucose tolerance tests (GTTs). Low-dose OCs were shown to cause mild insulin resistance but do not affect the oral GTT.[24] The effect of OCs on serum lipid levels depends on the dose and the type of progesterone used.[25] Lipid changes associated with the low-dose estrogen OC preparations are not thought to be clinically relevant.

Malignancies. Studies of OC users demonstrate markedly lower risks of ovarian and endometrial cancers. The effect of OC use on breast cancer risk remains controversial despite over 60 epidemiologic studies dedicated to this topic. A pooled data analysis from 54 studies demonstrated a small but statistically significant 1.25 relative risk in breast cancer with current OC use.[26] A recent study involving 4,575 women younger than 64 years with breast cancer showed no increase in the risk of breast cancer among women using OCs or among those who had ever used OCs, even with long-term use.[27] OC use greater than

5 years may be associated with a slightly, but significantly, increased risk of breast cancer in *BRAC1* mutation carriers. This increased risk is not seen in OC users who carry *BRAC2* mutations.[28]

There is evidence that long-term use of OCs (10 or more years) may be associated with an increased risk of cancer of the cervix. However, until recent years, human papillomavirus (HPV) infection was not accounted for in these studies. Some studies suggest that OC users may acquire HPV infection easier and have higher HPV persistence rate, which would be consistent with a cancer-promoting effect.[29] A 2003 analysis by the International Agency for Research on Cancer found an increased risk of *cervical* cancer with longer use of OCs. Researchers analyzed data from 28 studies that included 12,531 women with cervical cancer. The findings suggest that the risk of cervical cancer may decrease after discontinuation of OC use. More research is needed to determine the extent women remain at risk of cervical cancer after they cease using OCs.[31]

The long-term safety data of the new hormonal delivery systems including transdermal and transvaginal preparations are limited, yet the risks are thought similar to those of OCs. The long-term risks of continuous versus cyclical OCs have yet to be determined. The contraindications for depomedroxyprogesterone acetate (DMPA) are: known or suspected pregnancy, breast cancer, and undiagnosed vaginal bleeding.[30] A WHO Collaborative study concluded that DMPA is not associated with an increase in cardiovascular risk, making the injectable contraceptive a choice for women in whom cardiovascular risk prohibits OC use.[31] Screening tests should be employed as recommended for all women of reproductive age; no additional testing is required.

What are the sequelae of the condition that are of interest in clinical medicine?

Major medical complications reported to be associated with *oral* OC use include myocardial infarction, venous thromboembolic events, such as deep-vein thrombosis or pulmonary embolism, stroke, and hypertension. The magnitude of risk for each condition in otherwise healthy women using low-dose OCs is very low. The association between OC use and breast cancer and cervical cancer is controversial. Contraindications identified by the WHO for the use of OCs include deep venous thrombosis, pulmonary embolism, stroke, coronary artery disease, ischemic heart disease, or histories of any of these conditions. Uncontrolled hypertensive patients, heavy smokers (> 15 cigarettes/day) older than 35 years, or women with migraines complicated by focal neurologic symptoms should also be excluded from OC use. Women with diabetes greater than 20 years' duration or those with vascular disease such as retinopathy or nephropathy should not take OCs. Breast cancer, pregnancy, active liver disease, and immobilization due to surgery comprise the remainder of contraindications.[13]

■ The Tests

What is the purpose of the tests?

The purpose of screening OC users is to identify women at increased risk of venous thrombosis and the related complications that preclude the use of hormonal contraception.

What is the nature of the tests?

Laboratory tests for thrombophilia and a detailed history.

The first edition of this book stated that "there are no screening tests for potential thrombosis." Since then, multiple laboratory tests have been designed to detect many of the inherited thrombophilias. Factor V Leiden mutation is the most common of the inherited thrombophilias (see also Chapter 26). It is a genetic mutation that leads to resistance to activated C protein (APC), enhancing susceptibility to thrombosis. Screening tests have been developed to measure APC resistance. There is also polymerase chain reaction (PCR) testing to determine the specific factor V mutation.

A detailed history is necessary to determine the contraindications for OC use outlined above. Blood pressure should be measured. Some studies suggest a pelvic examination and a Pap smear should not be required for the initiation of OC use, provided the history and blood pressure measurements reveal no contraindications. Although there is little evidence to support this recommendation, it is often suggested that all sexually active, young women should have a physical examination, a Pap smear, and routine screening for sexually transmitted infections, regardless of their contraceptive choice. The woman's weight may also be important, as recent studies suggest a decrease in the efficacy of OCs in overweight women.[32] Now that the literature demonstrates low-dose OCs have little impact on lipid and carbohydrate metabolism, routine blood testing of these parameters is not indicated. Routine biochemical measurements yield insufficient information to warrant the expense.[33]

What are the implications of testing?

What does an abnormal test result mean? APC resistance would suggest an increased risk of thrombosis should OCs be initiated. However, the screening tests have very low predictive values due to the very low absolute risk of thrombosis among OC users, estimated to be 1.4/10,000. In one analysis, an estimated 61,991 would test positive if one million women were screened for all thrombophilias, yet only 140 of these would suffer from a venous thromboembolism.[32] Fewer than 50 of the 140 women at risk could be identified by a general screening protocol. Moreover, the probability of suffering from OC-associated venous thromboembolism is less than 1/1,000 for women screened positive for APC resistance or for the factor V Leiden mutation and less than 1/500 for women screened positive for any of the inhibitor deficiencies. Thus, the predictive value of these tests for venous thromboembolism would be less than 0.2%. Another analysis concluded that more than 500,000 women would need to be screened for factor V Leiden to avoid a single death since the mutation carrier rate is only 5%, and the mortality associated with venous thromboembolism in young women is low.[33]

Women with a history of deep venous thrombosis, pulmonary embolism, stroke, coronary artery disease, ischemic heart disease or histories of any of these conditions should not receive an OC. The same holds true for women with uncontrolled hypertension, heavy smokers (> 15 cigarettes/day) older than 35 years, and for women with migraines complicated by focal neurological symptoms. Women with diabetes greater than 20 years' duration or those with vascular disease, such as retinopathy or nephropathy, should not receive OCs.

What does a normal test result mean? An estimated two thirds of all women who experience a thrombotic event on OCs will have a negative thrombophilia screen.[33] A normal test is reassuring; but so is the low prevalence of the disease (about 1.4/10,000).

What is the cost of the testing?

Given the rarity of fatal venous thromboembolism in young women, it is likely that more than one million OC users would need to be screened to prevent two OC-associated deaths. More than 60,000 of the screened women identified would be falsely positive (i.e., in spite of a positive test they will not develop thromboembolic disease).[34] The charge for screening tests that measure APC resistance in our hospital is $215. The charge at our institution for the more specific PCR test for the factor V Leiden mutation is $317. Given the above considerations, generalized screening of the entire OC user population is clearly not cost-effective. The risks, benefits, and financial implications of targeted screening are unknown at this time.

■ Conclusions and Recommendations

OC use may increase the risk of serious health conditions including myocardial infarction, venous thromboembolism, stroke, and hypertension. However, the magnitude of risk overall and the likelihood of these conditions occurring in otherwise healthy women using low-dose OC are extremely low. In addition to numerous therapeutic uses, OC use appears to reduce the risk of endometrial and ovarian cancer. A thorough history and a blood pressure check may be the most helpful tools in assessing whether the benefit of OC use outweighs the risks to a particular individual. Physical examination and the performance of a Pap smear may comprise important parts of an overall assessment of reproductive age women, but do not provide essential information leading to the identification of women who should avoid hormonal contraceptives. A consensus developed during the last 10 years supports the opinion that OCs can be safely provided on the basis of the history and blood pressure alone.[34] Indeed, requiring a physical examination and a Pap smear may actually create a barrier, especially for young women where the risks are so low. No blood screening tests should routinely be ordered in OC users, including generalized screening for thrombophilias. The value of screening for thrombophilias in women with positive family histories of venous thromboembolism has yet to be determined.

■ Summary

1 ■ What Is the Problem that Requires Screening?

Conditions that might be exacerbated by oral contraceptive (OC) use.

a. What is the incidence/prevalence of the target condition?
The prevalences of ischemic stroke, hypertension, diabetes, hyperlipidemia, and hormone-sensitive malignancy in low-dose OC users are similar to those in the noncontraceptive population. There is a small, but clinically relevant increased risk of thromboembolism among women using OCs containing third-generation progestins. Furthermore, there is an increased risk of deep-vein thrombosis among women who have an inherited thrombophilia that in majority of cases is caused by a mutation of factor V Leiden

b. What are the sequelae of the condition that are of interest in clinical medicine?
Major medical complications associated with OC use include myocardial infarction, venous thromboembolic events, such as deep-vein thrombosis or pulmonary embolism, stroke, and hypertension. However, the magnitude of risk overall and the likelihood of these conditions occurring in otherwise healthy women using low-dose OC are extremely low.

2 ■ The Tests

a. What is the purpose of the tests?

To identify women with an increased risk of complications from OC use.

b. What is the nature of the tests?

Laboratory tests for thrombophilia and a detailed family and medical history.

c. What are the implications of testing?

1. What does an abnormal test result mean?

   One out of 500 women who test positive for thrombophilia will develop thromboembolic disease. Women screened positive for thrombophilia should be counseled about the benefits and risks of alternative contraception.

   Contraindications identified by the WHO for the use of OCs include deep venous thrombosis, pulmonary embolism, stroke, coronary artery disease, ischemic heart disease, or histories of any of these conditions. Uncontrolled hypertensive patients, heavy smokers (> 15 cigarettes/day) older than 35 years, or women with migraines complicated by focal neurologic symptoms should also be excluded from OC use. Individuals with diabetes greater than 20 years' duration or those with vascular disease, such as retinopathy or nephropathy, should not receive OCs.

2. What does a normal test result mean?

   A normal test is reassuring, but so is the low prevalence of the disease (about 1.4/10,000).

d. What is the cost of testing?

Generalized screening for thrombophilia of the entire OC user population is clearly not cost-effective because of the low prevalence of complications in affected women. The risks, benefits, and financial implications of targeted screening are unknown at this time.

3 ■ Conclusions and Recommendations

The risk associated with the use of OCs appears to act synergistically with thrombophilic conditions. However, general screening

Continued

■ **Summary—cont'd**

for thrombophilia before prescribing OCs cannot be recommended at this time. One option proposed to lower the false positive rate associated with any test for thrombophilia is to pre-select women for screening based on a positive family history. Further research is needed to evaluate such targeted screening. A detailed history is necessary to determine the contraindications for OC use.

INTRAUTERINE DEVICE (IUD)

Despite being used by over 100 million women worldwide, intrauterine devices (IUDs) are used by only several hundred thousand women in the United States,[35] due in part to inaccurate information about the risks of infection and in part because of physician reluctance associated with the past litigation history. IUD use is currently increasing after studies that document only very low risks of infection attributable to the IUD itself. Another factor underlying the growth is the introduction and marketing of the levonorgestrel-containing intrauterine device, which can provide noncontraceptive benefits.

■ What Is the Problem that Requires Screening?

Pelvic inflammatory disease.

What is the incidence/prevalence of the target condition?

The IUD was associated with the development of upper genital tract infection, also known as pelvic inflammatory disease (PID), but failure to control for important confounding variables greatly exaggerated the risk of infection.[37] In the early 1980s, the annual occurrence of PID in IUD users was estimated at 2%. A large randomized controlled trial of antibiotic prophylaxis before IUD insertion in a low-risk population in the US reported that the prevalence of salpingitis following IUD insertion was 1/1,000 women, regardless of antibiotic usage.[36] The greatest risk of developing PID occurs within the first 20 days after insertion. The estimated incidence is 9.7/1,000 woman-years during the first 20 days, compared with 1.4/1,000 woman-years during later times. The risk remains low after up to 8 years of follow-up. The early, insertion-related infections are typically polymicrobial in nature and are derived from the patient's endogenous vaginal flora.[37] Infections occurring after 3 months after insertion are typically due to acquired sexually transmitted infections and are not attributable to the IUD.[38] Even in countries such as Africa with a high prevalence of sexually transmitted diseases (STDs), only eight cases of PID were diagnosed in 1,292 woman-years of follow-up.[39] Women with asymptomatic gonorrhea and chlamydial infections have a higher risk of PID than uninfected women, but the risk is similar to that of women not having an IUD inserted.[39] It has been suggested that progesterone-medicated IUDs may have an even lower risk of PID, perhaps due to progesterone-induced cervical mucous thickening,[40] but data to support this assertion are conflicting.[39,43]

What are the sequelae of the condition that are of interest in clinical medicine?

Potential medical complications of PID include infertility, chronic pelvic pain, ectopic pregnancy, recurrent PID, and tuboovarian abscess. With effective selection of candidates and proper insertion technique, both the copper and the medicated IUDs are not associated with increased risk of infertility after removal.

■ The Tests

What is the purpose of the tests?

To identify women at risk of developing PID after IUD insertion.

What is the nature of the tests?

Perhaps the most important technique to reduce the risk of PID development in an IUD user is through appropriate selection of women. Current, recent (within 3 months) or recurrent episodes of PID are contraindications for IUD insertion. A current history of multiple sex partners or a current partner with multiple sex partners should be reasons to seek an alternative form of birth control. Women who are drug-and/or alcohol-dependent and who are not in a stable relationship are not good candidates for IUD use. Age and parity were traditionally important in patient selection, but recent studies revealed that when sexual behaviors are not risky, there are no increased risks of PID and subsequent infertility in young or nulligravid women.[41] A history of HIV was traditionally a relative contraindication for IUD use. However, at least one study concluded that HIV infected women who use an IUD for contraception do not have an increased risk of PID.[42]

There is very limited evidence that screening for and treating *Chlamydia* organisms before insertion of an IUD can reduce the risk of PID.[43] As a result, some experts suggest that attempts to identify women with *Chlamydia* organisms or gonorrhea at the time of IUD insertion may be justified. However, chlamydial infection can be successfully treated with an IUD in place. In one randomized trial of 445 women, 13 participants had *Chlamydia* at insertion; all were treated and none developed PID.[44] Two case series, one from Norway and one from the United Kingdom, found no cases of PID in 14 women who had an IUD inserted despite the presence of chlamydial infection.[45,46] However, without a comparison group, these studies cannot draw cause-and-effect conclusions.

Two other tests have been considered as potential screens before IUD insertion to reduce the risk of upper tract infection: visual inspection of the cervix and microscopic examination of a saline preparation of vaginal secretions. Inspection may identify women with mucopurulent cervicitis, and examination of a wet mount of vaginal secretions can identify women with either bacterial vaginosis or trichomoniasis. In addition, a Gram stain could be added to identify clue cells or gram-negative intracellular diplococci suggestive of gonorrhea. Bacterial vaginosis has been shown to increase the risk of postabortal infection and, therefore, may increase the risk of upper genital tract infection after IUD insertion.[47] In addition, 25% to 50% of all women with mucopurulent cervicitis or positive testing for gonorrhea or *Chlamydia* species will have concurrently upper genital tract infection based a simultaneously obtained endometrial biopsy.[48,49]

There have been four randomized clinical trials using either doxycycline or azithromycin as antibiotic prophylaxis prior to IUD insertion as an alternative to screening for STDs.[41,50,51] PID was uncommon regardless of antibiotic usage. A Cochrane review concluded that the prophylactic administration of oral antibiotics prior to IUD insertion confers little benefit. Prophylaxis does provide a significant, but small reduction (odds ratio [OR], 0.82; 95% confidence interval [CI] 0.70, 0.98) in unscheduled visits to the provider.[52]

What are the implications of testing?

What does an abnormal test result mean? An abnormal result indicates the increased likelihood, or the possible presence, of an STD. The positive predictive value of current tests for *Chlamydia* or gonorrhea is low in general screening settings with population prevalences of 2% to 3% when compared with targeted screening or diagnostic settings with high prevalence populations (see related information in Chapter 1). For example, if the prevalence of *Chlamydia* is 2%, and the test has a sensitivity of 99% and specificity of 99%, the positive predictive value is 67%. The positive predictive value is over 86% when the prevalence of *Chlamydia* is 6%. Regardless of the setting, it is recommended antibiotic treatment be started when a woman is screen positive for gonorrhea or *Chlamydia* species. Male sex partners of infected women must also be treated to prevent reinfection, and infected women should be screened for other sexually transmitted diseases. Moreover, the woman should be counseled about the benefits and risks of alternative contraception.

What does a normal test result mean? The risk of postinsertion PID in a woman with no evidence of lower genital tract infection is very low provided the woman does not have a history of risky sex behaviors.

What is the cost of testing?

Assuming universal screening in the United States of 700,000 IUD users for gonorrhea and *Chlamydia* at a cost $85 per woman screened, the total cost of testing would be $59.5 million. Assuming a 2% prevalence of endocervical infection, test sensitivity of 99% and specificity of 99%, the positive predictive value would be 67%. One third of positive cases would be falsely positive; women would be incorrectly informed that they had an STD and undergo unnecessary treatment. Only a small percentage of the true positives would have developed PID if undetected. The cost of screening is likely to be higher than the cost of the disease it seeks to prevent. This does not consider the emotional costs to the thousands of women who would be incorrectly informed that they were positive for an STD.

Screening would appear to have a greater potential in a high-risk setting with a relatively high prevalence of disease. The U.S. Preventative Task Force reviewed the evidence for *Chlamydia* screening and concluded that all sexually active women age 25 and younger and other asymptomatic women at increased risk of infection should be routinely screened.[53] Thus, screening for *Chlamydia* should be performed as currently recommended for young women, regardless of contraceptive method (see Chapter 13).

Visual inspection and saline wet-mount preparations in search of mucopurulent cervicitis and vaginitis are cheaper than culture or nucleic amplification methods to identify lower genital tract infection. A Gram stain adds cost and time, but increases the specificity of the diagnosis of gonorrhea or bacterial vaginosis should either gram negative intracellular diplococci or clue cells be identified. If any of these tests are positive, the clinician could consider IUD insertion after the treatment of cervicitis or bacterial vaginosis is completed. A cost analysis of this approach has not been published.

Antibiotic prophylaxis with doxycycline costs approximately $0.63, but has questionable benefit.

■ Conclusions and Recommendations

One of the best ways to minimize risk of PID after IUD insertion is to screen potential candidates with a detailed history of current, recurrent, or recent episodes of sexually transmitted infections. A history of sexual behaviors is also important in identifying women at risk of PID. it is unclear whether additional testing is beneficial. clinical inspection of the cervix and saline wet-mount preparation of vaginal secretions may help to identify women at risk of PID without incurring large costs. Screening for gonorrhea and Chlamydia may only be efficacious in a high prevalence population. Routine screening for Chlamydia is recommended for all sexually active women under age 25 (and other women at increased risk of PID), regardless of whether an IUD is their choice for contraception.[54] If gonorrhea or Chlamydia testing is positive, and an IUD is placed prior to receiving the results of the test, it would be prudent to treat with the IUD in place. Antibiotic prophylaxis prior to IUD insertion does not prevent cases of PID.[55]

■ Summary

1 ■ What Is the Problem that Requires Screening?

Pelvic inflammatory disease (PID).

a. What is the incidence/prevalence of the target condition?

The greatest risk of developing PID occurs within the first 20 days after insertion. The estimated incidence is 9.7/1,000 woman-years during the first 20 days, compared with 1.4/1,000 woman-years during later times.

b. What are the sequelae of the condition that are of interest in clinical medicine?

Potential medical complications of PID include infertility, chronic pelvic pain, ectopic pregnancy, recurrent PID, and tuboovarian abscess.

2 ■ The Tests

a. What is the purpose of the tests?

To identify women at risk of developing PID after IUD insertion.

b. What is the nature of the tests?

Selection of women by obtaining the history of sexual behavior, relationship(s), and lifestyle, gonorrhea and *Chlamydia* testing, visual inspection of the cervix, and microscopic examination of a saline preparation of vaginal secretions.

c. What are the implications of testing?

1. What does an abnormal test result mean?

If gonorrhea or *Chlamydia* testing is positive, antibiotic treatment should be instituted. Male sex partners of infected women must also be treated to prevent reinfection, and infected women should be screened for other sexually transmitted diseases. Moreover, the woman should be counseled about the benefits and risks of alternative contraception. The clinician could consider IUD insertion after the treatment of cervicitis or bacterial vaginosis is completed.

2. What does a normal test result mean?

The risk of postinsertion PID in a woman with no evidence of lower genital tract infection is very low, provided that the woman is not engaged in risky sex behaviors.

d. What is the cost of testing?

The cost of screening is likely to be higher than the cost of the disease it seeks to prevent. This does not consider the emotional costs to the thousands of women who would be incorrectly informed they were positive for an STD.

3 ■ Conclusions and Recommendations

One of the best ways to minimize risk of PID after IUD insertion is to screen potential candidates with a detailed history of current, recurrent, or recent episodes of sexually transmitted infections. General screening for gonorrhea and *Chlamydia* species before insertion of an IUD is not recommended. However, sexually active women age 25 and younger and other asymptomatic women at increased risk of infection should be routinely tested for *Chlamydia*. Antibiotic prophylaxis prior to IUD insertion does not prevent cases of PID.

References

1. Hatcher RA, Trussel J, Stewart F, et al. *Contraceptive Technology*, 18th ed. New York: Ardent Media, 2004:222.
2. Abma JC, Chandra A, Mosher WD, et al. Fertility, family planning and women's health: new data from the 1995 National Survey of Family Growth. *Vital Health Stat* 1997;23:1–114.
3. Burkman R, Schlesselman JJ, Zieman M. Safety concerns and health benefits associated with oral contraception. *Am J Obstet Gynecol* 2004;190:S5–22.
4. Pettiti DB. Combination Estrogen-Progestin Oral Contraceptives. *N Engl J Med* 2003;349: 443–450.
5. Lewis MA, Heinemann LA, Spitzer WO, et al. The use of oral contraceptives and the occurrence of acute myocardial infarction in young women: results from the Transnational Study on Oral Contraceptives and the Health of Young Women. *Contraception* 1997;56:129–140.

6. WHO Collaborative Study of Cardiovascular Disease and Steroid Hormone Contraception. Acute myocardial infarction and combined oral contraceptives: results of an international multicentre case-control study. *Lancet* 1997;349:1202–1209.

7. Sidney S, Siscovick DS, Pettiti DB, et al. Myocardial Infarction and use of low-dose oral-contraceptives: a pooled analysis of 2 US studies. *Circulation* 1998;98:1058–1063.

8. Dunn N, Thorogood M, Faragher B, et al. Oral contraceptives and myocardial infarction: results of the MICA case-control study. *BMJ* 1999;318:1579–1683.

9. Rosenberg L, Palmer JR, Rao RS, et al. Low-dose oral contraceptive use and the risk of myocardial infarction. *Arch Intern Med* 2001;161:1065.

10. Croft P, Hannaford PC. Risk factors for acute myocardial infarction in women: evidence from the Royal College of General Practioners' oral contraception study. *BMJ* 1989;298:165–168.

11. Hatcher RA, Trussel J, Stewart F, et al. *Contraceptive Technology*, 17th ed. New York: Ardent Media, 1990:420.

12. Spizter WO, Lewis MA, Heinemann LAJ, et al. Third generation oral contraceptives and risk of venous thromboembolic disorders: An international case-control study. *BMJ* 1996;312:83–88.

13. Effect of different progestagens in low oestrogen oral contraceptives on venous thromboembolic disease. World Health Organization Collaborative Study of Cardiovascular Disease and Steroid Hormone Contraception. *Lancet* 1995;346:1582–1588.

14. Jick H, Jick SS, Gurewich V, et al. Risk of idiopathic death and non-fatal venous thromboembolism in women using oral contraceptives with differing progestagen components. *Lancet* 1995;346:1589–1593.

15. Leblanc ES, Laws A. Benefits and risks of the third-generation oral contraceptives. *J Gen Intern Med* 1999;14:625–632.

16. Hannaford P. Cardiovascular events associated with different combined oral contraceptives: a review of the current data. *Drug Safety* 2000;22:361–371.

17. Kemmeren JM, Algra A, Grobbee DE. Third generation oral contraceptives and the risk of venous thrombosis: meta-analysis. *BMJ* 2001;323:131–134.

18. Endrikat J, Noah M, Gerlinger C, et al. Impact of oral contraceptive use on APC resistance: a prospective, randomized trial with three low-dose preparations. *Contraception* 2001:64:217–222.

19. Vandenbroucke JP, Koster T, Briet E, et al. Increased risk of venous thrombosis in oral contraceptive users who are carriers of factor V Leiden mutation. *Lancet* 1994;344:1453–1457.

20. Schwartz SM, Siscovick DS, Longstreth,WT Jr, et al. Use of low dose contraceptives and stroke in young women. *Ann Intern Med* 1997;127:596–603.

21. Gillum LA, Mamipudi SK, Johnston SC. Ischemic stroke risk with oral contraceptives: a meta-analysis. *JAMA* 2000;284:72–78.

22. Ischemic stroke and combined oral contraceptives: results of an international, multicentre, case-control study. WHO Collaborative Study of Cardiovascular Disease and Steroid Hormone Contraception. *Lancet* 1996;348:498–505.

23. Chasan-Taber L, Willett WC, Manson JE, et al. Prospective study of oral contraceptives and hypertension among women in the United States. *Circulation* 1996;94:483–489.

24. Krauss, RM, Burkman, RT. The metabolic impact of oral contraceptives. *Am J Obstet Gynecol* 1992;167:1177–1184.

25. Lobo RA, Skinner JB, Lippman JS, et al. Plasma Lipids and desogestrel and ethinyl estradiol: a meta-analysis. *Fertil Steril* 1996;65:1100–1119.

26. Collaborative Group on Hormonal Factors in Breast Cancer. Breast cancer and hormonal contraceptives: collaborative reanalysis of individual data on 53,297 women with breast cancer and 100,239 women without breast cancer from 54 epidemiological studies. *Lancet* 1996; 347:1713–1727.

27. Marchbanks PA, Mc Donald JA, Wilson HG, et al. Oral contraceptives and the risk of breast cancer. *N Engl J Med* 2002;346:2025–2032.

28. Narod SA, Dube MP, Klijn J, et al. Oral contraceptives and the risk of breast cancer in BRAC1 and BRAC2 mutation carriers. *J Natl Cancer Inst* 2002;94:1773–1779.

29. Thomas DB, Ray RM, Koetsawang A, et al. Human papilloma viruses and cervical cancer in Bangkok. I. Risk factors for invasive cervical carcinomas with human papillomavirus types 16 and 18 DNA. *Am J Epidemiol* 2001;153:723–731.

30. National Cancer Institute. Oral contraceptives and cancer risk. Available at http://cis.nci.nih.gov/fact/3_13.htm#cervix. Date reviewed: 11/03/2003. Accessed: December 22, 2004.
31. World Health Organization. Improving access to quality care in family planning: medical eligibility criteria for contraceptive use. Geneva: World Health Organization, 1996.
32. World Health Organization Collaborative Study of Cardiovascular Disease and Steroid Hormone Contraception. Cardiovascular disease and use of oral and injectable progesterone-only contraceptives and combined injectable contraceptives. Results of an international, multicenter, case-control study. *Contraception* 1998;57:314–324.
33. Winkler U. Blood coagulation and oral contraceptives: a critical review. *Contraception* 1998;57:203–209.
34. Vandenbroucke JP, van der Meer FJ, Helmerhorst, FM, et al. Factor V Leiden: should we screen oral contraceptive users and pregnant women? *BMJ* 1996;313:1127–1130.
35. Stewart FH, Harper CC, Ellertson CE, et al. Clinical breast and pelvic examination requirements for hormonal contraception: Current practice vs. evidence. *JAMA* 2001;285:2232–2239.
36. Speroff L, Darney PA. *A Clinical Guide for Contraception*. Baltimore: Williams and Wilkins, 2001:221.
37. Walsh T, Grimes D, Frezieres R, et al. Randomised controlled trial of prophylactic antibiotics before insertion of intrauterine devices. *Lancet* 1998;351:1005–1008.
38. Mishell DR Jr, Bell JH, Good RG, et al. The intrauterine device: a bacteriologic study of the endometrial cavity. *Am J Obstet Gynecol* 1966;96:119–126.
39. Huggins GR, Cullins VE. Fertility after contraception or abortion. *Fertil Steril* 1990;54:559–573.
40. Farley TM, Rosenburg MJ, Rowe PJ, et al. Intrauterine devices and pelvic inflammatory disease: an international perspective. *Lancet* 1992;339:785–788.
41. Toivonen J, Luukkainen T, Alloven H. Protective effect of intrauterine release of levonorgestrel on pelvic infection: three years' comparative experience of levonorgestrel and copper-releasing devices. *Obstet Gynecol* 1991;77:261–264.
42. Hubacher D, Lara-Ricalde R, Taylor DJ , et al. Use of copper intrauterine devices and the risk of tubal infertility among nulligravid women. *N Engl J Med* 2001;345:561–567.
43. Sinei SK, Morrison CS, Sekadde-Kiogondu C, et al. Complications of use of intrauterine devices among HIV-1 infected women. *Lancet* 1998;351:1238–1241.
44. Sprague DS, Bullough CHW, Rashid S, et al. Screening for and treating chlamydia before contraceptive use and subsequent pelvic inflammatory infection. *Br J Fam Plann* 1990;16:54.
45. Pap-Akeson M, Solhein F, Thorbert G, et al. Genital tract infections associated with the intrauterine contraceptive device can be reduced by inserting the threads inside the uterine cavity. *Br J Obstet Gynaecol* 1992;99:676–679.
46. Skeldestad FE, Halvorsen HK, Norbo SA, et al. IUD users in Norway are at low risk for genital C. trachomatis infection. *Contraception* 1996;54:209–212.
47. James NJ, Wilson S, Hughes S. A pilot study to incorporate chlamydial testing in the management of women anticipated IUD insertion in community clinics. *Br J Fam Plann* 1997; 23:16–19.
48. Larsson PG, Platz-Christensen JJ, Theljs H, et al. Incidence of pelvic inflammatory disease after first-trimester legal abortion in women with bacterial vaginosis after treatment with metronidazole: a double-blind, randomized study. *Am J Obstet Gynecol* 1992;166:100–103.
49. Paavonen J, Kiviat N, Brunham RC, et al. Prevalence and manifestations of endometritis among women with cervicitis. *Am J Obstet Gynecol* 1985;152:280–286.
50. Wiesenfeld HC, Hillier SL, Krohn MA, et al. Lower genital tract infection and endometritis: insight into subclinical pelvic inflammatory disease. *Obstet Gynecol* 2002;100:456–463.
51. Walsh TL, Bernstein GS, Grimes DA, et al. Effect of prophylactic antibiotics on morbidity associated with IUD insertion: results of a pilot randomized controlled trial: IUD Study Group. *Contraception* 1994;50:319–327.
52. Sinei SK, Schulz KF, Lamptey PR, et al. Preventing IUCD-related pelvic infection: the efficacy of prophylactic doxycycline at insertion. *J Obstet Gynaecol* 1990;97:412–419.
53. Grimes DA, Schulz KF. Antibiotic prophylaxis for intrauterine contraceptive device insertion [Cochrane Review]. In: The Cochrane Library, Issue 4, 2000. Oxford: Update Software.
54. U.S. Preventative Services Task Force. Screening recommendations for *Chlamydia* infection: recommendations and rationale. *Am J Prevent Med* 2001;20:90–94.
55. Peipert J. Clinical practice: genital chlamydial infections. *N Engl J Med* 2003;349:2425–2430.

Genetic Predisposition to Gynecologic Cancers

Hanne Meijers-Heijboer

■ What Is the Problem that Requires Screening?

Familial cancer of the breast and ovary.

What is the incidence/prevalence of the target condition?

Evidence that inherited susceptibility plays a role in the risk of breast, ovarian, and other tumors of the female genital organs stems from two observations. First, there is a strong clustering of these cancers within certain families; second, at the population level, first-degree relatives of cases are at increased risk of the same tumor, and sometimes tumors at other anatomic sites. The proof came with the identification of susceptibility genes for breast, ovarian, and other cancers.

The risk of a first-degree relative of a patient with breast cancer is on average increased twofold. However, the risk may be higher depending on family history (i.e., the number of affected first-degree relatives and their ages at diagnoses). Above all, the identification of a pathogenic mutation in a breast cancer associated gene (*BRCA1* or *BRCA2)* confers on women a very high lifetime risk of breast cancer, up to 85%.

Prevalence of mutations and carrier probabilities. The prevalence rates of *BRCA1* and *BRCA2* mutations differ among countries and populations. Although the frequency of *BRCA2* mutations in the United Kingdom and Iceland exceeds the frequency of *BRCA1* mutations, it is the opposite in the United States and The Netherlands. In Western populations, the prevalence of *BRCA1* and *BRCA2* mutation is 0.2% among the general population at birth, about 3% in breast cancer patients diagnosed before age 70 years, and 6% in women diagnosed with breast cancer prior to age 50 years.[1] The prevalence of mutations in specific populations may, however, differ considerably from these figures. For instance, the prevalence of the founder mutations of *BRCA1* and *BRCA2* in the general Ashkenazi Jewish population is 2.4%,[2,3] whereas 0.6% of the general Icelandic population carries the BRCA2 999del5.[4,5]

Several models have been derived to estimate the probability that an individual carries a mutation, given their personal and family history of cancer. In general, strong predictors for the presence of a BRCA1 or BRCA2 mutation within a family are multiple cases of breast cancer diagnosed at young age and multiple cases of ovarian cancer. Cooccurrence of male breast cancer in a family, and Ashkenazi Jewish ancestry substantially enhances the probability of finding a BRCA1 or BRCA2 mutation. Based on these parameters, the probability of identifying a mutation may exceed 50%.

Although genetic testing for BRCA1 and BRCA2 mutations is laborious and expensive, careful case selection is desirable. Many clinics use a 10% probability threshold to identity women for screening. In clinical settings, the probability of finding a mutation can be quickly delineated from the periodically updated probability tables produced by the clinical testing service of Myriad Genetics Laboratories (http:/www.myriadtests.com/provider/mutprev.htm). A computer program may also be used (e.g., BRCAPRO, http:/astor.som. jhmi.edu/brcapro). The BRCAPRO model considers the complete structure of the family pedigree including the number of breast, ovarian, male breast, and bilateral breast cancers; the ages at diagnosis; and Ashkenazi Jewish ancestry. These models should be used with caution in certain situations when marked discrepancies exist between current models and tables.

BRCA1 and BRCA2: Most families with a clustering of breast and ovarian cancers harbor mutations in BRCA1 or BRCA2. In families with two cases of ovarian cancer and no cases of breast cancer, the BRCA1 or BRCA2 mutations account for one fifth, whereas in families with three cases of ovarian cancer, 70% are BRCA1- or BRCA2-mutation positive.[6] In unselected ovarian cancer cases from the United Kingdom or North America, frequencies of BRCA1 and BRCA2 mutations of about 5% to 10% are reported. Of note, in some ethnic groups, such as the Jewish Ashkenazi population, this figure may rise to 30% for specific founder mutations.

What are the sequelae of the condition that are of interest in clinical medicine?

Breast cancers arising in carriers of a BRCA1 mutation are different from those in noncarriers.[7,8] They have higher mitotic counts, continuous pushing margins, and a lymphocytic infiltrate. They are less likely to be lobular or to be associated with ductal or lobular carcinoma in situ. Breast cancer in BRCA1 is more likely to be estrogen- and progesterone-receptor negative, is more likely to have somatic TP53 mutations, is less likely to be c-erb-b2 positive, and stains positive for basal keratins.[9–12] In line with these pathologic differences, gene expression profiling of breast cancers shows a distinct BRCA1-associated signature if compared with BRCA2-associated and sporadic breast cancers.[13]

Breast cancers arising in carriers of a BRCA2 mutation show less tubule formation, fewer mitoses, and continuous pushing margins.[7] Otherwise, the pattern of the pathology of *BRCA2*-associated breast cancers is more similar to that in sporadic breast cancers.

Most studies on the prognosis of *BRCA1*-associated breast cancer conclude either no difference or a poorer prognosis.[14–16] Some suggest that patients with relatively small, node-negative *BRCA1*-associated tumors may have a worse prognosis.[17] It is suggested that this phenomenon reflects an increased sensitivity for chemotherapy of *BRCA1*- and *BRCA2*-associated tumors.[18] The prognosis of *BRCA2*-associated breast cancer does not seem to differ markedly from their sporadic counterparts.[19]

Hormonal and reproductive risk factors seem to modify *BRCA1*- and *BRCA2*-associated cancer risks. Mutation carriers with children have an increased risk of breast cancer by age 40 years compared with mutation carriers without children.[20] *BRCA1* mutation carriers whose use oral contraceptive for more than 5 years before age 30 years probably have a modestly increased risk of breast cancer.[21] It appears that the short-term use of modern contraceptives poses no increase in risk, but further studies are needed. Breast-feeding is reported to have a greater protective effect in *BRCA1* mutation carriers than in the general population.[22] It is unknown whether hormonal replacement therapy (HRT) increases the risk of breast cancer in *BRCA1* and *BRCA2* mutation carriers.

First-degree relatives of women with ovarian cancer have a threefold increase risk of ovarian cancer. In absolute terms, this risk equates to a cumulative risk of 4% by age 70 years in Western populations. Unaffected women from families with two first-degree relatives with ovarian cancer are estimated to have a cumulative risk of 11% by the age of 70 years. The large majority of genetic susceptibility to ovarian cancer relates to *BRCA1*, *BRCA2*, or HNPCC (hereditary nonpolyposis colorectal cancer syndrome)–associated gene mutations (the mismatch repair genes [MMR]).

Ovarian cancers associated with *BRCA1* mutations are more often serous type,[23] more likely to be of a high grade,[24] and occur at earlier ages compared with ovarian cancers unassociated with *BRCA1* mutations. It is unclear whether *BRCA1* and *BRCA2* mutations influence outcome in ovarian cancer.

■ The Tests

What is the purpose of the tests?

To identify women at high risk of breast or ovarian cancer.

What is the nature of the tests?

The following breast cancer susceptibility genes are recognized as of 2004: the high-penetrance genes *BRCA1*, *BRCA2*, *TP53*, *PTEN*, *STK11*, and the low-penetrance genes *ATM* and *CHEK2* (Table 47–1). Mutations of these genes confer autosomal dominantly inherited breast cancer susceptibility and account for

Table 47-1	**Specific inherited syndromes involving cancers of the breast and female genital organs**		
Syndrome	**Gene**	**Location**	**Associated sites/tumors**
BRCA1 syndrome	*BRCA1*	17q	Breast, ovary, endometrium, cervix, fallopian tube, peritoneum, pancreas, prostate below age 65
BRCA2 syndrome	*BRCA2*	13q	Breast, ovary, fallopian tube, prostate, pancreas, gallbladder, stomach, melanoma, peritoneum, buccal cavity, pharynx
Li-Fraumeni syndrome	*TP53*	17p	Breast, sarcoma, brain, adrenal, leukemia
Cowden syndrome	*PTEN*	10q	Skin, breast, thyroid, endometrium
Peutz-Jeghers syndrome	*STK11*	19p	Small intestine, ovary, cervix, breast, testis, pancreas
HNPCC syndrome	*MLH1* *MSH2*	3p 2p	*For all three genes*: colorectum, endometrium, ovary, small bowel
	MSH6	2p	Ureter/renal pelvis, brain, stomach
Ataxia telangiectasia	*ATM*	11q	Breast (heterozygotes)

HNPCC, hereditary nonpolyposis colorectal cancer.

about one fourth of familial breast cancer; the remaining mechanisms await elucidation.[25]

***BRCA1* and *BRCA2* genes.** The *BRCA1* and *BRCA2* genes, and the encoded proteins of 1863 and 3418 amino acids in length, were identified in 1994 and 1995, respectively.[26,27] Both proteins are implicated in multiple biologic processes including DNA repair and recombination. The mutations are evenly scattered throughout both genes, and hundreds of distinct pathogenic mutations are reported per gene (http://research.nhgri.nih.gov/bic/). Certain mutations observed multiple times have been shown to originate from a common ancestor. These mutations, called founder mutations, are described in Askenazi Jews (*BRCA1* 185delAG, 5382insC; *BRCA2* 6174delT), Iceland (*BRCA2* 999del5), The Netherlands, and several other countries.

A few genetic variants have been proposed that modify *BRCA1*- and *BRCA2*-associated cancer risks. These include, for breast cancer, the lengths of triplet repeats in the androgen-receptor and AIB1 genes, and polymorphisms in the progesterone-receptor and (for *BRCA2*) the *RAD51* genes.[28–32] Rare alleles at the *HRAS1* microsatellite locus were also suggested to be associated with ovarian cancer risk in *BRCA1* mutation carriers.[33]

TP53. Breast cancers are the most frequent cancers in families with a *TP53* germline mutation, in particular in women aged 16 to 45 years.

Breast cancers account for 80% of tumors encountered in patients with the Li-Fraumeni syndrome (LFS). LFS is characterized by multiple primary cancers in children and young adults, with a predominance of soft-tissue sarcoma, osteosarcomas, breast cancers, brain tumors, leukemias, and adrenocortical cancers. Seventy-five percent of LFS families are associated with a *TP53* germline mutation.[34,35] The criteria for the diagnosis of LFS are (a) occurrence of sarcoma before the age of 45 years; (b) at least one first-degree relative with any tumor before age 45; and (c) a second-(or first-) degree relative with cancer before age 45 years or a sarcoma at any age.[36–38] In women with a *TP53* germline mutation, the penetrance of any cancer is estimated at 12%, 84%, and 100% for ages 16, 45, and 85 years, respectively.[35] Conversely, the frequency of *TP53* germline mutations is low in patients with unselected breast cancer, or breast cancer diagnosed in patients younger than 40 years, namely 0.25% and 1%, respectively.[39–43] LFS is rare, and worldwide only a few hundreds of families with a *TP53* mutation have been registered. Genetic testing for *TP53* germline mutations requires extensive counseling in view of the high cancer risks from childhood onward and the lack of risk-reducing strategies for several of LFS-associated tumors.

PTEN. Cowden syndrome is caused by mutations of the *PTEN* gene.[44] It is characterized by multiple hamartomas involving organs derived from all three germ cell layers and a high risk of breast, uterine, and nonmedullary thyroid cancers. The classic hamartoma is the trichilemmoma; it is pathognomonic for Cowden syndrome. The prevalence of *PTEN* germline mutations has been estimated to be at least 1/300.000.[45] It is suggested that some two thirds of women with Cowden syndrome develop benign breast disease, while 25% to 50% develop invasive breast cancer.[46–48] The majority of Cowden syndrome–associated breast cancer occurs after age 30 to 35 years (range from 14 years to as old as the 60s).

Endometrial cancer was only recently suggested to be part of Cowden syndrome.[47] Neither the frequency among mutation carriers nor the age distribution are known. Uterine leiomyomas are believed to occur in half of the affected women, and occur at young ages, even in the 20s.

STK11 or LKB1. Peutz-Jeghers syndrome is characterized by hamartomatous polyposis of the gastrointestinal tract and is caused by mutations of *STK11* gene (also named *LKB1*).[49,50] The hallmark feature in 95% of affected subjects is melanin spots on the lips and buccal mucosa. There is also an increased risk of gastrointestinal, pancreatic, testis, ovarian, breast, uterine, and cervical cancers.[51] Peutz-Jeghers syndrome is rare, and mutations of *STK11* are not found in patients with one of the associated cancer types in the absence of other clinical stigmata of the syndrome.

CHEK2. The *CHEK2* gene is involved in low-penetrance breast cancer susceptibility.[52–54] The *CHEK2* 1100delC variant, which has a prevalence of about 1% in

Western populations, confers a twofold increase in breast cancer risk in women. Other *CHEK2* mutations are found in breast cancer families, but their overall contribution to breast cancer risk is likely to be small.[55,56]

ATM. Ataxia-telangiectasia (A-T) is an autosomal recessive disorder associated with a high incidence of cancer, in particularly lymphoma and leukemia. The causative gene is known as *ATM.* Approximately 0.2% to 1% of the general population are estimated to be heterozygous carriers of a type of germline mutation in the *ATM* gene that in the homozygous state causes the A-T syndrome. Heterozygous female carriers are at an increased risk of breast cancer.[57,58] There is controversy regarding the magnitude of the increased risk,[59–61] but evidence is emerging that female heterozygotes do indeed have a small increase in the risk of breast cancer.

What are the implications of testing?

What does an abnormal test result mean? Asymptomatic women with either a *BRCA1* or *BRCA2* mutation have a high risk of breast and/or ovarian cancer at a young age. These women should be counseled, closely monitored, and treated by prophylactic surgery and chemoprevention, where indicated. Furthermore, genetic counseling and testing should be offered to relatives of affected women. The overall life expectancy of women with a *BRCA1* or *BRCA2* mutation clearly is decreased due to the high cancer mortality.

Counseling: Knowledge of the age-specific cancer risks (or penetrance) associated with *BRCA1* and *BRCA2* mutations are central to the counseling of mutation carriers. Current estimates are based on retrospective studies. In general, cancer risks have been higher in studies based on high-risk families compared with population studies based on relatives of unselected mutation carriers.[62–65] The cumulative risk of breast and ovarian cancers for *BRCA1* and *BRCA2* mutation carriers using either method are shown in Figure 47–1. The cumulative risks of both breast and ovarian cancer are higher in *BRCA1* carriers than in *BRCA2* carriers, but the difference is more marked for ovarian cancer. The difference is also more marked for breast cancer at younger ages that at older ages. This is a consequence of the fact that *BRCA1* breast cancer prevalence rate rises steeply to approximately 3% to 4% per annum in the 40- to 49-year age group, and is constant thereafter, whereas the *BRCA2* rates show a pattern similar to the general population (just tenfold higher), rising steeply up to age 50 years and more slowly thereafter. By age 70 years, the cumulative risk of breast cancer is estimated in carriers of a *BRCA1* mutation to be 85% and 65% within family-based studies and population-based studies, respectively; likewise, it is 84% and 45% respectively in carriers of a *BRCA2* mutation, (Figure 47–1).

The ovarian cancer risks differ markedly for *BRCA1* and *BRCA2* mutation carriers. In *BRCA1* mutation carriers, ovarian cancer risks are low in absolute terms below age 40 years, rising thereafter to 1% to 2% per annum. Ovarian cancer risks in *BRCA2* carriers are, in contrast, very low below age 50 years, but

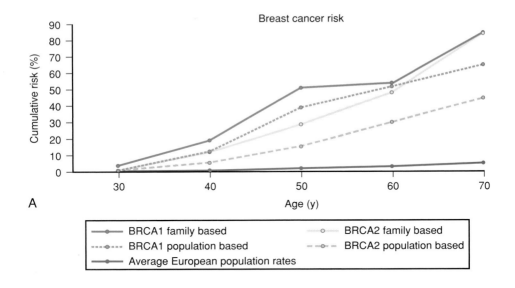

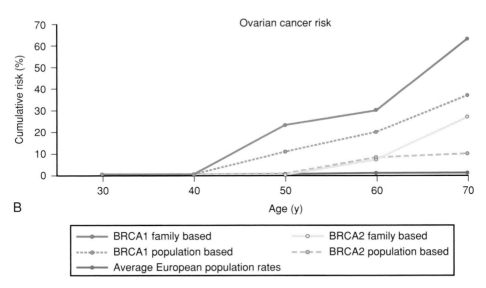

Figure 47-1   Cumulative risks of breast cancer **(A)** and ovarian cancer **(B)** in women with a *BRCA1* or *BRCA2* mutation according to family-based studies (from Easton DF, Ford D, Bishop DT. Breast and ovarian cancer incidence in *BRCA1*-mutation carriers: Breast Cancer Linkage Consortium. *Am J Hum Genet* 1995;56:265–271; Ford D, Easton DF, Stratton M, et al. Genetic heterogeneity and penetrance analysis of the BRCA1 and BRCA2 genes in breast cancer families: the Breast Cancer Linkage Consortium. *Am J Hum Genet* 1998;62:676–689) and a meta-analysis of population-based studies (Antoniou A, Pharoah PD, Narod S, et al. *Am J Hum Genet* 2003; 72:1117–1130).

then increase sharply. By age 70 years, the cumulative risk of ovarian cancer in carriers of a *BRCA1* mutation is estimated to be 63% and 39% by family-based and population-based studies, respectively; likewise it is 27% and 11%, respectively, in carriers of a *BRCA2* mutation (Figure 47–1).

The position of the mutation within the *BRCA1* and *BRCA2* gene affects the breast and ovarian cancer risks to some degree.[66–69] This is most clear for mutations of the *BRCA2* "ovarian cancer cluster region" (OCCR, region between nucleotides 3059 and 6629). The cumulative ovarian cancer risk for women with mutations within the *BRCA2* OCCR is 20%, whereas it is only 11% for mutations outside this region.[70] This risk modification is too moderate, however, to be used in genetic counseling.

Women who are both carriers and affected with breast cancer have an increased risk of developing a contralateral breast cancer and ovarian cancer (Table 47–2). The risk of contralateral breast cancer in *BRCA1* carriers is about 4% per annum in women aged 30 to 39 years, and thereafter declining to about 1.5% per annum at ages 60 to 69 years. Annual rates of contralateral breast cancer in *BRCA2* mutation carriers are approximately 2% across the age range of 30 to 60 years. These rates contrast with a rate of about 0.7% in unselected breast cancer patients. The risks of ovarian cancer following breast cancer are comparable to the estimated incidence rates for a first ovarian cancer in women with a *BRCA1* and *BRCA2* mutation (Table 47–2).

In addition to the marked excess risk of breast and ovarian cancer in *BRCA1* and *BRCA2* mutation carriers, there is also evidence of slightly increased risk of other types of cancer in women. In a series of 699 families with a *BRCA1* mutation, the overall cancer risk in male carriers was close to the general population, whereas the risk of cancers other than breast or ovarian in female carriers was increased approximately twofold. Moderately elevated risks of cancer of the fallopian tube and peritoneum were observed. Small to moderately elevated

Table 47–2	**Estimates of the prevalence rates and cumulative risks (between parentheses) of a contralateral breast cancer or ovarian cancer following a breast cancer in women with *BRCA1* or *BRCA2* mutation**

	Contralateral breast cancer		Ovarian cancer	
Age group, y	*BRCA1*	*BRCA2*	*BRCA1*	*BRCA2*
30–39	4.0% (7)	1.7% (9)	1.4% (4)	—
40–49	2.8% (9)	2.6% (28)	2.4% (12)	0.2% (3)
50–59	2.3% (7)	1.9% (20)	1.3% (5)	0.7% (8)
60–69	1.5% (3)	0.8% (6)	1.0% (2)	0.8% (7)

Estimates derived from Ford et al. *Lancet* 1994;343:692–695; and the Breast Cancer Linkage Consortium. *Natl Cancer Inst* 1999;91:1310–1316.

cancer risks were observed in the corpus uteri, cervix, pancreas, male breast, and prostate in those younger than 65 years. In a series of 173 families with a *BRCA2* mutation, the risk of other cancers was approximately twofold greater for both male and female carriers than in the general population. Excess risks in *BRCA2* mutation carriers were observed for cancer of the prostate, male breast, pancreas, stomach, buccal cavity and pharynx, gallbladder, bile duct, and fallopian tube and for melanoma.

Surveillance: The value of mammography and clinical breast examination in young women with a *BRCA1* or *BRCA2* mutation is still uncertain.[71] However, two recent reports suggest that magnetic resonance imaging (MRI) is a better screening modality in *BRCA1* and *BRCA2* mutation carriers compared with mammography.[72,73] The identification of breast cancers at earlier stages by MRI than that for mammography fuels hope that mortality rates for these women will diminish over time. Several family cancer clinics have added a yearly MRI from age 25 years onward to the regular surveillance of *BRCA1* and *BRCA2* mutation carriers.

Prophylactic surgery: Bilateral oophorectomy at premenopausal ages lowers the risk of breast cancer by 50% in the general population, as it does in *BRCA1* and *BRCA2* mutation carriers.[74] Bilateral salpingo-oophorectomy is the preferred method in mutation carriers in view of the increased risk of ovarian cancer *and* cancer of the fallopian tubes. A long-term risk of 4% of peritoneal cancer remains after bilateral salpingo-oophorectomy.[75,76] Prophylactic bilateral salpingo-oophorectomy is often performed around age 40 years in *BRCA1* and *BRCA2* carriers.

Prophylactic bilateral mastectomy in carriers of a *BRCA1* or *BRCA2* mutation reduces the risk of breast cancer by more than 90%.[77–79] The risk of contralateral breast cancer is also greatly reduced in women who have already had breast cancer and carry a *BRCA1* and *BRCA2* mutation.[80,81] Total mastectomy, which removes the total breast gland, including the nipple–areolar complex, is the preferred method.[82] Subcutaneous mastectomy preserves the nipple–areolar complex, and therefore leaves a substantial amount of breast tissue behind. Although breast cancer after prophylactic mastectomy is rare, nearly all of those cases reported occurred in patients with subcutaneous mastectomy.[83] Most women who undergo prophylactic mastectomy prefer an immediate breast reconstruction. Several techniques are available, like subpectoral implantation of silicone prosthesis, or autologous tissue transfer, such as a TRAM (transverse rectus abdominis muscle) flap or a free flap grafting. Nipple-areola reconstruction can be performed immediately or as a second-stage procedure, using a variety of techniques including grafting and skin tattooing. However, these are not simple procedures. Prophylactic mastectomy has a complication rate up to 50%, depending on the type of surgery and follow-up period.[84,85] Fortunately, women who chose prophylactic mastectomy do not normally develop a significant mental health or body image problem[86,87] and only rarely indicate regretting this procedure. A proportion of women do report negative changes in feelings of sexual attractiveness, femininity, and looks.

Worldwide, large variation exists in the appreciation of prophylactic bilateral mastectomy by women with a mutation of *BRCA1* and *BRCA2* and their doctors.[88–90] At present, the usage by unaffected mutation carriers ranges from about zero to 50% in The Netherlands and the United Kingdom, but figures may change over time when the efficacy of surveillance, chemoprevention or treatment improves.

Medical prevention: Tamoxifen, a selective estrogen receptor modulator (SERM), was the first drug shown to reduce (by 50%) the risk of breast cancer in healthy women. The results are conflicting for high-risk women, in particular *BRCA1* mutation carriers.[91–93] Chemoprevention trials are currently under way, but low interest in participation is hampering these studies.[89]

The combined estrogen-progestin oral contraceptive pill decreases the risk of ovarian cancer in the general population, women with a family history of ovarian cancer, and women with *BRCA1* or *BRCA2* mutations. The benefit of oral contraceptive use for *BRCA1* and *BRCA2* mutation carriers, however, may be outweighed by an enhancement of the breast cancer risk. The impact of hormone replacement therapy on the prevalence of breast cancer in women with *BRCA1* and *BRCA2* mutations after premenopausal bilateral salpingo-oophorectomy is unknown.

Option for relatives to undergo genetic testing: Once a pathogenic *BRCA1* or *BRCA2* mutation has been identified within a member of the family, relatives can be given the option to be tested for that mutation. The management of families at high-risk of breast cancer requires a multidisciplinary approach in view of its complex clinical genetic, oncologic, surgical, gynecologic, and psychological aspects. At present, multidisciplinary care is provided by several family cancer clinics throughout the Western world. Patients' support groups, if available, often also play a significant role in the decision-making processes of women at high-risk. The interest in genetic testing for *BRCA1* and *BRCA2* mutations by women with a pretest risk of 50% of carrying such a mutation is high in most countries (i.e., above 50%).[88,94–97] The use of this test is, however, much lower in countries where mutation carrier status may result in financial or social discrimination.[97]

What does a normal test result mean? Women without *BRCA1* or *BRCA2* mutation can be reassured that their likelihood of breast or ovarian cancer approximates that of the general population.

What is the cost of testing?

The charge for commercial BRCA testing is $2,580. This includes the full sequence of the large genes. A recent cost-effectiveness study from Spain demonstrated that costs of a familial breast cancer genetic counseling and screening program were 4,294 euros per life-year gained. The model was sensitive to the prevalence of mutation carriers, the lifetime risk of breast cancer, and the effectiveness of the screening.[98]

■ Conclusions and Recommendations

It is increasingly clear that many diseases reflect a genetic predisposition, either alone or in conjunction with environmental changes that may have greater effects on certain genetic backgrounds. Genetic predisposition to disease is also starting to influence strategies of prevention, early detection, and treatment. In oncology, such new knowledge has already impacted on the care of common cancers. Today, it is known that single genes are responsible for breast/ovarian cancers, and some of these genes (e.g., *BRCA1* and *BRCA2*) can be identified by genetic testing. Genetic information on breast cancer is, however, still limited.

Currently available screening programs for familial breast cancer include the assessment of high-penetrance genes *BRCA1* and *BRCA2* or other breast cancer susceptibility genes, where indicated. Asymptomatic women with a *BRCA1* or *BRCA2* mutation have a high risk of breast cancer and ovarian cancer at a young age. Knowledge of the age-specific cancer risk associated with *BRCA1* and *BRCA2* mutations is critical for genetic counseling of mutation carriers. These women should also be closely monitored and treated by prophylactic surgery and chemoprevention, where indicated. Close monitoring of women with *a BRCA1* or *BRCA2* mutation includes clinical breast examination and mammography (see Chapter 48). The value of mammography and clinical breast examination in young women with a *BRCA1* or *BRCA2* mutation is still uncertain. Recently, two reports suggest that MRI is a superior screening modality for *BRCA1* and *BRCA2* mutation carriers compared with mammography. Several family cancer clinics have now added to the regular surveillance a yearly MRI from age 25 years onwards in *BRCA1* and *BRCA2* mutation carriers.

Prophylactic mastectomy is associated with a complication rate of up to 50%, depending on the type of surgery and follow-up period. However, women only rarely indicate they regret having had the procedure, though a proportion of women report negative changes in feelings of sexual attractiveness, femininity, and looks.

Currently available screening strategies for ovarian cancer consist of transvaginal ultrasound and measurement of serum levels of cancer antigen 125 (CA-125). The efficacy of these methods in high-risk women is as yet unproven (see Chapter 52). However, most family cancer clinics offer screening for ovarian cancer to women with a cumulative lifetime risk of 10%. In women with mutations of *BRCA1* or *BRCA2*, or *MMR* gene mutations, bilateral salpingo-oophorectomy is offered after the age of 40 years or earlier depending on the family history.

Once a pathogenic *BRCA1* or *BRCA2* mutation has been identified in a member of the family, relatives should be offered the option to be tested. The management of families at high-risk of breast cancer requires a multidisciplinary approach in view of its complex clinical genetic, oncologic, surgical, gynecologic, and psychological aspects.

■ **Summary**

1 ■ **What Is the Problem that Requires Screening?**

Familial breast and ovarian cancer.

a. What is the incidence/prevalence of the target condition?

The prevalence of mutations of *BRCA1* and *BRCA2* differs between countries and populations. In Western populations, the prevalence of *BRCA1* and *BRCA2* mutation is 0.2% among the general population at birth, about 3% in breast cancer patients diagnosed before the age of 70 years, and 6% in women diagnosed with breast cancer before the age of 50 years.

b. What are the sequelae of the condition that are of interest in clinical medicine?

Asymptomatic women with a *BRCA1* or *BRCA2* mutation have a high risk of breast cancer and ovarian cancer at young ages.

2 ■ **The Tests**

a. What is the purpose of the tests?

To identify women at high risk of breast cancer and ovarian cancer.

b. What is the nature of the tests?

In 2004, the following breast cancer susceptibility genes were identified: the high-penetrance genes *BRCA1, BRCA2, TP53, PTEN, STK11,* and the low-penetrance genes *ATM* and *CHEK2.* Mutations of these genes confer autosomal dominantly inherited breast cancer susceptibility, and account for about one fourth of familial occurrence of breast cancer, the remaining still awaiting elucidation.

c. What are the implications of testing?

1. What does an abnormal test result mean?
   Asymptomatic women with a *BRCA1* or *BRCA2* mutation should be counseled, closely monitored, and treated by prophylactic surgery and chemoprevention, when indicated. Furthermore, genetic counseling and testing should be offered to relatives of the affected woman.

Continued

■ **Summary—cont'd**

2. What does a normal test result mean?
Women without *BRCA1* or *BRCA2* mutation can be reassured as the likelihood of breast or ovarian cancer approximates that of the general population.

d. *What is the cost of testing?*
Depending on prevalence of mutation carriers, the lifetime risk of breast cancer and the effectiveness of the screening, a genetic counseling and screening program targeted at women with familial breast cancer is cost-effective.

3 ■ Conclusions and Recommendations

Today it is known that single genes are also responsible for breast cancer and some of these genes (e.g., *BRCA1* and *BRCA2*) can be identified by genetic testing. Genetic information on breast cancer is, however, still limited. Currently available screening programs for familial breast cancer include a careful assessment of the family history and laboratory assessment of women deemed to be at increased risk of breast or ovarian cancer. Laboratory assessment includes the analysis of high-penetrance genes *BRCA1* and *BRCA2* or other specific breast cancer susceptibility genes, where indicated. Once a pathogenic *BRCA1* or *BRCA2* mutation has been identified, a multidisciplinary approach is advocated in view of its complex clinical genetic, oncologic, surgical, gynecologic, and psychological aspects.

References

1. Peto J, Collins N, Barfoot R, et al. Prevalence of BRCA1 and BRCA2 gene mutations in patients with early-onset breast cancer. *J Natl Cancer Inst* 199;91:943–949.
2. Struewing JP, Abeliovich D, Peretz T, et al. The carrier frequency of the BRCA1 185delAG mutation is approximately 1 percent in Ashkenazi Jewish individuals. *Nat Genet* 1995;11:198–200.
3. Roa BB, Boyd AA, Volcik K, et al. Ashkenazi Jewish population frequencies for common mutations in BRCA1 and BRCA2. *Nat Genet* 1996;14:185–187.
4. Thorlacius S, Olafsdottir G, Tryggvadottir L, et al. A single BRCA2 mutation in male and female breast cancer families from Iceland with varied cancer phenotypes. *Nat Genet* 1996;13:117–119.
5. Thorlacius S, Sigurdsson S, Bjarnadottir H, et al. Study of a single BRCA2 mutation with high carrier frequency in a small population. *Am J Hum Genet* 1997;60:1079–1084.

6. Gayther SA, Russell P, Harrington P, et al. The contribution of germline BRCA1 and BRCA2 mutations to familial ovarian cancer: no evidence for other ovarian cancer-susceptibility genes. *Am J Hum Genet* 1999;65:1021–1029.

7. Lakhani SR, Jacquemier J, Sloane JP, et al. Multifactorial analysis of differences between sporadic breast cancers and cancers involving BRCA1 and BRCA2 mutations. *J Natl Cancer Inst* 1998;90:1138–1145.

8. Pathology of familial breast cancer: differences between breast cancers in carriers of BRCA1 or BRCA2 mutations and sporadic cases: Breast Cancer Linkage Consortium. *Lancet* 1997;349:1505–1510.

9. Lakhani SR, Van De Vijver MJ, Jacquemier J, et al. The pathology of familial breast cancer: predictive value of immunohistochemical markers estrogen receptor, progesterone receptor, HER-2, and p53 in patients with mutations in BRCA1 and BRCA2. *J Clin Oncol* 2002;20:2310–2318.

10. Verhoog LC, Brekelmans CT, Seynaeve C, et al. Survival and tumour characteristics of breast-cancer patients with germline mutations of BRCA1. *Lancet* 1998;351:316–321.

11. Johannsson OT, Idvall I, Anderson C, et al. Tumour biological features of BRCA1-induced breast and ovarian cancer. *Eur J Cancer* 1997;33:362–371.

12. Foulkes WD, Brunet JS, Stefansson IM, et al. The prognostic implication of the basal-like (cyclin E high/p27 low/p53+/glomeruloid-microvascular-proliferation+) phenotype of BRCA1-related breast cancer. *Cancer Res* 2004;64:830–835.

13. Hedenfalk I, Duggan D, Chen Y, et al. Gene-expression profiles in hereditary breast cancer. *N Engl J Med* 2001;344:539–548.

14. Chappuis PO, Rosenblatt J, Foulkes WD. The influence of familial and hereditary factors on the prognosis of breast cancer. *Ann Oncol* 1999;10:1163–1170.

15. Phillips KA, Andrulis IL, Goodwin PJ. Breast carcinomas arising in carriers of mutations in BRCA1 or BRCA2: are they prognostically different? *J Clin Oncol* 1999;17:3653–3663.

16. Robson M. Are BRCA1- and BRCA2-associated breast cancers different? Prognosis of BRCA1-associated breast cancer. *J Clin Oncol* 2000;18:113S–118S.

17. Foulkes WD, Chappuis PO, Wong N, et al. Primary node negative breast cancer in BRCA1 mutation carriers has a poor outcome. *Ann Oncol* 2000;11:307–313.

18. Chappuis PO, Goffin J, Wong N, et al. A significant response to neoadjuvant chemotherapy in BRCA1/2 related breast cancer. *J Med Genet* 2002;39:608–610.

19. Verhoog LC, Berns EM, Brekelmans CT, et al. Prognostic significance of germline BRCA2 mutations in hereditary breast cancer patients. *J Clin Oncol* 2000;18:119S–124S.

20. Jernstrom H, Lerman C, Ghadirian P, et al. Pregnancy and risk of early breast cancer in carriers of BRCA1 and BRCA2. *Lancet* 1999;354:1846–1850.

21. Narod SA, Dube MP, Klijn J, et al. Oral contraceptives and the risk of breast cancer in BRCA1 and BRCA2 mutation carriers. *J Natl Cancer Inst* 2002;94:1773–1779.

22. Jernstrom H, Lubinski J, Lynch HT, et al. Breast-feeding and the risk of breast cancer in BRCA1 and BRCA2 mutation carriers. *J Natl Cancer Inst* 2004;96:1094–1098.

23. Werness BA, Ramus SJ, Whittemore AS, et al. Histopathology of familial ovarian tumors in women from families with and without germline BRCA1 mutations. *Hum Pathol* 2000;31:1420–1424.

24. Rubin SC, Benjamin I, Behbakht K, et al. Clinical and pathological features of ovarian cancer in women with germ-line mutations of BRCA1. *N Engl J Med* 1996;335:1413–1416.

25. Easton DF. How many more breast cancer predisposition genes are there? *Breast Cancer Res* 1999;1:14–17.

26. Miki Y, Swensen J, Shattuck-Eidens D, et al. A strong candidate for the breast and ovarian cancer susceptibility gene BRCA1. *Science* 1994;266:66–71.

27. Wooster R, Bignell G, Lancaster J, et al. Identification of the breast cancer susceptibility gene BRCA2. *Nature* 1995;78:789–792.

28. Rebbeck TR, Kantoff PW, Krithivas K, et al. Modification of BRCA1-associated breast cancer risk by the polymorphic androgen-receptor CAG repeat. *Am J Hum Genet* 1999;64:1371–1377.

29. Kadouri L, Easton DF, Edwards S, et al. CAG and GGC repeat polymorphisms in the androgen receptor gene and breast cancer susceptibility in BRCA1/2 carriers and non-carriers. *Br J Cancer* 2001;85:36–40.

30. Anzick SL, Kononen J, Walker RL, et al. AIB1, a steroid receptor coactivator amplified in breast and ovarian cancer. *Science* 1997;277:965–968.
31. Levy-Lahad E, Lahad A, Eisenberg S, et al. A single nucleotide polymorphism in the RAD51 gene modifies cancer risk in BRCA2 but not BRCA1 carriers. *Proc Natl Acad Sci U S A* 2001; 98:3232–3236.
32. Wang WW, Spurdle AB, Kolachana P, et al. A single nucleotide polymorphism in the 5′ untranslated region of RAD51 and risk of cancer among BRCA1/2 mutation carriers. *Cancer Epidemiol Biomarkers Prev* 2001;10:955–960.
33. Phelan CM, Rebbeck TR, Weber BL, et al. Ovarian cancer risk in BRCA1 carriers is modified by the HRAS1 variable number of tandem repeat (VNTR) locus. *Nat Genet* 1996;12:309–311.
34. Malkin D, Li FP, Strong LC, et al. Germ line p53 mutations in a familial syndrome of breast cancer, sarcomas, and other neoplasms. *Science* 1990;250:1233–1238.
35. Chompret A, Brugieres L, Ronsin M, et al. P53 germline mutations in childhood cancers and cancer risk for carrier individuals. *Br J Cancer* 2000;82:1932–1937.
36. Birch JM, Hartley AL, Blair V, et al. Cancer in the families of children with soft tissue sarcoma. *Cancer* 1990;66:2239–2248.
37. Garber JE, Goldstein AM, Kantor AF, et al. Follow-up study of twenty-four families with Li-Fraumeni syndrome. *Cancer Res* 1991;51:6094–6097.
38. Li FP, Fraumeni JF Jr, Mulvihill JJ, et al. A cancer family syndrome in twenty-four kindreds. *Cancer Res* 1988;48:5358–5362.
39. Rapakko K, Allinen M, Syrjakoski K, et al. Germline TP53 alterations in Finnish breast cancer families are rare and occur at conserved mutation-prone sites. *Br J Cancer* 2001;84:116–119.
40. Zelada-Hedman M, Borresen-Dale AL, Claro A, et al. Screening for TP53 mutations in patients and tumours from 109 Swedish breast cancer families. *Br J Cancer* 1997;75:1201–1204.
41. Sidransky D, Tokino T, Helzlsouer K, et al. Inherited p53 gene mutations in breast cancer. *Cancer Res* 1992;52:2984–2986.
42. Prosser J, Porter D, Coles C, et al. Constitutional p53 mutation in a non-Li-Fraumeni cancer family. *Br J Cancer* 1992;5:527–528.
43. Borresen AL, Andersen TI, Garber J, et al. Screening for germ line TP53 mutations in breast cancer patients. *Cancer Res* 1992;52:3234–3236.
44. Liaw D, Marsh DJ, Li J, et al. Germline mutations of the PTEN gene in Cowden disease, an inherited breast and thyroid cancer syndrome. *Nat Genet* 1997;16:64–67.
45. Nelen MR, Kremer H, Konings IB, et al. Novel PTEN mutations in patients with Cowden disease: absence of clear genotype-phenotype correlations. *Eur J Hum Genet* 1999;7:267–273.
46. Starink TM, van der Veen JP, Arwert F, et al. The Cowden syndrome: a clinical and genetic study in 21 patients. *Clin Genet* 1986;29:222–233.
47. Eng C. Will the real Cowden syndrome please stand up: revised diagnostic criteria. *J Med Genet* 2000;37:828–830.
48. Longy M, Lacombe D. Cowden disease: report of a family and review. *Ann Genet* 1996;39:35–42.
49. Jenne DE, Reimann H, Nezu J, et al. Peutz-Jeghers syndrome is caused by mutations in a novel serine threonine kinase. *Nat Genet* 1998;18:38–43.
50. Hemminki A, Avizienyte E, Roth S, et al. A serine/threonine kinase gene defective in Peutz-Jeghers syndrome. *Nature* 1998;391:184–187.
51. Giardiello FM, Welsh SB, Hamilton SR, et al. Increased risk of cancer in the Peutz-Jeghers syndrome. *N Engl J Med* 1987;316:1511–1514.
52. Meijers-Heijboer H, Wijnen J, Vasen H, et al. The CHEK2 1100delC mutation identifies families with a hereditary breast and colorectal cancer phenotype. *Am J Hum Genet* 2003;72:1308–1314.
53. Vahteristo P, Bartkova J, Eerola H, et al. A CHEK2 genetic variant contributing to a substantial fraction of familial breast cancer. *Am J Hum Genet* 2002;71:432–438.
54. CHEK2*1100delC and susceptibility to breast cancer: a collaborative analysis involving 10,860 breast cancer cases and 9,065 controls from 10 studies. *Am J Hum Genet* 2004;74:1175–1182.
55. Schutte M, Seal S, Barfoot R, et al. Variants in CHEK2 other than 1100delC do not make a major contribution to breast cancer susceptibility. *Am J Hum Genet* 2003;72:1023–1028.
56. Sodha N, Bullock S, Taylor R, et al. CHEK2 variants in susceptibility to breast cancer and evidence of retention of the wild type allele in tumours. *Br J Cancer* 2002;87:1445–1448.

57. Swift M, Morrell D, Massey RB, et al. Incidence of cancer in 161 families affected by ataxia-telangiectasia. *N Engl J Med* 1991;325:1831–1836.
58. Olsen JH, Hahnemann JM, Borresen-Dale AL,et al. Cancer in patients with ataxia-telangiectasia and in their relatives in the nordic countries. *J Natl Cancer Inst* 2001;93:121–127.
59. Chenevix-Trench G, Spurdle AB, Gatei M, et al. Dominant negative ATM mutations in breast cancer families. *J Natl Cancer Inst* 2002;94:205–215.
60. FitzGerald MG, Bean JM, Hegde SR, et al. Heterozygous ATM mutations do not contribute to early onset of breast cancer. *Nat Genet* 1997;15:307–310.
61. Szabo CI, Schutte M, Broeks A, et al. Are ATM mutations 7271T→G and IVS10-6T→G really high-risk breast cancer-susceptibility alleles? *Cancer Res* 2004;64:840–843. histopathology. *Int J Cancer* 2000;86:60–66.
62. King MC, Marks JH, Mandell JB. Breast and ovarian cancer risks due to inherited mutations in BRCA1 and BRCA2. *Science* 2003;302:643–646.
63. Antoniou A, Pharoah PD, Narod S, et al. Average risks of breast and ovarian cancer associated with BRCA1 or BRCA2 mutations detected in case series unselected for family history: a combined analysis of 22 studies. *Am J Hum Genet* 2003;72.
64. Easton DF, Ford D, Bishop DT. Breast and ovarian cancer incidence in BRCA1-mutation carriers: Breast Cancer Linkage Consortium. *Am J Hum Genet* 1995;56:265–271.
65. Ford D, Easton DF, Stratton M, et al. Genetic heterogeneity and penetrance analysis of the BRCA1 and BRCA2 genes in breast cancer families: the Breast Cancer Linkage Consortium. *Am J Hum Genet* 1998;62:676–689.
66. Thompson D, Easton D. Variation in BRCA1 cancer risks by mutation position. *Cancer Epidemiol Biomarkers Prev* 2002;11:329–336.
67. Gayther SA, Mangion J, Russell P, et al. Variation of risks of breast and ovarian cancer associated with different germline mutations of the BRCA2 gene. *Nat Genet* 1997;15:103–105.
68. Risch HA, McLaughlin JR, Cole DE, et al. Prevalence and penetrance of germline BRCA1 and BRCA2 mutations in a population series of 649 women with ovarian cancer. *Am J Hum Genet* 2001;68:700–710.
69. Thompson D, Easton DF. Cancer Incidence in BRCA1 mutation carriers. *J Natl Cancer Inst* 2002;94:1358–1365.
70. Thompson D, Easton D. Variation in cancer risks, by mutation position, in BRCA2 mutation carriers. *Am J Hum Genet* 2001;68:410–419.
71. Brekelmans CT, Seynaeve C, Bartels CC, et al. Effectiveness of breast cancer surveillance in BRCA1/2 gene mutation carriers and women with high familial risk. *J Clin Oncol* 2001;19:924–930.
72. Warner E, Plewes DB, Hill KA, et al. Surveillance of BRCA1 and BRCA2 mutation carriers with magnetic resonance imaging, ultrasound, mammography, and clinical breast examination. *JAMA* 2004;292:1317–1325.
73. Kriege M, Brekelmans CT, Boetes C, et al. Efficacy of MRI and mammography for breast-cancer screening in women with a familial or genetic predisposition. *N Engl J Med* 2004;351:427–437.
74. Rebbeck TR, Levin AM, Eisen A, et al. Breast cancer risk after bilateral prophylactic oophorectomy in BRCA1 mutation carriers. *J Natl Cancer Inst* 1999;91:1475–1479.
75. Rebbeck TR, Lynch HT, Neuhausen SL, et al. Prophylactic oophorectomy in carriers of BRCA1 or BRCA2 mutations. *N Engl J Med* 2002;346:1616–1622.
76. Kauff ND, Satagopan JM, Robson ME, et al. Risk-reducing salpingo-oophorectomy in women with a BRCA1 or BRCA2 mutation. *N Engl J Med* 2002;346:1609–1615.
77. Meijers-Heijboer H, van Geel B, van Putten WL, et al. Breast cancer after prophylactic bilateral mastectomy in women with a BRCA1 or BRCA2 mutation. *N Engl J Med* 2001;345:159–164.
78. Hartmann LC, Sellers TA, Schaid DJ, et al. Efficacy of bilateral prophylactic mastectomy in BRCA1 and BRCA2 gene mutation carriers. *J Natl Cancer Inst* 2001;93:1633–1637.
79. Rebbeck TR, Friebel T, Lynch HT, et al. Bilateral prophylactic mastectomy reduces breast cancer risk in BRCA1 and BRCA2 mutation carriers: the PROSE Study Group. *J Clin Oncol* 2004;22:1055–1062.

80. McDonnell SK, Schaid DJ, Myers JL, et al. Efficacy of contralateral prophylactic mastectomy in women with a personal and family history of breast cancer. *J Clin Oncol* 2001;19:3938–3943.

81. Peralta EA, Ellenhorn JD, Wagman LD, et al. Contralateral prophylactic mastectomy improves the outcome of selected patients undergoing mastectomy for breast cancer. *Am J Surg* 2000;180:439–445.

82. van Geel AN. Prophylactic mastectomy: the Rotterdam experience. *Breast* 2003;12:357–361.

83. Eisen A, Rebbeck TR, Wood WC, et al. Prophylactic surgery in women with a hereditary predisposition to breast and ovarian cancer. *J Clin Oncol* 2000;18:1980–1995.

84. Contant CM, Menke-Pluijmers MB, Seynaeve C, et al. Clinical experience of prophylactic mastectomy followed by immediate breast reconstruction in women at hereditary risk of breast cancer (HB(O)C) or a proven BRCA1 and BRCA2 germ-line mutation. *Eur J Surg Oncol* 2002;28:627–632.

85. Zion SM, Slezak JM, Sellers TA, et al. Reoperations after prophylactic mastectomy with or without implant reconstruction. *Cancer* 2003;98:2152–2160.

86. Metcalfe KA, Esplen MJ, Goel V, et al. Psychosocial functioning in women who have undergone bilateral prophylactic mastectomy. *Psychooncology* 2004;13:14–25.

87. Frost MH, Schaid DJ, Sellers TA, et al. Long-term satisfaction and psychological and social function following bilateral prophylactic mastectomy. *JAMA* 2000;284:319–324.

88. Meijers-Heijboer EJ, Verhoog LC, Brekelmans CT, et al. Presymptomatic DNA testing and prophylactic surgery in families with a BRCA1 or BRCA2 mutation. *Lancet* 2000;355:2015–2020.

89. Evans D, Lalloo F, Shenton A, et al. Uptake of screening and prevention in women at very high risk of breast cancer. *Lancet* 2001;358:889–890.

90. Eisinger F, Geller G, Burke W, et al. Cultural basis for differences between US and French clinical recommendations for women at increased risk of breast and ovarian cancer. *Lancet* 1999;353:919–920.

91. Powles T, Eeles R, Ashley S, et al. Interim analysis of the incidence of breast cancer in the Royal Marsden Hospital tamoxifen randomised chemoprevention trial. *Lancet* 1998;352:98–101.

92. Veronesi U, Maisonneuve P, Costa A, et al. Prevention of breast cancer with tamoxifen: preliminary findings from the Italian randomised trial among hysterectomised women: Italian Tamoxifen Prevention Study. *Lancet* 1998;352:93–97.

93. Narod,SA, Brunet JS, Ghadirian P, et al. Tamoxifen and risk of contralateral breast cancer in BRCA1 and BRCA2 mutation carriers: a case-control study. Hereditary Breast Cancer Clinical Study Group. *Lancet* 2000;356:1876–1881.

94. Lerman C, Narod S, Schulman K, et al. BRCA1 testing in families with hereditary breast-ovarian cancer. A prospective study of patient decision making and outcomes. *JAMA* 1996;275:885–892.

95. Wagner TM, Moslinger R, Langbauer G, et al. Attitude towards prophylactic surgery and effects of genetic counselling in families with BRCA mutations. Austrian Hereditary Breast and Ovarian Cancer Group. *Br J Cancer* 2000;82:1249–1253.

96. Julian-Reynier C, Sobol H, Sevilla C, et al. Uptake of hereditary breast/ovarian cancer genetic testing in a French national sample of BRCA1 families: the French Cancer Genetic Network. *Psychooncology* 2000;9:504–510.

97. Lee SC, Bernhardt BA, Helzlsouer KJ. Utilization of BRCA1/2 genetic testing in the clinical setting: report from a single institution. *Cancer* 2002;94:1876–1885.

98. Balmana J, Sanz J, Bonfill X, et al. Genetic counseling program in familial breast cancer: analysis of its effectiveness, cost and cost-effectiveness ratio. *Int J Cancer* 2004;112:647–652.

48

Screening for Breast Cancer

Jacques Fracheboud

Harry J. de Koning

■ What Is the Problem that Requires Screening?

Breast cancer.

What is the incidence/prevalence of the target condition?

In 2000, breast cancer was the second most common cancer site in the world with an estimated 1 million incident cases each year and 3.9 million prevalent cases within 5 years of diagnosis.[1] In 2000, 373,000 women died of breast cancer worldwide.[1] The highest incidence (100–125/100,000 women) is found in North America and the European Union; the lowest (13–23/ 100,000 women) in China, South Central Asia and Africa.[2] Table 48–1 illustrates the breast cancer annual incidence rates of several countries.[3] Incidence differences between countries for premenopausal breast cancer are usually smaller than for postmenopausal breast cancer.[3] More than 50% of all breast cancers are diagnosed in women aged 65 years and over, and almost 75% are in postmenopausal women.[4] In young women, breast cancer is often associated with a hereditary/genetic predisposition or family history. Women with mutations of the *BRCA1* and *BRCA2* genes have a considerably higher lifetime risk for breast cancer than the general population (see related material in Chapter 47).[5] Other known risk factors include early menarche, late first pregnancy, nulli- or low parity, and oral contraceptive use, all representing a moderate relative risk.[6]

Mortality rates for the different countries follow a pattern similar to that for incidence.[7] The incidence/mortality ratio varies between countries, depending on many factors including different stage at diagnosis and survival. However, survival differences should be interpreted with caution, as they often are biased by differences in tumor stage at diagnosis.[8] Although survival has improved in most countries during the last two decades, 5-year relative survival rates still vary considerably from 55% to 74% in Europe and to 89% in the United States.[9] In The Netherlands the average relative survival is approximately 70%, 55%, and 50% for 5 years, 10 and 20 years, respectively.[10]

Table 48-1	**Age-standardized world annual incidence rates (per 100,000 women), 1993–1987**		
Northern America		**Latin America**	
United States, SEER White)	92.1	Uruguay, Montevideo	114.9
United States, SEER (Black)	83.1	Argentina, Bahia Blanca	86.1
Canada	78.5	Argentina, Concordia	55.1
		Colombia, Cali	37.3
Australia, Oceania		Cuba, Villa Clara	28.9
Australia, Victoria	81.4	Ecuador, Quito	26.5
New Zealand	75.8		
Australia, Northern Territory	59.3	**Asia**	
		Singapore (Chinese)	44.7
Europe		China, Hong Kong	36.2
The Netherlands	85.6	Japan, Nagasaki Prefecture	29.8
Sweden	76.5	India, Madras	23.9
UK, England	74.4	Korea, Busan	18.6
Germany, Saarland	71.4	Thailand, Chiang Mai	16.1
Italy, Romagna	71.1	Oman (Omani)	12.7
Spain, Tarragona	59.3	China, Qidong County	10.0
		Africa	
Poland, Warsaw City	53.7	Algeria, Algiers	21.3
Lithuania	37.7	Zimbabwe, Harare (African)	20.3
		The Gambia	7.0

From Parkin DM, Whelan SL, Ferlay J, et al, eds. Cancer Incidence in Five Continents, Vol. VIII. Lyon: IARC Press, 2000:1–781.

What are the sequelae of the condition that are of interest in clinical medicine?

In the past, breast cancer was typically diagnosed after the woman felt a lump in the breast or observed visible changes. Such tumors generally have a diameter of at least 2 cm when diagnosed. Since the 1990s, mammography screening has become common in many countries, either in the form of organized screening programs[11] or as widespread opportunistic (spontaneous) screening. This has led to a gradual decline in the average tumor size and an increasing proportion of incident ductal carcinoma in situ.[6]

■ The Tests

What is the purpose of the tests?

The detection of a malignant tumor in asymptomatic women before it has metastasized.

Breast cancer is treated either by surgery, radiotherapy, adjuvant systemic treatment, or any combination of these modalities. Early detection increases the likelihood that primary therapy will result in a complete cure. In addition, both the size of the primary tumor at initial treatment and degree of angiogenesis are strongly related to the probability of metastases.[12,13] Classically, primary therapy consists of a surgical treatment, either breast-conserving therapy or mastectomy, with removal of the axillary lymph nodes. The latter can be avoided if the sentinel node is free from tumor tissue. The surgery is intended to be curative, but is often followed by radiotherapy. In the recent years, surgery has been preceded by radiotherapy or (neoadjuvant) chemotherapy to reduce the size of the primary tumor (downstaging) so that breast-conserving therapy can be considered.[14-16] Adjuvant systemic hormonal and chemotherapy treatment, introduced in the 1980s, improves survival. It is also claimed that chemotherapy has a beneficial effect in women with breast cancer without evidence of axillary lymph node metastasis.[17] The average survival after the diagnosis of distant metastases in the 1980s was approximately 20 months[18] and may have slightly improved since then.

What is the nature of the tests?

Breast self-examination. Most breast masses in a nonscreened population are discovered by the women. The breast self-examination is best performed during the first few days after menstruation in premenopausal women and monthly in postmenopausal women. The examination begins with an inspection of the breasts in the mirror, looking for changes in shape and contour. It should then continue in the shower, where tactile sensation is increased. After showering, the woman should lie on her side and, using the second through fourth fingers, systematically palpate the contralateral breast. Typically, the examination begins with the nipples and works away from them in a circular fashion. The process is repeated on the other side.

Clinical breast examination. Clinical breast examination (CBE) has the potential to detect smaller tumors than BSE and some tumors that are not detected by mammography. It requires highly trained examiners who take enough time for a thorough visual inspection and systematic palpation. Although a Canadian trial did not find a significant difference in breast cancer mortality reduction between CBE alone and CBE combined with mammography, the debate continues as to whether screening by CBE alone could be a serious alternative to mammography screening in developing countries.[19,20]

Mammography. Mammography consists of a radiographic examination of each breast, often from two different directions. The compression that occurs when the breasts are placed between two radiographic film plates can be painful to some women.[21] Screening mammography requires high-quality, specially calibrated equipment and experienced radiographers and radiologists who have been trained in screening mammography. Preferably, two radiologists read the films independently. Certain abnormalities on the mammogram may indicate early malignant lesions that are not yet clinically apparent.

The conventional x-ray mammography is more and more often being replaced by (full-field) digital mammography, in which a digital image is generated instead of one on the screen-film. Digital mammography has several advantages in the logistics of the mammogram handling, including the potential use of computer-aided detection (CAD) software. Potentially, the latter may count as a second reading, but it is not yet used in large-scale screening programs. However, despite a higher resolution and the improved possibility of image processing, the effects of digital mammography on the sensitivity and specificity remain unclear.[22]

Magnetic resonance imaging. Magnetic resonance imaging (MRI) produces three-dimensional images of the breast and provides information on newly formed vascular structures based on the administration of an intravenous contrast medium. MRI is time-consuming and expensive and cannot be performed in women with claustrophobia or with pacemakers.[23] For these reasons, MRI is not an appropriate screening test in unselective populations, but is of value in the screening of high-risk women because of its high sensitivity.[24]

Ultrasonography. Ultrasonography (US) is a noninvasive and nonionizing technique, but cannot serve as primary screening method. One of the reasons is that US is a dynamic examination and the documentation of the entire examination of both breasts is difficult, which makes a second reading practically impossible. Sensitivity depends mainly on expertise of the examiners.[25] US is useful for the assessment of breast abnormalities and as an adjunct to mammography for the screening of asymptomatic women with dense breasts.

At the moment, other imaging techniques such as mammoscintigraphy and positron emission tomography (PET) have at the most an additional role in diagnosis and have not yet been tested as a screening instrument in larger populations.[6]

What are the implications of testing?

What does an abnormal test result mean? An abnormal test means further investigation is necessary. Many randomized controlled screening trials confirm that screening women aged 50 to 69 years using mammography reduces breast cancer mortality by 24%.[6,26,27] Figure 48–1 summarizes the results of the different randomized controlled screening trials as assessed in a Cochrane meta-analysis for women aged 50 and over.[28] Although it seems the Canadian trial shows smaller benefit, the trial also included screening in the control arm. The researchers recently concluded that it is likely the mammography screening also decreased breast cancer mortality in the Canadian trial from 13% to 34%.[29]

Also shown in nationwide programs is that the observed reduction in breast cancer mortality is strongly related to mammography screening. We examined 30,560 women who died of breast cancer from 1980 to 2001. The mortality trends were studied by calendar year and time since the introduction of screening. For all 650 municipalities, the exact month and year in which screening began was taken into account. Breast cancer mortality rates fell significantly from 1997 onward, reaching a 20% reduction in 2001. When the data were analyzed by time since the start of screening instead of calendar time, there was a

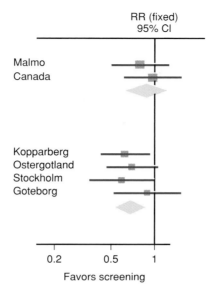

RR (fixed)
95% CI

Malmo
Canada

Kopparberg
Ostergotland
Stockholm
Goteborg

0.2   0.5   1

Favors screening

Figure 48-1 Relative risk and 95% confidence interval of dying from breast cancer in randomized mammography screening trials, women aged 50 years and older, after 7 years of follow-up. From Olsen O, Gotzsche PC. Screening for breast cancer with mammography. Cochrane Database Syst Rev: CD001877, 2001.

continuous increase of 0.3% per year in the breast cancer mortality rates until screening was introduced; thereafter an annual 1.7% decline was noted.[30] In premenopausal women, active glandular tissue makes the interpretation of the mammogram more difficult. The results of screening trials are less convincing in premenopausal women than in postmenopausal women, and therefore, the introduction of mammography screening for this group is still debated.[31,32]

Although programs in which women are trained in periodic breast self-examination are associated with somewhat earlier detection of breast cancers, the effect achieved is not sufficient to reduce mortality by a clinically significant degree.[32–34] Women are better advised to participate regularly in a mammography program where available.

The sensitivity and specificity of mammography for the detection of breast cancer in women aged 50 to 69 years are approximately 80% and 95%, respectively.[6] In younger women, the sensitivity is estimated to be less than 60% to 80% of the former value.[35] The positive predictive value of an abnormal test result in a population with a high prevalence of breast cancer, such as The Netherlands, is at best about 50%.[36] This means that half of the women with an abnormal test result have no proven malignancy. However, in most other screening programs, the positive predictive values are much lower because of high recall rates and vary from 5% to 15%.[37,38] To limit the consequences of a false-positive screening test result, a standardized sequential diagnostic workup should be available without delay to the woman. As the suspect lesion will not be palpable in 40% of instances, this further diagnostic assessment should be done at breast centers with the required equipment and expertise. Breast-conserving therapy is more often an option because the lesions discovered by screening are smaller on average.

The natural history of very small or very early breast cancer lesions is only partly known. The inevitable uncertainty about the prognostic improvement of major primary therapy must be weighed against its risks and drawbacks. Ductal carcinoma in situ (DCIS) constitutes 15% to 20% of all breast cancers detected in some mammography screening series. In some instances, this may result in overtreatment, although there is a growing understanding of prognostic factors in DCIS.[39]

The balance between benefits and harms of mammography screening is subtle. Thirty of every 100 women aged 50 to 69 with screen-detected breast cancer will benefit in the sense that they will be cured instead of dying from their disease. The remaining 70 will not benefit from the earlier diagnosis and must live more years with the knowledge of having breast cancer: More than 50 would have been cured anyway given the cure rate after primary therapy for symptomatic breast cancer, another 15 will die of breast cancer despite the earlier diagnosis, and about five will die from an unrelated problem before the breast cancer would have become clinically manifest without the screening. These five women represent an "artificial" increase in the incidence of breast cancer owing to screening.[40] However, it is generally agreed that the benefit, about 15 life-years gained per prevented breast cancer death, outweighs the unfavorable effects.[41] Table 48–2 provides an overview of favorable and unfavorable effects per 1,000,000 screens.

What does a normal test result mean? Nearly 20% of all breast cancers go undetected by mammography screening, the so-called interval cancers.[6] It is important to explain to women that they should not postpone a visit to the doctor or wait until the next round of screening if they feel or see an abnormality in their breasts after having a normal test result. Interval cancers are inevitable in a cancer-screening program. From site visits within the Dutch breast cancer screening program, it is known that 55% of the screening mammograms that precede interval cancers show no abnormalities retrospectively.[42] Minimal signs not considered a reason to refer the woman for assessment according to the common practice were present in 23% of the preceding screening mammograms. Twenty-one percent of the screening mammograms preceding the interval cancer have retrospectively suspect lesions that would have justified a referral recommendation by the screening. Women with dense breasts and women using hormonal replacement therapy have a higher risk of interval cancer.[43,44]

What is the cost of testing?

The costs and cost-effectiveness of breast cancer screening were examined in several countries.[45–47] The costs vary with the type of screening organization and the characteristics of the health care system. Table 48–3 offers some key figures on

Table 48-2 Favorable and unfavorable effects when implementing nationwide breast cancer screening of women aged 50–69 every 2 years[1]

Unfavorable effects		Favorable effects	
Screens	1 million	Life-years gained	16,500
Screen false positives that have led to biopsy	2,100	Breast cancer deaths prevented	1,080
Increase in life-years after known diagnosis (earlier diagnosis without extra survival)	17,500	Breast-conserving therapy instead of mastectomy	750
Additional number of primary surgical treatments	590	Decrease in biopsies outside program with benign result	3,200
Additional number of primary radiation treatments	650	Decrease in adjuvant hormonal treatment	525
		Decrease in treatment of advanced disease	1,080

[1]Numbers are based on population screening 1990–2017 in The Netherlands (total of 15.8 million screens) and follow-up of effects until 2090.
From de Koning HJ, van Ineveld BM, van Oortmarssen GJ, et al. Breast cancer screening and cost-effectiveness; policy alternatives, quality of life considerations and the possible impact of uncertain factors. *Int J Cancer* 1991;49:531–537.

Table 48-3 Mortality effects, cost, and cost-effectiveness of two scenarios: no breast screening, screening with nlbb as diagnostic workup

	Scenario (A) (no screening)		Scenario (B) (NLBB) (difference with no screening)	
Discount rate	0%	3%	0%	3%
Effectiveness				
Deaths from breast cancer	351,364	140,520	–31 195	– 16 180
Per year of screening	6,374	2,395	–1 155	– 202.6
Life years lost from breast cancer (× 1,000)			–513.9	
Costs (× 10⁶ £)				
Screening	0	0	+ 635	+ 432
Diagnostics	1,802	910	– 70	– 40
Primary treatment	3,059	1,296	+ 87	+ 81
Follow up	1,136	454	+ 56	+ 30
Palliative care	4,272	1,708	– 379	– 197
Total	10,269	4,369	+ 328	+ 307
Cost-effectiveness[1] (£)				
Costs per life-year gained	-	-	639	1 515

NLBB, Nederlandse Luister - en Braille bibliotheek; £, pound sterling.
[1]To calculate the cost-effectiveness, the difference in costs between the situation without mass screening and that with mass screening is divided by the difference in effects.
From Groenewoud JH, Pijnappel RM, van den Akker-Van Marle ME, et al. Cost-effectiveness of stereotactic large-core needle biopsy for nonpalpable breast lesions compared to open-breast biopsy. *Br J Cancer* 2004;90:383–392.

cost and cost-effectiveness for the centralized mammography screening program in The Netherlands.[48] The cost per screen per woman in an organized large-scale screening program approximates $55. The cost of further diagnostic evaluation will increase owing to the extra prevalence (Table 48-3) and the false positives. This increase may be partly offset by a decrease in preventive activity outside the screening program. The increased prevalence will also increase the frequency of primary therapy and follow-up. However, major savings result from prevented cases of advanced disease.[18] Cost-effectiveness ratios show a wide variation among countries because they are not only sensitive to health care differences including attendance rates, but also to the effect of size, which is directly related to the incidence and prevalence of the disease.[49] Cost-effectiveness ratios are generally more favorable in countries with higher prevalence.

■ Conclusions and Recommendations

Systematic screening for breast cancer by mammography in women aged 50 to 69 years reduces the mortality from breast cancer by 25%, and probably is beneficial up to age 74. The effect of mammography screening for women aged 40 to 49 years is less certain. MRI is likely to be particular useful in the detection of early stage tumors in *BRCA1/2* carriers. CBE may be effective, but is in most countries no alternative for mammography.

The balance between the favorable and unfavorable effects of breast cancer screening is fragile. A favorable balance is achieved only in a systematic program with high-quality equipment, well-trained radiographers and radiologists, and a system of continuous quality and effect control. Therefore, occasional clinical mammography for preventive purposes outside a systematic screening program is not recommended.

When mass screening is introduced, clinicians should be aware that the population of referred women differs fundamentally from the population that presents with symptoms. Such awareness is necessary not only to prevent overdiagnosis and overtreatment but also underdiagnosis and undertreatment.

■ Summary

1 ■ What Is the Problem that Requires Screening?
Breast cancer.

a. What is the incidence/prevalence of the target condition?
The highest annual incidence (100–125/100,000 women) is found in North America and the European Union. In Asia, the

incidence is typically three to five times lower. In The Netherlands the prevalence of breast cancer is estimated to be about seven times the incidence rate. This is likely to be a typical prevalence/incidence ratio in other, similar countries.

b. *What are the sequelae of the condition that are of interest in clinical medicine?*

Breast cancer is the most common form of cancer among women in many industrialized countries. The typical length of survival after diagnosis without treatment is 3 years. Both surgery that conserves the breast and mastectomy with or without radiotherapy/chemotherapy are intended to be curative. The average survival after diagnosis of distant metastases is 20 months.

2 ■ The Tests

a. *What is the purpose of the tests?*

To detect a malignant breast tumor before metastasis.

b. *What is the nature of the tests?*

Mammography consists of a radiograph of each breast, often viewed from two different directions. Screening mammography requires specially calibrated equipment and experienced radiologists who have been trained in screening mammography. Breast self-examination is performed monthly in a standing and supine position.

c. *What are the implications of testing?*

1. What does an abnormal test result mean?

   The sensitivity and specificity of mammography for the detection of breast cancer in women aged 50 to 69 years are approximately 80% and 95%, respectively. In younger women, the sensitivity is estimated to be less than 60% to 80% of the former value. The positive predictive value of an abnormal test result in a population with a high prevalence of breast cancer, such as The Netherlands, is at best about 50%. This means that half of the women with an abnormal test result have no proven malignancy. About 30 of every 100 women aged 60 to 69 years with a screen-detected breast cancer will benefit in the sense that they will be cured

Continued

■ **Summary—cont'd**

instead of dying from their disease. The remaining 70 will not benefit from the earlier diagnosis; about 50 would have been cured anyway, another 15 will die of breast cancer despite early diagnosis, and five will die from an unrelated problem before their breast cancer had become clinically apparent without screening.

2. What does a normal test result mean?
   About 20% of all breast cancers are still missed by screening with mammography.

d. ***What is the cost of testing?***
The costs and cost-effectiveness of breast cancer screening with mammography varies with the type of screening organization and the characteristics of the health care system. The cost per screen per woman approximates $55.

3 ■ Conclusions and Recommendations

Systematic screening for breast cancer by mammography in women aged 50 to 69 years reduces the mortality from breast cancer by 25%, and probably is beneficial up to age 74. The effect of mammography screening for women aged 40 to 49 years is less certain.

References

1. Parkin DM, Bray F, Ferlay J, et al. Estimating the world cancer burden: Globocan 2000. *Int J Cancer* 2001;94:153–156.
2. Pisani P, Bray F, Parkin DM. Estimates of the world-wide prevalence of cancer for 25 sites in the adult population. *Int J Cancer* 2002;97:72–81.
3. Parkin DM, Whelan SL, Ferlay J, et al. *Cancer Incidence in Five Continents, Vol. VIII.* Lyon: IARC Press, 2000:1–781.
4. Fracheboud J, Otto SJ, van Dijck JAAM, et al. Decreased rates of advanced breast cancer due to mammography screening in the Netherlands. *Br J Cancer* 2004;91:861–867.
5. Liberman L. Breast cancer screening with MRI: what are the data for patients at high risk? *N Engl J Med* 2004;351:497–500.
6. *IARC Handbooks of Cancer Prevention: Breast Cancer Screening. Vol. 7.* IARC Press: Lyon, 2002.
7. Botha JL, Bray F, Sankila R, et al. Breast cancer incidence and mortality trends in 16 European countries. *Eur J Cancer* 2003;39:1718–1729.
8. de Koning HJ. Why improvement in survival of screen-detected cases is not necessarily equivalent to benefit? *Breast* 2003;12:299–301.

9. Sant M, Allemani C, Berrino F, et al. Breast carcinoma survival in Europe and the United States. *Cancer* 2004;100:715–722.

10. Nab HW. Trends in incidence and prognosis in female breast cancer since 1955. Thesis. Erasmus University Rotterdam: Rotterdam, 1995.

11. Shapiro S, Coleman EA, Broeders M, et al. Breast cancer screening programmes in 22 countries: current policies, administration and guidelines: International Breast Cancer Screening Network (IBSN) and the European Network of Pilot Projects for Breast Cancer Screening. *Int J Epidemiol* 1998;27:735–742.

12. Horak ER, Leek R, Klenk N, et al. Angiogenesis, assessed by platelet/endothelial cell adhesion molecule antibodies, as indicator of node metastases and survival in breast cancer. *Lancet* 1992;340:1120–1124.

13. Guidi AJ, Berry DA, Broadwater G, et al. Association of angiogenesis in lymph node metastases with outcome of breast cancer. *J Natl Cancer Inst* 2000;92:486–492.

14. Legorreta AP, Chernicoff HO, Trinh JB, et al. Diagnosis, clinical staging, and treatment of breast cancer: a retrospective multiyear study of a large controlled population. *Am J Clin Oncol* 2004;27:185–190.

15. Lerouge D, Touboul E, Lefranc JP, et al. Combined chemotherapy and preoperative irradiation for locally advanced noninflammatory breast cancer: updated results in a series of 120 patients. *Int J Radiat Oncol Biol Phys* 2004;59:1062–1073.

16. Mano MS, Awada A. Primary chemotherapy for breast cancer: the evidence and the future. *Ann Oncol* 2004;15:1161–1171.

17. Abrams JS. Adjuvant therapy for breast cancer: results from the USA consensus conference. 2001. *Breast Cancer* 2001;8:298–304.

18. de Koning HJ, van Ineveld BM, de Haes JC, et al. Advanced breast cancer and its prevention by screening. *Br J Cancer* 1992;65:950–955.

19. Miller AB, To T, Baines CJ, et al. Canadian National Breast Screening Study-2: 13-year results of a randomized trial in women aged 50-59 years. *J Natl Cancer Inst* 2000;92:1490–1499.

20. Mittra I, Baum M, Thornton H, et al. Is clinical breast examination an acceptable alternative to mammographic screening? *BMJ* 2000;321:1071–1073.

21. Aro AR, Absetz-Ylostalo P, Eerola T, et al. Pain and discomfort during mammography. *Eur J Cancer* 1996;32A:1674–1679.

22. Irwig L, Houssami N, van Vliet C. New technologies in screening for breast cancer: a systematic review of their accuracy. *Br J Cancer* 2004;90:2118–2122.

23. Morris EA. Screening for breast cancer with MRI. *Semin Ultrasound CT MR* 2003;24:45–54.

24. Kriege M, Brekelmans CT, Boetes C, et al. Efficacy of MRI and mammography for breast-cancer screening in women with a familial or genetic predisposition. *N Engl J Med* 2004;351: 427–437.

25. Teh W, Wilson AR. The role of ultrasound in breast cancer screening. A consensus statement by the European Group for Breast Cancer Screening. *Eur J Cancer* 1998;34:449–450.

26. Nyström L, Andersson I, Bjurstam N, et al. Long-term effects of mammography screening: updated overview of the Swedish randomised trials. *Lancet* 2002;359:909–919.

27. de Koning HJ. Mammographic screening: evidence from randomised controlled trials. *Ann Oncol* 2003;14:1185–1189.

28. Olsen O, Gotzsche PC. Screening for breast cancer with mammography. Cochrane Database Syst Rev: CD001877, 2001.

29. Rijnsburger AJ, van Oortmarssen GJ, Boer R, et al. Mammography benefit in the Canadian National Breast Screening Study-2: a model evaluation. *Int J Cancer* 2004;110:756–762.

30. Otto SJ, Fracheboud J, Looman CW, et al. Initiation of population-based mammography screening in Dutch municipalities and effect on breast-cancer mortality: a systematic review. *Lancet* 2003;361:1411–1417.

31. de Koning HJ, Boer R, Warmerdam PG, et al. Quantitative interpretation of age-specific mortality reductions from the Swedish breast cancer-screening trials. *J Natl Cancer Inst* 1995;87:1217–1223.

32. Humphrey LL, Helfand M, Chan BK, et al. Breast cancer screening: a summary of the evidence for the U.S. Preventive Services Task Force. *Ann Intern Med* 2002;137:347–360.

33. Semiglazov VF, Moiseyenko VM, Bavli JL, et al. The role of breast self-examination in early breast cancer detection (results of the 5-years USSR/WHO randomized study in Leningrad). *Eur J Epidemiol* 1992;8:498–502.

34. Thomas DB, Gao DL, Ray RM, et al. Randomized trial of breast self-examination in Shanghai: final results. *J Natl Cancer Inst* 2002;94:1445–1457.

35. Brekelmans CT, Collette HJ, Collette C, et al. Breast cancer after a negative screen: follow-up of women participating in the DOM Screening Programme. *Eur J Cancer* 1992;28A:893–895.

36. Fracheboud J, de Koning HJ, Boer R, et al. Nationwide breast cancer screening programme fully implemented in The Netherlands. *Breast* 2001;10:6–11.

37. Lynge E, Olsen AH, Fracheboud J, et al. Reporting of performance indicators of mammography screening in Europe. *Eur J Cancer Prev* 2003;12:213–222.

38. Yankaskas BC, Klabunde CN, Ancelle-Park R, et al. International Comparison of Performance Measures for Screening Mammography: Can it be done? *J Med Screen* 2004;11:187–193.

39. Yen MF, Tabar L, Vitak B, et al. Quantifying the potential problem of overdiagnosis of ductal carcinoma in situ in breast cancer screening. *Eur J Cancer* 2003;39:1746–1754.

40. Boer R, Warmerdam P, de Koning H, et al. Extra incidence caused by mammographic screening. *Lancet* 1994;343:979.

41. de Haes JC, de Koning HJ, van Oortmarssen GJ, et al. The impact of a breast cancer screening programme on quality-adjusted life-years. *Int J Cancer* 1991;49:538–544

42. National Expert and Training Centre for Breast Cancer Screening. Visitaties 2001-2002. Landelijk Referentiecentrum voor bevolkingsonderzoek op Borstkanker (LRCB): Nijmegen, 2003.

43. Banks E. Hormone replacement therapy and the sensitivity and specificity of breast cancer screening: a review. *J Med Screen* 2001;8:29–34.

44. Greendale GA, Reboussin BA, Slone S, et al. Postmenopausal hormone therapy and change in mammographic density. *J Natl Cancer Inst* 2003;95:30–37.

45. de Koning HJ, van Ineveld BM, van Oortmarssen GJ, et al. Breast cancer screening and cost-effectiveness; policy alternatives, quality of life considerations and the possible impact of uncertain factors. *Int J Cancer* 1991;49:531–537.

46. Brown ML, Fintor L. Cost-effectiveness of breast cancer screening: preliminary results of a systematic review of the literature. *Breast Cancer Res Treat* 1993;25:113–118.

47. Beemsterboer PM, de Koning HJ, Warmerdam PG, et al. Prediction of the effects and costs of breast-cancer screening in Germany. *Int J Cancer* 1994;58:623–628.

48. Groenewoud JH, Pijnappel RM, van den Akker-Van Marle ME, et al. Cost-effectiveness of stereotactic large-core needle biopsy for nonpalpable breast lesions compared to open-breast biopsy. *Br J Cancer* 2004;90:383–392.

49. de Koning HJ. Breast cancer screening; cost-effective in practice? *Eur J Radiol* 2000;33:32–37.

Pap Smear

Clare Wilkinson

Roy Farquharson

■ What Is the Problem that Requires Screening?

Cervical cancer.

What is the incidence/prevalence of the target condition?

Cervical cancer is the second most common female cancer worldwide; the incidence peaks at about age 50. In 2000, there were over 471,000 new cases diagnosed, and 288,000 deaths. Most cases (80%) occurred in the developing world where women do not have access to screening programs.[1] The incidence of abnormal cytology or histological evidence of cervical intraepithelial neoplasia (CIN) is substantially higher than that of invasive cervical cancer due to regression of the precursor lesion. Most of these lesions do not progress to invasive cancer, even without treatment.[2] Recent analyses and projection of U.K. trends, however, suggest that 40% of high-grade precursor lesions (CIN3) will progress to invasive cancer over a lifetime. Given that the peak incidence of CIN3 is at age 40 years, approximately 1% of CIN3 will convert to invasive cancer per year.[3] Based on this modeling exercise, the cervical screening program has prevented an epidemic of cervical cancer.

The annual incidence of cervical cancer fell by 42% between 1988 and 1997 in the United Kingdom to 9.3/100,000 by 1999.[4] This is attributed to the screening program.[5] The annual incidence rates have also decreased steadily in the United States over the past two decades to 8.1/100,000.[6] In Europe, the highest incidence is observed in Portugal at 19/100,000 and the lowest in Luxembourg at 4/100,000.

On the other hand, the cervical cancer incidence is unaltered in developing countries unless they have transitioned to industrialization and relative affluence. The World Health Organization (WHO) refers to the latter group as the "middle-income"category.[1] The highest annual incidences are found in some countries of Central and South America, with an incidence of 923.8/100,000 in Haiti.[7]

There is increasing evidence that high-risk types of the human papillomavirus[16,18][31,33] cause invasive cervical cancer, with high-risk genotypes detected in virtually 100% of cervical cancers.[8,9] Women who are not infected with a high-risk HPV infection and have mild or borderline smear results are very unlikely to develop invasive cancer; therefore, triage with human papillomavirus (HPV) testing has been the subject of recent research (also see Chapter 50). One health technology assessment (HTA) review concluded that HPV testing cannot be recommended for widespread testing.[10] Further information will become available from the U.K. Medical Research Council-funded TOMBOLA study by 2005. The U.S. Preventive Services Task Force has also concluded that the evidence for HPV as a primary screening test was too weak for implementation.[11] The Dutch Ministry of Health will await the outcome of the POBAS-CAM trial (Population Based Screening Study Amsterdam), which includes a cost-effectiveness study, to decide whether cervical screening should combine HPV and cytology tests or be based on cytology alone.[12]

What are the sequelae of the condition that are of interest in clinical medicine?

The precursor lesions (CIN or squamous intraepithelial neoplasia [SIL]) are asymptomatic and can only be detected through screening. CIN is easily treated and prevents invasive cancer in most cases. Therefore, the sequelae are those associated with colposcopy, biopsy, and local treatment; these processes have minimal physical and potential psychological sequelae. In terms of local treatment, only cold-knife cone biopsy requires a general or regional anesthetic; other treatments are carried out during colposcopy examination.

Invasive cervical cancer, if left untreated, generally advances by extensive local invasion and spread via the lymphatic system. It is fatal. The prognosis of treated invasive cancer depends on the stage at the time of diagnosis. The prognosis is excellent after treatment for early-stage disease. Microinvasive (<3 mm) stage 1A cervical cancer can be treated conservatively with conization in women wishing to preserve fertility; otherwise, the treatment is simple hysterectomy. Stages 1B and IIA can be treated with either radical hysterectomy or radiotherapy. Chemoirradiation is the current treatment for stages IIB, III, and IVA. Some clinicians also use this in patients with stage IB disease who choose radiotherapy as their primary treatment.[13] Novel treatments may include tumor-specific gene therapy[14] and vaccination against oncogenic HPV types.[15]

■ The Tests

What is the purpose of the tests?

Identification of abnormal cells at the transition zone of the uterine cervix that could indicate CIN.

What is the nature of the tests?

The standard screening test for cancer of the cervix is the Pap or cervical smear test. This is performed by speculum examination allowing direct visualization of the cervix. The smear is taken from the transition zone or at the junction of the squamous and glandular epithelium. A wooden spatula is rotated 360 degrees and the scraped cells spread onto a glass slide with fixative applied. Most cervical screening tests are carried out in primary care settings.

Liquid-based cytology (LBC) is currently being introduced as an alternative to conventional cervical cytology testing in a number of developed countries with full screening programs. This method is designed to reduce the rate of inadequate tests and improve sensitivity. It involves using a brushlike device to obtain the sample, which is then suspended in buffer and processed so that a thin layer of cells is produced without contamination. The National Institute for Clinical Excellence recommended a pilot of LBC in the United Kingdom. The appraisal was published in 2003[16] and the process of implementation begun.

Targeted screening with colposcopy examination may be recommended in some developed countries for women at highest risk of invasive cancer, including those who are immunosuppressed due to transplant therapy and those with HIV infection.

Alternative and more limited screening programs are undergoing evaluation in low-income countries where no program presently exists, for example, visual inspection of the cervix with acetic acid (VIA). This involves nonmagnified visualization of the cervix soaked with 3-5% acetic acid. HPV tests also have a possible primary screening (or triage) role in middle-income countries.[1]

What are the implications of the test?

What does an abnormal test mean? There are a number of different systems for classifying cervical cytology and histology; these are derived from the original Papanicolaou system. The WHO divides cervical dysplasia into mild, moderate, and severe, with a separate category for cancer in situ (CIS).[17] The Richart system subsequently followed in North America and is still often used for histologic classification. This system classifies lesions into three grades of CIN, with CIN1 corresponding to mild dysplasia, CIN2 to moderate dysplasia, and CIN3 to severe dysplasia and CIS combined.[18]

The Bethesda system (United States) was designed to simplify cytologic diagnosis. This system reports abnormal cytology results as low- and high-grade squamous intraepithelial neoplasia (LSIL and HSIL, respectively).[19] LSIL correlates with mild dysplasia/CIN1, and HSIL correlates with moderate to severe dysplasia/CIN2–3. Milder abnormalities are described as atypical squamous cells of undetermined significance (ASCUS; correlates with "atypical" OR "borderline" cytology results).

The management of abnormal tests is either by cytologic surveillance for milder abnormalities or by colposcopy examination leading to histologic diagnosis and local ablative treatment for more significant abnormalities. Careful follow-up regimes are implemented following initial treatment of high-grade lesions. The exact nature of the management and treatment guidelines varies according to geography, but the patterns are broadly similar.

Management of abnormal cytology tests. The optimum management of mildly abnormal results is not clear and is the subject of a significant research program in the United Kingdom, the United States, and The Netherlands. Women who have borderline smears (also known as atypical or ASCUS) should be referred for colposcopy after three tests with this result in a series. Women with one test reported as borderline changes in the endocervical cells should be referred for colposcopy. Ideally, one mildly dyskaryotic smear (equivalent to CIN1 or LSIL) should generate a referral for colposcopy, but it remains acceptable to repeat the test. Although women should be referred and assessed, to avoid overtreatment of CIN1, a '"see and treat" policy is often adopted. Patient choice over these management plans does not appear to have a significant impact on psychological outcome.[20] Management of cytology suggestive of CIN2 or CIN3 (HSIL), or persistent milder abnormalities, is by referral for colposcopy with histologic sampling and treatment based on the histologic finding. Women with invasive cells or cells indicating glandular neoplasia must be referred urgently for assessment.

Treatment of high-grade lesions. Commonly used treatments for premalignant lesions include laser vaporization or excision, cryosurgery, cold-knife conization, loop electrosurgical excision, or simple hysterectomy. Some strategies such as loop electrosurgical excision procedure (LEEP) combine diagnosis and treatment. All of these treatments are considered curative for CIN and are followed by a period of surveillance.

What does a normal test result mean? A normal test means that there is no evidence of CIN. However, the false-negative rate of the test is significant and variable and may be up to 30%.[21] A recent systematic review concluded that the sensitivity of the conventional test ranged from 30% to 87% and the specificity from 86% to 100%.[22]

Women who have a normal test are expected to adhere to screening schedules with wide international variation. The U.S. Preventive Services Task Force and the Centers for Disease Control and Prevention (CDC) recommend that women commence screening at 21 and after three annual normal tests increase to a 2- to 3-year interval until age 65; however, annual screening is common.[11] In the United Kingdom, the National Screening Committee recommends that screening commences at 25, with a 3-year interval from ages 25 to 49 years, and a 5-year interval from ages 50 to 64 years.[23] Most U.K. areas have implemented a 3-year interval and there is evidence that this may improve adherence.[24] The European Union recommends that screening is commenced at not less than 20 years and ceased at not less than 60.[25] The literature suggests that women with a normal cytology history could potentially cease screening at age 50 rather than 65 years. A recent prospective study confirmed that those with

Table 49-1	Risk reduction offered against cervical cancer by a single negative smear: effect of age group		
	20–39 y	**40–54 y**	**55–69 y**
3-yearly screening	41%	69%	73%
5-yearly screening	30%	63%	73%

From National Health Service Cervical Screening Programme Web site (http: www.cancerscreening.nhs.uk/cervical/risks.html).

previous mild abnormalities should continue until age 64.[26] There is a strong argument for interval variation at different ages, given the differing performance statistics of the test (Table 49–1).[27]

What is the cost of testing?

The National Health Service Clinical Screening Program (CSP) has estimated that the total cost of cervical screening including treating cervical abnormalities in England is £150 million per year, or £37.50 per woman screened.[28] The main costs of the cervical screening program are the costs of taking and processing the smears. In the United Kingdom, during 1994 to 1995 the total cost of a 5-year recall program was £476,768 per 100,000 eligible women.[29] In developed countries, the cost of decreasing the interval below 3 to 5 years outweighs gains in effectiveness, with an additional cost per life saved of £250,000.[30] A recent study in The Netherlands supports a 5-year program as the most cost-effective option.[31] A recent U.S. study concluded that in well-screened women, 3-yearly screening would prevent virtually all cancers prevented by annual screening, yet an additional 70,000 smears and 4,000 colposcopies would be needed to prevent one extra cancer,[32] other authors suggest this generates psychological sequelae.[33]

The cost of converting from traditional cervical screening to LBC in the United Kingdom is about £10 million, but modeling has demonstrated that LBC is always the more cost-effective method in the long run.[34]

The costs of alternative programs such as VIA or HPV triage are not known, but modeling work is under way. Work from South Africa suggests that both could be good options for those countries where the opportunity costs of a full CSP are too high.

■ Conclusions and Recommendations

Although there has never been randomized controlled trial evidence for the effectiveness and cost-effectiveness of cervical screening programs, there is substantial observational evidence of effectiveness. Indeed, it may be that an epidemic of cancer of the cervix related to increasing rates of oncogenic HPV infection has been prevented by successful screening programs.[3] In global

Table 49–2	**Essential components for a successful cervical screening program**

Leadership
Management of all phases of the process
Linkages between all program levels
Realistic budgeting
Training of relevant health professionals
Smear takers
Smear readers (cytotechnologists)
Cytopathologists
Histopathologists
Colposcopists
Gynecologists
Program managers
An agreed decision on the priority age group to be screened
Adequately taken and fixed smears and their preparation
Efficient and high-quality laboratory services
Quality control of cytology reading
A means to transport smears rapidly to the laboratory
A mechanism to inform screened women of the test results in an understandable form
A mechanism to ensure that women with an abnormal test result attend for management
   and treatment
Trained and licensed colposcopists
An accepted definition of an abnormality
A mechanism to follow up treated women
Decision on frequency of subsequent smears
A mechanism to invite women with negative smears for a subsequent smear

terms, the first priority for countries that already have an established CSP is to ensure successful functioning of that program in its entirety. Well-organized call and recall is probably always more cost-effective than opportunistic screening.[35] The establishment of either affordable triage or screening programs in those countries with no programs would have the greatest effect on global mortality from this preventable disease (Table 49–2).

Consideration should be given to avoiding intervals of less than 3 years for women with normal cytology histories, given the minimal gain in effect.

■ Summary

1 ■ What Is the Problem that Requires Screening?

Cervical cancer.

a. What is the incidence/prevalence of the target condition?

The annual incidence of invasive cervical cancer varies by geography and the presence of a screening program from 4/100,000 to 923/100,000.

b. **What are the sequelae of the condition that are of interest in clinical medicine?**

Precursor lesions are asymptomatic and easily treated, invasive cervical cancer is fatal if left untreated.

2 ■ The Tests

a. **What is the purpose of the tests?**

To identify abnormal cells from the uterine cervix that may indicate cervical intraepithelial neoplasia.

b. **What is the nature of the tests?**

A Pap smear is taken with a wooden spatula or brush from the cervix during a speculum examination.

c. **What are the implications of testing?**

1. What does an abnormal test result mean?
   Cytologic surveillance is necessary if mildly abnormal; a colposcopic examination, biopsy, and treatment are necessary if higher grade. Ideally, one mildly dyskaryotic smear should generate a referral for colposcopy.
2. What does a normal test result mean?
   There is no evidence of CIN and women should seek retesting at an interval determined by their local program.

c. **What is the cost of testing?**

About £37.50 per woman screened when all program costs are included.

3 ■ Conclusions and Recommendations

Existing screening program should be of high quality. The establishment of full or limited programs in developing countries would have the greatest global effect on the disease.

References

1. WHO. *Cervical Cancer Screening in Developing Countries; Report of a WHO Consultation.* Geneva: WHO, 2002.

2. Holowaty P. The natural history of dysplasia of the uterine cervix. *J Natl Cancer Inst* 1999;91:252–258.
3. Peto J, Gilham C, Fletcher O, et al. The cervical cancer epidemic that screening has prevented in the UK. *Lancet* 2004;364:249–256.
4. Registrations of cancer diagnosed in 1999. National Statistics MB1 No 30.
5. Health Quarterly Statistics 07, Autumn 2000. National Statistics (UK).
6. American Cancer Society Cancer Facts and Figures 2003.
7. *IARC Monographs on the Evaluation of Carcinogenic Risks to Humans and their Supplements: Human Papillomaviruses,* Vol. 64, Paris: IARC, 1995.
8. Bekkers RL, Massuger LF, Bulten J, et al. Epidemiological and clinical aspects of human papillomavirus detection in the prevention of cervical cancer. *Rev Med Virol* 2004;14:95–105.
9. Plummer M, Herrero R, Francheschi S, et al. Smoking and cervical cancer: pooled analysis of the IARC multi-centre case control study. *Cancer Causes Control* 2003;14:805–814.
10. Cuzick J, Sasieni P, Davies P, et al. A systematic review of the role of human papillomavirus testing within a cervical screening programme. *Health Technol Assess* 1999;3:1–96.
11. U.S. Preventive Services Task Force. *Guide to Clinical Preventive Services,* 2nd ed. Washington, DC: U.S. Department of Health and Human Services, 1996.
12. Bulkmans NW, Rozendaal L, Snijders PJ, et al. POBASCAM, a population-based randomized controlled trial for implementation of high-risk testing in cervical screening: design, methods and baseline data of 44,102 women. *Int J Oncol* 2004;110:94–101.
13. Holtz DO, Dunton C. Traditional management of invasive cervical cancer. *Obstet Gynecol Clin North Am* 2002;29:645–657.
14. Lim HY, Ahn M, Chung HC, et al. Tumor-specific gene therapy for uterine cervical cancer using MN/CA9-directed replication competent adenovirus. *Cancer Gene Ther* 2004;11:532–538.
15. DePalo G. Cervical precancer and cancer, past, present and future. *Eur J Gynaecol Oncol* 2004;25:269–278.
16. National Institute for Clinical Excellence. *Liquid Based Cytology for Cervical Screening Review,* No. 69. 2003–5.
17. Riotton G, Christopherson WM. Cytology of the female genital tract. In: World Health Organization, ed. *International Histological Classification of Tumors.* Geneva, Switzerland: WHO, 1973.
18. Richart RM. The patient with an abnormal Pap smear: screening techniques and management. *N Engl J Med* 1980;302:332–334.
19. Bethesda Workshop Group. The revised Bethesda System for reporting cervical/vaginal cytologic diagnosis: report of the 1991 Bethesda workshop. *J Reprod Med* 1992;37:383–386.
20. Kitchener HC, Burns S, Nelson L, et al. A randomised controlled trial of cytological surveillance versus patient choice between surveillance and colposcopy in managing mildly abnormal cervical smear tests. *Br J Obstet Gynaecol* 2004;111:63–70.
21. Coste J, Cochand-Priollet B, Cremoux P, et al. Cross sectional study of conventional cervical smear, monolayer cytology and HPV DNA testing for cervical cancer screening. *BMJ* 2003;326:732–733.
22. Nanda K, McCrory DC, Myers ER, et al. Accuracy of the Papanicolaou test in screening for and follow-up of cervical cytologic abnormalities: a systematic review. *Ann Intern Med* 2000; 132:810–819.
23. http://www.cancerscreening.nhs.uk/cervical/index.html
24. Howe A, Owen-Smith V, Richardson J. Health authority cervical screening policies and time since last smear: a retrospective cohort analysis in north west England. *J Med Screen* 2003; 10:184–188.
25. Advisory Committee on Cancer Prevention in the European Union. *Recommendations on Cancer Screening in the European Union.* Vienna, 1999.
26. Flannelly G, Monaghan J, Cruickshank M, et al. Cervical Screening in women over the age of 50: results of a population based multicentre study. *Br J Obstet Gynaecol* 2004;111:362–368.
27. Sasieni P, Adams J, Cuzick J. Benefit of cervical screening at different ages: evidence from the UK audit of screening histories. *Br J Cancer* 2003;89:88–93.
28. National Health Service Cervical Screening Programme Web site. Available at www.cancerscreening.nhs.uk/cervical/risks.html.

29. Grant CM. Cervical screening interval: costing the options in one health authority. *J Public Health Med* 1999;21:140–144.

30. Waugh N, Robertson A. Costs and benefits of cervical screening II. Is it worthwhile reducing the screening interval from 5 to 3 years? *Cytopathology* 1996;7:241–248.

31. Siemens FC, Boon ME, Kuypers JC, et al. Population-based cervical screening with a five year interval in the Netherlands. Stabilization of the incidence of squamous cell carcinoma and its precursor lesions in the screened population. *Acta Cytologica* 2004;48:348–354.

32. Sawaya GF, McConnell KJ, Kulasingam SL, et al. Risk of cervical cancer associated with extending the interval between cervical-cancer screenings. *N Engl J Med* 2003;349:1501–1509.

33. Wilson S, Lester H. How can we develop a cost-effective quality cervical screening programme? *Br J Gen Pract* 2002;52:485–490.

34. Karnon J, Peters J, Platt J, et al. Liquid based cytology in cervical screening: an updated rapid and systematic review and economic analyses. *Health Technol Assess* 2004;8:1–78.

35. Kim JJ, Leung GM, Woo PP, et al. Cost-effectiveness of organised versus opportunistic cervical cytology screening in Hong Kong. *J Public Health* 2004;26:130–137.

High-Risk Human Papillomavirus Testing in Cervical Cancer Screening

Mariëlle A. E. Nobbenhuis

Theo J. M. Helmerhorst

■ What Is the Problem that Requires Screening?

Cervical cancer.

What is the incidence/prevalence of the target condition?

Cervical cancer is the second most common cancer among women worldwide. There are approximately 450,000 new cases of invasive cancer of the cervix diagnosed annually worldwide; 80% occur in developing countries. The age-adjusted annual incidence rate varies from 4–15/100,000 women in countries with well-organized screening programs, compared with 20–54/100,000 in developing countries.[1]

What are the sequelae of the condition that are of interest in clinical medicine?

Human papillomavirus (HPV). The concept cervical cancer was related to sexual activity began more than a century ago. Various candidates like *Neisseria gonorrhea, Trichomonas,* and *Treponema* species passed in review. Zur Hausen[2] was the first to suggest a wart virus may be involved since cervical cancer shows a similar epidemiologic pattern as papillomavirus-induced condylomata acuminata. Potentially oncogenic (high risk) HPV types could be isolated from cervical cancers. Following this discovery, numerous epidemiologic studies demonstrated the relationship between an infection with high-risk HPV and the development of cervical cancer and its precursors.[3–5] High-risk HPV DNA can be identified in nearly all cervical carcinomas[6,7] and in case-control studies around the world, a strong association between cervical carcinomas and the presence of high-risk HPV types (odds ratios [ORs] up to 200) is found.[4,5,8,9]

Eighteen high-risk types are identified so far, namely: HPV type 16, 18, 26, 31, 33, 35, 39, 45, 51, 52, 53, 56, 58, 59, 66, 68, 73, and 82. The most prevalent type found in cervical cancer is HPV type 16, followed by HPV type 18.[6]

Natural history of human papillomavirus. HPV is a ubiquitous virus. The lifetime risk of acquiring HPV approximates 80%.[10] transmission of high-risk HPV is associated with sexual intercourse.[11,12] A peak prevalence of a high-risk HPV infection of 20% is found among sexually active young women 20 to 29 years of age, which declines to about 4% in women older than 34 years.[13] More than 80% of these high-risk HPV infections are cleared.[14] They remain asymptomatic and do not cause epithelial alterations to the cervix. The median duration of a transient infection is 6 to 14 months.[15,16]

About 20% of a high-risk HPV infections lead to morphologic changes of the cervical epithelium (i.e., cervical epithelial neoplasia [CIN]). Only 1% to 2% of women ultimately develop invasive cervical cancer over 12 to 15 years if not treated.[17] Thus, most of the lesions regress spontaneously. Regression begins with the clearance of high-risk HPV, which depends on the severity of the lesion (see Figure 50–1). The cervical smear will become normal in nearly all women who clear their high-risk HPV infection.[18,19]

Risk factors. The most important risk factor for acquisition of high-risk HPV is the number of sexual partners. However, the risk factor for progressive CIN

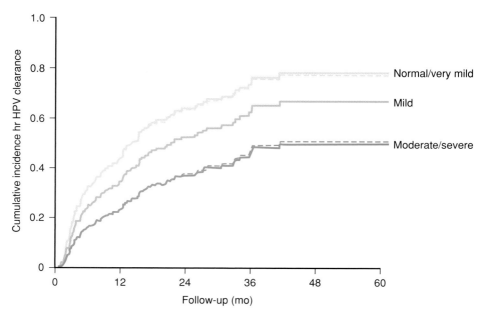

Figure 50–1   High-risk human papillomavirus (HPV) clearance stratified for normal cervical cytology and very mild (borderline) dyskaryosis; mild dyskaryosis; and moderate and severe dyskaryosis. (Cox regression; overall $p = 0.0248$).[23]

leading to cervical cancer is different. The only risk factor for CIN 3 or cervical cancer is the persistence of a high-risk HPV infection.[16,20] More than two sexual partners, age at first sexual intercourse, smoking and age are not independent risk factors for development of CIN 3 after adjusting for high-risk HPV.[16] Thus, cervical cancer is not directly a sexually transmitted disease, rather it is the HPV infection. Cervical cancer is a rare complication of a persistent infection with high-risk HPV.[21] There is growing evidence that, once a CIN lesion has developed, an increased viral load is predictive for viral persistence.[22]

■ The Test

HPV DNA testing for potentially high-risk types.

What is the purpose of the tests?

To identify women who are at risk of developing cervical cancer.

What is the nature of the tests?

Material for testing is obtained by a cervical swab or lavage. Tests that detect all known high-risk HPV types are sufficient because it is known that the risk of developing cervical cancer is not different for the different high-risk HPV types.[4,5,16,23] Individual HPV typing is only necessary in detailed epidemiologic studies or in studies evaluating the effectiveness of a certain preventive or therapeutic vaccine.

The tests most commonly used are the commercially available hybrid capture II (HCII) and consensus polymerase chain reaction (PCR) methods. The principle of the HCII test is based on direct HPV DNA detection with full-length RNA probes and signal amplification to detect captured RNA/DNA hybrid. Two cocktail probes comprising low-risk and high-risk types are available.[24] Thus, although HCII does not allow for individual typing, it is sufficient for diagnosis and direct management.

Consensus PCR methods are based on PCR amplification of HPV target DNA directed by so-called consensus or general primers that bind to highly conserved regions within the DNA of all genital HPV genotypes. Several read-out systems are used for these assays, but enzyme immunoassay (EIA) with the aid of a cocktail of type-specific probes and reversed line blot assays (e.g., LiPA) are most common.[25,26] By adapting the composition of the probes, these assays have the potency to detect all high-risk HPV types. However, these methods have been applied with different number of probes, which may in part explain the variable HPV detection rates described in the literature. General or consensus primers are used for primary screening of cervical cancer or clinical management of women with CIN.

What are the implications of testing?

Cervical cancer screening has important drawbacks including low attendance rates and the limited sensitivity of cytologic screening, resulting in high numbers of false-negative cases.[27,28] In an attempt to increase the sensitivity of cytology, its specificity was reduced to as low as 70%.[29,30] In screening programs, this resulted in a high number of women diagnosed with borderline or mildly dyskaryotic smears among women without CIN 2 or 3, leading to unnecessary costly follow-up and anxiety among women concerned. A more accurate screening tool is needed.

Another problem in screening is the high rate of spontaneous regression of CIN. Regression rates of 57%, 43%, and 32% have been reported in CIN 1, CIN 2, and CIN 3, respectively.[17] Natural history data for CIN have important implications in the formulation of treatment policy (i.e., whether to treat or follow-up). Therefore, there is a strong need for new and better progression markers to predict the clinical outcome of an individual woman. Selecting only those women with CIN at risk for progression could prevent overtreatment. Therefore, the use of high-risk HPV testing next to cervical cytology is proposed.

What does an abnormal test result mean?

Women with a normal cervical smear. In women with normal cervical cytology the prevalence of high-risk HPV is age-related. Figures of 20% are found in women between 20 and 29 years and 4% in women older than 35 years.[13] This decrease indicates that HPV infections are very common in young women and frequently resolve spontaneously. On the other hand, the cumulative risk of CIN 3 in women with a normal cervical smear and a positive high-risk HPV test is considerable: relative risk (RR), 116; 95% confidence interval (CI), 13–990.[31]

Women with an abnormal cervical smear. A positive high-risk HPV test in women with an abnormal cervical smear indicates a higher chance of having an underlying cervical lesion. When taking into account only the sensitive amplification methods like PCR and HCII, a wide range of high-risk HPV positive tests are found in CIN 1: 30% to 65%. There is a greater consistency regarding sensitivity rates for detecting CIN 3; these are in the range of 60% to 90%, with somewhat lower values for CIN 2: 40% to 70%.[32]

Numerous studies conclude that additional testing for high-risk HPV in cervical cancer screening will improve sensitivity and specificity of conventional cytology. There is a wide range of results, depending on the population under study, the assay used, and the quality of the study. Overall, the sensitivity of high-risk HPV testing to detect CIN 2 or 3 in studies of women with low-grade cytologic abnormalities ranges between 70% and 85%. When high-risk HPV testing was used as an adjunct to cytology, the detection rates for CIN 3 rose from 93% to 100%.[30,33] In another study, additional high-risk HPV testing identified 41% of women with CIN 2 or 3 who would have been missed by screening using only cytology.[34] The specificity of high-risk HPV testing can be improved with measurement of viral load.[22]

Women treated for CIN. Failure rates of 5% to 15% have been observed following treatment for CIN 2 or 3 (high-grade CIN). One of the drawbacks of close cytologic follow-up after treatment is that many women present with abnormal cervical cytology, but an underlying CIN lesion is present in only 40% to 60%, indicating high sensitivity but low specificity for residual or recurrent CIN.[35,36]

Effective treatment for CIN results in the eradication of high-risk HPV infection present before treatment. High-risk HPV is often present in residual or recurrent lesions. In one observational study, it appeared that a positive high-risk HPV test 6 months after treatment was more predictive of residual or recurrent CIN than abnormal cervical cytology (sensitivity 90% vs. 62%). When both cervical smear and high-risk HPV test were negative, the chance of recurrent or residual CIN was extremely low (negative predictive value after 6 months, 99%; after 24 months, 100%).[37] In one meta-analysis, the results of high-risk HPV testing next to cervical cytology showed a sensitivity and specificity for residual or recurrent disease of 98% versus 81%, respectively, with positive and negative predictive values of 46% and 99%, respectively.[38]

What does a normal test result mean?
Women with a normal cervical smear. No risk of underlying high-grade CIN or cervical cancer.

Women with an abnormal cervical smear. In most cases, the women have already cleared their high-risk HPV infection. In time, the lesion will regress and the cytology become normal.[18,19] Cytologic regression is seen in all women with moderate to severe dyskaryosis and a negative high-risk HPV compared with 85% in women with mild dyskaryosis.[18] False-negative results of high-risk HPV in women with CIN 3 are seen in about 2%.[16]

What is the cost of testing?

The cost-effectiveness of high-risk HPV screening in population-based cervical cancer screening depends on the test used and the age of women being screened. In The Netherlands, all women between 30 and 60 years are invited to participate every 5 years. Whether implementing high-risk HPV screening in conjunction with cervical cytology is cost-effective is now being investigated in a prospective, randomized study including 44,000 women. Inclusion data have been published recently.[39]

▪ Conclusions and Recommendations

The addition of high-risk HPV testing to cervical cancer screening in addition to cervical cytology, plays an important role in the identification of women at risk of developing high-grade cervical lesions and cervical cancer. In the US, high-risk HPV testing has already been incorporated in the management of women with CIN.[40] Other countries are still in the process of performing cost-effectiveness studies before high-risk HPV testing can be included as an adjunct to cervical cytology in cervical cancer screening programs.

A major problem with the addition of high-risk HPV testing is that it does not improve the low specificity of cytologic screening alone, especially when high-risk HPV testing is performed in young women with a high percentage of transient infections and no underlying lesion. Because most CIN regresses spontaneously, it is necessary to identify only those women with a persistent high-risk HPV infection. They are the ones who are "at risk" to develop cervical cancer. Women with one high-risk HPV positive test have a high chance of clearing the infection, with additional disappearance of possible epithelial changes. Since a high-risk HPV infection is common in women under the age of 30 years, additional testing will only be beneficial in women over 30 years of age.

In women with a normal cervical smear and a high-risk HPV negative test the screening interval can be prolonged.

Women with borderline to mild dyskaryosis will reach cytologic regression in about 50% after a wait-and-see period of 6 months.[18] About 30% of these women are high-risk–HPVpositive at their initial visit. Since progression to CIN 3 in women without high-risk HPV is not observed, the addition of colposcopy to the testing paradigm is not needed. Further, regression can be expected in those women with an abnormal cervical smear. Only women who are persistently positive for high-risk HPV with abnormal cytology should be referred for colposcopy because only these women are at risk of developing high-grade cervical lesions. A wait-and-see policy of 6 months is advocated in women with borderline to mild dyskaryosis.

In one Dutch study, similar regression and progression rates were seen in women with mild and moderate dyskaryosis.[18] To reduce costs, it may be worthwhile to initiate a wait-and-see policy in women with moderate dyskaryosis to allow for the clearance of the high-risk HPV infection. This means that a 4% risk of developing CIN 3 after retesting in 6 months must be weighed against a 20% chance of cytologic regression.

Women with severe dyskaryosis should be referred for colposcopy immediately, regardless of high-risk HPV test results. Regression rates are low in these women and the progression rates relatively high.

In women treated for CIN 2 and 3, additional high-risk HPV testing should be used in monitoring initial treatment. A decrease in frequency of screening post-treatment can be considered if negative. Testing only at 6 months appears to be sufficient. However, re-testing after 24 months as a safety net is a consideration to avoid missing severe lesions because of detection problems or newly acquired infections with high-risk HPV. If both the cervical smear and high-risk HPV test are negative, women may be referred to the routine screening program. Prospective studies investigating this regimen are underway.

■ Summary

1 ■ What Is the Problem that Requires Screening?

Cervical cancer.

a. What is the incidence/prevalence of the target condition?

The age-adjusted annual incidence rate varies from 4–15/100,000 women in countries with well-organized screening programs compared with 20–54/100,000 in developing countries.

b. What are the sequelae of the condition that are of interest in clinical medicine?

HPV is a ubiquitous virus. The lifetime risk of acquiring HPV is about 80%. Transmission of high-risk HPV is associated with sexual intercourse. About 20% of a high-risk HPV infection will lead to morphologic changes of the cervical epithelium (i.e., CIN). When not treated, only 1% to 2% of women ultimately develop invasive cervical cancer in about 12 to 15 years.

2 ■ The Tests

a. What is the purpose of the tests?

To identify women with a high risk of developing cervical cancer.

b. What is the nature of the tests?

The tests most commonly used are the commercially available HCII and consensus PCR methods. Eighteen high-risk types have been identified so far, namely: HPV type 16, 18, 26, 31, 33, 35, 39, 45, 51, 52, 53, 56, 58, 59, 66, 68, 73, and 82. The most prevalent type found in cervical cancer is HPV type 16, followed by HPV type 18.

c. What are the implications of testing?

1. What does an abnormal test result mean?

A woman who has a positive high-risk HPV test, but a normal cytologic smear, likely has a transient HPV infection. A woman who has a positive high-risk HPV test and an abnormal cytologic smear is at high risk of developing CIN, and if untreated, potentially cervical cancer.

2. What does a normal test result mean?
A woman with a negative HPV test and a normal cytologic smear does not have a high-grade CIN or cervical cancer. A woman with a negative HPV test but an abnormal cytologic smear has probably cleared her high-risk HPV infection and will subsequently revert to normal cervical cytology.

d. What is the cost of testing?
The cost-effectiveness of high-risk HPV screening is presently unknown.

3 ■ Conclusions and Recommendations

In cervical cancer screening, additional testing for high-risk HPV, next to cervical cytology, plays an important role in the identification of women at risk of developing high-grade cervical lesions and cervical cancer. Its role in a screening program remains unclear until further evidence of cost-effectiveness accrues.

References

1. Bosch FX, de Sanjose S, Castellsague X, et al. Geographical and social patterns of cervical cancer incidence. In: Franco E, Monsonego J, eds. *New Developments in Cervical Cancer Screening and Prevention,* 1997:23–30.
2. Zur Hausen H. Condylomata acuminata and human genital cancer. *Cancer Res* 1976;36:794.
3. IARC. *Monographs on the Evaluation of the Carcinogenic Risks to Human, Vol. 64, The Human Papillomavirus.* Lyon: International Agency for Research on Cancer, 1995.
4. Chicareon S, Herrero R, Muñoz N, et al. Risk factors for cervical cancer in Thailand: a case-control study. *J Natl Cancer Inst* 1998;90:43–49.
5. Ngelangel C, Muñoz N, Bosch FX, et al. The causes of cervical cancer in the Philippines: a case-control study. *J Natl Cancer Inst* 1998;90:50–57.
6. Bosch FX, Manos MM, Muñoz N, et al. Prevalence of human papillomavirus in cervical cancer: a world-wide perspective: International Biological Study on Cervical Cancer (IBSCC) Study group. *J Natl Cancer Inst* 1995;87:796–802.
7. Walboomers JMM, Jacobs MV, Manos MM, et al. Human papillomavirus is a necessary cause of invasive cervical cancer worldwide. *J Pathol* 1999;189:12–19.
8. Chaouki N, Bosch FX, Muñoz N, et al. The viral origin of cervical cancer in Rabat, Morocco. *Int J Cancer* 1998;75:546–554.
9. Rolon PA, Smith JS, Muñoz N, et al. Human papillomavirus infection and invasive cervical cancer in Paraguay. *Int J Cancer* 2000;85:486–491.
10. Schiffman MH. Recent progress in defining the epidemiology of human papillomavirus infection and cervical neoplasia. *J Natl Cancer Inst* 1992;84:394–398.

11. Kjaer SK, Chackerian B, van den Brule AJ, et al. High-risk human papillomavirus is sexually transmitted: evidence from a follow-up study of virgins starting sexual activity (intercourse). *Cancer Epidemiol Biomarkers Prev* 2001;10:101–106.

12. Winer RL, Lee SK, Hughes JP, et al. Genital human papillomavirus infection: incidence and risk factors in a cohort of female university students. *Am J Epidemiol* 2003;157:218–226.

13. Jacobs MV, Walboomers JMM, Snijders PJF, et al. Age-related distribution patterns of 37 mucosotropic HPV types in women with cytomorphologically normal cervical smears: decreased high/low risk ratio at older age. *Int J Cancer* 2000;87:221–227.

14. Hinchliffe SA, van Velzen D, Korporaal H, et al. Transience of cervical HPV infection in sexually active, young women with normal cervicovaginal cytology. *Br J Cancer* 1995;72:943–945.

15. Ho GYF, Bierman R, Beardsley L, et al. Natural history of cervicovaginal papillomavirus infection in young women. *N Engl J Med* 1998;338:423–428.

16. Nobbenhuis MAE, Walboomers JMM, Helmerhorst ThJM, et al. Relation of human papillomavirus status to cervical lesions and consequences for cervical-cancer screening: a prospective study. *Lancet* 1999;354:20–25.

17. Östör AG. The natural history of cervical intraepithelial neoplasia: a critical review. *Int J Gynecol Pathol* 1993;12:186–192.

18. Nobbenhuis MAE, Helmerhorst ThJM, van den Brule AJC, et al. Cytological regression and high-risk HPV clearance in women referred for colposcopy because of an abnormal cervical smear. *Lancet* 2001;358:1782–1783.

19. Zielinski GD, Snijders PJF, Rozendaal L, et al. High-risk HPV testing in women with borderline and mild dyskaryosis: long-term follow-up data and clinical relevance. *J Pathol* 2001;195:300–306.

20. Kjaer SK, van den Brule AJC, Paull G, et al. Type specific persistence of high risk human papillomavirus (HPV) is an indicator of high grade cervical squamous intraepithelial lesions in young women: population based prospective follow-up study. *BMJ* 2002;325:572–578.

21. Helmerhorst ThJM, Meijer CJLM. Cervical cancer should be considered as a rare complication of oncogenic HPV infection rather than a STD. *Int J Gynecol Cancer* 2002;12:235–236.

22. Schlecht NF, Trevisan A, Duarte-Franco E, et al. Viral load as an predictor of the risk of cervical intraepithelial neoplasia. *Int J Cancer* 2003;103:519–524.

23. Muñoz N, Bosch FX, de Sanjose S, et al. Epidemiologic classification of human papillomavirus types associated with cervical cancer. *N Engl J Med* 2003;348:518–527.

24. Lorincz A. Hybrid Capture method for detection of human papillomavirus DNA in clinical specimens. *Papillomavirus Report* 1996;7:1–5.

25. Jacobs MV, van den Brule AJC, Snijders PJF, et al. A general primer GP5+/6+ mediated PCR-EIA for rapid detection of high- and low-risk HPV DNA in cervical scrapes. *J Clin Microbiol* 1997;35:791–795.

26. Kleber B, van Doorn LJ, Schrauwen L, et al. Development and clinical evaluation of a highly sensitive PCR-reverse hybridization line probe assay for detection and identification of anogenital human papillomavirus. *J Clin Microbiol* 1999;37:2508–2517.

27. Koss LG. The Papanicolaou test for cervical cancer detection: a triumph and a tragedy. *JAMA* 1989;261:737–743.

28. Raffle AE, Alden B, Mackenzie EFD. Detection rates for abnormal cervical smears: what are we screening for? *Lancet* 1995;345:1469–1473.

29. Reid R, Greenberg MD, Lörincz A, et al. Should cervical cytologic testing be augmented by cervicography or human papillomavirus deoxyribonucleic acid detection? *Am J Obstet Gynecol* 1991;164:1461–1471.

30. Cox JT, Lörinzc AT, Schiffman MH, et al. Human papillomavirus testing by hybrid capture appears to be useful in triaging women with a cytologic diagnosis of atypical squamous cells of undetermined significance. *Am J Obstet Gynecol* 1995;172:946–954.

31. Rozendaal L, Walboomers JMM, van der Linden JC, et al. PCR-based high risk HPV test in cervical cancer screening gives objective risk assessment of women with cytomorphologically normal cervical smears. *Int J Cancer* 1996;68:766–769.

32. Cuzick J, Sasieni P, Davies P, et al. A systematic review of the role of human papillomavirus testing within a cervical screening programme. *Health Technol Assess* 1999;3:1–196.
33. Wright TC Jr, Sun XW, Koulos J. Comparison of management algorithms for the evaluation of women with low-grade cytologic abnormalities. *Obstet Gynecol* 1995;85:202–210.
34. Cuzick J, Swarewski A, Terry G, et al. Human papillomavirus testing in primary cervical screening. *Lancet* 1995;345:1533–1536.
35. Bigrigg A, Haffenden DK, Sheehan AL, et al. Efficacy and safety of large-loop excision of the transformation zone. *Lancet* 1994;343:32–34.
36. Bollen LJM, Tjong-A-Hung SP, Mol BW, et al. Prediction of recurrent cervical dysplasia by human papillomavirus detection among patients with abnormal cytology. *Gynecol Oncol* 1999;72:199–201.
37. Nobbenhuis MAE, Meijer CJLM, van den Brule AJC, et al. Addition of high-risk HPV testing improves the current guidelines on follow-up after treatment for Cervical Intraepithelial Neoplasia. *Br J Cancer* 2001;84:796–801.
38. Zielinski GD, Bais AG, Helmerhorst ThJM, et al. HPV testing and monitoring of women after treatment of CIN 3: review of the literature and meta-analysis. *Obstet Gynecol Survey* 2004;59:543–553.
39. Bulkmans NWJ, Rozendaal L, Snijders PJF, et al. POBASCAM a population-based randomized controlled trial for implementation of high-risk HPV testing in cervical cancer screening: design, methods and baseline of 44,102 women. *Int J Cancer* 2004;110:94–101.
40. Wright TC, Cox JT, Massad LS, et al. 2001 Consensus guidelines for the management of women with cervical intraepithelial neoplasia. *Am J Obstet Gynecol* 2003;189:295–304.

51

Transvaginal Ultrasound as a Screening Method for Ovarian Cancer

Paul D. DePriest

Frederick R. Ueland

John R. van Nagell, Jr.

■ What Is the Problem that Requires Screening?

Ovarian cancer.

What is the incidence/prevalence of the target condition?

There will be an estimated 25,580 new cases of ovarian cancer in the United States this year, and 16,000 women will die of their disease.[1] An estimated 165,000 women worldwide will develop ovarian cancer this year. Ovarian cancer rates are highest in the industrialized countries of Europe (13/100,000) and North America (11/100,000), and lowest in the developing countries of Asia and Africa (3/100,000).[2] The annual incidence of ovarian cancer in the general population increases to approximately 50/100,000 women over 50 years of age.[3] Other factors that increase the risk of ovarian cancer include family history, nulliparity, early menarche, and delayed childbearing.[4,5] Approximately 5% of ovarian cancer cases may be due to hereditary syndromes, which have a small but definite effect on risk.[6] As a result, the risk of ovarian cancer is higher in women with a family history. For example, the incidence of ovarian cancer in English women who have at least one close relative with the disease is 390/100,000 per year, or approximately ten times the risk of ovarian cancer in the general population.[7] In contrast, oral contraceptive pills and breast-feeding each have a protective effect on the development of ovarian cancer. It is unclear whether the use of fertility drugs alters the risk of ovarian cancer.[8]

What are the sequelae of the condition that are of interest in clinical medicine?

Despite effective tumor debulking and appropriate chemotherapy, the prognosis for the woman with ovarian cancer is poor. Five-year survival rates are typically 25% to 30% in patients with stage III and IV disease.[1] In contrast, cancer confined to the ovary itself (stage I disease) is highly curable, with 5-year survival rates approaching 90% to 95%.[1, 9] Any such comparison should acknowledge lead-time bias (see Chapter 1).

The economic burden of ovarian cancer is the highest of all gynecologic malignancies.[10] Many patients with stage I ovarian cancers do not require postoperative adjuvant chemotherapy, whereas advanced ovarian cancer requires both radical surgery and multiple courses of combination chemotherapy.[11] Advanced ovarian cancer often requires frequent and prolonged hospitalization, salvage chemotherapy, and additional surgeries. A cost analysis of ovarian cancer in California (1998) showed direct and indirect costs totaled $292,000 per patient.[10] Thus, the detection of ovarian cancer at an early stage could considerably reduce the cost associated with this disease.

■ The Tests

What is the purpose of the tests?

The identification of women at high risk of having ovarian cancer.

What is the nature of the tests?

Transvaginal sonography (TVS) is performed using a standard ultrasound unit with a high-resolution (5.0 Mhz or higher) vaginal transducer. Color Doppler capability may be a useful adjunct. The test is essentially painless, takes approximately 5 minutes to perform, and is well accepted by patients.[12] Each ovary is measured in three dimensions, and the ovarian volume calculated using the volume formula for an ellipsoid (length × height × width × 0.523). An ovarian volume more than 20 cm^3 in a premenopausal woman and more than 10 cm^3 in a postmenopausal woman is deemed abnormal based on volume measurements 2 standard deviations (SDs) above normal ovarian volumes for premenopausal and postmenopausal women.[13] In addition, any papillary projection from the tumor wall is classified as abnormal.

What are the implications of testing?

Who are the potential screening candidates? General screening of the premenopausal population is not advocated. Most screening protocols are open to postmenopausal women older than 50 years because the ovarian volume varies cyclically during the menstrual cycle[14] and the prevalence of ovarian cancer is highest in women over the age of 50 years. Screening may also be indicated in women older than 25 years when there is a documented family history of ovarian cancer.

Certain known germ line mutations are associated with ovarian cancer.[15] The hereditary breast-ovarian cancer (HBOC) syndrome is associated with *BRCA1* and *BRCA2* mutations. Hereditary nonpolyposis colorectal cancer (HNPCC) of the Lynch II variant is associated with numerous mismatch repair mutations (*hMSH2, hMLH1, hPMS2, hMSH3, and hMSH6*).[16,17] DNA testing is available for both syndromes but should be preceded by genetic counseling. The susceptibility for cancer is inherited as an autosomal dominant trait in each of these syndromes. Therefore, the siblings and children of an affected individual from an ovarian cancer family each have a 50% chance of inheriting the disease trait. Epidemiologic studies suggest that in such families, gene carriers have a 40% lifetime risk of developing invasive ovarian cancer.[18, 19] The age of onset for familial ovarian cancer is much earlier than for ovarian cancer not genetically associated. Some women contract the disease as early as the third decade of life.

The 1995 National Institutes of Health (NIH) Consensus Conference concluded that it may be useful to screen women with two or more affected first-degree relatives using a combination of TVS and serum cancer antigen 125 (CA-125) testing.[11] However, widespread screening with TVS and CA-125 for ovarian cancer is not currently recommended.

After 12 years of TVS screening at the University of Kentucky, 14,500 women have received annual screens. Seventeen ovarian cancers (11 epithelial ovarian cancers) were detected in 180 persistently abnormal screens: 11 stage I, three stage II, and three stage III. All patients with stage I and II disease were alive and well without evidence of recurrence at 1.9 to 9.8 years (median, 4.5 years) after diagnosis. TVS screening for ovarian cancer was associated with the following statistical parameters: sensitivity 81%, specificity 98.9%, positive predictive value (PPV) 9.4%, and negative predictive value (NPV) 99.9%. The calculated ovarian cancer survival rate in the annually screened population was 95% at 2 years and 88.2% at 5 years.[20]

Morphology scoring systems are now used to further improve the PPV of sonography.[21] A recent modification of the Kentucky morphology index (MI) combines tumor volume and structure and is illustrated in Figure 51–1.[22] An MI score below 5 is associated with a very low risk of malignancy (< 1%), whereas a score of five or greater is associated with a 41% risk of malignancy. These findings are age independent.

What does an abnormal test result mean? Women with an abnormal sonogram have a repeated TVS in 4 to 6 weeks. If the repeated sonogram findings are abnormal, the patient undergoes morphologic indexing of the tumor, Doppler assessment of tumor blood flow, and a serum CA-125 determination. The tumor is removed either laparoscopically or by laparotomy.

What does a normal test result mean? A normal test indicates there is no sonographic evidence of abnormal ovarian size or morphology. High-risk women with a normal test are screened annually because of the potential for a fast-growing tumor.

	Tumor volume	Tumor structure
0	<10 cm^3	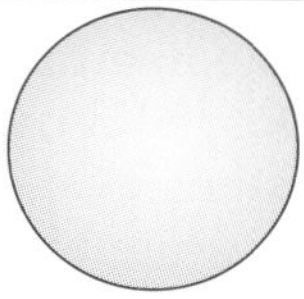
1	10–50 cm^3	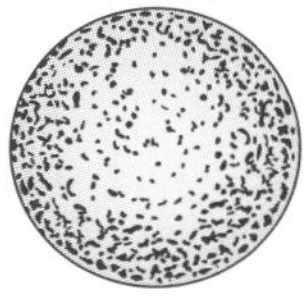
2	>50–100 cm^3	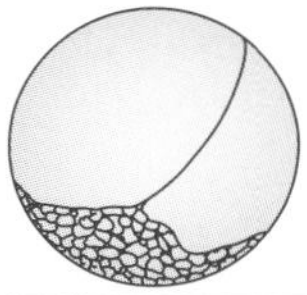
3	>100–200 cm^3	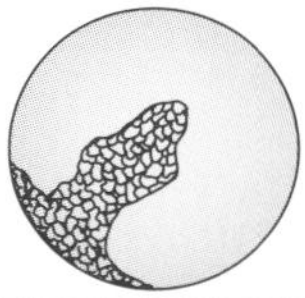
4	>200–500 cm^3	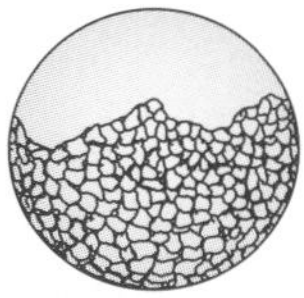
5	>500 cm^3	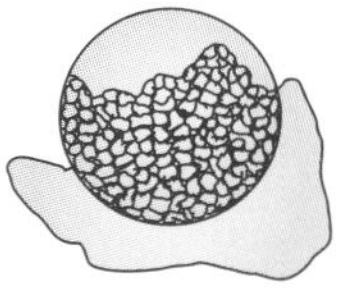

Figure 51-1 Morphology index.

What is the cost of testing?

The cost-effectiveness of screening for ovarian cancer by transvaginal ultrasound has not been evaluated.

■ Conclusions and Recommendations

Because ovarian cancer produces no symptoms until it is advanced, most women are virtually incurable at the time they present to a physician. Despite advances in surgery and chemotherapy, there has been only slight improvement in the 5-year survival rate from 1970s (37%) to the 1990s (53%).[1] Ovarian cancer is now the fourth leading cause of female cancer mortality in the United States. Clearly, methods for the early detection of ovarian cancer are highly desirable.

Data from existing ovarian cancer screening studies indicate that sonographic screening can reduce the stage at detection, and has the potential to reduce ovarian cancer mortality.[23] Not all centers have met with the same success. A properly designed, multicenter, randomized controlled trial (RCT) is needed to determine the effect of ovarian cancer screening on site-specific ovarian cancer mortality. Such a trial would also provide valuable data concerning the cost of screening, as well as the optimal population to be screened. Until such a screening trial is completed, it is premature to proceed with routine ovarian cancer screening.

■ Summary

1 ■ What Is the Problem that Requires Screening?

Ovarian cancer.

a. What is the incidence/prevalence of the target condition?

It is estimated that over 140,000 women worldwide will develop ovarian cancer this year. The annual incidence of ovarian cancer in the general population increases with age to approximately 1/2,000 women over 50 years of age.

b. What are the sequelae of the condition that are of interest in clinical medicine?

Five-year survival rates are typically 15% to 20% in women with stage III and IV disease; thus, death is a major concern.

2 ■ The Tests

a. What is the purpose of the tests?

To detect ovarian cancer in a high-risk population at an early stage.

b. What is the nature of the tests?

Transvaginal ultrasonography of the ovaries.

c. What are the implications of testing?

1. What does an abnormal test result mean?

   In most protocols, patients with an abnormal sonogram have a repeated TVS in 4 to 6 weeks. If still abnormal, the patient undergoes morphologic indexing of the tumor and may have additional adjuvant tests such as Doppler flow assessment of tumor blood flow or a serum CA-125 determination. The patient undergoes operative removal of a persisting abnormality either through the laparoscope or by open laparotomy.

2. What does a normal test result mean?

   A normal test indicates there is no sonographic evidence of an ovarian abnormality. Women are screened annually.

d. What is the cost of testing?

Cost of testing depends on the acceptable level of surgery for benign ovarian disorders. The cost ranges between $40,000 and $100,000 per case of ovarian cancer identified including the cost of surgery for benign lesions. These costs should be examined in the context of the medical costs required for a patient with stage III or IV ovarian cancer (over $200,000/case) versus the costs for a patient with stage I ovarian cancer ($10,000/case).

3 ■ Conclusions and Recommendations

A properly designed national RCT is needed to determine the effect of ovarian cancer screening on site-specific ovarian cancer mortality. Such a trial would also provide valuable data concerning the cost of screening and the optimal population to be screened.

References

1. Jemal A, Tiwari R, Murray T, et al. Cancer statistics 2004. *CA Cancer J Clin* 2004;54:8–29.
2. Ferlay J, Bray F, Pisani P, et al. *Cancer Incidence, Mortality and Prevalence Worldwide,* version 1.0. Lyon: IARC Press, 2001.
3. The Surveillance Program, Division of Cancer Prevention and Control. *Cancer Statistics Review 1973–1987,* Pub. no. 90-2789. Washington DC: National Cancer Institute, 1988.

4. Greene M, Clark J, Blayney D. The epidemiology of ovarian cancer. *Semin Oncol* 1984;11:209–226.
5. Koch M, Jenkins H, Gaedke H. Risk factors of ovarian carcinoma of epithelial origin: a case control study. *Cancer Detect Prevent* 1988;13:131–136.
6. Ponder BAJ, Easton DF, Peto J. Risk of ovarian cancer associated with a family history. In: Sharp F, Mason WP, Leake RE, eds. *Ovarian Cancer*. London: Chapman & Hall, 1989:3–6.
7. Bourne TH, Whitehead M, Campbell S, et al. Ultrasound screening for familial ovarian cancer. *Gynecol Oncol* 1991;43:92–97.
8. Shoham Z. Epidemiology, etiology, and fertility drugs in ovarian epithelial carcinoma: where are we today? *Fertil Steril* 62:433–448.
9. Young RC, Walton LA, Ellenberg SS, et al. Adjuvant therapy in stage I and stage II epithelial ovarian cancer: results of two prospective randomized trials. *N Engl J Med* 1990;322:1021–1027.
10. Max W, Rice D, Sung H, et al. The economic burden of gynecologic cancers in California, 1998. *Gynecol Oncol* 2003;88:96–103.
11. NIH consensus conference. Ovarian cancer: screening, treatment and follow-up—NIH Consensus Development Panel on Ovarian Cancer. *JAMA* 1995;273:491–497.
12. van Nagell JR, Higgins RV, Donaldson ES, et al. Transvaginal sonography as a screening method for ovarian cancer: a report of the first 1000 cases screened. *Cancer* 1990;65:573–577.
13. Pavlik E, DePriest P, Gallion H, et al. Ovarian volume related to age. *Gynecol Oncol* 2000;77:410–412.
14. van Nagell JR, DePriest PD, Puls LE, et al. Ovarian cancer screening in asymptomatic postmenopausal women by transvaginal sonography. *Cancer* 1991; 68:458–462.
15. Schildkraut JM, Risch N, Thompson WD. Evaluating genetic association among ovarian, breast and endometrial cancer: evidence for a breast/ovarian relationship. *Am J Hum Genet* 1989;45:521–529.
16. Lynch H, Casey M, Shaw T, Lynch J. Hereditary Factors in Gynecologic Cancer. *The Oncologist* 1998;3:319–338.
17. Lynch HT, Lynch J. Genetic predictability and minimal cancer clues in Lynch syndrome II. *Dis Colon Rectum* 1987;30:243–246.
18. Thompson D, Easton D (on behalf of the Breast Cancer Linkage Consortium). Variation in cancer risks, by mutation position, in BRCA2 mutation carriers. *Am J Hum Genet* 2001;68:410–419.
19. Antoniou A, Pharaoh PD, Narod SA. Average risk of breast and ovarian cancer associated with BRCA1 or BRCA2 mutations detected in case series unselected for ovarian cancer: a combined analysis of 22 studies. *Am J Hum Genet* 2003;72:1117–1130.
20. van Nagell JR, DePriest P, Reedy M, et al. The efficacy of transvaginal sonographic screening in asymptomatic women at risk for ovarian cancer. *Gynecol Oncol* 2000;77:350–356.
21. DePriest PD, Varner E, Powell J, et al. The efficacy of a sonographic morphology index in identifying ovarian cancer: a multi-institutional investigation. *Gynecol Oncol* 1994;55:174–178
22. Ueland F, DePriest P, Pavlik E, et al. Preoperative differentiation of malignant from benign ovarian tumors: the efficacy of morphology indexing and doppler flow sonography. *Gynecol Oncol* 2003;91:46–50.
23. DePriest PD, van Nagell JR. Transvaginal ultrasound screening for ovarian cancer. *Clin Obstet Gynecol* 1992;35:40–44.

52

Serum CA-125 Screening for Ovarian Cancer

Kees A. Yedema

Peter Kenemans

■ What Is the Problem that Requires Screening?

Ovarian carcinoma.

What is the incidence/prevalence of the target condition?

Approximately 1/70–80 female newborns in the United States will develop ovarian cancer during their lifetime.[1,2] The lifetime risk for ovarian cancer in the general population is approximately 1.4%. Ovarian cancer can occur at any age. The median age of detection is 53 years.[3]

The incidence of ovarian cancer increases with age, from 15.7/100,000 women per year in the 40- to 44-year age group, to an estimated 40/100,000 women per year over age 50.[1,4] Fewer than 25% of affected women have ovarian tumors confined to the ovaries at diagnosis.[5,6]

Familial cases of ovarian cancer account for 3% to 10% of all women with the disease.[2,7] Overall, these women have at least a threefold risk of developing ovarian cancer.[8,9] The relative risk among women with a single first-degree relative with ovarian cancer is 3.1, whereas *BRCA1* or *BRCA2* mutation carriers have a lifetime risk of ovarian cancer between 16% and 65%.[10,11]

What are the sequelae of the condition that are of interest in clinical medicine?

Ovarian cancer is the most common cause of death in women with genital tract malignancies in Europe and North America.[12,13] Since women with early stage disease (stage I or II) do not usually have obvious clinical signs or symptoms, most women with ovarian cancer are detected after their disease has progressed to stage III or IV.

Despite appropriate therapy including cytoreductive surgery and combination chemotherapy, the 5-year survival rates of women with stage III to IV disease are poor, ranging from 5% to 20%.[14,15] Although complete clinical response is achieved in about 50% of women with advanced disease, only 25% have evidence of complete pathologic response at second-look procedures.[16] Moreover, high relapse rates are encountered in women with histologically proven complete remission.[16] In contrast, the reported 5-year survival rates after diagnosis of women with stage I or II disease are much better, ranging from 50% (stage II) to 90% (stage I) (see related information in Chapter 5).

■ The Tests

Serum cancer antigen 125 (CA-125) measurement.

What is the purpose of the tests?

To identify women with ovarian cancer at an early stage and to differentiate between benign and malignant ovarian disease in women with a pelvic mass.

What is the nature of the tests?

The standard serum CA-125 assay (Centocor CA-125 immunoradiometric assay, Horsham, PA) was introduced in the early 1980s.[17] The OC125 monoclonal antibody was generated by immunizing BALB/c mice with the OVCA 433 cell line derived from the ascitic fluid of a woman with a serous papillary cystadenocarcinoma of the ovary.[18]

Subsequently, various antibodies have been raised against the CA-125 antigen. A double-determinant immunoassay was developed using the M11 antibody as a catcher and OC125 as a tracer.[19] Using different commercially available CA-125 assay systems, reference values differ substantially from those found with the original OC125-based homologous two-site sandwich assay, described by Bast et al.,[17] which was used in the earlier studies.[20–25]

The CA-125 antigen has been partially cloned[26,27] and is encoded for by a mucin gene designated *MUC16*. The function of the CA-125 is still not understood.[28] It is postulated that the basement membrane in the normal ovary and the peritoneum prevent access of CA-125 to the circulation.[29,30] Both benign and malignant growth disturbs these natural borders and may lead to elevated CA-125 serum levels. Moreover, abdominal surgery, ascites, pleural effusions, and inflammatory processes can all elevate CA-125 serum levels, possibly as a consequence of serosal irritation and increased production by the peritoneum.[31–36]

In recent years, it has become clear that most ovarian carcinomas arise from monoclonal single cells in the ovary and not from multiple primary tumors in both the ovaries and peritoneum.[85,86] However, the duration of stage I disease is still unknown. This time interval should be sufficiently long enough to permit screening for curable early ovarian cancer should an effective technique be available.

It is yet not clear whether advanced ovarian carcinomas are always proceeded by clinical detectable stage I disease or that a significant proportion of ovarian carcinomas, which present with metastasized disease, have tumor spread to the peritoneal cavity before the ovarian tumor itself has grown large enough to be clinically detected. The survival advantage is primarily due to the detection of early stage I ovarian cancer.

Elevated levels of CA 125 are typically defined as in excess of 35 U/mL. The exact sensitivity and specificity of the CA-125 test is difficult to estimate because ovarian cancer is a relatively rare disease and consequently large patient numbers are required to obtain reliable data. Elevated levels have been observed from 10 months to more than 5 years before any clinical manifestation of ovarian cancer.[47,48] On the other hand, only 41% of women with stage I disease have a serum CA-125 level greater than 35 U/mL.[33]

What are the implications of testing?

What does an abnormal test result mean?

Asymptomatic women at average risk. An elevated serum CA-125 level (> 35 U/mL) is found in 80% of women with ovarian cancer, but elevated levels are found in up to 5.8% of apparently healthy women.[17,19,,23,25,33] Premenopausal women are more often falsely positive (8.8% > 35 U/mL) than postmenopausal women (0.7% > 35 U/mL).[23] Benign circumstances and diseases are often associated with an elevated CA-125 serum level. Both pregnancy and menstruation can cause elevated CA-125 levels. Other benign gynecologic diseases that frequently lead to an elevation include pelvic inflammatory disease and endometriosis.[24,25] An estimated 36% of women with endometriosis have CA-125 levels exceeding 35 U/mL.[33] Other well-known nongynecologic causes of an elevated serum CA-125 level include congestive heart failure, pancreatitis, hepatitis, and liver cirrhosis.[19,32,37-45]

Malignancies other than ovarian cancer are often associated with an elevated serum CA-125 level. More than half of the women with nonovarian pelvic malignancies have CA-125 levels exceeding 35 U/mL, particularly tumors metastatic to the ovaries and those originating from the endometrium or the colon.[33] Sjovall et al.[46] found a difference in cancer risk between women who participated in an ovarian cancer screening trial and were found to have an elevated CA-125 level as opposed to women with normal CA-125 levels at screening. Malignancies were detected in 6.9% of women with an elevated level compared with 1.6% of women with normal levels. It was concluded that asymptomatic women with an elevated CA-125 level should be investigated for lung or breast cancer after ovarian cancer has been ruled out.[46]

An elevated CA-125 serum screening is usually followed by ultrasound. In one systematic review of prospective screening tests for ovarian cancer in asymptomatic women, 25 studies were identified: Sixteen studies concerned women at average risk and nine were in women at high risk of ovarian cancer.[49] Various large screening studies are summarized in Table 52–1 (women at average risk) and Table 52–2 (women at high risk).

Einhorn et al.[50] identified six women with ovarian cancer using CA-125 as a first-line screening test in a study of 5,550 women 40 years of age and over. Women with an elevated CA-125 level underwent serial CA-125 measurements, pelvic examination, and ultrasound. Two patients had stage I disease,

Table 52-1	Ovarian cancer screening studies in asymptomatic women based on CA125 in combination with ultrasound						
Author	No. screened	Patient characteristics	Screening strategy	No. of primary ovarian cancer detected	No. of primary epithelial ovarian cancer missed	No. of months detected after screen	Follow-up
Einhorn 1992[50]	5.500	≥40 y	CA125, then AUS if CA125 >35 U/ml; later: > 30 U/ml	6 (2 stage I, 2 stage II, 2 stage III)	3 (1 stage I, 2 stage III)	12–22 mo	median 32 mo range 32–46 mo
Jacobs 1993[51]	22.000	≥45 y and postmenopausal	CA125, then AUS CA125 >30 U/ml	11 (3 stage I, 1 stage II, 5 stage III, 2 stage IV)	8 (5 stage I, 3 stage III)	6–22 mo	12-24 mo
Grover 1995[52]	2.550	≥40 y and 3% familial ovarian cancer	CA125, then AUS or VUS if CA125 >35 U/ml on repeat testing	0	1 (1 stage III)	10 mo	12 mo
Adonakis 1996[53]	2.000	≥45 y	CA125, then VUS if CA125 >35 U/ml	2 (2 stage I, including 1 borderline ovarian cancer)	0	-	"at least" 12 mo
Total	32.050			19	12		

AUS, abdominal ultrasound; VUS, vaginal ultrasound; mo, month; y, year.

Table 52–2 **Screening trials in high-risk women using ultrasound and CA125**

Author	No. screened	No. of ovarian cancer detected	No. of ovarian cancer missed
Muto 1993[54]	386	0	0
Bourne 1994[55]	1502	7 (5 stage I, 1 stage II, 1 stage III)	unknown
DePriest 1997[56]	6470	6 (5 stage I, 1 stage III)	1 (1 stage II)
Karlan 1999[57]	1261	7 (3 stage I, 4 stage III[1])	3 (3 stage III[2])
Laframboise 2002[58]	311	1 (1 stage I)	0
Tailor 2003[59]	2550	11 (8 stage I, 1 stage II, 2 stage III)	9 (9 stage III[3])
Total	12.480	32	13

[1]including 4 peritoneal cancers.
[2]including 3 peritoneal cancers.
[3]including 2 peritoneal cancers.

two stage II, and two stage III. Three women with ovarian carcinoma were missed, including one patient with stage I and two with stage III disease. All three patients were younger than 50 years. Specificity was calculated for women above and under 50 years. For a CA-125 cutoff of 30 U/mL, the specificity was 91% under 50 years and 97% above 50 years. For the higher cutoff level of 35 U/mL, specificities were 94.5% and 98.5%, respectively. The highest reported specificity in premenopausal women (98.8%) was achieved using a CA-125 threshold of 65 U/mL.[77] If 16/100,000 women screened have ovarian cancer, the positive predictive value (PPV) of an elevated CA-125 level for ovarian malignancy would be 1.3% at a sensitivity of 100% using the CA-125 assay for screening. Given a specificity of 98.8%, 1,200 of the 100,000 women screened would be falsely positive, implying that 75 surgical procedures would be performed per year to detect a single case of ovarian cancer. If one applies a 35 U/mL cutoff instead, the specificity decreases below 95%, and as a result, the number of false positives will increase dramatically.[50]

Jacobs et al.[51] studied 22,000 postmenopausal women 45 years of age and older. CA-125 was used as the first-line screening test, followed by ultrasound examination if the CA-125 levels were above 30 U/mL. Eleven of 19 ovarian carcinomas were detected, three patients with stage I, one patient with stage II, five patients with stage III disease, and two patients with stage IV disease. Of the eight patients missed, five had stage I and three stage III disease 6 to 22 months after the initial screening. The sequential combination of CA-125 measurement and ultrasound examination achieved a specificity of 99.9%, a positive predictive value of 26.8%, and an apparent sensitivity of 78.6%. By the 2-year follow-up, sensitivity had declined to 57.9%.

In an attempt to circumvent the problem of low specificity, some investigators have combined serial CA-125 measurements for "screen positive" with an ultrasound.[50,78] Indeed elevated CA-125 levels usually remain stable or regress to normal over time if associated with benign conditions.

The specificity of CA-125 for ovarian cancer screening could be further improved by the inclusion of new tumor markers, such as the CA-15.3 and TAG 72.3 assay but at the cost of lower sensitivity, particularly in women with stage I disease.[66,79,80]

A PPV of 10% is commonly considered reasonable. Assuming a specificity of 99.6%, a sensitivity of 100%, and a prevalence of 40 ovarian carcinomas per 100,000 women annually (1/2,500 per year), ten surgical interventions would be necessary to find one case of ovarian cancer.[35] But in reality, sensitivity will be considerably lower, especially in early stage I disease.

The specificity for CA-125 measurements tends to be better for post-menopausal women.

Table 52–1 summarizes data derived from screening trials in asymptomatic women. Overall, 19 (61%) of 31 ovarian cancers were detected. Although the aim of screening with CA-125 was to detect women with ovarian cancer at an early and curable stage, only seven of the 19 women with ovarian cancer detected by screening had stage I disease at surgery.

Women at high risk. CA-125 may also be used for targeted screening of women considered to be at high risk of ovarian cancer. Muto at al.[54] studied the combination of repeated CA-125 measurements and ultrasound examinations in 386 women with a family history of ovarian cancer. If elevated, the CA-125 measurement was repeated in 3 months. A doubling over 3 months or a rise above 95 U/mL prompted further evaluation. Initially, 42 women (11%) had a CA-125 level above 35 U/mL. Forty-one of these 42 women were premenopausal. Eventually, 15 had surgery, and no malignancies were found. Bourne et al.[55] assessed the value of CA-125 measurement as an adjunct to an ultrasound-based screening program for ovarian cancer in women with a history of ovarian cancer. Sixty percent of the women were premenopausal. A vaginal ultrasound was performed and CA-125 levels measured at the first visit. Abnormal initial scans were repeated 3 to 8 weeks later. Of the 1,502 women evaluated, 62 (4.1%) had an abnormal repeated ultrasound scan and were surgically evaluated. Ovarian cancer was found in seven women, six of whom were premenopausal. Five patients had stage I disease including three borderline malignancies, one patient had stage II and one patient had advanced stage III disease. Only three of the even patients had elevated CA-125 levels above 35 U/mL. In fact, all women with ovarian cancer were detected using ultrasound alone. These authors concluded that CA-125 measurements were not helpful for screening purposes in a high-risk population.

From 1987 to 1993, 6,470 women with a mean age of 58 years were enrolled in an ovarian cancer screening project of which the clinical outcome was reported by DePriest et al.[56] (see Chapter 51). Both pre- and postmenopausal women were included and 24% had a history of familial ovarian cancer. Vaginal ultrasound was the first-line screening method. If a repeated ultrasound was persistently abnormal, CA-125 levels were measured. Normal screens were repeated on a yearly basis. Six ovarian carcinomas were detected by ultrasound including five stage I cancers and one stage III ovarian cancer. None of these women had an elevated CA-125 level and only one had a palpable abnormality. One stage II ovarian cancer was missed and found 11 months after the last screen.[56]

Karlan et al.[57] found ten cases of ovarian cancer or peritoneal serous papillary carcinoma in 1,261 patients aged 35 years and older seen in a familial ovarian cancer screening clinic. Screening was initially offered biannually, and from 1995 on, annually. The screening program consisted of ultrasound assessment and CA-125 measurement. Three stage I ovarian cancers were found by ultrasound, whereas the CA-125 levels were normal. Peritoneal cancers were found in two of seven women by ultrasound and two by CA-125 elevations despite normal ultrasound findings. Peritoneal carcinomas in three women were only detected by clinical symptoms 5, 6, and 16 months after the last visit.[57] The authors concluded that women with papillary serous peritoneal carcinomas cannot rely on ultrasound and CA-125 testing. Laframboise et al.[58] studied 311 high-risk women with a mean age of 47 years using CA-125 and ultrasound biannually. In 7 years of screening, only one stage I ovarian carcinoma was detected by ultrasound when the CA-125 was normal. Of the CA-125 results, 2.7% were abnormal as opposed to 17% of the ultrasound findings.[58]

In a recent report, 11 ovarian carcinomas were detected among 2,550 predominantly premenopausal women participating in a familial ovarian cancer screening program with a mean age of 48 years.[59] This targeted screening program was ultrasound-based and CA-125 levels were measured retrospectively. The screened group showed eight stage I ovarian cancers (including four borderline tumors), one stage II, and two stage III ovarian cancers. Seven ovarian malignancies were missed, as were two peritoneal carcinomas, all presenting with stage III disease. All these cases were found 9 to 46 months after the last scan. If CA-125 had been used as a first-line screen, most ovarian carcinomas would have been missed. The sensitivity was only 33% at the 35-U/mL cutoff level.

In summary, annual screening comprising pelvic examination, transvaginal ultrasound, and CA-125 determination is recommended for women with a hereditary ovarian cancer syndrome.

Table 52–2 summarizes the results of various screening trials based on ultrasound and CA-125 levels measured simultaneously, if only ultrasound results were abnormal, or retrospectively. In total, 45 ovarian cancers were reported, of which 32 (71%) were detected by screening, whereas 13 were missed (29%) including some cases of peritoneal cancer.

These targeted screening programs for familial ovarian cancer are encouraged to contribute data on the women to large randomized controlled trials comparing regular physical examination, ultrasound, and CA-125 levels alone or in combinations and at varying intervals to obtain more evidence for the most effective screening strategy in high-risk women. False-positive rates are calculated to range between 1.2% and 2.5% for gray-scale ultrasound, 0.3% and 0.7% for color Doppler ultrasound, and between 0.1% and 0.6% for CA-125 assay followed by ultrasound screening.[49]

Women with a palpable pelvic mass. The serum CA-125 assay has been used to discriminate between benign and malignant pelvic masses. The differential diagnosis of a pelvic mass varies widely and includes both benign diseases such as benign ovarian neoplasms, pseudocysts, fibroids, hydrosalpinges, tubo-ovarian abscesses, and diverticulitis as well as malignant diseases originating from the ovary, uterus, bowel, or urinary tract. Adequate discrimination between benign and malignant pelvic masses could facilitate optimal preoperative planning, rendering the likelihood of inadequate surgery lower.

Eighty-five percent of women with ovarian cancer have an elevated CA-125 level (>35 U/mL) compared with 26% of women with benign ovarian tumors.[33] If 65 U/mL is considered the upper limit of normal in premenopausal women with a pelvic mass, approximately 50% to 60% of all patients with malignant disease still have elevated CA-125 levels with a specificity of about 90% (Table 52–3). In postmenopausal women, the use of the lower 35-U/mL cutoff level seems justified, with a higher sensitivity of about 80% and a specificity around 85% (Table 52–3).

The additive value of combinations of tumor markers such as CA-15.3 or CA72-4 next to CA-125 for the discrimination between benign from malignant disease is limited. If a positive test result is defined as "all diagnostic tests being positive," sensitivity will decrease whereas specificity increases. If a positive test result is defined as "only one of the tumor markers being elevated," sensitivity increases but specificity declines.[66–68] Schutter et al.[68] evaluated 412 pre- and postmenopausal women with a pelvic mass. Specificity was as high as 99% when a positive test was defined as three concomitantly elevated serum tumor markers. However, sensitivity was as low as 28% using this criteria.[68] If CA-125 was elevated in combination with elevated CA-15-3 or CA-72-4, sensitivity rose

Table 52–3   Performance of the CA125 test in discriminating a benign mass from a malignant mass in premenopausal and postmenopausal patients

Author	N Total	Sens	Spec	PPV	NPV
Premenopausal (cut-off level 65 U/ml)					
Malkasian 1988[60]	66	60	89	49	93
Gadduci 1992[61]	213	50	87	24	96
Postmenopausal (cut-off level 35 U/ml)					
Finkler 1988[62]	32	84	92	94	80
Malkasian 1988[60]	92	81	91	94	74
Patsner 1988[63]	125	77	81	87	68
Schutter 1994[64]	228	72	80	73	79
Maggino 1994[65]	290	78	82	78	83

Sens, sensitivity, the percentage of patients with malignant disease having a positive test result; Spec, specificity, the percentage of patients with benign disease having a negative test result; PPV, positive predictive value, the percentage of patients with a positive test result having malignant disease; NPV, negative predictive value, the percentage of patients with a negative test result having benign disease.

to 48% and specificity decreased to 93%. Sensitivity for the CA-125 assay as a single test at the 35-U/mL cutoff level was 60% with a specificity of 76%. The resulting PPV was 77% and negative predictive value (NPV), 59%. Even if all three markers showed normal levels, malignancy could not be excluded.[68]

Jacobs et al.[69] devised a risk of malignancy index (RMI) incorporating several parameters including CA-125 as a continuous variable, ultrasound features, and menopausal status.[69] For the ultrasound segment, one point is given for features such as multilocular disease, solid areas, abdominal metastases, ascites, or bilateral lesions. The ultrasound score is 0 for 0 points, 1 for 1 point or 3 for 2 to 5 points. For menopausal status, a score of 1 is given if premenopausal and a score of 3 if postmenopausal. The RMI is the product of the ultrasound score (U), the menopausal score (M) and the absolute value of CA-125 serum levels:

$$RMI = U \times M \times CA\text{-}125$$

A score above 200 suggests malignant disease. The RMI was a superior discriminator to individual parameters such as CA-125, menopausal status, or ultrasound score. Sensitivity was around 80% and specificity around 90%, and the RMI is applicable to both premenopausal and postmenopausal women. The RMI has been validated in both retrospective and prospective series and seems a simple but practical method to differentiate between benign and malignant pelvic masses. Cumulative data are summarized in Table 52–4. Tingulstad et al.[70, 71] modified the original RMI by changing the scoring of U (ultrasound) and M (menopausal status). They found the RMI II performed significantly better than the RMI I, an observation confirmed by Morgante et al.[72] Both methods were more accurate than menopausal status, CA-125, or ultrasound separately. Aslam et al.[73] found no differences among the performances of RMI I II and III.[73,74]

Andersen et al.[75] reported limitations of the RMI II in borderline tumors and stage I invasive ovarian cancers.[75] Forty-four percent of patients with stage I ovarian cancer and 83% patients with borderline tumors had RMI scores below 200, although the clinical relevance of these findings seems limited.

Overall, applying the RMI, sensitivity is around 75%, and specificity around 90% in the differentiation of benign from malignant pelvic masses. Which of the three RMI methods gives the best results is still a matter of debate. However, reported sensitivities in more recent studies reveal consistently lower sensitivities compared with the earlier reports of Jacobs et al.[69] and Davies et al.[76]

Schutter et al.[64] combined CA-125 measurement, physical examination, and ultrasound in a group of 228 postmenopausal patients to discriminate benign from malignant disease. One point was given for CA-125 35 U/mL or lower, 2 for CA-125 above 35 U/mL. A benign clinical impression at physical examination was given 1 point, suspected malignancy was given 2 points; ultrasound score was given 1 point if the Finkler score was below 7 and 2 points if the Finkler score was 7 or higher. The ultrasound criteria used by Finkler et al.[62] are

Table 52-4   **Performance of the risk of malignancy index (RMI, cut-off level > 200)**

Author	Total	No. malig-nant	No. benign	RMI method	Sens %	Spec %	PPV %	NPV %
Jacobs 1990[69]	143	42	101	RMI I[1]	85	97	—	—
Davies 1993[76]	124	37	87	RMI I	87	89	75	—
Tingulstad 1996[70]	173	56	117	RMI I	71	96	89	88
				RMI II[2]	80	92	83	91
Tingulstad 1999[71]	365	75	290	RMI III[3]	71	92	69	92
Morgante 1999[72]	124	31	93	RMI I	58	95	78	87
				RMI II	74	93	77	92
Aslam 2000[73]	61	23	38	RMI I	74	92	—	—
				RMI II	74	89		
Manjunath 2001[74]	148	93	55	RMI I	73	91	93	67
				RMI II	76	82	88	67
				RMI III	74	91	93	68
Andersen 2003[75]	402	102	300	RMI II	71	88	66	90

Sens, sensitivity, the percentage of patients with malignant disease having a positive test result; Spec, specificity, the percentage of patients with benign disease having a negative test result; PPV, positive predictive value, the percentage of patients with a positive test result having malignant disease; NPV, negative predictive value, the percentage of patients with a negative test result having benign disease.
[1]RMI I (Jacobs et al.[69]): U × M × CA125, where a total ultrasound score of 0 gave U=0, a score of 1 gave U=1, and a score of ≥2 gave U=3; premenopausal status gave M=1and postmenopausal M=3. The serum level of CA125 was applied as a continuous variable to the calculation.
[2]RMI II (Tingulstad et al.[70]): U × M × CA125, where a total ultrasound score of 0 or 1 gave U=1, and a score of ≥2 gave U=4; premenopausal status gave M=1 and postmenopausal M=4. The serum level of CA125 was applied as a continuous variable to the calculation.
[3]RMI III (Tingulstad et al.[71]): U × M × CA125, where a total ultrasound score of 0 or 1 gave U=1, and a score of ≥2 gave U=3; premenopausal status gave M=1 and postmenopausal M=3. The serum level of CA125 was applied as a continuous variable to the calculation.

described elsewhere in detail.[62] It is a 1- to 10-point scale starting with a clear smooth cyst scoring (1 point) ending with a highly suspicious mass and ascites (10 points). Overall single tests gave similar results in discriminating pelvic masses. The most sensitive single test was physical examination with 93%, but this was paired to a low specificity of 63%. The best specificity was found for CA-125 with 80%, paired to a sensitivity of 72%. Sensitivity decreased to 64% using CA-125 plus ultrasound in combination, but specificity increased till 89%. The best combination of two tests was physical examination in combination with ultrasound with a sensitivity of 83% and a specificity of 79%. If all three test results were positive, the sensitivity was 62% and specificity 92%. Malignancy was not found if all three tests were negative. The authors concluded that the combined use of two or three diagnostic methods had opposite effects on the sensitivity and specificity. If all tests were positive, sensitivity was low but specificity high. If only one of the three tests was positive, sensitivity was high but specificity low.

In a later study CA72-4 was added as an extra test to aid discrimination between benign and malignant pelvic tumors.[67] In that study, 155 postmenopausal women were selected from their previous study.[64] Again, the overall test performances of single tests were equal. CA72-4 showed the highest specificity with 93%, but this was paired with a low sensitivity of 61%. If all four tests were positive, specificity rose to 100% but sensitivity was not higher than 46%. Again, no malignancies were found when all tests scored negative. This result was found in almost half of the benign pelvic masses.[67]

What does a normal test result mean?

Asymptomatic women at average risk. Menopausal status must be considered. A negative CA-125 in the premenopausal woman effectively rules out ovarian carcinoma. A negative test in postmenopausal women is reassuring. Ultrasound could be used as a secondary screening test in postmenopausal women to improve specificity to 99.9% (Jacobs et al.,[51] Table 52–1). Given that 35 of 100,000 screened postmenopausal women have ovarian cancer, and assuming a sensitivity of 100% and a specificity of 99.9%, the PPV would only be 26%. Hence, 100 of the 100,000 screened will be falsely positive, implying that four surgical procedures should be performed to detect one case of ovarian cancer. Einhorn and co-workers[81] reported their long-term follow-up of their screened study population. Twenty ovarian carcinomas were identified through the Swedish Cancer Registry during the 10-year follow-up after the initial screening. CA-125 levels all had been in the normal range during the initial screening period for all women subsequently found to have ovarian carcinoma.[81] Ovarian cancer was diagnosed a median of 91 (range, 8–142 months) months after the initial screening. Median survival of the patients with ovarian cancer in the originally screened group was significantly better than median survival in the control group.

A negative test and a palpable mass necessitate further evaluation and potentially surgical intervention. High-risk women with a normal test result are unlikely to have ovarian carcinoma.

Women at high risk. There are limited data on CA-125 measurements in combination with ultrasound screening in women with a family history of ovarian cancer. Bourne et al.[55] found seven ovarian carcinomas, all detected by ultrasound alone. Only three women had concomitantly elevated CA-125 levels.[55] In one recent study, 11 ovarian cancers were found by an ultrasound screening program in a high-risk population. Seven of these 11 women had normal CA-125 levels. Nine stage III ovarian cancers were missed by ultrasound screening, two of these nine women had elevated CA-125 levels detected retrospectively. It was concluded that CA-125 is of limited value compared with ultrasound screening in patients with familial ovarian cancer.[59]

Hensley et al.[82] studied the consequences of false-positive screens in 147 high-risk patients who were either *BRCA1/2* mutation carriers, members of a family with the HNPCC (hereditary nonpolyposis colorectal cancer) syndrome, or with a strong family history of breast and/or ovarian cancer. All participants were offered biannual ultrasound and CA-125 measurement and repeated screening tests 4 to 6 weeks after an abnormal first ultrasound or CA-125. Among premenopausal women, 34% required repeated screens compared with 25% of postmenopausal women. CA-125 required repeat measurements in 10.8% of premenopausal women and in 4.6% of postmenopausal women. Repeated ultrasound was respectively necessary in 23.3% and 20.6%. All but one repeated screen was normal. One woman underwent surgery, but no malignancy was found. Five women underwent prophylactic surgery. The authors concluded that premenopausal women perceived higher cancer risks and anxiety while they are more likely to have false-positive screening results. Since serial screening is recommended, the lifetime risk of having a false-positive screening result is extremely high.

What is the cost of testing?

The cost-effectiveness of screening has yet to be established in a large population. Two randomized controlled screening trials in women aged 50 or more have been initiated to obtain data on the impact of screening on ovarian cancer mortality and cost-effectiveness of such programs. We eagerly await their results.

■ Conclusions and Recommendations

In asymptomatic women, the role of serum CA-125 measurement for screening purposes remains controversial. Skates and Singer[83] developed a putative model using CA-125 in a screening for women aged 50 to 75 years. Survival was prolonged by 3.4 years per case detected if the women were screened annually. Fitting serial CA-125 levels obtained from patients participating in a screening trial, the estimated mean interval between the initiation of tumor growth and clinical detection was 1.9 ± 0.4 years.[84]

There is concern about the relatively high false-positive rates particularly in premenopausal women. Even in a high-risk predominantly premenopausal population, only four of 11 ovarian cancers detected by ultrasound had CA-125 levels above 35 U/mL. Eight of these 11 ovarian cancers were early stage I, including four borderline tumors.[59] Even in women with a family history of ovarian cancer, the usefulness of CA-125 and ultrasound for the early detection of ovarian cancer remains unclear. A drawback for CA-125 targeted screening in these women is that a relatively large proportion of these women are premenopausal. Efficacy and survival data in these high-risk groups are lacking. As a result, the CA-125 assay is not suitable as a single screening test for ovarian cancer in asymptomatic premenopausal women. Recently, three new putative biomarkers for ovarian cancer were identified suggesting a potential to improve the detection of early stage ovarian cancers using serum proteomic analysis when combined with CA-125.[87]

However, in postmenopausal women, the combination of CA-125 measurement as a primary screening test with an ultrasound scan as a secondary test yields high specificities up to 99.9%. Preliminary data shown in Table 52–1 suggest that two thirds of the ovarian cancers could be identified. Unfortunately, only approximately one third of the ovarian carcinomas found are stage I.

Jacobs reported a survival benefit in a randomized controlled trial involving 22,000 postmenopausal women aged 45 years and older. Survival was significantly prolonged for the screened group compared with a control group.[88] Mortality from ovarian cancer, however, did not differ between both groups. Screening included three annual CA-125 determinations and an ultrasound examination if the CA 125 levels exceeded 30 U/mL. In the screened group, six ovarian carcinomas were found at the first screening and ten ovarian carcinomas were found during 8 years of follow-up. In the control group 20 ovarian carcinomas were identified. A long-term follow-up study in Sweden showed a better median survival in a group of ovarian cancer women detected by screening compared with women identified by clinical symptoms.[81] These two studies may be explained by lead-time bias.

Currently two randomized controlled trials for ovarian cancer screening are in progress. One study, the U.K. Collaborative Trial for Ovarian Cancer Screening (UKCTOCS), includes around 200,000 postmenopausal women aged 50 to 74 years. In this study, mortality at 7 years after randomization will be measured. Groups are randomized between ultrasound screening, ultrasound plus CA-125 screening, and a control group without screening. In the United States, the Prostate, Lung, Colon, Ovary (PLCO) trial has been started, in which 74,000 women aged 55 to 74 years will be enrolled in a 5-year randomized controlled trial. Women are included in a group with annual CA-125 and ultrasound screening and in a group without screening. Results include survival, mortality, and cost-effectiveness and are not expected for 4 to 6 years.[89]

Both studies may provide more definite answers as to whether ovarian cancer screening decreases mortality, is cost-effective, and is associated with unacceptable morbidity in women with false-positive screens undergoing unnecessary surgical procedures.

The measurement of CA-125 as a single test can be used in premenopausal women with a pelvic mass. About 85% of the pelvic masses in premenopausal women will be correctly classified if a cutoff of 65 U/mL is used. A cutoff level of 35 U/mL is advocated for postmenopausal women, where 80% will be correctly classified. A combination of tumor markers is of limited value in the discrimination of benign from malignant pelvic masses as specificity is increased at the cost of lower sensitivity. Single tumor markers or tumor marker panels seem to be less discriminative than the RMI or the combination of CA-125, physical examination, and ultrasound.

The RMI appears valuable for the preoperative evaluation of patients presenting with a pelvic mass of uncertain nature. It uses a relatively simple scoring system including ultrasound, menopausal status, and CA-125 levels. It is applicable to both pre- and postmenopausal patients. Overall sensitivity is around 75% paired to a specificity of approximately 90 %.

Since all ultrasound scoring systems are based on the interpretation of semiquantitative tumor appearance, the evaluation of which scoring system appears best remains a diagnostic challenge taking into account intra- and interobserver variability. To permit comparison of various ultrasound scores and tumor marker performance, patients should ideally be stratified for confounding variables as the distribution of malignant versus benign disease, ovarian cancer versus nonovarian cancer, the number of borderline malignancies, the number of early stage I ovarian cancers, and finally the number of nonepithelial ovarian cancers encountered in the study population.

In clinical practice, both falsely elevated CA-125 serum levels, especially in premenopausal women, and ultrasound features of malignancy shared by benign pathologies, are common. In addition, early-stage ovarian cancer is often accompanied by normal CA-125 serum levels as previously noted.

In conclusion, routine population screening for ovarian cancer is not yet a reality. However, considerable progress is being made and there are a number of modalities that appear useful to discriminate masses to screen elderly and high-risk women.

■ Summary

1 ■ What Is the Problem that Requires Screening?

Ovarian carcinoma.

a. *What is the incidence/prevalence of the target condition?*

Approximately 1/70–80 female newborns will develop ovarian cancer during their lifetime with a median age of 53 years at detection. The incidence increases with age from 15.7/100,000 women per year for the 40- to 44-year age group to an estimated 40/100,000 per year for higher age groups. Fewer than 25% of affected women have ovarian tumors confined to the ovaries at diagnosis. Familial cases of ovarian cancer account for 3% to 10% of all women with the disease. The lifetime risk for the general population is 1.4%. In contrast, it is estimated at 16-65% for *BRCA1* or *BRCA2* mutation carriers.

b. *What are the sequelae of the condition that are of interest in clinical medicine?*

Ovarian cancer is the most common cause of death in women with genital tract malignancies. Because women with stage I or II disease usually do not have clinical signs or symptoms, most women with ovarian cancer are detected after at stage III. Despite appropriate therapy, 5-year survival rates for stage III and IV disease are low (< 20%). In contrast, 5-year survival rates exceed 90% in early stage I disease.

2 ■ The Tests

a. *What is the purpose of the tests?*
To identify at an early stage women with ovarian cancer and to differentiate between benign and malignant disease in women with a pelvic mass.

b. *What is the nature of the tests?*
Standard serum CA-125 assay using a double-antibody immunoassay.

c. *What are the implications of testing?*
1. What does an abnormal test result mean?
   An elevated CA-125 serum level (>35 U/mL) is found in 1% of postmenopausal healthy women, but in up to 8% to 9% of premenopausal healthy women. Eighty percent of ovarian cancer patients have an elevated CA-125 serum level. Screening trials in asymptomatic women report a 60% detection rate, of which only one third had early stage I disease. In patients with a family history of ovarian cancer, with a large proportion of premenopausal patients, CA-125 measurements are of limited value and ultrasound screening is at present the cornerstone. Seventy-one percent of ovarian cancers are detected using ultrasound in varying combinations with CA-125 measurements.

2. What does a normal test result mean?
   Twenty percent of the patients with ovarian cancer have normal CA-125 levels. Thus normal CA-125 levels do not preclude ovarian cancer. Some 40% of the ovarian cancers in asymptomatic patients are missed at screening. In high-risk patients with a family history of ovarian cancer, preliminary data reveals that 29% of ovarian cancers will be missed by the screening methods.

c. *What is the cost of testing?*
The cost-effectiveness of screening has yet to be established in a large population.

Continued

■ **Summary—cont'd**

3 ■ Conclusions and Recommendations

CA-125 as a single test is not suitable for screening asymptomatic premenopausal women.

In postmenopausal women, the combination of CA-125 and ultrasound can reach a high specificity. Preliminary results indicate that approximately 60% of ovarian cancers are detected.

So far, around 70% of ovarian cancers are detected in high-risk patients participating in screening trials when screened at 6-month intervals or annually.

Using CA-125 as a single test to discriminate benign from malignant pelvic masses, a cutoff level of 65 U/mL is advised, with a sensitivity of 50% to 60% and a specificity of about 90%.

In postmenopausal patients, the lower 35-U/mL cutoff can be used with a higher sensitivity of approximately 80% paired with an 85% specificity.

The RMI, based on ultrasound, menopausal status, and CA-125 levels as a continuous variable, is a simple and reproducible tool in the preoperative evaluation of patients with a pelvic mass. Overall, sensitivity is approximately 75% and specificity 90%. This method is applicable in both pre- and postmenopausal patients.

The potential cost-effectiveness of screening is not known for women within the normal population or for women with a family history of ovarian cancer. The real effect on disease-free survival and mortality has yet to be established. Because ovarian cancer is a disease with a relative low incidence, screening methods based on CA-125 levels, ultrasound, and physical examination are currently being evaluated in large groups of women allowing for more definite conclusions in the near future.

References

1. Disaia P, Creasman W. Advanced epithelial ovarian cancer. In: Disaia P, Creasman W, eds. *Clinical Gynecologic Oncology*. St. Louis: CV Mosby, 1989:325–416.
2. Petterson F. *Annual FIGO Report on the Results of Treatment in Gynaecological Cancer*. Stockholm: International Federation of Gynaecology and Obstetrics, 1995.
3. Katsube Y, Berg J, Silverberg S. Epidemiologic pathology of ovarian tumors. *Int J Gynecol Pathol* 1982;1:3–16.

4. Greenlee R, Hill-Harmon M, Murray T, et al. Cancer statistics 2001. *CA Cancer J Clin* 2001;51:15–36.

5. Petterson F, Kolstad P, Ludwig H. *Annual Report on the Results of Treatment in Gynecological Cancer, Vol. 20.* Stockholm: International Federation of Gynaecology and Obstetrics, 1988.

6. Ries L, Kosary C, Hankey B, et al. *SEER Cancer Statistics Review 1973-1996.* Bethesda, MD: National Cancer Institute, 1999.

7. Oram D, Jeyarajah A. The role of ultrasound and tumour markers in the early detection of ovarian cancer. *Br J Obstet Gynaecol* 1994;101:939–945.

8. Schiltkraut J, Thompson W. Familial ovarian cancer: a population-based case-control study. *Am J Epidemiol* 1988;128:456–466.

9. Houlston R, Bourne T, Davies A, et al. Use of family history in a screening clinic for familial ovarian cancer. *Gynecol Oncol* 1992;47:247–252.

10. Easton D, Ford D, Bishop D, et al. Breast and ovarian cancer incidence in BRCA1-mutation carriers. *Am J Hum Genet* 1995;56:265–271.

11. Whittemore A, Gong G, ltnyre J. Prevalence and contribution of BRCA1 mutations in breast cancer and ovarian cancer: results from three US-population based case-control studies of ovarian cancer. *Am J Hum Genet* 1997;60:496–504.

12. Parkin D, Laara E, Muir C. Estimates of the world wide frequency of sixteen major cancers in 1980. *Int J Cancer* 1988;41:184–197.

13. Henderson B, Ross R, Pike M. Towards the prevention of cancer. *Science* 1991;254:1131–1138.

14. Friedlander M, Dembo A. Prognostic factors in ovarian cancer. *Sem Oncol* 1991;18:205–212.

15. Neijt J, Bokkel Huinink W, Burg M, et al. Long-term survival in ovarian cancer. *Eur J Cancer* 1991;27:1367–1372.

16. Creasman W, Eddy G. Prognostic factors in relation to second look laparotomy in ovarian cancer. *Baillieres Clin Obstet Gynaecol* 1989;3:183–190.

17. Bast R, Klug T, St John E, et al. A radioimmunoassay using a monoclonal antibody to monitor the course of epithelial ovarian cancer. *N Engl J Med* 1983;309:883–887.

18. Bast R, Feeney M, Lazarus H, et al. Reactivity of a monoclonal antibody with human ovarian carcinoma. *J Clin Invest* 1981;68:1331–1337.

19. Kenemans P, Bon G, Kessler A, et al. Technical and clinical evaluation of a new fully automated enzyme immunoassay for the detection of CA125, a multicenter study. *Clin Chem* 199238:1466–1471.

20. Yedema C, Thomas C, Seger M, et al. Comparison of five immunoassay procedures for the ovarian-carcinoma-associated antigenic determinant CA 125 in serum. *Eur J Obstet Gynecol* 1992;47:245–251.

21. Kamp GJ van, Verstraeten AA, Kenemans P. Discordant serum CA 125 values in commercial immunoassays. *Eur J Obstet Gynecol Reprod Bio.* 1993;49:99–103.

22. Bonfrer JM, Korse CM, Verstraeten RA, et al. Clinical evaluation of the Byk LIA-mat CA125 II assay: discussion of a reference value. *Clin Chem* 1997;43:491–497.

23. Bon G, Kenemans P, Verstraeten R, et al. Serum tumor marker assays in gynecologic oncology: establishment of reference values. *Am J Obstet Gynecol* 1996;174:107–114.

24. Davelaar EM, Kamp GJ van, Verstraeten RA, et al. Comparison of seven immunoassays for the quantification of CA 125 antigen in serum. *Clin Chem* 1998;44:1417–1422.

25. Davelaar EM, Schutter EM, Mensdorff-Pouilly S, et al. Clinical and technical evaluation of the ACS:OV serum assay and comparison with three other CA125-detecting assays. *Ann Clin Biochem* 2003;40:663–673.

26. Yin B, Lloyd K. Molecular cloning of the CA125 ovarian cancer antigen: identification as a new mucin, MUC16. *J Biol Chem* 2001;276:27371–27375.

27. Yin B, Dnistrian A, Lloyd K. Ovarian cancer antigen CA125 is encoded by the MUC16 mucin gene. *Int J Cancer* 2002;98:737–740.

28. Whitehouse C, Solomon E. Current status of the molecular characterization of the ovarian cancer antigen CA125 and implications for its use in clinical screening. *Gynecol Oncol* 2003;88:S152–157.

29. Fleuren G, Nap M, Aalders J, et al. Explanation of the limited correlation between tumor CA125 content and serum CA125 antigen levels in patients with ovarian tumors. *Cancer* 1987;60:2437–2442.

30. Hilgers J, Zotter S, Kenemans P. Polymorphic epithelial mucin and CA125 bearing glycoprotein in basic and applied carcinoma research. *Cancer Rev* 1988;11/12:3–10.

31. Yedema C, Kenemans P, Thomas C, et al. CA125 serum levels in the early post-operative period do not reflect tumour reduction obtained by cytoreductive surgery. *Eur J Cancer* 1993;29A: 966–971.

32. Kenemans P, Yedema CA, Bon GG, et al. CA 125 in gynecological pathology–a review. *Eur J Obstet Gynecol Reprod Biol* 1993;49:115–124.

33. Yedema C, Mensdorff-Pouilly S, Kenemans P, et al. Update on the serum tumour marker CA125. In: Bruhat M, ed. *The Management of Adnexal Cysts*. Oxford: Blackwell, 1994:75–97.

34. Epiney M, Bertossa C, Weil A, et al. CA125 production by the peritoneum: in-vitro and in-vivo studies. *Hum Reprod* 2000;15:1261–1265.

35. Bast R, Urban N, Shridhar V, et al. Early detection of ovarian cancer: promise and reality. *Cancer Treat Res* 2002;107:61–97.

36. Sevinc A, Camci C, Turk H, et al. How to interpret serum CA125 levels in patients with serosal involvement? A clinical dilemma. *Oncology* 2003;65:1–6.

37. Ruibal A, Encabo G, Martinez-Miralles E, et al. CA125 serum levels in non-malignant pathologies. *Bull Cancer* 1984;71:145–146.

38. Mastropaolo W, Fernandez Z, Miller E. Pronounced increases in the concentration of an ovarian tumor marker CA125 in serum of a healthy subject during menstruation. *Clin Chem* 1986;32:2110–2111.

39. Pittaway D, Fayez J. Serum CA125 in the diagnosis and management of endometriosis. *Fertil Steril* 1986;46:790–795.

40. Pittaway D, Fayez J. Serum CA125 antigen levels increase during menses. *Am J Obstet Gynecol* 1987;156:75–76.

41. Seki K, Kikuchi Y, Uesatom T et al. Increased serum CA125 levels during the first trimester of pregnancy. *Acta Obstet Gynecol Scand* 1986;65:583–585.

42. Halila H, Stenman U, Seppala M. Ovarian cancer antigen levels CA125 in pelvic inflammatory disease and pregnancy. *Cancer* 1986;57:1327–1329.

43. Bergmann JF, Bidart JM, George M, et al. Elevation of CA 125 in patients with benign and malignant ascites. *Cancer* 1987;59:213–217.

44. Metzger J, Haussinger K, Wilmanns W, et al. Hohe CA125 serumspiegel bei benignem ascites oder pleuraerguss. *Geburtsh Frauenheilk* 1987;47:463–465.

45. Duk J, Kauer F, Fleuren G, et al. Serum CA125 levels in patients with a provisional diagnosis of pelvic inflammatory disease. *Acta Obstet Gynecol Scand* 1989;68:637–641.

46. Sjovall K, Nilsson B, Einhorn N. The significance of serum CA125 elevation in malignant and nonmalignant diseases. *Gynecol Oncol* 2002;85:175–178.

47. Bast R, Siegal F, Runowicz C, et al. Evaluation of serum CA125 prior to diagnosis of an epithelial ovarian carcinoma. *Gynecol Oncol* 1985;22:115–120.

48. Zurawski V, Orjaseter H, Andersen H, et al. Elevated serum CA125 levels prior to diagnosis of ovarian neoplasia: relevance for early detection of ovarian cancer. *Int J Cancer* 1988;42: 677–680.

49. Bell R, Petticrew M, Sheldon T. The performance of screening tests for ovarian cancer: results of a systematic review. *Br J Obstet Gynaecol* 1998;105:1136–1147.

50. Einhorn N , Sjovall K, Knapp R, et al. Prospective evaluation of serum CA125 levels for early detection of ovarian cancer. *Obstet Gynecol* 1992;80:14–18.

51. Jacobs I, Davies A, Bridges J et al. Prevalence screening for ovarian cancer in postmenopausal women by CA125 measurement and ultrasonography. *Br Med J* 1993;306:1030–1034.

52. Grover S, Quinn M, Weidman P, et al. Screening for ovarian cancer using serum CA125 and vaginal examination: report on 2550 females. *Int J Gynecol Cancer* 1995;5:291–295.

53. Adonakis G, Paraskevaidis E, Tsiga S, et al. A combined approach for the early detection of ovarian cancer in asymptomatic women. *Eur J Obstet Gynecol* 1996;65:221–225.

54. Muto M, Cramer D, Brown D, et al. Screening for ovarian cancer: the preliminary experience of a familial ovarian cancer center. *Gynecol Oncol* 1993;51:12–20.

55. Bourne T, Campbell S, Reynolds K, et al. The potential role of serum CA125 in an ultrasound-based screening program for familial ovarian cancer. *Gynecol Oncol* 1994;52:379–385.

56. DePriest P, Gallion H, Pavlik E, et al. Transvaginal sonography as a screening method for the detection of early ovarian cancer. *Gynecol Oncol* 1997;65:408–414.

57. Karlan B, Baldwin R, Lopez-Luevanos E, et al. Peritoneal serous papillary carcinoma, a phenotypic variant of familial ovarian cancer: implications for ovarian cancer screening. *Am J Obstet Gynecol* 1999;180:917–928.

58. Laframboise S, Nedelcu R, Murphy J, et al. Use of CA125 and ultrasound in high-risk women. *Int J Gynecol Cancer* 2002;12:86–91.

59. Tailor A, Bourne T, Campbell S, et al. Results from an ultra-sound based familial ovarian cancer screening clinic: a 10-year observational study. *Ultrasound Obstet Gynecol* 2003;21:378–385.

60. Malkasian G, Knapp R, Lavin P, et al. Pre-operative evaluation of serum CA125 levels in premenopausal and postmenopausal patients with pelvic masses: discrimination of benign from malignant disease. *Am J Obstet Gynecol* 1988;159:341–346.

61. Gadducci A, Ferdeghini M, Prontera C, et al. The concomitant determination of different tumormarkers in patients with epithelial ovarian cancer and benign ovarian masses: relevance for differential diagnosis. *Gynecol Oncol* 1992;44:147–154.

62. Finkler N, Benacerraf B, Lavin P, et al. Comparison of serum CA125 clinical impression and ultrasound in the pre-operative evaluation of pelvic masses. *Obstet Gynecol* 1988;72:659–664.

63. Patsner B, Mann W. The value of pre-operative serum CA125 levels in patients with a pelvic mass. *Am J Obstet Gynecol* 1988;159:873–876.

64. Schutter E, Kenemans P, Sohn C, et al. Diagnostic value of pelvic examination, ultrasound and serum CA125 in postmenopausal women with a pelvic mass; An international multicenter study. *Cancer* 1994;74:1398–1406.

65. Maggino T, Gadducci A, D'Addario V, et al. Prospective multicenter study on CA125 in postmenopausal pelvic masses. *Gynecol Oncol* 1994;54:117–123.

66. Yedema C, Massuger L, Hilgers J, et al. Preoperative discrimination between benign and malignant ovarian tumors using a combination of CA125 and CA15.3 serum assays. *Int J Cancer* 1988;S3:61–67.

67. Schutter E, Sohn C, Kristen P, et al. Estimation of probability of malignancy using a logistic model combining physical examination, ultrasound, serum CA125 and serum CA72-4 in postmenopausal women with a pelvic mass, an international multicenter study. *Gynecol Oncol* 1998;69:56–63.

68. Schutter E, Davelaar E, van Kamp G, et al. The differential diagnostic potential of a panel of tumor markers (CA125, CA15-3, and CA72-4) in patients with a pelvic mass. *Am J Obstet Gynecol* 2002;187:385–392.

69. Jacobs I, Oram D, Fairbanks J, et al. A risk of malignancy index incorporating CA125, ultrasound and menopausal status for the accurate pre-operative diagnosis of ovarian cancer. *Br J Obstet Gynaecol* 1990;97:922–929.

70. Tingulstad S, Hagen B, Skjeldestad F, et al. Evaluation of a risk of malignancy index based on serum CA125, ultrasound findings and menopausal status in the pre-operative diagnosis of pelvic masses. *Br J Obstet Gynaecol* 1996;103:826–831.

71. Tingulstad S, Hagen B, Skjeldestad F, et al. The risk of malignancy index to evaluate potential ovarian cancers in local hospitals. *Obstet Gynecol* 1999;93:448–452.

72. Morgante G, la Marca A, Ditto A, et al. Comparison of two malignancy risk indices based on serum CA125, ultrasound score and menopausal status in the diagnosis of ovarian masses. *Br J Obstet Gynaecol* 1999;106:524–527.

73. Aslam N, Tailor A, Lawton F, et al. Prospective evaluation of three different models for the pre-operative diagnosis of ovarian cancer. *Br J Obstet Gynaecol* 2000;107:1347–1353.

74. Manjunath A, Pratapkumar M, Sujatha K, et al. Comparison of three risk of malignancy indices in evaluation of pelvic masses. *Gynecol Oncol* 2001;81:225–229.

75. Andersen E, Knudsen A, Rix P, et al. Risk of malignancy index in the pre-operative evaluation of patients with adnexal masses. *Gynecol Oncol* 2003;90:109–112.

76. Davies A, Jacobs I, Woolas R, et al. The adnexal mass: benign or malignant? Evaluation of a risk of malignancy index. *Br J Obstet Gynaecol* 1993;100:927–931.

77. Zurawski V, Broderick S, Pickens P, et al. Serum CA125 levels in a group of non-hospitalized women: relevance for the early detection of ovarian cancer. *Obstet Gynecol* 1987;69:606–611.

78. Zurawski V, Sjovall K, Schoenfeld D, et al. Prospective evaluation of serum CA125 levels in a normal population, phase I: the specificities of single and serial determinations in testing for ovarian cancer. *Gynecol Oncol* 1990;36:299–305.

79. Bast R, Knauf S, Epenetos A, et al. Coordinate elevation of serum markers in ovarian cancer but not in benign disease. *Cancer* 1991;68:1758–1763.

80. Jacobs I, Oram D, Bast R. Strategies for improving the specificity of screening for ovarian cancer with tumor-associated antigens CA125, Ca15.3 and TAG 72.3. *Obstet Gynecol* 1992;80:396–399.

81. Einhorn N, Bast R, Knapp R, et al. Long-term follow-up of the Stockholm screening study on ovarian cancer. *Gynecol Oncol* 2000;79:466–470.

82. Hensley M, Robson M, Kauff N, et al. Pre- and postmenopausal high-risk women undergoing screening for ovarian cancer: anxiety, risk perceptions, and quality of life. *Gynecol Oncol* 2003;89:440–446.

83. Skates S, Singer D. Quantifying the potential benefit of CA125 screening for ovarian cancer. *J Clin Epidemiol* 1991;44:365–380.

84. Skates S, Jacobs I, Macdonald N, et al. Estimated duration of pre-clinical ovarian cancer from longitudinal CA125 levels. *Proc Am Assoc Cancer Res* 1999;40:43.

85. Jacobs I, Kohler M, Wiseman R, et al. Clonal origin of epithelial ovarian cancer: Analysis by loss of heterozygosity, p53 mutation and chromosome inactivation. *J Natl Cancer Inst* 1992;84:1793–1798

86. Mok C, Tsao S, Knapp R, et al. Unifocal origin of advanced human epithelial ovarian cancers. *Cancer Res* 1992;52:5119–5122.

87. Zhang Z, Bast RC Jr, Yu Y, et al. Three biomarkers identified from serum proteomic analysis for the detection of early stage ovarian cancer. *Cancer Res* 2004;64:5882–5890.

88. Jacobs I, Skates S, Macdonald N et al. Screening for ovarian cancer: a pilot randomised controlled trial. *Lancet* 1999;353:1207–1210.

89. Szucs T, Wyss P, Dedes K. Cost-effectiveness studies in ovarian cancer. *Int J Gynecol Cancer* 2003;13S2:212–219.

53

Screening for Colorectal Cancer

Mehul Lalani

Robert E. Schoen

■ What Is the Problem that Requires Screening?

Colorectal cancer.

What is the incidence/prevalence of the target condition?

In 2003, there were 148,000 new cases of colorectal cancer in the United States and more than 57,000 will die, accounting for approximately 10% of cancer deaths.[1] colorectal cancer is a disease of aging, rarely diagnosed before age 40 year. The prevalence of colorectal cancer increases significantly after age 50 year, with further increases in each subsequent decade. Colorectal cancer ranks second to lung cancer as a cause of cancer death in the United States. A family history of colorectal cancer in a first-degree relative (mother, father, sibling, or child) increases an individual's risk of colorectal cancer by about twofold. If the family member is diagnosed at a young age, for example, younger than age 50, the risk of colorectal cancer is increased by three- to fivefold.[2] Other risk factors implicated in colorectal cancer include a history of inflammatory bowel disease, obesity, and a host of dietary factors including meat and saturated fat intake. Protective factors include physical activity, a high-fiber diet, calcium intake, and ingestion of aspirin or nonsteroidal anti-inflammatory medications.[3] The death rates from colorectal cancer have declined in the United States since the mid 1980s with overall 5-year survival now 61%.[4] However, whether this decline is due to screening or to modifications in etiologic factors is unclear.

What are the sequelae of the condition that are of interest in clinical medicine?

There is a marked survival difference depending on cancer stage at diagnosis. The 5-year survival rate for localized cancer (cancer confined to wall of colon) is over 90%, for regional cancer (cancer spread to regional lymph nodes) the survival is 64%, but for metastatic cancer (spread to liver or other organs), 5-year survival is only 8%.[5] In the United States, approximately 37% of colorectal cancers are detected at the localized stage, 38% at the regional stage, and 20% at the metastatic stage.[5]

Colorectal cancer arises from a premalignant precursor, the adenomatous polyp, in a progression known as the adenoma–carcinoma sequence. The evolution of adenoma to carcinoma occurs over a 7- to 10-year time frame.[6] This long period allows ample clinical opportunity to detect and remove premalignant adenomas. Studies of early detection demonstrate that screening, by detecting cancer at an earlier stage, reduces the mortality from colorectal cancer.[7] Furthermore, if adenomas do evolve into cancer, removing them before spread should also reduce cancer incidence. Data suggest that removing adenomatous polyps can reduce subsequent colorectal cancer incidence.[8] Thus, colorectal cancer is a public health problem for which there is substantial proof of the effectiveness of screening in both reducing cancer occurrence and death. The U.S. Preventive Services Task Force recently bestowed a grade A recommendation on colorectal cancer screening, indicating that the task force "strongly recommends that clinicians routinely provide screening to eligible patients."[9] Despite the evidence supporting the effectiveness of colorectal cancer screening, fewer than 45% of eligible subjects in the United States are screened.[10]

■ The Tests

What is the purpose of the test?

The detection of colorectal cancer at an early clinical stage.

What is the nature of the tests? Available modalities for colorectal cancer screening include fecal occult blood testing (FOBT), endoscopic testing with flexible sigmoidoscopy or colonoscopy, radiologic testing with barium enema, and newer methodologies such as virtual colonoscopy with computed tomography (CT) scanning and fecal DNA testing. Each of these modalities has unique characteristics, benefits, and liabilities. The current consensus is that any of a number of tests can be used to screen for colorectal cancer. The most important issue is that screening should not await symptoms, but be implemented on the basis of age-related risk. All individuals should begin screening at age 50. Individuals with a family history of colorectal cancer in a first-degree relative should begin screening at age 40, or 10 years before the age of diagnosis in the relative (whichever comes first). Some individuals may require screening even earlier based on more extensive family history risk or other genetic factors.[11]

Fecal occult blood testing. FOBT is the only screening test for which randomized, controlled trials evidence is available. Three trials conducted in England, Denmark, and Minnesota enrolled more than 258,000 patients and followed them for colorectal cancer mortality.[7,12,13] In the Minnesota trial, there was a 33% reduction in mortality in the annually screened group and 21% in the biannually screened group after 18 years of follow-up. In England and Denmark, biannual screening achieved a 15% and 18% reduction in mortality, respectively. These data confirm the efficacy of FOBT in reducing mortality to colorectal cancer. But the use of fecal blood has inherent limitations as a screening tool. Cancers may bleed intermittently, limiting sensitivity. As a single test, the sensitivity of FOBT is a relatively poor 25%,[14] although program sensitivity with repeated yearly applications may be 80% to 90%.[15] In addition, most gastrointestinal (GI) bleeding is from causes other than cancer, which increases the number of false-positive examinations and reduces specificity.

FOBT involves collecting stool samples from *three* spontaneously passed bowel movements and then smearing them on test cards. Individuals are advised to abstain from consuming foods that contain peroxidases, rare red meat, and aspirin or other nonsteroidal anti-inflammatory agents because these may lead to false-positive results. The current guidelines for FOBT recommend yearly use.[11] A positive result returned on any sample mandates colonoscopy. The inconvenient sampling process and the need for yearly repeat examinations limit compliance with FOBT. Immunochemical fecal occult blood tests work through antibodies that detect the intact globin portion of human hemoglobin. They do not require dietary modification and, in some cases, offer far simpler sampling techniques, such as brushing the toilet water.[16] Studies evaluating these tests are under way.

Flexible sigmoidoscopy. Flexible sigmoidoscopy allows direct visualization, identification of adenomatous polyps, and tissue sampling of the colorectal mucosa. After patient preparation with enemas, sigmoidoscopy detects lesions in the distal one third to one half of the colon. The major risk involved is perforation, with an incidence of 1/30,000 examinations.[17] Case control studies reveal a 60% to 95% reduction in colorectal cancer mortality due to cancers within the reach of the sigmoidoscope.[18,19] There are no randomized trials, although several large scale studies in the United Kingdom, Italy, and the United States are under way.[20–22] The major limitation of sigmoidoscopy is that it may miss lesions in the proximal colon. This is estimated to occur in 1% to 2% of individuals.[23] Repeated screening sigmoidoscopy at a 5-year interval is recommended.

Fecal occult blood testing in combination with flexible sigmoidoscopy. Given the limitations of flexible sigmoidoscopy in detecting proximal lesions, investigators have wondered whether the combination of FOBT with flexible sigmoidoscopy would be better than either alone. In a study of screening colonoscopy from the VA cooperative group, the authors determined that FOBT would add only 5% additional detection of advanced adenomas over that of flexible sigmoidoscopy.[24] FOBT plus sigmoidoscopy is an option for screening, but it is not clear whether FOBT plus sigmoidoscopy substantially improves the detection of proximal colon pathology.

Screening colonoscopy. Colonoscopy is the only technique that allows detection and removal of premalignant lesions throughout the colon. Colonoscopy requires a vigorous bowel preparation, a constrained diet for 24 hours before examination, and sedation that generates the need for a driver to escort the patient home. The main risks include those related to sedation, bleeding, and perforation. Respiratory depression occurs in 5/1,000 patients. Approximately 3/1,000 patients have marked bleeding and 1–3/10,000 patients die as a result. The risk of bowel perforation approximates 1–2/1,000 patients.[11] The American College of Gastroenterology endorses colonoscopy every 10 years as its preferred screening strategy,[25] but the U.S. Preventive Services Task Force has concluded that the available evidence does not permit endorsement of one screening strategy over another.[9] In particular, it is unclear whether the increased accuracy of colonoscopy offsets the additional complications, inconvenience, and costs. There are no trials evaluating colonoscopy for its impact on reducing mortality to colorectal cancer. Its efficacy is extrapolated from the case control studies of sigmoidoscopy and from the National Polyp Study that showed removal of adenomatous polyps resulted in a 76% to 90% reduction in colorectal cancer incidence compared with historical controls.[26]

Barium enema. Air-contrast barium enema has been recommended as a screening strategy for colorectal cancer although there are scant data to support it. The sensitivity of barium enema for colon cancer is 82.9% in comparison with 95% for colonoscopy.[25] A number of studies have documented a high adenoma miss rate for barium enema, including a miss rate of 87% for polyps between 0 and 9 mm and 67% for polyps larger than 9 mm.[27] Based on data from the National Polyp Study, double-contrast barium enema examination compared with paired colonoscopy detected 39% of all adenomas and only 48% of large adenomas greater than 10 mm.[28] For these reasons, barium enema is not currently widely used as a screening modality.

Virtual colonoscopy. Virtual colonoscopy uses imaging from spiral CT scanning to create three-dimensional (3D) simulated endoluminal images of the colon. In a landmark study by Pickhardt et al.[29] using a 3D scanning technique, virtual colonoscopy had a sensitivity greater than 92% for 9-mm adenomas, a rate that exceeds colonoscopy. However, a recent multicenter study of virtual colonoscopy was disappointing, reporting sensitivity for 10-mm adenomas of only 55%.[30] Clearly, greater standardization of technique and proficiency in interpretation are needed before widespread use can be advocated. Furthermore, virtual colonoscopy is expensive, and if a positive test occurs, the subject still needs a colonoscopy to remove the lesion. Virtual colonoscopy will probably only be useful in settings where the chance of finding a lesion is low, such as in surveillance of low-risk individuals who have already had a colonoscopy.

Molecular screening methods. Because malignant cancer cells have a different molecular mutational profile than normal colonocytes, researchers have developed a means of isolating human DNA from stool and assaying it for mutations. A number of potential mutational targets are identified including *K-ras,* APC, p53, microsatellite instability, and long DNA (a marker of abnormal apoptosis).[31] Preliminary studies have demonstrated sensitivity for cancer of around 64%, but large-scale studies are nearing completion.[32] A commercially available stool DNA test is available, but the cost is high and patients are required to collect an entire bowel movement, pack it in a special mailing crate, and send it to a central laboratory. Patient acceptance and compliance with stool DNA testing will need further study.

What are the implications of testing?

A range of sensitivity and specificity for adenoma and cancer is provided in Table 53–1.[33]

What does an abnormal test result mean? The most comprehensive test is colonoscopy, in that adenomas can be removed during the procedure. Thus, colonoscopy is both diagnostic and therapeutic. Any abnormal result from one of the other tests should prompt a colonoscopy.

What does a normal test result mean? A normal test must be put in context with the test sensitivity. For example, a normal sigmoidoscopy does not exclude the presence of a proximal colon cancer. However, even within the range of the sigmoidoscope, lesions can be missed or develop rapidly. A large study found a 3.1% prevalence rate for distal adenoma 3 years after a negative sigmoidoscopy, including a nearly 1% rate of advanced adenoma or cancer.[34] Colonoscopy can miss lesions too. Adenomas smaller than 10 mm are missed 15% of the time, and cancers after recent colonoscopy can occur.[35] The recommended interval for a repeat colonoscopy after a negative exam is 5 to 10 years.

What is the cost of testing?

Table 53–2 shows the approximate cost of available test. Any cost-effectiveness analysis must account for positive tests that prompt additional testing. For example, a positive FOBT, sigmoidoscopy, or radiology study would require a subsequent colonoscopy. Compared with no screening, cost-effectiveness ratios for screening with FOBT, sigmoidoscopy, or colonoscopy generally cost $10,000

Table 53–1	**Performance of common screening tests**			
Test	Sensitivity adenomas, %	Specificity adenomas, %	Sensitivity cancer, %	Specificity cancer, %
Fecal occult blood	4–89	62–98	20–100	63–100
Flexible sigmoidoscopy	33–78	84	67–90	85–95
Colonoscopy	75–100	90–98	79–100	90–96
Barium enema	48–100	67–100	62–100	90–100
Virtual Colonoscopy	32–96	63–98	90–100	90–100
Stool DNA	10–82	95	52–91	90–100

From Economic Models of Colorectal Cancer Screening in Average-Risk Adults: A Workshop. Institute of Medicine National Cancer Policy Board. January 2004.

Table 53–2 **Approximate costs of available tests**	
Tests	**Cost, $**
Fecal occult blood	10
Screening sigmoidoscopy	200
Sigmoidoscopy with biopsy	375
Screening colonoscopy	625
Colonoscopy with polypectomy	900
Prototype radiology procedure	200
Stool DNA (PreGenPlus) (Exact Science, Marlborough,MA)	795

to 25,000 per life-year saved. Although many studies show that colorectal cancer screening is cost-effective, they disagree over which test is most cost-effective.[36] These differences are due to differences in the assumptions made about the effectiveness and costs of a screening program.

■ Conclusions and Recommendations

Consensus guidelines endorsed by all major organizations support routine colorectal cancer screening for average risk individuals beginning at age 50. All screening tests are likely to be effective. The decision about which test to use depends on patient preference, availability, cost, risk, and emphasis on efficacy. Balancing these concerns is not an easy task. As the data supporting colorectal cancer screening have emerged, greater emphasis on screening will ensue. Offering colorectal cancer screening is likely to become a measure of quality of care, and not offering screening will expose physicians to the risk of malpractice litigation. Medical science has found an effective means of reducing death to and incidence of colorectal cancer, a major public health problem. It is now the responsibility of physicians to encourage their patients to get tested.

■ Summary

1 ■ What Is the Problem that Requires Screening?

a. What is the incidence/prevalence of the target condition?

The annual age-adjusted colorectal cancer incidence rates among females in the U.S. approximate 50 per 100,000. The prevalence of colorectal cancer increases significantly after age 50, with further increases in each subsequent decade. A family history of colorectal cancer in a first degree relative (mother, father, sibling, or child) increases an individual's risk of colorectal cancer by about 2-fold. Following cancer of the lung and bronchus and breast cancer, colorectal cancer is the most common cause of cancer death among women in the U.S. Overall, colorectal cancer accounts for approximately 10% of cancer deaths.

b. *What are the sequelae of the condition which are of interest in clinical medicine?*

Colorectal cancer arises from a pre-malignant precursor, the adenomatous polyp, in a progression known as the adenoma-carcinoma sequence. The evolution of adenoma to carcinoma occurs over a 7–10 year time frame. This long period allows ample clinical opportunity to detect and remove pre-malignant adenomas. There is a marked survival difference depending on cancer stage at diagnosis. The 5-year survival for localized cancer is over 90% and for regional cancer the survival is 64%, but for metastatic cancer the 5 year survival is only 8%.

c. *What is the purpose of the tests?*

To detect adenomatous polyps or colorectal cancer at an early stage.

d. *What is the nature of the tests?*

Fecal occult blood testing, endoscopic testing with flexible sigmoidoscopy or colonoscopy, radiological testing with barium enema and newer methodologies such as virtual colonoscopy with CT scanning and fecal DNA testing.

e. *What are the implications of testing?*

1. What does an abnormal test result mean?

   Any abnormal result from one of the other tests should prompt a colonoscopy or sigmoidoscopy. These procedures are both diagnostic and therapeutic.

2. What does a normal test result mean?

   Both sigmoidoscopy and colonoscopy do not exclude the presence of disease. With coloscopy, adenomas smaller than 10 mm are missed 15% of the time, and cancers after recent colonoscopy can occur. The recommended interval for a repeat colonoscopy after a negative exam is 5–10 years.

Continued

■ **Summary—cont'd**

f. What is the cost of testing?

Although many studies show that colorectal cancer screening is cost effective, they disagree over which test is most cost-effective.

■ **Conclusions and recommendations**

All screening tests are likely to be effective. Consensus guidelines endorsed by all major organizations support routine colorectal cancer screening for average risk individuals beginning at age 50. The decision about which test to use depends on patient preference, availability, cost, risk, and emphasis on efficacy.

References

1. Jemal A, Murray T, Samuels A, et al. Cancer statistics, 2003. *CA Cancer J Clin* 2003;53:5–26.
2. Schoen RE. Families at risk for colorectal cancer: risk assessment and genetic testing. *J Clin Gastroenterol* 2000;31:114–120.
3. Potter JD, Slattery ML, Bostick RM, et al. Colon cancer: a review of the epidemiology [review]. *Epidemiol Rev* 1993;15:499–545.
4. Ries LA, Wingo PA, Miller DS, et al. The annual report to the nation on the status of cancer, 1973-1997, with a special section on colorectal cancer. *Cancer* 2000;88:2398–2424.
5. Ries LAG, Eisner MP, Kosary CL, et al. *SEER Cancer Statistics Review, 1975-2001*. Bethesda, MD: National Cancer Institute, 2004. Available at: http://seer.cancer.gov/csr/1975_2001/.
6. Bond JH. Polyp guideline: diagnosis, treatment, and surveillance for patients with colorectal polyps. Practice Parameters Committee of the American College of Gastroenterology. *Am J Gastroenterol* 2000;95:3053–3063.
7. Mandel JS, Church TR, Ederer F, et al. Colorectal cancer mortality: effectiveness of biennial screening for fecal occult blood [see comments]. *J Natl Cancer Inst* 1999;91:434–437.
8. Mandel JS, Church TR, Bond JH, et al. The effect of fecal occult-blood screening on the incidence of colorectal cancer [letter; comment]. *N Engl J Med* 2000;343:1603–1607.
9. U.S. Preventive Services Task Force. Screening for colorectal cancer: recommendation and rationale. *Ann Intern Med* 2002;137:129–131.
10. Trends in screening for colorectal cancer: United States, 1997 and 1999. *MMWR Morb Mortal Wkly Rep* 2001;50:162–166.
11. Winawer S, Fletcher R, Rex D, et al. Colorectal cancer screening and surveillance: clinical guidelines and rationale: update based on new evidence. *Gastroenterology* 2003;124:544–560.
12. Hardcastle JD, Chamberlain JO, Robinson MH, et al. Randomised controlled trial of faecal-occult-blood screening for colorectal cancer [see comments]. *Lancet* 1996;348:1472–1477.
13. Kronborg O, Fenger C, Olsen J, et al. Randomised study of screening for colorectal cancer with faecal-occult-blood test [see comments]. *Lancet* 1996;348:1467–1471.
14. Ransohoff DF, Lang CA. Screening for colorectal cancer with the fecal occult blood test: a background paper: American College of Physicians [see comments] [review]. *Ann Intern Med* 1997;126:811–822.
15. Church TR, Ederer F, Mandel JS. Fecal occult blood screening in the Minnesota study: sensitivity of the screening test [see comments]. *J Natl Cancer Inst* 1997;89:1440–1448.
16. Young GP, St John DJ, Cole SR, et al. Prescreening evaluation of a brush-based faecal immunochemical test for haemoglobin. *J Med Screen* 2003;10:123–128.

17. Schoen RE, Levin TR. Re: Risk of perforation after colonoscopy and sigmoidoscopy: a population-based study [comment]. *J Natl Cancer Inst* 2003;95:830–831.

18. Selby JV, Friedman GD, Quesenberry CPJ, et al. A case-control study of screening sigmoidoscopy and mortality from colorectal cancer [see comments]. *N Engl J Med* 1992;326:653–657.

19. Newcomb PA, Norfleet RG, Storer BE, et al. Screening sigmoidoscopy and colorectal cancer mortality [see comments]. *J Natl Cancer Inst* 1992;84:1572–1575.

20. UK Flexible Sigmoidoscopy Screening Trial Investigators. Single flexible sigmoidoscopy screening to prevent colorectal cancer: baseline findings of a UK multicentre randomised trial [comment]. *Lancet* 2002;359:1291–1300.

21. Prorok PC, Andriole GL, Bresalier RS, et al. Design of the Prostate, Lung, Colorectal and Ovarian (PLCO) cancer screening trial. *Control Clin Trials* 2000;21[6 Suppl]:309S.

22. Segnan N, Senore C, Andreoni B, et al. Baseline findings of the Italian multicenter randomized controlled trial of "once-only sigmoidoscopy"—SCORE [see comment]. *J Natl Cancer Inst* 2002; 94:1763–1772.

23. Schoen RE. Prevalence of isolated advanced proximal neoplasia [comment]. *Arch Intern Med* 2003;163:2103–2104.

24. Lieberman DA, Weiss DG, Veterans Affairs Cooperative Study Group. One-time screening for colorectal cancer with combined fecal occult-blood testing and examination of the distal colon [see comments]. *N Engl J Med* 2001;345:555–560.

25. Rex DK, Johnson DA, Lieberman DA, et al. Colorectal cancer prevention 2000: screening recommendations of the American College of Gastroenterology. *Am J Gastroenterol* 2000;95:868–877.

26. Winawer SJ, Zauber AG, Ho MN, et al. Prevention of colorectal cancer by colonoscopic polypectomy: the National Polyp Study Workgroup [see comments]. *N Engl J Med* 1993; 29: 1977–1981.

27. Cheong Y, Farrow R, Frank CS, et al. Utility of flexible sigmoidoscopy as an adjunct to double-contrast barium enema examination. *Abdom Imaging* 1998;23:138–140.

28. Winawer SJ, Stewart ET, Zauber AG, et al. A comparison of colonoscopy and double-contrast barium enema for surveillance after polypectomy. National Polyp Study Work Group [see comments]. *N Engl J Med* 2000;342:1766–1772.

29. Pickhardt PJ, Choi JR, Hwang I, et al. Computed tomographic virtual colonoscopy to screen for colorectal neoplasia in asymptomatic adults [see comment]. *N Engl J Med* 2003;349:2191–2200.

30. Cotton PB, Durkalski VL, Pineau BC, et al. Computed tomographic colonography (virtual colonoscopy): a multicenter comparison with standard colonoscopy for detection of colorectal neoplasia [see comment]. *JAMA* 2004;291:1713–1719.

31. Ahlquist DA, Skoletsky JE, Boynton KA, et al. Colorectal cancer screening by detection of altered human DNA in stool: feasibility of a multitarget assay panel. *Gastroenterology* 2000;119:1219–1227.

32. Tagore KS, Lawson MJ, Yucaitis JA, et al. Sensitivity and specificity of a stool DNA multitarget assay panel for the detection of advanced colorectal neoplasia. *Clin Colorectal Cancer* 2003;3:47–53.

33. Economic Models of Colorectal Cancer Screening in Average-Risk Adults: A Workshop. Institute of Medicine National Cancer Policy Board. January 2004.

34. Schoen RE, Pinsky PF, Weissfeld JL, et al. Results of repeat sigmoidoscopy 3 years after a negative examination [comment]. *JAMA* 2003;290:41–48.

35. Schoen RE. Surveillance after positive and negative colonoscopy examinations: issues, yields, and use. *Am J Gastroenterol* 2003;98:1237–1246.

36. Pignone M, Saha S, Hoerger T, et al. Cost-effectiveness analyses of colorectal cancer screening: a systematic review for the U.S. Preventive Services Task Force. *Ann Intern Med* 2002;137:96–104.

54

The Electrocardiogram

Rudolph W. Koster

Patrick M. M. Bossuyt

■ What Is the Problem that Requires Screening?

Asymptomatic disturbances of cardiac rhythm or conduction and ischemic heart disease.

What is the incidence/prevalence of the target condition?

The prevalence of coronary heart disease (CHD) increases with age. The incidence of all CHD in adults is 14.3/1,000 per year for men and 7.2/1,000 per year for women (morbidity) and mortality is 3.1/1,000 per year for men and 1.4/1,000 per year for women. This is true for all manifestations of CHD including angina pectoris, myocardial infarction (Figure 54–1), and sudden death. However, the gender ratio is not constant with advancing age.[1] After menopause, the male to female ratio of coronary heart disease declines from 7:1 to 3:1. It becomes equal by the sixth and seventh decades, and finally reverses slightly in the eighth and ninth decades. The proportions of silent (i.e., asymptomatic) myocardial infarction are more less equal over the age groups: 35% in women, 28% in men (Figure 54–1).[2] Atrial fibrillation may occur at any age, but its prevalence increases with age from 2/1,000 women aged 25 to 34 years to 30/1,000 of women aged 55 to 64 years.[3]

What are the sequelae of the condition that are of interest in clinical medicine?

Disturbances of rhythm. Most people are aware of occasional palpitations and skipped beats, which are not generally clinically significant. True arrhythmias rarely go unnoticed. Paroxysmal tachycardias are generally sensed immediately, but occasionally a patient may be unaware of a paroxysmal or persistent tachycardia. Atrial fibrillation is the single most important paroxysmal tachycardia. It can occur in the presence or absence (lone atrial fibrillation) of organic heart disease. Atrial fibrillation impairs the circulatory response to blood pressure changes during surgery, may cause congestive heart failure, and is often the source of arterial or pulmonary emboli. The management of atrial fibrilla-

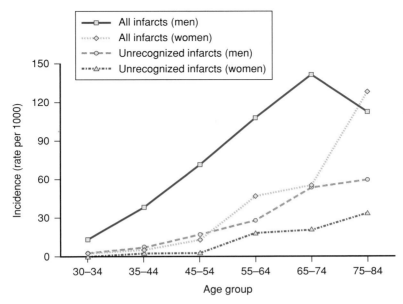

Figure 54–1   Ten-year incidence of myocardial infarction in the Framingham cohort. Unrecognized infarcts are those infarcts identified on the biannual electrocardiogram without previous clinical symptoms. In all age groups the proportion of unidentified infarcts is about one third of all infarcts. (From Kannel WB, Abbott RD. Incidence and prognosis of unrecognized myocardial infarction: an update of the Framingham study. *N Engl J Med* 1984;311:1144–1147.)

tion includes heart rate control, possibly by conversion to sinus rhythm, and prevention of thrombosis development in the atria with subsequent embolism.

Premature atrial beats are usually benign and do not require medical intervention. Premature ventricular beats, especially when frequent, may be associated with ischemic myocardial disease and can trigger ventricular tachycardia. Ventricular tachycardia rarely goes unnoticed and is almost always associated with important heart disease. Other supraventricular tachycardias—such as the tachycardia associated with the Wolff-Parkinson-White syndrome and atrioventricular junction tachycardia—are not associated with organic heart disease, with rare exceptions.

Conduction disturbances. First-degree and second-degree atrioventricular nodal blocks are occasionally observed especially during sleep and are not necessarily associated with heart disease. A third-degree conduction block is usually associated with complaints of dizziness and fainting (Adams-Stokes attack) but may occasionally be found in asymptomatic individuals. The consequences of complete heart block depend on the location of the block, the ability of the heart to increase its rate with exercise, and the absence of disturbances in pump function. In general, complete heart block is considered an indication for implantation of a permanent pacemaker.

Ischemic heart disease. Ischemic heart disease (IHD) is the most important reason for preoperative screening, as it is associated with much of the perioperative morbidity and mortality. The diagnosis of a silent myocardial infarction can only be made by electrocardiogram (ECG), usually after the demonstration of pathologic Q waves. In some patients chest pains have been absent, whereas in others the manifestations were mild or were perceived as another, self-limiting problem. Silent myocardial infarction is associated with recurrent infarction, congestive heart failure, and (sudden) death. The prognosis of a silent myocardial infarction is similar to that of a symptomatic myocardial infarction.

■ The Tests

What is the purpose of the tests?

The preoperative identification of patients with potentially lethal cardiac pathology, including rhythm and conduction disturbances and IHD, so that medical therapy may be initiated and nonemergency surgery avoided.

What is the nature of the tests?

The ECG yields information on several, essentially independent functions of the heart. These include disturbances of rhythm, disturbances of impulse transmission through the conduction system, the presence of ischemic heart disease and congenital or acquired abnormalities of the heart chambers, and electrolyte disturbances. Disturbances of rhythm and conduction and ischemic manifestations can be present in apparently healthy people and thus detected for the first time at a preoperative screening. Throughout this chapter, it is assumed that a detailed history and physical examination have not revealed any important abnormal findings.

The ECG is a standardized, 12-lead recording of the electrical activity of the heart, lasting 12 to 60 seconds. It is simple and noninvasive. Since abnormalities of the heart such as ischemia, arrhythmias, and conduction disturbances are typically intermittent, the likelihood of one of these being recorded during this short interval is small. In general, routine ECG findings cannot show myocardial ischemia in the absence of angina pectoris. Prolonged (24-hour) ECG recordings or recordings made during exercise improve the detection rate. On the other hand, if an abnormality is observed during this short period, it probably occurs frequently and is thus a more serious disorder.

What are the implications of testing?

What does an abnormal test result mean? The ECG diagnosis of acute myocardial infarction of more than trivial size is relatively simple during the first weeks after occurrence, especially when serial ECGs are available. In most patients, pathologic Q waves remain visible. However, pathologic Q waves may be absent in smaller infarcts making a diagnosis based solely on the ECG difficult. The timing of a myocardial infarction cannot be determined with any certainty after the first 2 to 3 months, as the pathologic Q waves become less obvious or even disappear, yielding a false-negative rate of 33% to 62%.[4,5] Other myocardial or neurologic disorders may mimic an old myocardial infarction leading to the unjustified diagnosis of an acute myocardial infarction. Misinterpretation of a pathologic Q wave is also possible. Although the frequency of false-positive readings has not been studied in the context of screening, it is probably low.

Goldman et al.[6] identified three preoperative cardiac risk factors for noncardiac surgery that could not be identified by either history of physical examination: (a) a myocardial infarction less than 6 months before surgery; (b) a rhythm other than sinus rhythm or premature atrial beats on the preoperative ECG; and (c) more than five premature ventricular beats per minute at any time before surgery. The risk of surgery after a recent (under 6 months) symptomatic myocardial infarction was reviewed in detail by Haagensen and Steen.[7] The risks of perioperative reinfarction ranged from 1.9% to 15.9%; subsequent mortality ranged from 28% to 72%.[7] In general, the diagnosis of recent acute myocardial infarction is made by history and confirmed by a preoperative ECG.

It is unclear if the finding of a silent myocardial infarction has the same prognosis during the perioperative period as a documented recent acute myocardial infarction. Nevertheless, many consider the finding of a silent myocardial infarction on a routine preoperative ECG a contraindication to elective surgery for a 6-month period. It is assumed that postponement of surgery will reduce the excess risk of a perioperative cardiac complication to nil. Even if true, such a policy has a sizable impact on the patient and society. As illustrated in Table 54–1, 260 of every 100,000 women aged 35 to 44 years screened preoperatively with an ECG would have their operation postponed for

Table 54-1	**Likelihood of silent MI by age, together with the possible impact of ECG testing on mortality**		
Age group, y	No. silent MIs detected (per 100,000 ECGs)	No. silent MIs occurring in the 6 months before ECG (per 100,000 ECGs)	Reduction in mortality when all patients with silent MI are recognized and their operation postponed (per 100,000 ECGs)
30–34	0	0	0
35–44	260	13	0.6
45–54	550	15	0.7
55–64	2,330	90	4.5
65–74	4,410	108	5.4
75–84	7,660	173	8.6

ECG, electrocardiogram; MI, myocardial infarction.

6 months because of the diagnosis of a silent myocardial infarction. Statistically, only 13 (5%) of the 260 would have actually suffered their myocardial infarction in the preceding 6 months. As a result, the *maximum* reduction in perioperative mortality achieved by delaying surgery would be less than one for every 100,000 women screened (Table 54–1). In older age groups, these numbers are even less favorable in terms of number of women falsely labeled with myocardial infarction in the preceding 6 months. For every 100,000 screened people of 60 years, 2,330 would have their operation postponed for 6 months, yet only 90 patients (3.8%) would have had their myocardial infarction in the preceding 6 months. The maximum reduction in mortality from this screening policy would be 4.5/100,000 women screened.

The most important arrhythmia is atrial fibrillation, which by itself is a concern if the ventricular rate is very high or very low. In addition, arrhythmias may reflect underlying heart disease (ischemia, congestive heart failure), which should be identified and treated, preferably before surgery.

First-degree or second-degree heart block needs no precautions prior to surgery. Neither is bundle branch block an independent risk factor for perioperative complications, even in the case of bifascicular bundle branch block.[8] A temporary, transvenous pacemaker is indicated if a complete, third-degree heart block is diagnosed. However, it can be argued that definitive pacemaker implantation should be considered first in women who do not require emergency surgery. Complete heart block should be identifiable as a significant arrhythmia on physical examination.

What does a normal test result mean? The likelihood of perioperative cardiac complications in women with an uneventful medical history and normal ECG tracing is very small.

What is the cost of testing?

The direct costs of a routine ECG comprise use of equipment, personnel, and the fee for the cardiologist for assessment of the ECG tracing. In The Netherlands, these costs total approximately 22 euros ($29). In many hospitals, the tracing is screened first by computer. The cost rises considerably should a consultation be needed in the case of abnormal findings on the ECG. The need for such a consultation largely depends on the age of the patient, as the likelihood of unexpected pathology, old or recent, increases with age.

The chance of finding a silent myocardial infarction is given in Table 54–1. In The Netherlands the consultant fee is 57 euros ($76). Thus, in the range 45 to 54 years, routine preoperative ECG screening would cost $4.1 million per life saved using these conservative Dutch estimates. In the United States, the typical ECG with interpretation approximates $45. Thus, the total cost per life saved by routine preoperative ECG screening approximated $6.7 million if no additional consultant is used. It exceeds $500,000 even after age 75 years. Further assessment including exercise testing or nuclear scintigraphic studies only increase the costs.

■ Conclusions and Recommendations

Before surgery, rhythm and conduction disturbances can be detected by careful history and routine physical examination. The most important contributor to perioperative cardiac complications is a recent myocardial infarction (within 6 months). The diagnosis of a silent myocardial infarction is based on typical ECG changes. The timing of a silent myocardial infarction cannot be determined from the ECG findings. Thus, it is impossible to differentiate a silent myocardial infarction that occurred during the preceding 6 months from one that occurred more than 6 months previously. This inability has immense consequences. Based on the findings of Kannel and Abbott,[3] the calculated cost-benefit ratio for routine ECG screening in terms of deaths prevented is very high. The costs are even higher if one considers the negative medical effects and the costs to society of delaying surgery for 6 months.

It can be concluded that preoperative ECG screening is not warranted in gynecologic surgery at any age, if history and physical examination do not give any evidence of the presence of heart disease.

■ Summary

1 ■ What Is the Problem that Requires Screening?
Asymptomatic disturbances of cardiac rhythm or conduction, and ischemic heart disease.

a. What is the incidence/prevalence of the target condition?
The incidence of CHD in adults is 14.3/1,000 per year for men and 7.2/1,000 per year for women (morbidity) with mortality of 3.1/1,000 per year for men and 1.4/1,000 per year for women. The incidence rises with age. This is true for all manifestations of CHD including angina pectoris, myocardial infarction, and sudden death.

b. What are the sequelae of the condition that are of interest in clinical medicine?
Atrial fibrillation impairs the circulatory response to blood pressure changes during surgery, may cause congestive heart failure, and is often the source of arterial or pulmonary emboli. Ventricular tachycardia rarely goes unnoticed and is in almost all instances associated with important heart disease. Coronary

Continued

■ **Summary—cont'd**

heart disease is the most important reason for preoperative screening, as it is associated with much of the perioperative morbidity and mortality.

2 ■ The Tests

Electrocardiogram (ECG).

a. *What is the purpose of the tests?*
   The preoperative identification of patients with potentially lethal cardiac pathology, including rhythm and conduction disturbances and ischemic heart disease, so that medical therapy may be initiated and nonemergency surgery avoided.

b. *What is the nature of the tests?*
   The ECG is a standardized, 12-lead recording of the electrical activity of the heart, lasting 12 to 60 seconds.

c. *What are the implications of testing?*
   1. What does an abnormal test result mean?
      Surgery should be delayed. There are three preoperative cardiac risk factors for noncardiac surgery not identifiable by either history or physical examination: (a) a myocardial infarction within 6 months before surgery; (b) a rhythm other than sinus rhythm or premature atrial beats on the preoperative ECG; and (c) more than five premature ventricular beats per minute at any time before surgery. The risk of surgery within 6 months of a symptomatic myocardial infarction is perioperative reinfarction (1.9% to 15.9%) and death in the case of perioperative reinfarction (28% to 72%). The diagnosis of atrial fibrillation will lead to medical therapy. The discovery of complete heart block could end with the placement of a permanent pacemaker.
   2. What does a normal test result mean?
      The likelihood of perioperative cardiac complications in women with an uneventful medical history and normal ECG tracing is very small.

d. *What is the cost of testing?*
   The cost is $4 to $7 million per life saved in women aged 45 to 54 years. The cost exceeds $500,000 even after age 75 years.

3 ■ Conclusions and Recommendations

Preoperative ECG screening is not warranted in gynecologic surgery at any age, if the history and physical examination do not give any evidence of the presence of heart disease.

References

1. Lerner DJ, Kannel WB. Patterns of coronary heart disease morbidity and mortality in the sexes: 26-year follow-up of the Framingham population. *Am Heart J* 1986;111:383–390.
2. Kannel WB, Abbott RD. Incidence and prognosis of unrecognized myocardial infarction: an update of the Framingham study. *N Engl J Med* 1984;311:1144–1147.
3. Kannel WB, Abbott RD, Savage DD, et al. Epidemiologic features of chronic atrial fibrillation: the Framingham study. *N Engl J Med* 1982;306:1018–1022.
4. Smith S, Hayes WL. The prognosis of complete left bundle branch block. *Am Heart J* 1965;70: 157–159.
5. Uusitupa M, Pyörälä K, Raunio H, et al. Sensitivity and specificity of Minnesota Code Q-QS abnormalities in the diagnosis of myocardial infarction verified at autopsy. *Am Heart J* 1983;106: 753–757.
6. Goldman L, Caldera DL, Nussbaum SR, et al. Multifactorial index of cardiac risk in noncardiac procedures. *N Engl J Med* 1977;297:845–850.
7. Haagensen R, Steen PA. Perioperative myocardial infarction. *Br J Anaesthesiol* 1988;61:24–37.
8. Pastore JO, Yurchak PM, Janis KM, et al. The risk of advanced heart block in surgical patients with right bundle branch block and left axis deviation. *Circulation* 1978;57:677–680.

55

Intravenous Pyelography

Michelle L. Kush

Joanne T. Piscitelli

David L. Simel

■ What Is the Problem that Requires Screening?

Anomalies and anatomic distortion of the urinary tract that may increase the risk of ureteral injury during benign gynecologic surgery.

What is the incidence/prevalence of the target condition?

Benign gynecologic procedures account for 80% to 90% of all surgical ureteral injuries[1] occurring in 0.1% to 2.5% of procedures.[2–12] The injury rate is similar for abdominal, vaginal, and laparoscopic procedures. Pathologic processes such as pelvic masses, endometriosis, pelvic adhesive disease, prior pelvic surgery, or urinary tract anomalies that alter, distort, or obscure normal anatomic relationships may place the patient at a greater risk of intraoperative ureteral injury.[5,13] Knowledge of the anatomic course of the ureter and any urinary tract distortion before a procedure may be useful to the surgeon.

What are the sequelae of the condition that are of interest in clinical medicine?

Ureteral injury. Ureteral injury may result in longer operative time, greater operative blood loss, and more frequent transfusions.[7] In addition, ureteral injuries can lead to pyelonephritis, sepsis, ileus, fistula formation, urinoma formation with subsequent intrapelvic abscess formation, unilateral or bilateral urinary obstruction, and loss of renal function.[10,14,15] Further surgical procedures may be required entailing further morbidity for the patient.

■ The Tests

What is the purpose of the tests?

The purpose of the preoperative intravenous pyelogram is to determine the course of the ureter and identify any preexisting distortion or anomalies.

What is the nature of the tests?

Intravenous pyelography is a sequenced examination that consists of abdominal radiographs obtained at timed intervals after the administration of intravenous iodinated contrast material. The serial films provide morphologic information only, and outline the kidneys, renal calyces, ureters, and bladder. Congenital anomalies such as ureteral duplication and pelvic kidneys, as well as ureteral dilation, compression, and deviation will be seen. Bladder compression from pelvic masses can also be visualized.

Preoperative screening of the urinary tract with ultrasound has been compared with intravenous pyelography.[16] Each modality identified hydronephrosis equally, but ultrasound failed to identify two of five duplicated ureters. Little information about the ureteral course can be obtained through ultrasound, so despite the lower cost and absence of contrast reactions, ultrasound cannot provide the same preoperative evaluation as intravenous pyelography.

Magnetic resonance pyelography has been compared with intravenous pyelography for the evaluation of dilated[17] and nondilated urinary tracts.[18] Both modalities equally identify morphologic abnormalities. However, information about renal function, in addition to anatomic information, can be obtained with magnetic resonance pyelography and patients with iodine allergies avoid contrast exposure. However, the cost of magnetic resonance pyelography is approximately ten times that of an intravenous pyelogram.

What are the implications of testing?

What does an abnormal test result mean? An abnormal test result demonstrates an abnormal anatomic course for one or both ureters.

The rationale for preoperative intravenous pyelography has been that the recognition of anatomic abnormalities prior to surgery would reduce the occurrence of surgical injury. This remains unproven. Retrospective studies revealed similar ureteral injury rates for patients undergoing preoperative intravenous pyelography versus those who do not.[19,20] Since intraoperative ureteral injuries occur infrequently, a randomized controlled trial to prove the effectiveness of a preoperative intravenous pyelogram in reducing ureteral injuries would require multiple study sites at prohibitive costs.

The likelihood of finding an abnormality of the urinary tract with a preoperative intravenous pyelogram is known. In 455 patients undergoing major pelvic surgery, 5.2% had genitourinary anomalies, 7% had hydronephrosis, and 3.1% had ureteral deviation.[21] In another series, 1.8% had congenital anomalies and 11.6% had ureteral dilation or deviation.[22] Both studies included patients with gynecologic malignancies. In the largest study of routine preoperative intravenous pyelograms for gynecologic procedures, a prevalence of 2% congenital anomalies, 5.2% ureteral deviation, and 7% hydronephrosis was reported.[23]

A relevant question for the surgeon is "are there any features from the patient's history or physical examination that identify them as having an increased risk of a urinary tract abnormality warranting a preoperative pyelogram?" Several studies have investigated this relationship. Ureteral dilation or displacement was present in 82% of patients with ovarian cysts, 71% with leiomyomata above the pelvic brim, 55% with leiomyomata below the pelvic brim, and 25% with uterine prolapse.[24]

A 20% prevalence of ureteral dilation and 10% prevalence of ureteral deviation was found in women with a uterine size 12 weeks' gestation or larger. In contrast, there were no intravenous pyelograms revealing ureteral dilation and only 2.5% showing ureteral deviation when the uterus was less than 12-weeks' size.[20] In women with an adnexal mass, 21% had dilation and 9% had deviations of the ureters.[20] Uterine prolapse is associated with obstructive uropathy in 4% to 80% of patients, with the degree of urinary obstruction increasing as the degree of prolapse increases.[20,25,26] Tubo-ovarian abscesses are associated with ureteral dilation in 39% and deviation in 36% of patients.[27]

In 16 women with the diagnosis of endometriosis, the preoperative intravenous pyelogram identified ureteral duplication in 12% and ureteral dilation in 18%.[20] However, a similar study with 63 patients found subtle abnormalities on the intravenous pyelogram in 15.9% of patients, but no cases of ureteral dilation or obstruction.[28] Previous abdominal surgery does not appear to increase the likelihood of an abnormal intravenous pyelogram.[20]

The surgeon should be interested in screening tests that increase the likelihood of detecting an abnormality. In this context, the patient's history and physical examination findings do function as a screening test for urinary tract abnormalities. No retrospective study adequately allows for the precise estimation of the sensitivity and specificity of these features. However, reanalysis of the data to correct for verification bias does permit and estimation of the sensitivity and specificity from data presented by Piscitelli et al.[20] Virtually all retrospective studies of diagnostic tests are affected by verification bias where patients with the abnormality of interest (e.g., uterine enlargement) are more likely to be referred for the reference test (e.g., intravenous pyelography) than those with normal examinations. These uncorrected biases result in an overestimated sensitivity and an underestimated specificity. Since the data of Piscitelli et al.[20] were derived from consecutive patients and the results included for those with normal findings, we can mathematically correct for the verification bias (Table 55–1).

Table 55–1 **Gynecologic pathways and IVP abnormalities**

Finding	Sensitivity, %	Specificity, %	LRpos (95% CI)	LRneg (95% CI)
Adnexal mass	14	92	1.8 (1.1, 3.2)	0.9 (0.8, 1.0)
Leiomyomata ≥ 12 wk	35	78	1.6 (1.2, 2.2)	0.6 (0.7, 0.9)
Endometriosis	6	96	1.3 (0.5, 2.9)	1.0 (0.9, 1.0)
Uterine prolapse	5	95	0.9 (0.4, 2.0)	1.0 (0.9, 1.0)

CI, confidence interval; LRpos, positive likelihood ratio; LRneg, negative likelihood ratio.

A likelihood ratio approaching 1.0 indicates the test has no value. From these results, the presence of either an adnexal mass or a leiomyomata greater than 12 weeks' gestational size increases the likelihood of finding a urinary tract abnormality and is the only positive finding where the confidence interval around the estimate excludes 1.0. Smaller leiomyomas or normal uterine size decreases marginally the likelihood of an abnormality by a factor of 0.6 and is the only negative finding where the confidence interval around the estimate excludes 1.0. The presence of endometriosis or uterine prolapse does not increase the underlying risk of a urinary tract abnormality. The absence of an adnexal mass, endometriosis, or uterine prolapse does not alter the chance of finding an abnormality beyond the baseline prevalence.

What does a normal test result mean? A normal preoperative intravenous pyelogram reduces the likelihood of preexisting urinary tract anatomic distortion. It does not obviate the need for direct intraoperative ureteral identification.

What is the cost of the testing?

The cost of an intravenous pyelogram is approximately $200 (2001) and magnetic resonance pyelography costs approximately $1,900 (2001). Minor reactions to the intravenous contrast occur in 0.4% to 2% of patients, with severe life-threatening reactions occurring in 0.04% to 0.2% of patients. Nephrotoxicity occurs in about 0.6% of patients without preexisting renal disease.[29–31] The use of low-osmolality intravascular contrast agents reduces these risks markedly, but is more expensive.[32]

Simel et al.[33] applied decision analysis techniques to evaluate the cost-effectiveness of preoperative screening intravenous pyelograms. Approximately $166,600 would be spent to avoid one ureteral injury, assuming a baseline ureteral injury rate of 0.5%, test efficacy of 25% (i.e., a preoperative intravenous pyelogram reduces the risk of injury by 25%), and a $200 cost. Approximately $3.33 million would be spent to prevent a single death. As the probability of injury increases, the marginal cost-effectiveness ratio is less dependent on the test efficacy and is more modest.[33]

If abnormal ureteral anatomy increases the risk of injury and certain clinical findings correlate with the presence of abnormalities in ureteral anatomy, selective use of preoperative intravenous pyelograms would be more cost-effective. Unfortunately, the clinical findings of an adnexal mass or a leiomyoma greater than 12 weeks' gestational size only increased the likelihood of a ureteral abnormality by 1.8- and 1.6-fold, respectively. Even if the probability of an injury was as high as 2.5% when the ureters are abnormal, the cost is still approximately $31,700 to prevent a single injury.[33]

■ Conclusions and Recommendations

The preoperative intravenous pyelogram delineates the anatomy of urinary tract and identifies any anomalies or distortion. Ureteral abnormalities such as deviation, dilation, and duplication place the patient at increased risk of surgical injury. However, it remains unproven that preoperative intravenous pyelography reduces the risk of such injury. With the low probability of an intraoperative ureteral injury during a gynecologic procedure for benign disease, the intravenous pyelogram may be effective. However, it is expensive to perform. Its use can only be justified in women predicted on clinical grounds to have a high probability of abnormal findings. The only categories of women identified from the literature to have a greater likelihood of ureteral abnormalities are those with an adnexal mass or with uterine leiomyomata at least 12 weeks' gestational size. Unfortunately, the absence of any historical or physical examination finding does not rule out the presence of ureteral abnormalities, reminding the surgeon to use careful intraoperative techniques for visualizing the ureters.

■ Summary

1 ■ What Is the Problem that Requires Screening?

Urinary tract injury during benign gynecologic surgery.

a. *What is the incidence/prevalence of the target condition?*
Ureteral injuries occur during hysterectomy in 0.1% to 2.5% of procedures.

b. *What are the sequelae of the condition that are of interest in clinical medicine?*
Unrecognized ureteral injury may result in pyelonephritis, sepsis, ileus, fistula formation, and loss of renal function. Reoperation may be required.

2 ■ The Tests

a. *What is the purpose of the tests?*
To delineate the urinary tract anatomy and identify preexisting pathology.

b. *What is the nature of the tests?*
Intravenous pyelography sequences abdominal radiographs at timed intervals after intravenous injection of contrast agents. Ultrasound is less effective in identifying congenital duplication or an abnormal course of the ureter.

c. *What are the implications of testing?*

1. What does an abnormal test result mean?

   The assumption is that awareness of anatomic abnormalities prior to surgery reduces the risk of inadvertent injury. This has not been proven by any study to date.

2. What does a normal test result mean?

   A normal preoperative intravenous pyelogram reduces the likelihood of preexisting urinary tract disease and anatomic distortion. *It does not obviate the need for direct intraoperative ureteral identification.*

d. *What is the cost of testing?*

Approximately $166,600 would be spent to avoid one ureteral injury, assuming a baseline ureteral injury rate of 0.5%, test efficacy of 25% (i.e., a preoperative intravenous pyelogram reduces the risk of injury by 25%), and a $200 cost. Approximately $3.33 million would be spent to prevent a single death.

3 ■ Conclusions and Recommendations

Given the low risk of an intraoperative injury during a hysterectomy for benign disease, the intravenous pyelogram clearly is expensive even if it is effective. Its use can only be justified in patients predicted on clinical grounds to have a high probability of abnormal findings. The only such category of patients identified from the literature are those with an adnexal mass or uterine leiomyomata at least 12 weeks' gestational size.

References

1. Symmonds RE. Ureteral injuries associated with gynecologic surgery: prevention and management. *Clin Obstet Gynecol* 1976;19:623–644.
2. Drake MJ, Noble JG. Ureteric trauma in gynecologic surgery. *Int Urogynecol J Pelvic Floor Dysfunct* 1998;9:108–117.
3. Goodno JA Jr, Powers TW, Harris VD. Ureteral injuries in gynecologic surgery: a ten-year review in a community hospital. *Am J Obstet Gynecol* 1995;172:1817–1820.
4. Harkki-Siren P, Sjöberg J, Tiitinen A. Urinary tract injuries after hysterectomy. *Obstet Gynecol* 1998;92:113–118.
5. Daly JW, Higgins KA. Injury to the ureter during gynecologic surgical procedures. *Surg Gynecol Obstet* 1988;167:19–22.
6. Liapis A, Bakas P, Giannopoulos V, et al Ureteral injuries during gynecological surgery. *Int Urogynecol J Pelvic Floor Dysfunct* 2001;12:391–393.
7. Carley ME, McIntire D, Carley JM, et al. Incidence, risk factors and morbidity of unintended bladder or ureter injury during hysterectomy. *Int Urogynecol J Pelvic Floor Dysfunct* 2002; 13:18–21.

8. Mathevet P, Valencia P, Cousin C, et al. Operative injuries during vaginal hysterectomy. *Eur J Obstet Gynecol Reprod Biol* 2001;97:71–75.
9. Tamussino KF, Lang PF, Breinl E. Ureteral complications with operative gynecologic laparoscopy. *Am J Obstet Gynecol* 1998;178:967–970.
10. Ostrzenski A, Radolinski B, Ostrzenska KM. A review of laparoscopic ureteral injury in pelvic surgery. *Obstet Gynecol Surv* 2003;58:794–799.
11. Saidi MH, Sadler Rk, Vancainllie TG, et al. Diagnosis and management of serious urinary complications after major operative laparoscopy. *Obstet Gynecol* 1996;87:272–276.
12. Harkki-Siren P, Sjoberg J, Makinen J, et al. Finnish national register of laparoscopic hysterectomies : a review and complications of 1165 operations. *Am J Obstet Gynecol* 1997;176:118–122.
13. Meirow D, Moriel EZ, Zilberman M, et al. Evaluation and treatment of iatrogenic ureteral injuries during obstetric and gynecologic operations for nonmalignant conditions. *J Am Coll Surg* 1994;178:144–148.
14. Rafique M, Arif MH. Management of iatrogenic ureteric injuries associated with gynecologic surgery. *Int Urol Nephrol* 2002;34:31–35.
15. Liapis A, Bakas P, Sykiotis K, et al. Urinomas as a complication of iatrogenic ureteric injury in gynecological surgery. *Eur J Obstet Gynecol Reprod Biol* 2000;91:83–85.
16. Aslaksen A, Gothlin JH, Geitung JT, et al. Ultrasonography versus urography as preoperative investigation prior to hysterectomy. *Acta Obstet Gynecol Scand* 1989;68:443–445.
17. Catalano C, Pavone P, Laghi A, et al. MR pyelography and conventional MR imaging in urinary tract obstruction. *Acta Radiol* 1999;40:198–202.
18. El-Diasty T, Mansour O, Farouk A. Diuretic contrast-enhanced magnetic resonance urography versus intravenous urography for depiction of nondilated urinary tracts. *Abdom Imaging* 2003;28:135–145.
19. Sack Ra. The value of intravenous urography prior to abdominal hysterectomy for gynecologic disease. *Am J Obstet Gynecol* 1979;143:208–212.
20. Pitcitelli JT, Simel DL, Addison WA. Who should have intravenous pyelograms before hysterectomy for benign disease? *Obstet Gynecol* 1987;68:541–545.
21. Roden JS, Haugen HM, Hall DG, et al. The value of intravenous pyelography prior to elective gynecologic operations. *Am J Obstet Gynecol* 1961;82:568–571.
22. Schwartz WR, Hofmeister FJ, Mattingly RF. The value of intravenous pyelogram in pelvic surgery. *Obstet Gynecol* 1964;23:1049–1053.
23. Klissaristos AA, Manouelides NS, Comninos AC. Preoperative intravenous pyelography in gynecology. *Inter Surg* 1974;59:31–32.
24. Kretschmer HL, Kanter AE. Effect of certain gynecologic lesions on the upper urinary tract: a pyelographic study. *JAMA* 1937;109:1097–1101.
25. Rodriguez AA, Gonzalez BA, Cachay A, et al. Obstructive anuria secondary to uterine prolapse. *Actas Urol Esp* 2002;26:703–707.
26. Beverly CM, Walters MD, Weber AM, et al. Prevalence of hydronephrosis in patients undergoing surgery for pelvic organ prolapse. *Obstet Gynecol* 1997;90:37–41.
27. Philips JC. A spectrum of radiologic abnormalities due to tubo-ovarian abscess. *Radiology* 1974;110:307–311.
28. Maxson WS. Hill GA, Herbert CM, et al. Ureteral abnormalities in women with endometriosis. *Fertil Steril* 1986;46:1159–1161.
29. Mushlin AI, Thornbury JR. Intravenous pyelography: the case against its routine use. *Ann Intern Med* 1989;111:58–70.
30. Thomsen HS, Bush WH Jr. Adverse effects of contrast media: incidence, prevention, and management. *Drug Saf* 1998;19:313–324.
31. Caro JJ, Trindade E, McGregor M. The risks of death and of severe nonfatal reactions with high- vs. low-osmolality contrast media: a meta-analysis. *Am J Roentgenol* 1991;156:825–832.
32. American College of Radiology Committee on Drugs and Contrast Media. Practice Guideline for the use of intravascular contrast media. *ACR* Reston, Virginia, 2001.
33. Simel DL, Matchar DB, Piscitelli JT. Routine intravenous pyelograms before hysterectomy in cases of benign disease: possibly effective, definitely expensive. *Am J Obstet Gynecol* 1988;159:1049–1053.

Osteoporosis

Susan R. Johnson

■ What Is the Problem that Requires Screening?

Postmenopausal osteoporosis.

Osteoporosis is a condition characterized by low bone mass and disordered microarchitecture that results in an increased risk of fracture

What is the incidence/prevalence of the target condition?

Osteoporosis is defined by the World Health Organization (WHO) as a bone density of either the hip or spine of more than 2.5 standard deviations (SDs) below the mean compared with healthy young women. It is estimated to affect 13% to 18% of postmenopausal women over age 50 in the United States.[7] There are considerable racial, ethnic, and geographic differences in the rates of osteoporosis, with white women having the highest rates in the United States.[8] The prevalence increases with age; white women lose on average 40% of their bone mass between menopause and age 90. *Osteopenia*, defined as a bone density between 1 and 2.5 SDs below the mean, is also associated with an increased risk of fracture and is found in up to half the women over 50.[7]

Although loss of estrogen coupled with advancing age is the most common cause of osteoporosis in women, there are many conditions associated with bone loss that lead to so-called "secondary" osteoporosis. Some of the more common causes include chronic corticosteroid use, hyperparathyroidism, hyperthyroidism, multiple myeloma, eating disorders, and long-term use of other drugs such as phenytoin, phenobarbital, heparin, or excessive thyroid replacement.[7]

What are the sequelae of the condition that are of interest in clinical medicine?

The primary sequelae of low bone mass are fractures. Osteoporosis related fractures are among the most common morbid conditions in postmenopausal women; half of the white women over the age of 50 years will sustain a fracture at some time during the remainder of their life.[9] The most common sites are the vertebral compression fractures, Colles type fracture of the wrist, and the femoral neck of the hip. Vertebral fractures are most common, with a prevalence of roughly 70/10,000 women; multiple vertebral fractures are common. Wrist and hip fractures occur with roughly the same frequency, approximately 40/10,000 women, but the relationship to age differs. Wrist fractures begin to occur in the late 50s, peaks early, and then remains constant. Hip fractures are uncommon until after age 70, when the incidence increases linearly.

The sequelae that occur as a result of a fracture depend on the site. Colles fractures may heal completely, but recovery can take up to a year. Some women lose full mobility of their wrist or grip strength or develop chronic joint pain. In addition, posttraumatic arthritis, reflex sympathetic dystrophy, and median nerve damage leading to carpal tunnel syndrome may occur. After 10 years, approximately 15% of women have continued problems related to the fracture.[10]

Vertebral body fractures are a cause of acute and chronic back pain, loss of height, and kyphosis (the so-called "dowager hump"). Difficulty bending or lifting and walking down stairs are increased.[11] Multiple compression fractures of the thoracic spine can lead to compromised cardiopulmonary and gastrointestinal function. Mortality and hospitalization rates are also increased among women with vertebral fracture compared to those without.[12] Finally, the presence of a vertebral fracture is associated with a fivefold increase in risk of hip fracture.

Hip fracture is the most feared consequence of osteoporosis. The mortality rate is approximately 20% the year after hip fracture, with 25% requiring admission to a nursing home; 50% do not fully recover.[8] Even women who fall, but do not fracture, experience loss of independence due to fear of fracturing their hip in a subsequent fall. In one study, most older women surveyed preferred death to survival after hip fracture. The economic cost of osteoporosis-related fractures, most of which are due to hip fracture care, is estimated at $17 billion annually in the United States and exceeds the cost of cardiovascular conditions in older women[13]

■ The Tests

What is the purpose of the tests?

To identify low bone mass.

Low bone mass can be accurately identified by using measurements of bone mineral density (BMD). BMD is highly predictive of future fracture risk and is as predictive as elevated blood pressure is for risk of stroke and more predictive than the cholesterol level for myocardial infarction.[14] There is no practical test for the disordered microarchitecture.

What is the nature of the tests?

Dual-energy x-ray absorptiometry (DEXA) is the gold standard test for the diagnosis of osteoporosis, and the test that is recommended for monitoring therapy.[7,15] Although BMD can be measured by DEXA at a peripheral site (e.g., wrist or heel) or centrally (hip and spine), the central measurements are the most useful. DEXA involves an extremely small dose of radiation (1/100th the dose of a single chest radiograph). Operators must be specially trained to perform and interpret the test.

The direct measurement of the hip is most predictive of hip fracture risk (relative risk [RR], 2.6 for each additional SD below the mean) and that of the spine, most accurate for fractures of the spine (RR, 2.0).[14,16] Because these two fractures account for most morbidity and mortality associated with osteoporosis, DEXA of the hip and/or spine is preferred when available and technically feasible. If only one measurement is taken, the hip is preferred because it has the highest predictive value for hip fracture if abnormal and a low value predicts risk at other sites.[17] DEXA measurements have variability in precision, some 2% to 3% for an individual measurement, and there is also variation among machines. Because the rate of loss per year may be less than the variability of the measurement, follow up testing should not be done more often than two years after the first test.[17,18] Because of machine variability, results are most accurately interpreted if the follow up tests are performed on the exact same machine as the original reading.

The primary result of the DEXA test is bone mineral density measured in grams per centimeter squared. This value is then converted to an SD from the mean for either women of the same age and race (the "z-score") or for young healthy women (the "t-score"). The t-score is currently considered the preferred method of reporting scores by most expert practice guidelines, including the WHO, North American Menopause Society, and National Osteoporosis Society.

What are the implications of testing?

What does an abnormal test result mean? The BMD t-score is used to predict risk of fracture and is primarily used to identify women who might benefit from drug therapy to reduce further bone loss and risk of fracture. Each additional SD reduction in density below the mean is associated with a twofold increase of risk. Fracture prediction is complex and not simply a matter of knowing the t-score.[19] A major challenge is that bone loss begins soon after menopause (an average age of 50 years), whereas fracture risk does not begin until many years later (e.g., 30 years after menopause for hip fracture).[20] Fracture risk is independently related to bone density, increasing age, prior fracture,[21] and the presence of additional risk factors such as smoking, low weight, a first-degree relative with a hip fracture, menopause before age 45, and glucocorticoid use. The risk of hip fracture is also related to factors that increase the risk of falls, such as visual problems, frailty, and use of medications that impair balance. Approximately half the women over the age of 85 experience at least one fall, accounting for the sharp increase in hip fractures as women reach old age.[8] The absolute risk of fracture depends on the woman's age, and each 5-year increase in age after 50 increases the relative risk of hip fracture by a factor 1.4 independent of BMD. As an example the annual probability of hip fracture for the next 5 years associated with a t-score of −2.5 is 0.24% for a 55-year-old woman, 0.45% for a 65-year-old, 1.24% for a 75-year-old, and 2.9% for an 85-year-old.[16]

Postmenopausal women with no additional historical risk factors should consider antiresorptive therapy when the DEXA-based t-score of either the hip or spine reaches −2.0 (two SDs below the mean for a healthy young population of women) and for women with at least one additional risk factor, when the t-score is −1.5 or lower. All postmenopausal women with a DEXA-based t-score in the hip or spine of −2.5 or who have already sustained a fragility fracture at any site should use antiresorptive therapy. Until the mid 1990s, the only effective antiresorptive drug was estrogen; and, long-term estrogen therapy was believed to have multiple benefits. Although BMD testing was available, most experts recommended testing *only* of women who needed BMD information to make a decision on long-term hormone therapy. Women who agreed to estrogen for other reasons were felt to not need bone density information, and there seemed to be no point testing women who refused to take estrogen under any circumstance. The landscape has since changed dramatically. First, the availability of other antiresorptive drugs made osteoporosis risk assessment a reasonable choice for women whether or not they were interested or able to take estrogen. These drugs, each of which has been shown in placebo-controlled trials to reduce the fracture risk, include alendronate,[1] risedronate,[2] raloxifene,[3] and to a lesser extent, calcitonin.[4] Second, and more profoundly, the conclusions of the Women's Health Initiative clinical trials of estrogen plus progestin and estrogen alone have dramatically altered the way hormone therapy is used such that long-term estrogen therapy solely for osteoporosis prevention in asymptomatic postmenopausal women is not generally recommended.[5,6]

What does a normal test result mean? A normal BMD (t-score higher than −1.0 [i.e., no more than 1 SD below the mean for young healthy women]) suggests that bone mass is adequate and the likelihood of fracture is low. The ability to predict future bone density is less clear, and depends to some extent on the "stage" of menopause and the presence of other risk factors. Peak bone density in women is achieved by the early 30s and remains relatively stable until at least the onset of the climacteric phase. After the final menstrual period, most women enter a phase of accelerated bone lost (2% to 5% per year) for several years, after which the rate of loss usually slows. If a bone density is obtained at the beginning of menopause, typically around the age of 50, a normal value may not predict bone density at age 65 as this woman could lose substantial bone if she is a rapid bone loser in the early post menopause; further screening by age 65 would be recommended. On the other hand, a healthy 65-year-old woman with a normal BMD who is 15 years postmenopausal and in the slow phase of bone loss may not need further screening.

Falsely reassuring elevations of bone density can result from arthritis or bone spurs, both of which are common in the spine but not hip. Thus, if both hip and spine BMD are determined, the clinical response is based on the lower of the two. If one value only is measured, the hip is preferred.

What is the cost of testing?

The cost of a single central DEXA reading is approximately $200. The lower the intervention cost and the higher the effectiveness, the lower the age at which intervention will be cost-effective. In one study with the base case ($500 per year; 35% efficacy) treatment in women was cost-effective with a 10-year hip fracture probability ranging from 1.4% at the age of 50 years to 4.4% at the age of 65 years.[28] The exclusion of osteoporotic fractures other than hip fracture would increase the threshold to 9% to 11% 10 year probability because of the substantial morbidity from fractures other than hip fracture, particularly at younger ages.

■ Conclusions and Recommendations

Osteoporosis prevention in women begins with strategies to optimize peak bone density in early life. Adequate calcium and vitamin D intake, weight-bearing exercise, and avoidance of factors that adversely affect bone mass, like smoking, constitute the essentials. Endogenous estrogen production is also key to optimizing and preserving bone mass in premenopausal women. When estrogen deficiency occurs, for example with hypothalamic pituitary dysfunction–associated amenorrhea, antiresorptive therapy, usually in the form of exogenously administered estrogen, is now considered routine. However, bone density testing is not generally necessary in this situation, as the consequences of estrogen deficiency are clear.

BMD testing with DEXA is the most valuable test for the identification of postmenopausal candidates for osteoporosis prevention and treatment. Although there are not yet randomized prospective trials of any screening approach, most expert groups agree on the following guidelines.[7,15,17,22–24] All women who are 65 years or older should be screened. Younger postmenopausal women should be screened if they have one or more additional risk factors. The cost effectiveness of routine screening for women under 65 who have no additional risk factors for osteoporosis (other than being postmenopausal) has not been established, although these women may pay more attention to their bone health after having a BMD test regardless of the results.

Most postmenopausal women are not yet screened or treated according to these guidelines.[19,25] Even women who have sustained clinical fragility fractures of the wrist, spine and hip are often neither tested nor treated with antiresorptive or anabolic agents.[26,27] BMD testing predicts osteoporotic fractures with the same power as other more frequently used screening tests such as cholesterol and blood pressure, and there are several established treatments that have been shown to reduce the risk of fracture by at least half. The current guidelines for screening should be applied to all postmenopausal women.[25]

■ Summary

1 ■ What Is the Problem that Requires Screening?

Postmenopausal osteoporosis.

Osteoporosis is a condition characterized by low bone mass and disordered microarchitecture which results in an increased risk of fracture.

a. What is the incidence/prevalence of the target condition?

It is estimated to affect 13% to 18% of postmenopausal women over age 50 in the United States.[7] There are considerable racial, ethnic, and geographic differences in the rates of osteoporosis, with white women having the highest rates in the United States.[8] The prevalence increases with age; white women lose on average 40% of their bone mass between menopause and age 90.

b. What are the sequelae of the condition that are of interest in clinical medicine?

The primary sequelae of low bone mass are fractures. Osteoporosis-related fractures are among the most common morbid conditions in postmenopausal women; half of the white women over the age of 50 years will sustain a fracture at some time during the remainder of their life. The most common types are vertebral compression fractures, Colles-type fracture of the wrist, and the fractures of the femoral neck of the hip.

2 ■ The Tests

a. What is the purpose of the tests?

To identify low bone mass.

b. **What is the nature of the tests?**
Bone mineral density (BMD) measurement by dual-energy x-ray absorptiometry (DEXA).

c. **What are the implications of testing?**
1. What does an abnormal test result mean?
Each additional standard deviation reduction in BMD t-score below the mean is associated with a twofold increased risk of fracture. Fracture prediction is complex and not simply a matter of knowing the t-score. Postmenopausal women with no additional historical risk factors should consider antiresorptive therapy when the DEXA based t-score of either the hip or spine reaches −2.0 (2 SDs below the mean for a healthy young population of women) and when the t-score is −1.5 or lower for women with at least one additional risk factor. All postmenopausal women with a DEXA-based t-score in the hip or spine of −2.5 or who have already sustained a fragility fracture at any site should use antiresorptive therapy.
2. What does a normal test result mean?
A normal BMD (t-score higher than −1.0 [i.e., no more than 1 SD below the mean for young healthy women]) suggests that bone mass is adequate and the likelihood of fracture is low.

d. **What is the cost of testing?**
The cost of a single central DEXA reading is approximately $200.

3 ■ Conclusions and Recommendations

Osteoporosis prevention in women begins with strategies to optimize peak bone density in early life. Adequate calcium and vitamin D intake, weight-bearing exercise, and avoidance of factors that adversely affect bone mass, like smoking, constitute the essentials. Long-term estrogen therapy solely for osteoporosis prevention in asymptomatic postmenopausal women is not generally recommended.

Continued

■ **Summary—cont'd**

BMD testing with DEXA is the most valuable test for the identification of postmenopausal candidates for osteoporosis prevention and treatment. All women who are 65 years or older should be screened. Younger postmenopausal women should be screened if they have one or more additional risk factors. The cost-effectiveness of routine screening for women younger than 65 who have no additional risk factors for osteoporosis (other than being postmenopausal) has not been established, although these women may pay more attention to their bone health after having a BMD test regardless of the results.

References

1. Black DM, Thompson DE, Bauer DC, et al. Fracture risk reduction with alendronate in women with osteoporosis: the Fracture Intervention Trial. FIT Research Group [erratum appears in *J Clin Endocrinol Metab* 2001;86:938]. *J Clin Endocrinol Metab* 2000;85:4118–4124.
2. Cranney A, Waldegger L, Zytaruk N, et al. Risedronate for the prevention and treatment of postmenopausal osteoporosis. Cochrane Database of Systematic Reviews. 2003:4CD004523.
3. Delmas PD, Ensrud KE, Adachi JD, et al. Efficacy of raloxifene on vertebral fracture risk reduction in postmenopausal women with osteoporosis: four-year results from a randomized clinical trial. *J Clin Endocrinol Metab* 2002;87:3609–3617.
4. Kanis JA. Calcitonin in osteoporosis. *Bone* 2002;30[5 Suppl]:65S–66S.
5. Anderson GL, Limacher M, Assaf AR, et al. Effects of conjugated equine estrogen in postmenopausal women with hysterectomy: the Women's Health Initiative randomized controlled trial [see comment]. *JAMA* 2004;291:1701–1712.
6. Rossouw JE, Anderson GL, Prentice RL, et al. Risks and benefits of estrogen plus progestin in healthy postmenopausal women: principal results from the Women's Health Initiative randomized controlled trial [see comment]. *JAMA* 2002;288:321–333.
7. American College of Obstetricians and Gynecologists. Osteoporosis. ACOG Practice Bulletin No. 50. *Obst Gynecol* 2004;103:203–216.
8. Cummings SR, Melton LJ. Epidemiology and outcomes of osteoporotic fractures [see comment]. *Lancet* 2002;359:1761–1767.
9. Chrischilles EA, Butler CD, Davis CS, et al. A model of lifetime osteoporosis impact [erratum appears in *Arch Intern Med* 1922 Mar;152:3655]. *Arch Intern Med* 1991;151:2026–2032.
10. Warwick D, Field J, Prothero D, et al. Function ten years after Colles' fracture. *Clin Orthopaed Rel Res* 1993:270–274.
11. Greendale GA, Barrett-Connor E, Ingles S, et al. Late physical and functional effects of osteoporotic fracture in women: the Rancho Bernardo Study. *J Am Geriatr Soc* 1995;43:955–961.
12. Ensrud KE, Thompson DE, Cauley JA, et al. Prevalent vertebral deformities predict mortality and hospitalization in older women with low bone mass: Fracture Intervention Trial Research Group. *J Am Geriatr Soc* 2000;48:241–249.
13. Keen R. Burden of osteoporosis and fractures. *Curr Osteopor Rep* 2003;1:266–270.
14. Marshall D, Johnell O, Wedel H. Meta-analysis of how well measures of bone mineral density predict occurrence of osteoporotic fractures [see comment]. *BMJ* 1996;312:1254–1259.

15. Hodgson SF, Watts NB, Bilezikian JP, et al. American Association of Clinical Endocrinologists 2001 medical guidelines for clinical practice for the prevention and management of postmenopausal osteoporosis. *Endocr Pract* 2001;7:293–312.

16. Kanis JA, Brazier JE, Stevenson M, et al. Treatment of established osteoporosis: a systematic review and cost-utility analysis. *Health Technol Assess* 2002;6:291–346.

17. Berg AO. Screening for osteoporosis in postmenopausal women: recommendations and rationale. *AJN* 2003;103:173–180.

18. Cummings SR, Palermo L, Browner W, et al. Monitoring osteoporosis therapy with bone densitometry: misleading changes and regression to the mean. *JAMA* 2000;283:1318–1321.

19. Bates DW, Black DM, Cummings SR. Clinical use of bone densitometry: clinical applications. *JAMA* 2002;288:1898–1900.

20. Black DM, Cummings SR, Melton LJ 3rd. Appendicular bone mineral and a woman's lifetime risk of hip fracture. *J Bone Min Res* 1992;7:639–646.

21. Klotzbuecher CM, Ross PD, Landsman PB, et al. Patients with prior fractures have an increased risk of future fractures: a summary of the literature and statistical synthesis. *J Bone Min Res* 2000;15:721–739.

22. North American Menopause S. Management of postmenopausal osteoporosis: position statement of the North American Menopause Society. *Menopause* 2002;9:284–301.

23. Osteoporosis: review of the evidence for prevention, diagnosis and treatment and cost-effectiveness analysis: executive summary. *Osteoporos Int* 1998;8[Suppl 4]:S3–S6.

24. National Osteoporosis Foundation. Physician's guide to prevention and treatment of osteoporosis. National Osteoporosis Foundation. Available at http://www.guideline.gov/summary/summary.aspx?view_id=1&doc_id=3862. Accessed November 1, 2004.

25. Mazanec D. Osteoporosis screening: time to take responsibility [comment]. *Arch Intern Med* 2004;164:1047–1048.

26. Feldstein AC, Nichols GA, Elmer PJ, et al. Older women with fractures: patients falling through the cracks of guideline-recommended osteoporosis screening and treatment. *J Bone Joint Surg Am* 2003;85-A:2294–2302.

27. Gunter MJ, Beaton SJ, Brenneman SK, et al. Management of osteoporosis in women aged 50 and older with osteoporosis-related fractures in a managed care population. *Dis Manag* 2003;6:283–291.

28. Kanis JA, Johnell O, Oden A, et al. Intervention thresholds for osteoporosis. *Bone* 2002; 31:126–131.

Index

A

A/B ratio. *See* Systolic to diastolic ratio
Abdominal circumference (AC), 434
Abdominal radiographs, intravenous
    pyelogram and, 666–69
Abdominal wall defects, 232
    summary for, 240–41
ABE. *See* Acute bilirubin encephalopathy
Aberrant placental implantation,
    tests for, 272–74
Abnormal test result
    AFP MoM values and, 236–38
    amniotic fluid embolism and, 470
    antithrombin deficiencies and, 272–73
    APS and, 295
    asymptomatic bacteriuria in pregnancy
        and, 41
    BPS and, 451–52
    cervical cytology and, 605
    CF and, 125–29, 515
    Chlamydia infection, 106
    chromosomal abnormalities and,
        206–8, 259
    CMV and, 69
    CO and, 398
    for congenital rubella infection, 57
    congenital toxoplasmosis and, 66
    criteria for, uterine fundus measurement,
        329
    CRS and, 59
    Doppler imaging and, fetal hypoxia and,
        439
    early-onset genetic diseases and, 157–58
    ECG and, 660
    fasting plasma glucose and, 552
    fetal arterial system, Doppler studies of,
        442–43
    fetal movement and, 450
    fetal structural anomalies and, 246–48
    fetal two-dimensional ultrasound and,
        435–36
    fetal venous circulation and, 443
    FHM and, 350–51, 354
    FHM v. dating and, 336
    FHR and, 448
    fragile X syndrome and, 169
    GDM and, 307–10
    gene mutation and, 579
    gestational age dating and, 194–95
    gonorrhea and, 99
    hemoconcentration plasma volume and,
        35
    hemoglobinopathies and, 143
    hepatitis A virus infection and, 76

hepatitis B during pregnancy and, 80
hepatitis C virus infection and, 85
HIV and, 115
Huntington disease and, 182
hyperthyroidism and, 281–82
infectious syphilis and, 91–92
IUFD and, 470
IUGR and, 362–63
low birth weight infants and, maternal
    height screening and, 322
mammography and, 594
maternal thyroid function tests and, 285
maternal weight, low birthweight infants
    with, *323*
MCAD and, 512
meaning of, 17–18, 20
neonatal hypoglycemia and, 486–87
neonate GBS and, 51, 53
ovarian cancer and, 630
peripheral vascular resistance and,
    preeclampsia and, 400
placental abruption and, 470
preeclampsia and, 397, 471
preterm birth and, 384–85
PTD and, 381
serum uric acid concentration and,
    preeclampsia and, 423–24
sexually transmitted disease and, IUDs
    and, 568
SLE in pregnancy and, 291
thrombosis, 272–73
toxoplasma infection and, 62–64
trisomy 18 and, 224
trisomy 21 fetus, 224
TVS and, 624
uterine artery waveforms and, 412
ABO grouping tests, 16
    costs of, 18–19
    normal test results for, 18
ABS. *See* Biophysical Profile Score
Absent end-diastolic velocity (AEDV),
    growth restricted fetuses and, 375
Absent nasal bone, second trimester, aneu-
    ploidy and, 220
Absolute velocities, Doppler ultrasound and,
    361
Acetic acid, HPV and, 605
Acid base balance
    abnormal test result and, 450
    fetal hypoxia and, 430
Acidemia, 443
    fetal movements and, 451
    hypoxemia v., 448
aCLs. *See* Anticardiolipin antibodies

ACOG. *See* American College of Obstetrics and Gynecology
Acquired immunodeficiency syndrome (AIDS), 112. *See also* Human immunodeficiency virus
Acquired thrombophilias, costs for, assay method and, *274*
ACTH. *See* Adrenal corticotrophin hormone
Activated C protein (APC), OC users and, screening tests and, 562
Activated partial thromboplastin time (APTT), 468
  APS and, 294
  DIC and, 471
Acute bilirubin encephalopathy (ABE), 492
Acute disseminated intravascular coagulation (DIC)
  abnormal test result for, 471
  normal test result for, 471
  recommendations for, 472
Acute myocardial infarction, ECG and, 660
Acylcarnitines, MCAD and, 512
ADA. *See* American Diabetes Association
Addison disease, 298
Adenoma-carcinoma sequence, colorectal cancer and, 650
Adenomatous polyp, colorectal cancer and, 650
Adnexal mass
  differential diagnosis of, 532
  pyelogram and, 668
Adrenal corticotrophin hormone (ACTH), CAH and, 509
Adverse perinatal outcome, SGA v., *349*
AFP screening test. *See* α-fetoprotein screening test
Age
  CHD and, 658
  osteoporosis and, 673
  silent MI, *661*
Agglutination tests, ABO grouping and, 16
Air-contrast barium enema. *See* Barium enema
Alkaline electrophoresis
  hemoglobin variants, 142
  hemoglobinopathies and, 140
Allele, Huntington disease and, 183
Alloimmunization, Rh negative women and, 477
Alloimmunization to Rh, 476
Alpha gene phenotypes, *142*
Alzheimer dementia, trisomy 21 and, 202
Ambulatory BP monitoring, preeclampsia and, 397
American College of Obstetrics and Gynecology (ACOG), GDM and, 312, 313
American Diabetes Association (ADA)
  fasting criteria, 551
  GDM and, 303, *304, 312*

Amino acid transfer, 430
Amniocentesis
  chromosome abnormalities with, *258*
  CMV and, 70
  fetal cells and, 254
  hemoglobinopathies and, 140
  HIV and, 115
  Huntington disease and, 179
  karyotyping v., 254
  screening tests and, 225
  second trimester, maternal age and, 217–18
  toxoplasma infection and, 63
  trisomy 21 and, 206, 221
  ultrasonography v., 237
Amniotic fluid
  assessment, 451
  embolism
    abnormal test result for, 470
    intrapartum coagulopathy and, 466
    normal test result for, 470
    peripartum coagulopathy and, 466
  fetal cells and, 254
  fFN and, 380
  GBS and, 48
  quantification, fetal hypoxia and, 432
  volume
    BPS and, 452
    FHM and, 345
    IUGR and, 436
A-mode ultrasound, aortic diameter and, 398
Analgesia, preeclampsia and, 469
ANAs. *See* Antinuclear antibodies
Anemia during pregnancy, 22, 27. *See also* Hematocrit levels
  abnormal test result and, 35
  health sequelae and, 34–35
  summary regarding, 37–38
  treatment for, 26
Anemia screening, abnormal test result and, 25
Anemia secondary to delivery
  incidence/prevalence of, 34
  screening problem and, 34
  summary regarding, 37–38
Anemia secondary to pregnancy
  incidence/prevalence of, 34
  screening problem and, 34
Anencephaly, 232
  high resolution ultrasound and, 237
  sequelae of, 233–34
Anesthesia, preeclampsia and, 469
Aneuploidy, 246
  fetal NT and, 205, *205,* 206
  first-trimester
    screening for, 201–13
    summary, 212–13
  IUGR and, 433, *433*
  test costs for, 225–26
Aneuploidy markers, trisomy 21 and, 222, 223

Angle of insonation, Doppler ultrasound and, 361–62
Antenatal care
fetal growth restriction and, 345, *346*
FHM and, 337
Antenatal diagnosis
congenital rubella infection and, 57
fetal structural anomalies and, 244
neural tube defects and, 237
Antenatal exclusion-definitive test, Huntington disease and, 182
Antenatal FHR monitor, testing costs for, 449
Antenatal maternal blood grouping, testing for, 16
Antenatal period, birthweight and, 349
Antenatal screening. *See also* Screening summary
CF carrier, 125
chromosomal abnormalities and, 204
clinician and patient choice in, flowchart for, *262*
disadvantages of, CF and, 127, 128, 129
fetal hypoxemia and, conclusions and recommendations for, 452–55, *453*
first trimester, 210–11
fragile X syndrome and, 168
hemoglobinopathies and, 140
Huntington disease and, 178, 181
neonatal GBS and, 50
nonsyndromic hearing loss and, 156
protocols for, chromosome abnormalities and, 261, *261*
trisomy 18 and, 217
trisomy 21 and, 220
ultrasound, 339
test costs of, 415
Antenatal sonography, trisomy 18 and, 223
Antenatal spiramycin, toxoplasma infection and, 63
Antepartum screening, testing costs and, 36
Antibiotic prophylaxis
IUDs and, 566
SCD and, 518
Antibiotic therapy
asymptomatic bacteriuria in pregnancy and, 44
maternal GBS and, *49*
neonatal GBS and, 50
positive fFN and, 380
Antibody screen, maternal red blood cell group and, 15–21
Anticardiolipin antibodies (aCLs), APS and, 294
Anticoagulant pathways, venous thrombosis and, 270
Anticoagulant therapy, pregnancy and, 273
Anti-D immunoglobulin, Rh (D)-negative typing and, 478

Anti-double-stranded DNA (anti-dsDNA), SLE and, 290
Antiembolic stockings, pregnancy and, 275
Antigen expression, 17
Antiglobulin test, 17
Anti-HBs (hepatitis B surface antibody), 80
Anti-La antibodies (SSB), 290, 291
Antimicrobial agents, asymptomatic bacteriuria in pregnancy and, 43, *43*
Antinuclear antibodies (ANAs), SLE and, 290
Antiphospholipid antibodies, APS and, 293
Antiphospholipid syndromes (APSs), 289
incidence/prevalence of, 293–94
maternal circulation and, 437
sequelae of, 294
summary of, 296–97
Anti-RBC antibodies, testing for, 19
Antiretroviral therapy, HIV and, 113
Anti-Ro antibodies (SSA), 290, 291
Antithrombin deficiencies
pregnancy-related thrombosis and, 272
tests for, 272
Antithyroid medication, Graves disease and, 280
Aortic diameter measurement, A-mode ultrasound and, 398
APC. *See* Activated C protein
Apgar scores, Doppler screening and, 367
Appropriate for gestational age (AGA) neonates, transient hypoglycemia and, 484
APSs. *See* Antiphospholipid syndromes
APTT. *See* Activated partial thromboplastin time
Arrhythmias, 658, 662
Arterial blood oxygen, fetal hypoxia and, 430
Arterial emboli, atrial fibrillation and, 658–59
Arterial thrombosis, APS and, 293
Arthralgia, congenital rubella infection and, 57
ASA. *See* Appropriate for gestational age neonates
Aspirin
APS and, 294
Doppler waveforms and, 414
IUGR and, 368
Asymptomatic bacteriuria in pregnancy, 40–46
abnormal test result meaning and, 41
antimicrobial agents for, 43, *43*
incidence of, 40
sequelae of, 40
summary for, 45–46
testing costs for, 43
tests for, 41, 43–44
treatment of, 43
Ataxia-telangiectasia (A-T), 579
Atenolol, preeclampsia and, 399
Atherogenic lipid profile, preeclampsia and, 543

ATM gene, 579
Atoacoustic emissions (OAEs), hearing impairment, 521–22
ATP III classification, *540*
Atrial fibrillation, 658, 662
Atrioventricular nodal blocks, 659
Auditory brainstem response, hearing impairment, 521–22
Auditory disturbances, CBE and, 493
Australian pregnancy hypertension guidelines, 397
Autoantibodies, 279
Autoimmune diseases, pregnancy and, 279–98
Autoimmune hemolytic anemia, pregnancy and, 298
Autoimmune thrombocytopenia, 298
Autosomal dominant inheritance
  FH and, 537
  Huntington disease and, 175
Autosomal trisomies, 201
  maternal age and, 201, 217
Azithromycin
  infectious syphilis and, 92
  IUDs and, 568

B
Bacterial vaginosis
  IUDs and, 568
  PTD and, 380
Barium enema, colorectal cancer and, 652
Basal ganglia, kernicterus and, 491, 492
Bayes theorem, 9
Bed rest
  IUGR and, 368
  PTD and, 380
Bedside clotting assessment, DIC and, 471
Bedside glucose meters, errors with, 485
Betamethasone
  fetal movement and, 450
  FHR and, 448
Bethesda system, cervical cytology and, 605
BH4. *See* Tetrahydrobiopterin
BiliChek device, neonatal hyperbilirubinemia and, 496
Bilirubin. *See also* Hour-specific bilirubin nomogram
  ABE and, 492
  levels, hearing impairment and, 520
  measurement, neonatal hyperbilirubinemia and, 494, *495*
Bilirubin nomogram. *See* Hour-specific bilirubin nomogram
Bilirubin reduction approach, hyperbilirubinemia and, *499*
Bilirubin-induced neurologic dysfunction (BIND)
  incidence/prevalence of, 491
  recommendations for, 500
  summary for, 500–501

Bimanual examination
  gynecologic malignancy and, 529–34
  ovarian cancer and, 530–33
Biochemical hypothyroidism, 280
Biochemical markers, chromosomal abnormalities and, 204
Biochemical tests
  anencephaly and, 233
  chromosomal abnormalities and, 204–6
  costs, 209
  fetal abnormalities and, 232–41
Biophysical Profile Score (BPS), 365, 433
  costs of, 452
  nature of test, 451
Biparietal diameter, gestational age dating and, 194
Birth, chromosomal abnormalities at, 201, *202*
Birth trauma, post term pregnancy and, 192
Birthweight, 321, *323,* 327
  antenatal period and, 349
  IUGR and, 360
  SGA and, 360
  TPR and, 400
Bishop's score, cervical examination and, 383, *383*
Bleeding
  colonoscopy and, 652
  spontaneous, maternal thrombocytopenia and, 471
Blood, hepatitis C virus infection and, 83
Blood clotting, laboratory assessment of, 468
Blood flow velocity, Doppler ultrasound and, *361,* 361–65
Blood glucose measurement, neonatal hypoglycemia and, *487, * 488
Blood grouping, tests for, 16
Blood loss at delivery, 34, 36
Blood phenylalanine level, normal, 505
Blood pressure (BP). *See also* Home BP monitoring; Hypertension; Preeclampsia; Second trimester; Third trimester
  preeclampsia and, 396
Blood spot immunoreactive trypsinogen, CF and, 514, 515
Blood tests, hyperthyroidism and, 281
Blood transfusion
  iron deficiency anemia and, 26
  postpartum anemia and, 36
Bloom syndrome, 151–52
  test for, 156
BMD. *See* Bone mineral density
Bone loss, causes of, 673
Bone marrow, FA and, 151
Bone mineral density (BMD), 673
  low bone mass and, 674–75
  t-score
    fracture prediction and, 675–76
    normal test result with, 676

Bowel preparation, colonoscopy
and, 651–52
BP. *See* Blood pressure
BPS. *See* Biophysical profile score
Brachial plexus injury, 311
GDM and, 309
Brain
Huntington disease and, 176
injury, hypoglycemia and, 484
neonatal hypoglycemia and, 487
sparing, 365
BRCA1 gene, 577
mutation carriers, 561
ovarian cancer and, 579, 629
mutations, prevalence of, 574–75
BRCA1/2 gene mutation carriers, false
positive screens and, 639
BRCA2 gene, 577
mutation carriers, ovarian cancer
and, 629
mutations
families with, 582
prevalence of, 574–75
BRCA2-associated breast cancer, 576
Breast cancer. *See also* Familial breast cancer
BRCA1 mutations and, 574
carriers v. noncarriers, 575
incidence/prevalence of, 591
inherited syndromes and, 577
OCs and, 560–61
screening for, 591–600
sequelae of, 592
serum CA-125 screening and, 631
summary, 598–600
tests for, 576–84, 592–98
Breast cancer mortality rates, mammography
and, 594
relative risk and, *595*
Breast cancer screening
conclusions and recommendations for,
598
costs of, 596, *597*, 598
favorable v. unfavorable effects of, *597*
mortality effects of, *597*
Breast cancer susceptibility genes, recognized, 576, *577*
Breast examination, clinical, 593
Breast self-examination, 593
Breast-conserving therapy, 596
breast cancer and, 593
Breast-fed infants, PKU and, 505
Breast-feeding
hypertriglyceridemia and, 542–43
neonatal hypoglycemia and, 485
Bundle branch block, 662

C

CA-15.3. *See* Cancer antigen 15.3 tumor
markers
CA72-4. *See* Cancer antigen 72-4
CA-125. *See* Cancer antigen-125

Cesarean section delivery
fetal macrosomia and, 305
GDM and, 308, 311
hepatitis C virus infection and, 87
HIV and, 115
placental dysfunction and, 433
ultrasound and, 196
CAG trinucleotide repeat, Huntington
disease and, 176, *177*, 178
CAH. *See* Congenital adrenal hyperplasia
Canavan disease, 150
test for, 155
Cancer. *See* specific type Cancer i.e. Breast
Cancer
Cancer antigen 15.3 (CA-15.3) tumor
markers, 634
Cancer antigen 72-4 (CA72-4), malignant
pelvic tumors and, 638
Cancer antigen-125 (CA-125), 532, 624
combined with ultrasound, ovarian
carcinomas and, 639
high-risk women and, 634
measurement, conclusions and recommendations on, 640–42
ovarian cancer and, 584
screening, ovarian cancer and, 629–42,
629–44
Cancer in situ (CIS), cancer categories
and, 605
Carbimazole
fetal hyperthyroidism and, 280
maternal hyperthyroidism in pregnancy
and, 282
Cardiac malformations, trisomy 18 fetuses
and, 220
Cardiac metabolism, fetal hypoxia and, 431
Cardiac output (CO)
measurement of, preexisting hypertension
and, 402–3
test purpose for, preeclampsia and, 399
Cardiac pathology
summary of, 663–65
tests for, 660–62
Cardiac rhythm screening, 658-665
Cardiotocography (CTG), 433
Cardiovascular compromise, chronic hypoxemia and, 429
Cardiovascular disease (CVD)
dyslipidemia and, 536
primary dyslipidemia and, 544
Carrier screening, nonsyndromic hearing
loss and, 156
Cascade screening
CF and, 124
fragile X syndrome and, 170
CBE. *See* Chronic irreversible bilirubin
encephalopathy
CCHB. *See* Complete congenital
heart block
CDC. *See* Centers for Disease Control
Cefazolin, neonatal GBS and, 51

Ceftriaxone, infectious syphilis and, 92
Cellular transport systems, fetal, 437
Centers for Disease Control (CDC)
  Chlamydia infection and, 105, 106
  CIN and, 606
  hepatitis B and, 80
  HIV and, 112, 113, 114, 116
  infectious syphilis and, 91, 92, 93
  perinatal HIV transmission and
Central nervous system (CNS) maturation, hypoxic IUGR fetuses and, 446
Cephalo-caudal progression, bilirubin levels and, *494*
Cerebral resistance, ultrasound and, 365
Cervical canal, fFN and, 380
Cervical cancer. *See also* Pap smear
  abnormal cervical smear and, 615
  high-risk HPV infection and, 614
  HPV testing in, 612–19
  incidence/prevalence of, 603–4
  OCs and, 561
  pap smear and, 605
  positive test result in, 615
  summary for, 608–9, 618–19
  tests, 614–16
Cervical cerclage, 387
  PTD and, 380
Cervical dilation, internal os and, 384
Cervical dysplasia
  categories for, 605
  HIV and, 113
Cervical epithelium, high risk HPV and, 613
Cervical examination, nature of, 383–84
Cervical insufficiency, 378
Cervical intraepithelial neoplasia (CIN), 603
  failure rates and, 616
  grades of, 605
  sequelae of, 604
  spontaneous regression of, 615
  tests for, 604–7
  treatment for, 606
Cervical intraepithelial neoplasia 3 (CIN3), high-risk HPV infection and, 614
Cervical length
  implications of testing, 385, *385*
  transvaginal ultrasonography and, *386*
Cervical screening
  components of, 608, *608*
  conclusions and recommendations for, 607
Cervical smear
  abnormal, 616
  cervical cancer and, 605
  negative test result and, 616
Cervix
  imaging of, 385, *385*
  normal test result and, 384–85
CESDI classifications, stillbirths and, 345
CF. *See* Cystic fibrosis
CFTR. *See* Cystic fibrosis transmembrane regulator

CHD. *See* Congenital hip dysplasia
CHEK2 gene, breast cancer and, 578
Chemoirradiation, invasive cervical cancer and, 604
Child Health and Development Study, low birth weight and, 320–21
Children
  congenital Toxoplasma infection and, 61–62
  CRS in, 58
  Huntington disease and, 179
  toxoplasma infection and, 64
CHIPS (Control of Hypertension in Pregnancy Study), 399
Chlamydia infection, 103–11, 569
  incidence/prevalence of, 103–4
  IUDs and, 567–68
  recommendations for, 107
  sequelae of, 104
  summary for, 108–9
  tests, 104–6, 104–7, 108–9
    costs, 107
    nature of, 104
Cholesterol, 539
  ATP III classification of, *540*
  measurement of, 538–39
Cholestyramine, pregnancy and, 544
Choroid plexus cysts (CPCs), trisomy 18 and, 224
Chromosomal abnormalities
  antenatal testing for, protocols for, 261, *261*
  at birth, 201, *202*
Chromosomal aneuploidies, incidence/prevalence of, 201
Chromosomal anomalies
  marker patterns for, 207, *207*
  test costs, 260
Chromosome 21, trisomy 21 and, 202
Chronic active hepatitis, pregnancy and, 298
Chronic anemia, 23
Chronic carrier state, hepatitis B infection and, 78
Chronic hepatitis, 83
Chronic hypoxemia
  global fetal activity and, 452
  stillbirth and, 429
Chronic irreversible bilirubin encephalopathy (CBE), excessive hyperbilirubinemia and, 492–93
CIN. *See* Cervical intraepithelial neoplasia
CIN3. *See* Cervical intraepithelial neoplasia 3
Cirrhosis, hepatitis C virus infection and, 83
Clindamycin, neonatal GBS and, 51
Clotting. *See* Blood clotting
CMV. *See* Congenital cytomegalovirus infection
CO. *See* Cardiac output

Coagulation abnormalities, tests for, 468–72
Coagulopathy, abnormal test results
    and, 470
Cochrane Collaboration, gestational
    age dating and, 194
Cochrane database, 442
Cognitive deficits, CBE and, 493
Colonoscopy, 651–52
    colorectal cancer and, 650
Color Doppler imaging, 362, 410
    fetal hypoxia and, 432
    ovarian cancer and, 623
Color-coded Doppler ultrasonography,
    fetal structural anomalies and, 248
Colorectal cancer, 649–56
    incidence/prevalence of, 649
    screening tests for, 654–56
        performance of, 653, 653
    sequelae of, 649–50
    tests for, 650–54
Colorectal cancer screening, summary of,
    654–56
Colposcopy, 605
    cervical cancer and, 605
Coma, ABE and, 492
Complete congenital heart block (CCHB),
    291
    SLE and, 290
Complete heart block, 659
Compliance, 13
Compound heterozygous disease, 518
Compression fractures of thoracic spine,
    674
Computer-aided detection (CAD) software,
    breast and, 594
Conception, FH and, 453
Conduction blocks, 659
Congenital adrenal hyperplasia (CAH)
    incidence/prevalence of, 509
    recommendations for, 511
    screening for, 509–11
    sequelae of, 509
    tests for, 510
Congenital cytomegalovirus infection
    (CMV), 68–73
    incidence/prevalence of, 68
    recommendations for, 71
    sequelae of, 68–69, 71
    summary for, 71–73
    tests for, 72
Congenital heart defects, trisomy 21 and, 202
Congenital heart disease, test costs for, 248
Congenital hip dysplasia (CHD), screening
    for, 516–18
Congenital hyperinsulinism, neonates and,
    484
Congenital hypothyroidism (CH), 284
    incidence/prevalence of, 506
    recommendations for, 508–9
    sequelae of, 507
    tests for, 507–8

Congenital malformations, fetal movement
    and, 450
Congenital nonsyndromic hearing loss
    (DFNB1), screening for, 148
Congenital rubella infection. See Congenital
    rubella syndrome
Congenital rubella syndrome (CRS)
    incidence/prevalence of, 55–56, 56
    sequelae of, 56
    tests, 56–58
Congenital syphilis
    incidence/prevalence of, 90, 93
    sequelae of, 90–91, 94
    tests for, 94–95
Congenital Toxoplasma infection
    incidence/prevalence of, 61
    screening and, 61–64
    sequelae of, 61–62
    tests for, 61, 62–64
Continuous wave (CW) Doppler, 362,
    410
    fetal hypoxia and, 432–36
Control of Hypertension in Pregnancy
    Study. See CHIPS
Cooley anemia (thalassemia major), 152
    sequelae of, 140
Coombs Test, HDN and, 477
Cordocentesis, 451
    fetal hyperthyroidism, 283
Coronary heart disease (CHD),
    incidence/prevalence of, 658
Corticosteroid replacement therapy
    Addison disease and, 298
    IUGR and, 453
Cost-benefit analysis, 12
    asymptomatic bacteriuria in pregnancy
        and, 44
    chromosomal screening, 209–10
    Doppler ultrasonography and,
        414–15
    iron supplementation and, 28
Cost-effectiveness, screening and, 10–11
Cost-effectiveness analysis. See Cost-benefit
    analysis
Cost-minimization analysis, 11–12
Costs. See Testing costs
Cost-utility analysis, 12
Counseling. See also Genetic counseling
    Chlamydia infection and, 109
    chromosomal anomalies and, 211
    emergent cerclage and, 384
    GDM and, 307
    HIV and, 115, 118
    MoM values and, 234
    mutation carriers and, 579
    neural tube defects and, 237
    screening and, 13
Couple screening
    CF carrier status and, 125, 127, 134
    counseling and, 126
    validity of, CF and, 131

Cowden syndrome, PTEN and, 578
CPCs. *See* Choroid plexus cysts
CRS. *See* Congenital rubella syndrome
Cry, ABE and, 492
CTG. *See* Cardiotocography
Customized antenatal growth chart, 353
Customized assessment of fetal growth, 348–50
Cutaneous flares, SLE and, 290
CVD. *See* Cardiovascular disease
CW. *See* Continuous wave Doppler
Cystic fibrosis (CF)
    abnormal test result for, 125–29
    carrier status, 121–35
    conclusions for, 515
    gene mutation, CF and, 123
    incidence/prevalence of, 121, 513
    recommendations for, 132–33
    screening for, 148, 513–15
        life cycle stages and, 125, *126*
    sequelae of, 121–23, 513–14
    summary, 133–35
    tests, 123–32, 514–15
Cystic fibrosis transmembrane regulator
    (CFTR), gene, 121
    CF and, 514
Cytology tests, abnormal, management
    of, 606

D

Dacron swab, fFN and, 380
DAT. *See* Direct antiglobulin test
Dating of pregnancy, post term pregnancy
    and, 337
DDH. *See* Developmental dysplasia
    of hip
Deafness, CH and, 507
Deep vein thrombosis, factor V Leiden
    mutation and, 273
Defective placentation, preeclampsia and,
    408–9
Degree of error, FHM and, 350
Delivery
    fetal acidemia and, 453, *454*
    IUGR and, 453
    timing, high risk fetus and, 364
Depomedroxyprogesterone acetate
    (DMPA), OCs and, 561
Dermatitis-tenosynovitis syndrome, gonor-
    rhea and, 98
Developmental dysplasia of hip (DDH)
    conclusions for, 517–18
    screening for, 516–18
    sequelae of, 516
    tests, 516–17
Developmental scores, IUGR and, 361
DEXA. *See* Dual-energy x-ray absorptiometry
DFA test. *See* Direct fluorescent antibody test
DFNBI. *See* Congenital nonsyndromic
    hearing loss

Diabetes mellitus. *See also* Gestational
    diabetes mellitus
    conclusions and recommendations
        for, 553–54
    incidence/prevalence of, 549
    IUGR and, 361
    serum uric acid and, 422
    tests for, 550–53
Diabetes mellitus type 1, sequelae
    of, 549–50
Diabetes mellitus type 2
    GDM and, 312
    risk factors for, *553*
    sequelae of, 550
Diagnostic test, 1
Diastolic BP, Korotkoff phase V
    and, 396
Diastolic flow, IUGR and, 368
Diastolic notching
    Doppler and, 410–11
    maternal circulation and, 439
Diastolic velocities
    fetal compromise and, 365
    uterine artery and, 363, *363*
DIC. *See* Disseminated intravascular
    coagulation
Diet therapy, GDM and, 307
Digital mammography, x-ray
    mammography v., 593–94
Dilute Russell viper venom time (DRVVT),
    APS and, 294
Dimeric inhibin A,, trisomy 21 and, 220
Dipstick testing, 41
    costs for, 43
Direct antiglobulin test (DAT), 477–78
    test costs, 479
    testing implications for, 478
    umbilical cord blood and, 477
Direct fluorescent antibody (DFA) test,
    Chlamydia infection and, 104, 105
Disseminated intravascular coagulation
    (DIC), 466, 468
    intrapartum coagulopathy and, 466
    IUFD and, 467
    peripartum bleeding abnormalities
        and, 466
    testing for, 471
DMPA. *See* Depomedroxyprogesterone
    acetate
DNA amplification, fetal aneuploidy
    and, 254
DNA analyzer, fetal aneuploidy
    and, 255
DNA mutation analysis, Huntington
    disease and, 178
DNA sequencing, FH and, 544
DNA tests
    CF and, 124, 514
    fragile X syndrome and, 163
    hemoglobinopathies and, 519
    TSD and, 154

Doppler flow velocimetry
  IUGR and, 360–73
  IUGR fetus and, 354, 355
  perinatal death v., 442
  stillbirth and, 443–44
Doppler resistance index, IUGR and, 362
Doppler ultrasound
  cost-benefit analysis of, 414–15
  fetal hyperthyroidism, 282
  fetal vessels and, 254
  indices, preeclampsia and, 409
  IUGR and, 361, 361–65
  maternal circulation and, 438–39
  ovarian cancer syndrome and, 635
  principle, preeclampsia and, 409
  screening
    consequences of, 368
    economic evaluation of, IUGR and,
      370
    mixed risk population and, 370
  technique, CO and, 399
  waveform analysis, fetal arterial system
    and, 442
Dot-blot immunobinding assay (HIV
  CHEK), HIV and, 113
Down syndrome. See Trisomy 21
Doxycycline, IUDs and, 568
DRVVT. See Dilute Russell viper venom time
Dry toxemia, 402
Dual-energy x-ray absorptiometry (DEXA),
  BMD and, 674
Ductal carcinoma in situ (DCIS), breast and,
  596
Ductus venosus
  Doppler index and, delivery and, 453, 454
  fetal growth restriction and, 363
  waveform, 444
Dysbetalipoproteinemia, 541
Dyskaryosis, 617
Dyslipidemia
  incidence/prevalence of, 536
  screening for, 545–47
  secondary causes of, 537
  sequelae of, 536–38, 537
  tests for, 538–45
Dystonia, CBE and, 492

E

Early-onset genetic diseases
  conclusions and recommendations for,
    159
  incidence/prevalence of, 148, 148–49, 149
  screening for, 147–60
  summary for, 159–60
  tests for, 154–58
Early-onset preeclampsia, APS and, 294
Early-onset septicemia
  GBS and, 48
  prevention of, 51–52
Eclampsia, 270
  excessive weight gain and, 401

Economic costs, screening and, 10–11
Economic evaluation
  needs for, 12–13
  strategies used for, 11–12
Edema, 402
  excessive weight gain and, 401
EDTA-anticoagulated blood,
  hemoglobinopathies and, 141
Edwards syndrome. See Trisomy 18
Effacement, 384
EIAs. See Enzyme-linked immunoassays
Either-or-testing option, 263–64
Electrocardiogram (ECG), 658–65
  cardiac pathology and, 660–62
  silent MI and, age and, 661
  testing implications and, 660–61
11-hydroxylase deficiency, CAH and, 509
ELISA. See Enzyme-linked immunosorbent
  assay
Emergent cerclage, contraindications
  for, 384
Encephalocele, 232
Encephalopathy, MCAD and, 511
Endocervix, fFN and, 380
Endocrine compromise, chronic hypoxemia
  and, 429
Endometriosis
  pyelogram and, 668
  serum CA-125 screening and, 631
Endoscopic testing, colorectal cancer and, 650
Endovaginal sonography, cervical length
  and, 385
Enzyme PAH, hyperphenylalaninemia and,
  505
Enzyme replacement therapy, genetic disor-
  ders and, 503
Enzyme-linked immunoassays (EIAs)
  21-hydroxylase deficiency test and, 510
  C. trachomatis antigens and, 105
  Chlamydia infection, 104, 105
  for congenital rubella infection, 56–57
  gonorrhea and, 98
  hepatitis A virus infection and, 76
  hepatitis C virus infection and, 84
  immunoglobulin G antibodies and, 56–57
Enzyme-linked immunosorbent assay
  (ELISA)
  APS and, 294
  congenital toxoplasmosis and, 66
  fFN and, 380
  hepatitis C virus infection and, 84, 86–87
  HIV and, 113, 114
Erroneous conception dating, gestational age
  v., 326
Erythromycin
  positive fFN and, 380
Escherichia coli, 41
Estimated date of confinement (EDC), 435
Estrogen, osteoporosis and, 673
Euroscan study, data from, fetal structural
  anomalies and, 247

Exclusion PGD, Huntington disease and, 182
Exclusion test, Huntington disease and, 181, *181*, 182
Exocrine glands, CFand, 513
Exocrine pancreatic insufficiency, CF and, 513–14
Exophthalmos, Graves disease and, 280–81
External validity (generalizability), 9

F
FA. *See* Fanconi anemia
Factor V Leiden mutation, 270, 272
    deep vein thrombosis and, 273
Factor XI deficiency, screening for, 148
False-negative test, TSH test, 508
False-positive screens
    CA-125 measurement and, 640
    FOBT and, 651
    GDM and, 312
    ovarian carcinomas and, 639
    PKU and, 506
Familial breast cancer
    cumulative risk of, gene mutation and, *580*
    gene mutation and, *581*
    incidence/prevalence of, 574
    summary for, 585–86
Familial combined hypercholesterolemia, 541
Familial dysautonomia, test for, 155
Familial history
    colorectal cancer and, 649
    Huntington disease and, 175
Familial hypercholesterolemia (FH), 536
    conception and, 453
    criteria for, 539, 541
    CVD mortality rates and, 538
    pregnancy and, 453
    summary of, 545–47
    survival in, *538*
Familial ovarian cancer, 634, 639
    cumulative risk of, gene mutation and, *580*
    incidence/prevalence of, 574
    summary for, 585–86
Family history of neural tube defects, AFP values and, 236
Fanconi anemia (FA), 151
    test for, 155
Fasting lipid profile, dyslipidemia and, 538
Fasting plasma glucose (FPG)
    diabetes mellitus and, 550–51
    GDM and, 309
Fatty acid oxidation, neonates and, 484
FDP. *See* Fibrin degradation product
Fecal DNA testing, colorectal cancer and, 650
Fecal occult blood testing (FOBT)
    colorectal cancer and, 650–51
    flexible sigmoidoscopy plus, 651
Feeding, ABE and, 492

Femur length, in second trimester, aneuploidy and, 220–21
Fetal abnormalities, biochemical screening for, 232–41
Fetal acidemia, 362, 432
    CTG and, 446
    Doppler and, 443
    fetal movements and, 451
Fetal activity, fetal hypoxia and, 432
Fetal adaptive responses, fetal hypoxia and, 432
Fetal and maternal arterial resistances, conclusions for, 370–71
Fetal anemia. *See also* Fetal hemolytic anemia
    absolute velocities and, 361
Fetal aneuploidy
    karyotyping and, 253–54, *254*
    molecular tests for, 253–66
    summary for, 265–66
    tests for, 255–68
Fetal anomaly scanning, 245
    approaches to, 245
Fetal apnea, IUGR and, 362
Fetal arterial system, Doppler studies of, 441–43
Fetal behavioral responses
    biophysical profile score, 451
    neurodevelopment status and, 445–46
Fetal biometry, fetal hypoxia and, 432
Fetal body fat, 437
Fetal brain development, thyroid hormone and, 285
Fetal breathing, 445
Fetal cardiac activity, 437
Fetal cells, testing of, 253–64
Fetal chromosome pattern, 246
Fetal compromise, fetal arterial system and, Doppler studies of, 442–43
Fetal crown-rump length, gestational age dating and, 194
Fetal distress, IUGR and, 368–69
Fetal dynamics, Doppler analysis of, 371
Fetal echocardiography, 291
Fetal fibronectin (fFN)
    PTD and, 388
    testing cost for, 382–83
    testing for, 380–83
Fetal growth, 344. *See also* Customized assessment of fetal growth
    from 26-28 weeks, 350, *351*
    hypertension reduction and, 399
    screening for, timing of, 350, *351*
    velocity, 360
Fetal growth curve, customized assessment, fetal growth and, 348
Fetal growth restriction, 344–57
    APS and, 294
    causes of, 345, *345*, 433
    incidence/prevalence of, 344
    sequelae of, 344–45
    summary of, 355–57

Fetal heart failure, venous indices and, 364
Fetal heart rate (FHR)
    aspects of, 447
    BPS and, 451
    characteristics of, 446
    continuous recording, fetal hypoxemia
        and, 446
    pattern, 433
    testing, 365
Fetal hemolytic anemia, IgG antibodies and,
    18
Fetal hypoglycemia, 430
Fetal hypothyroidism, 281
Fetal hypoxemia, 443
    CTG and, 446
    Doppler changes and
        early, 440
        late, 440–41
    summary of, 455–57
Fetal hypoxia
    diagnosis of, 429–30
    incidence/prevalence of, 429
    placental dysfunction and, 437
    predisposing conditions for, screening
        for, 433, 433–34
    screening for, 429–57
    tests for, 432–36
Fetal macrosomia, 310
    cesarean delivery and, 305
    glycemic control and, 309
Fetal malformation
    hydramnios and, 327
    ultrasound and, 191
Fetal monitoring, Doppler ultrasound screen-
    ing and, 368
Fetal movement, 449, 450
    abnormal test result for, 450
    fetal acidemia and, 451
Fetal neural defects, 232
Fetal NT, aneuploidy and, 205, 205, 206
Fetal origin of adult disease hypothesis,
    361
Fetal pH, BPS and, 452, 453
Fetal rest-activity cycles, 447, 448
Fetal size, IUGR and, 436
Fetal sonographic biometry, test purpose for,
    193
Fetal structural anomalies
    euroscan study data, 247, 247
    incidence/prevalence of, 244
    pregnancy and
        risk factors during, 246
        risk factors prior to, 245–46
    routine ultrasonography for, 244–50
    sequelae of, 244–45
    summary of, 249–50
    test costs for, 248
Fetal thrombocytopenia, maternal thrombo-
    cytopenia v., 471
Fetal thyrotoxicosis, 280
    maternal antithyroid medication and, 283

Fetal tone, 449
Fetal trisomy 21. See Trisomy 21
Fetal two-dimensional ultrasound
    abnormal test result with, 435–36
    fetal hypoxia and, 432
    purpose of, 435
Fetal ultrasound, hyperthyroidism
    and, 281
Fetal venous circulation, venous Doppler
    and, 443
Fetal vessels, test characteristics of, IUGR
    and, 364, 364
Fetal weight, customized assessment of fetal
    growth and, 348
Fetal weight curves, individual scan biome-
    try parameters v., 350
Fetomaternal hemorrhage (FMH), 17
    immunoglobulin and, 478
α-fetoprotein (AFP) screening test, 238, 239
    closed lesions and, 232
    measurement of, maternal serum and,
        234–36
Fetus
    CMV and, 70
    congenital rubella infection and, 56
    congenital Toxoplasma infection and, 61
    Graves disease and, 280
    infectious syphilis and, 94
    post term pregnancy and, 193
    preeclampsia and, 467
    RBC antigen and, 16
    second trimester, aneuploidy and, 220
    syphilis and, 91
    thalassemia and, 141
fFN. See Fetal fibronectin
FH. See Familial hypercholesterolemia
FHM. See Fundal height measurement
FHR. See Fetal heart rate
Fibrin, DIC and, 471
Fibrin degradation product (FDP)
    DIC and, 471
    placental abruption and, 467
    values for, 469
Fibrinogen, placental abruption and, 467
Fibrinogen level, 470
    pregnancy and, 469
Fibrinopeptide A, IUFD and, 470
First sign of delay testing, fragile X syn-
    drome and, 167
First-trimester
    cytotrophoblast in, 437
    fetal movement in, 449
    screening costs, studies of, 209
    uric acid excretion in, 422
    uterine artery blood flow velocity wave-
        forms in, 410
FISH. See Fluorescence in-situ hybridization
Flexible sigmoidoscopy
    colorectal cancer and, 650, 651
    FOBT plus, 651
    limitations aof, 651

Flow velocity waveform
  Doppler and, 409
  IUGR and, *361*
Fluorescence in-situ hybridization (FISH),
  246, 264
    antenatal diagnosis and, 254
    karyotyping fetal tissue, 206
    molecular testing v., *256*
Fluorescent treponemal antibody absorption
  (FTA-ABS), infectious syphilis and, 91
FMH. *See* Fetomaternal hemorrhage
FMRI gene, fragile X syndrome and, 165
FOBT. *See* Fecal occult blood testing
Folic acid
  deficiency, macrocytic anemia and, 27
  supplements, neural tube defects
    and, 233
47XXX karyotype, 203
Founder mutations, 577
FPG. *See* Fasting plasma glucose
Fractures, osteoporosis and, 673–74
Fragile X mental retardation 1 (FMR1) gene,
  166
Fragile X syndrome
  conclusions and recommendations for,
    169
  incidence/prevalence of, 163
  screening for, 148, 163–71
  sequelae, 163–65
  summary for, 170–71
  tests for, 165–70
Fragile X-associate tremor/ataxia syndrome,
  165
Framingham Heart Study, risk factors
  and, *537*
Free thyroxine, hyperthyroidism and, 281
Free triiodothyronine, hyperthyroidism
  and, 281
Friedenwald formula, 539
Fruit signs, neural tube defects and, 237
FTA-ABS. *See* Fluorescent treponemal antibody absorption
Full blood count, thalassemia and, 141
Fundal height measurement (FHM)
  conclusions and recommendations for,
    338–39
  gestational weight/age and, 328
  procedure for, *352*
  tests for
    predictive values for, 329, *331–35*
    sensitivity for, 329, *331–35*
    specificity for, 329, *331–35*
  timing of, 350
Furosemide, preeclampsia and, 399

G

Gastroschisis, 232
  prevalence of, 233
Gaucher disease
  forms of, 149–50
  test for, 155

Gaussian distribution, 205
Gaze, CBE and, 492
GBS. *See* Group B streptococcal disease
GCT. *See* Glucose challenge test
GDM. *See* Gestational diabetes mellitus
Gene expression, breast cancer
  and, 575
Gene mutation carriers, cancer
  and, 575, 576
Gene therapy, CF and, 123
ΔF508 gene mutation, CF and, 128
Generalizability. *See* External validity
Genetic amniocentesis, trisomy 18
  and, 220
Genetic carrier testing, models for, 124
Genetic counseling, 503
  FH and, 543
  fragile X syndrome and, 166
  Huntington disease and, 176
  neural tube defects and, 237
  trisomy 18 and, 224
  trisomy 21 fetus, 224–25
Genetic diseases, incidence/prevalence
  of, *148*, 148–49, *149*
Genetic drift, CF and, 513
Genetic linkage testing, Huntington
  disease and, 179
Genetic sonography
  aneuploidy markers, *221*
  cost effectiveness of, 227
  high-risk women and, 223
  predictive values of, 224
  second trimester aneuploidy
    and, 220–24
  trisomy 18 and, 220
  trisomy 21 and, 226
Genetic testing
  relative options for, 583
  TP53 and, 578
Genital organs, female, cancers of, inherited
  syndromes and, 577
Genital tract, HIV and, 113
GEN-PROBE. *See* Nucleic acid amplification
  tests
Germ line mutations, ovarian cancer
  and, 624
Gestation
  AFP at, 234
  FP and, 543
Gestational age dating, 435
  AFP values and, 235
  at delivery, neonatal complications and,
    445
  delivery and, 454, 455
  fetal sonographic biometry and, 193
  FHR and, 447
  fundal height measurement for, 328
  gold standard for, 193
  menstrual period and, 327
  third trimester and, 397
  ultrasound and, 193

Gestational diabetes mellitus (GDM), 303–14
   conclusions and recommendations for, 311–13
   incidence/prevalence of, 303
   offspring health outcomes, 304–5
   summary for, 313–14
   targeted v. universal screening for, 307
   test costs for, 310–11
Gestational hypertension, normal test result for, 397
Gestational pancreatitis, hypertriglyc-eridemia and, 542, 543
Gestational trophoblastic neoplasia, molar pregnancy and, 327
Gestational weight, fundal height measurement for, 328
Gestation-specific fetal death, 192–93
Global fetal activity, chronic hypoxemia and, 453
Glomerular endotheliosis, 421
Glucocorticosteroids, CAH and, 509
Gluconeogenesis, neonates and, 484
Glucose challenge test (GCT), GDM and, 307
Glucose intolerance
   during pregnancy
      incidence/prevalence of, 303
      screening for, 303–14
      testing for, 306–10
Glycemic control, GDM and, 308, 309
Glycogenolysis, neonates and, 484
Gonorrhea, 97–101
   incidence/prevalence of, 97
   sequelae of, 97–98
   summary for, 100–101
   tests, 100–101
      costs of, 99
      implications of, 99
      nature of, 98
      purpose for, 98
Gram stain testing
   costs for, 43
   gonorrhea and, 98
Graves disease, characteristics of, 280–81
Group B streptococcal disease (GBS), 48–53
Growth charts, customized assessment of fetal growth and, 348, *353*
Growth restrictions
   asymmetric v. symmetric, FHM and, 350–51
   FHM and, 350
   ultrasound and, 191
GTT. *See* Oral glucose tolerance test
Gut, CF and, 122
Guthrie inhibition assay, PKU and, 504
Gynecologic cancers
   genetic predisposition to, 574–86
   recommendations for, 584
Gynecologic pathways, IVP abnormalities and, *668*

H
Hamartomatous polyposis of gastrointestinal tract, Peutz-Jeghers syndrome and, 578
Hashimoto disease, 284
Hb H disease, 142
HbA2 levels, thalassemia and, 141
HBB alleles, sickle cell disease and, 153
HBOC. *See* Hereditary breast-ovarian cancer syndrome
HBsAg. *See* Hepatitis B surface antigen tests
hCG. *See* Serial human chorionic gonadotropin measurements
HDL. *See* High-density lipoprotein
HDN. *See* Hemolytic disease of newborn
Head circumference, gestational age dating and, 194
Health care programs, costs of, 11
Hearing impairment
   incidence/prevalence of, 520
   screening for, 520–22
   sequelae of, 520–21
   tests for, 521–22
Heart block, 662
Heart rate (HR), CO and, 399
HELLP syndrome, 467
   testing for, 469
Helsinki ultrasound randomized trial, fetal structural anomalies and, 248, 249
Hematocrit levels
   postpartum assessment of, 34–38
   pregnancy v., *23*, 26
   pregnant women and, 22
Hemoconcentration plasma volume, abnormal test result and, 35
Hemoglobin
   genes and, 138
   levels, pregnant women and, 22
   postpartum assessment of, 34–38
   variants, diagnosis of, 142
Hemoglobin A1, diabetes mellitus and, 551–52
Hemoglobin A1c, 551
Hemoglobinopathies
   clinically relevant, 138, *139*
   conclusions for, 143
   ethnic group and, *139*
   incidence/prevalence of, 138–40
   recommendations for, 145
   screening for, 138–45, 518–20
   sequelae of, 140
   summary of, 144–45
   tests, 140–41, 145
Hemolysis, sickle cell disease and, 153
Hemolytic anemia, SCD and, 518

Hemolytic disease of newborn (HDN)
  incidence/prevalence of, 19, 476
  newborn Rh status and, 480–81
  recommendations for, 20, 479
  screening for, 476
  screening of, 15–20
  sequelae of, 20, 476
  test costs and, 479
  tests for, 16, 20, 477–79
    implications of, 20
    nature of, 20
Hemorrhage, peripartum bleeding
  abnormalities and, 466
Heparin. *See also* Low-molecular-weight
  heparin
  APS and, 294
  hypertriglyceridemia and, 543
Hepatitis A virus infection
  incidence/prevalence of, 75
  sequelae of, 75–76
  summary for, 77–78
  tests for, 76
    costs of, 77
    implications of, 76
    nature of, 76
    purpose of, 76
Hepatitis B during pregnancy
  incidence/prevalence of, 79
  perinatal transmission at birth and
    prevention of, 81
    summary of, 81–83
  public health and, 62
  sequelae of, 79
  tests for, 79–81, 82
    costs of, 81
    implications of, 80
    nature of, 79–80
Hepatitis B surface antibody. *See* Anti-HBs
Hepatitis B surface antigen (HBsAg)
  tests, 79, 80
Hepatitis B virus infection
  e antigen, 80
  perinatal transmission of, 78–79
Hepatitis C virus infection, 83–87
  incidence/prevalence of, 83
  sequelae of, 83–84
  summary of, 86–87
  tests
    costs of, 85
    implications of, 85
    nature of, 84–85
    purpose for, 84
  tests for, 84–85
Hereditary breast-ovarian cancer (HBOC)
  syndrome, 624
Hereditary nonpolyposis colorectal cancer
  (HNPCC), 624
Heritable thrombophilias, costs for, assay
  method and, 274
HEXA enzyme-based testing, TSD and, 154
HEXA gene mutations, 149

Hexokinase method, neonatal hypoglycemia
  and, 485
High heart rate variation, 447
High performance liquid chromatography
  (HPLC), hemoglobinopathies and, 141
High resolution ultrasound, amnionic
  fluid AFP and, 237
High-density lipoprotein (HDL), dyslipi-
  demia and, 538
High-grade precursor lesions (CIN3),
  invasive cancer and, 603
High-performance liquid chromato-
  graphy (HPLC), hemoglobinopathies
  and, 519
Hip dislocation. *See also* Congenital hip
  dysplasia; Developmental dysplasia
  of hip
  incidence/prevalence of, 516
Hip fracture, osteoporosis and, 674
HIV CHEK. *See* Dot-blot immunobinding
  assay
HNPCC. *See* Hereditary nonpolyposis
  colorectal cancer
Home BP monitoring, pregnancy and, 397
Homocystine, 272
Homozygosity, 538
Hospital admission, IUGR and, 368
Hour-specific bilirubin nomogram
  abnormal test result with, 497
  as follow-up guide, 497–98, *498*
  pre-discharge TSB and, *498*
HPLC. *See* High performance liquid chromatography
HPV DNA testing, cervical testing and, 614
HPV. *See* Human papillomavirus
HR. *See* Heart rate
Human hair roots, fragile X syndrome and, 166
Human immunodeficiency virus (HIV),
  112–18
  adult transmission of, 112
  cervical cancer and, 605
  counseling for, 115, *115*
  hepatitis C virus infection and, 83, 85
  incidence/prevalence of, 112
  IUDs and, 567
  perinatal transmission of, 112
  recommendations, 116
  risk factors for, *114*
  sequelae of, infection spread and, 113
  summary for, 117–18
  tests for, 113–16
    costs, 116
Human papillomavirus (HPV), 607.
  See also Papillomavirus-induced
  condylomata acuminata
  cervical cancer screening and, 612–19
  conclusions and recommendations for,
    616–17
  DNA testing, 614
  high risk, normal cervical cytology and,
    613

natural history of, 613
OCs and, 561
oncogenic types of, 612–13, *613*
risk factors for, 613–14
testing, cervical cancer and, 604
Human placentation, preeclampsia
   and, 394
Humerus, second trimester, aneuploidy
   and, 220–21
Huntington disease
   couples and, reproduction choices
     for, *180*
   differential diagnosis for, 183
   incidence/prevalence of, 175
   recommendations for, 183–84
   screening for, 175–85
   sequelae of, 175–77
   summary for, 184–85
   test costs for, 183
Huntington disease gene, 176, *177*
   Huntington disease and, 177–78
Huntington protein, function of, 176
Hydralazine, preeclampsia and, 399
Hydramnios, 326
   fetal malformation and, 327
   monitoring, 337
Hyperbilirubinemia
   GDM and, 305
   tests for, 493–500
Hypercapnia, 362
Hypercoagulability, pregnancy
   and, 467
Hyperfusion, hemorrhage and, 36
Hyperhomocystinemia, 270, 272
   thromboembolic events v., 272
Hyperinsulinemia, insulin resistance
   and, 422
Hyperlipidemia, 536
   serum uric acid and, 422
Hyperphenylalaninemia, 505
Hypertension. *See also* White-coat
   hypertension
   diabetes mellitus and, 550
   excessive weight gain and, 401
   maternal uric acid and, 423
   OCs and, 560
   preeclampsia and, 394, 408
   in pregnancy, 396
   prepregnancy, preeclampsia and, 402
   serum uric acid and, 422
   third trimester and, 397, 398
Hyperthyroidism. *See also* Graves disease
   conclusions regarding, 282
   incidence/prevalence of, 280
   sequelae of, 280–81
   tests for, 281–82
Hypertonia, ABE and, 492
Hypertriglyceridemia, 542
   treatment
     breast-feeding and, 542–43
     pregnancy and, 542–43

Hyperuricemia, 422
   pregnancy-induced hypertension
     and, 421
Hypocalcemia, GDM and, 305
Hypofibrinogenemia, 468
Hypoglycemia. *See also* Neonatal
   hypoglycemia
   GDM and, 303, 305, 308
   MCAD and, 511
Hypothyroidism, 284–89
   incidence/prevalence of, 284
   screening for, 506–9
   trisomy 21 and, 202
Hypoxemia
   acidemia v., 448
   IUGR and, 360
Hypoxemic/acidemic fetuses
   growth restricted, 365
   nature of test for, 450
   test purpose for, 449
Hypoxic IUGR fetuses, CNS maturation
   and, 446

I

IEF. *See* Iso-electric focusing
IFA. *See* Indirect immunofluorescence
   assay
IgM antibodies
   CMV and, 69
   Toxoplasma infection and, 62
IgM assay, congenital rubella infection
   and, 57
Immune serologic tests, SLE and, 290
Immune thrombocytopenic purpura (ITP),
   467
   adult with, 468
Immunization, MCAD and, 511
Immunoassays, CMV and, 69
Immunoglobulin G (IgG) antibodies
   CMV and, 69
   congenital Toxoplasma infection
     and, 62
   fetal hemolytic anemia and, 18
Immunoreactive trypsinogen, CF
   and, 129
In utero fetal death, maternal risk
   and, 238
In utero repair, open spina bifida, 234
In vitro fertilization (IVF), CF and, 125
Incidence, characteristics of, 3, *4*
Increased lipoprotein A, 541–42
Indicated preterm delivery, 378
Indirect immunofluorescence assay (IFA),
   HIV and, 113
Individual scan biometry parameters,
   fetal weight curves v., 350
Individual screening, validity of, CF
   and, *131*
Induced labor
   gestational age dating and, 195
   post term pregnancy and, 192

Infantile GM2 gangliosidosis, 148–49
Infants. *See also* Low birth weight infants
  Chlamydia infection and, 104
  CMV and, 68
  congenital Toxoplasma infection
    and, 62
  deaths of, preeclampsia and, 394
  feeding practice with, neonatal
    hyperbilirubinemia and, 491
  fetal hypoxia and, 431
  GDM and, 305
  HIV/AIDS and
  size at birth, maternal height v., maternal
    weight v, 320
Infectious syphilis. *See* Syphilis
Inherited disorders of coagulation, 467
Inherited thrombophilias
  incidence of, *269*, 269–70
  summary for, 275–77
Insulin dependent diabetes mellitus,
  279, 550
Insulin resistance
  hyperinsulilnemia secondary to, 422
  OCs and, 560
Intelligence quotient (IQ), maternal
  hypothyroidism and, 285
Intermediate thalassemia, 152
Internal os, cervical dilation as, 384
Internal validity, screening test and, 5
Intrapartum chemoprophylaxis, neonatal
  GBS and, 50
Intrapartum coagulopathy
  primary screening tests for, cost of,
    472, 472
  sequelae of, 467–68
Intrapartum period, fetal growth restriction
  and, 345–46, *346*
Intrauterine devices (IUDs), 566–71
  contraindications for, 567
  insertion, recommendations for,
    569–70
  PID and, tests for, 567–69
Intrauterine fetal death (IUFD)
  abnormal test result with, 470
  coagulopathy associated with, 467
  peripartum coagulopathy and, 466
  sequelae of, 271
Intrauterine growth restriction (IUGR),
  329, 344, 443
  AC and, 436
  conclusions and recommendations for,
    370–71
  costs of, 337
  Doppler and, 360–73
    fetal hypoxia and, 439
  fetal hypoxia and, 431
  fetal movements and, 450
  FHM for, screening tool of, *331–35*
  gestational age and, 326
  hospital admission and, 368
  incidence/prevalence of, 360

low birthweight infants and, 327
maternal circulation and, 438–39
monitoring, 337
normal test result and, 436
perinatal mortality and, 244
placental dysfunction and, 429, 453
predisposing conditions for, screening
  for, *434*, 438
screening studies and, 366–67
sequelae, 361
single FHM and, *335*
summary for, 371–73
test costs for, *364*, 369–70
tests for, 361–70
uterine artery Doppler indices and,
  411–12, *412, 413*
Intravenous pyelogram (IVP), 666–71
  abnormal test, 667–69
  conclusions and recommendations
    for, 669–70
  nature of, 667
  screening summary for, 670–71
Intraventricular hemorrhage (IVH),
  443
  PTD and, 379
Invasive cervical cancer, 604
IQ. *See* Intelligence quotient
Iron chelation therapy, 140
Iron deficiency anemia, 23
  routines supplementation and, 28
Iron storage depletion, 23
Iron stores, cost of, 27–28
Iron supplementation, 27
  anemia screening and, 26
IRT. *See* Immunoreactive trypsinogen
Ischemic heart disease (IHD), 660
  screening, 658–65
Ischemic myocardial disease, 659
Ischemic stroke, OCs and, 560
Iso-electric focusing (IEF)
  hemoglobin variants, 142
  hemoglobinopathies and, 141, 519
ITP. *See* Immune thrombocytopenic
  purpura
IUDs. *See* Intrauterine devices
IUFD. *See* Intrauterine fetal death
IUGR. *See* Intrauterine growth restriction
IVF. *See* In vitro fertilization
IVH. *See* Intraventricular hemorrhage
IVP. *See* Intravenous pyelogram

J
Jarisch-Herxheimer reaction, infectious
  syphilis and, 92
Jaundice
  kernicterus and, 492
  visual assessment of, neonatal
    hyperbilirubinemia and, 493,
    494
Jewish community, disorders in, high-
  prevalence of, 147–48, *148*

K

Kaolin clotting time (KCT), APS and, 294
Karyotyping
  all cases, 263
  chromosome abnormalities with, *258*
    detection of, *259*
  comparing laboratory throughput for, *260*
  conclusions and recommendations for,
    264–65
  cost per case, *262, 263*
  disadvantages of, 254
  fetal aneuploidy and, 253–54
  fetal tissue, 225
    AFP MoM values and, 237
    trisomy 21 and, 206
  molecular tests plus, 261, *262, 263*
  molecular tests v., *256*
    panel specificity for, 257, *257*
  replacement of, molecular testing and, 261
KCT. *See* Kaolin clotting time
Kernicterus
  excessive hyperbilirubinemia and, 492–93
  incidence/prevalence of, 491
  neonatal jaundice and, 491
Kick count, fetal hypoxia and, 450
Klinefelter syndrome, 203
Korotkoff phase V, diastolic BP and, 396
Kyphosis, vertebral body fractures and, 674

L

LA. *See* Lupus anticoagulant
Labor. *See also* Induced labor
  FHM and, 336–37
  induction, 196
Lactate, 430
Lactating women, iron postpartum in, 38
Large gestational age infants (LGA)
  erroneous dating of pregnancy and, 328
  GDM and, 309
Latent syphilis, 92
Late-onset debilitating disease (FXTAS), 169
LBC. *See* Liquid-based cytology
LBW. *See* Low birth weight infants
LCR. *See* Ligase chain reaction
LDL. *See* Low density lipoprotein
Lead time, 5
Learning disabilities, PTD and, 379
LEEP. *See* Loop electrosurgical excision pro-
  cedure
Leiomyomata, pyelogram and, 668
Leukemia, trisomy 21 and, 202
Leukocyte esterase testing, 41
  costs for, 44
LFS. *See* Li-Fraumeni syndrome
LGA. *See* Large gestational age infants
Li-Fraumeni syndrome (LFS), breast cancer
  and, 578
Ligase chain reaction (LCR), Chlamydia
  infection, 104
Likelihood ratios (LRs), 8, *8*
  test and, 9

Lipid profile
  abnormal, 539
  FH and, 544
Liquid-based cytology (LBC), cervical cancer
  and, 605
Liver, CF and, 122
LMWH. *See* Low-molecular-weight heparin
Long bone length, gestational age dating
  and, 194
Loop electrosurgical excision procedure
  (LEEP), 606
Low birth weight (LBW) infants, 327, 378
  asymptomatic bacteriuria in pregnancy
    and, 40
  conclusions and recommendations for,
    324
  incidence/prevalence of, 320–21
  screening for, 26–27, 320–25
  sequelae of, 321
  summary for, 324–25
  test screening for, maternal height/
    weight and, 321–22, *322*
  third trimester and, 397
Low bone mass, BMD and, 674–75
Low density lipoprotein (LDL)
  receptor, 536
  receptor gene, 537, *538*
Low-molecular-weight heparin (LMWH),
  pregnancy and, 275
LRs. *See* Likelihood ratios
Lung cancer, serum CA-125 screening and,
  631
Lung disease, PTD and, 379
Lungs, CF and, 122
Lupus anticoagulant (LA), APS and, 294
Lupus nephritis, 290
Lupus nephropathy, 291
Lymphatic system, invasive cervical cancer
  and, 604

M

Macrocytic anemia, folic acid deficiency and,
  27
Macrosomia, GDM and, 305, 306, 308
Maculopapular rash, syphilis and, 90
Magnetic resonance imaging (MRI)
  breast and, 594
  gene mutation and, 582
  mammography v., breast cancer, 584
Malaria, 138
Malignancy
  gynecologic
    bimanual examination and, 529–34
    incidence/prevalence of, 529
    pelvic examination v. surgery, studies
      of, 530–31, *531*
    sequelae of, 529–30
    summary of, 533–34
  OCs and, 560–61
  RMI index score and, 637
  serum CA-125 screening and, 631

Malignant pelvic tumors, CA72-4 and, 638
Malignant tumors, pelvic examination and, 532
Mammography screening, 592, 593–94.
  See also Digital mammography; X-ray mammography
  breast cancer mortality rates, relative risk and, *595*
  conclusions and recommendations for, 598
  gene mutation and, *581*
Manual examination of cervix, 383
MAPA. *See* Multiplex ligation-dependent probe amplification
Marginal cost, 11
Mass spectrometry (TMS) screening, PKU and, 504
Maternal ABO group, HDN and, 477–78
Maternal age
  autosomal trisomies and, 201, 217
  second trimester and, 227
  trisomy 21 and, 219
Maternal age-specific risk, chromosomal abnormalities and, 204
Maternal antithyroglobulin autoantibodies, neonatal thyroid function and, 284
Maternal antithyroid medication, fetal thyrotoxicosis and, 283
Maternal biochemical serum screening, aneuploidy and, 219–20
Maternal blood, fFN and, 380
Maternal blood sample
  AFP in, 234
  pregnancy and, 19
Maternal body mass, euroscan study data and, *247, 248*
Maternal circulation, 437
  tests for, 438–41
Maternal complications during pregnancy, post term pregnancy and, 192
Maternal death, preeclampsia and, 394
Maternal diseases, bleeding risks and, 467
Maternal Fetal Medicine Unit (MFMU), PTD and, 379
Maternal glucose levels, pregestational diabetes and, 303
Maternal height, low birthweight infants with, screening for, 321
Maternal hypertension in pregnancy
  fetal growth restriction, 345
  implications of test for, 397, 398
Maternal hypertensive disorders, 437
Maternal hyperthyroidism, summary of, 283–84
Maternal hypothyroidism
  sequelae of, 284–85
  summary of, 286–87
Maternal IgG antibodies, 477
Maternal insulin-dependent diabetes, AFP values and, 235
Maternal morbidity, ultrasound during, 196

Maternal mortality
  obstetric hemorrhage and, 467
  preeclampsia and, 409
Maternal obesity, cesarean delivery and, 306
Maternal race, AFP values and, 235
Maternal red blood cell group, antibody screen and, 15–21
Maternal red blood cell mass
  antepartum abnormalities of, 22–31
    incidence/prevalence of, 22
    screening for, 22–31, 29
    sequelae of, 22–24
  antepartum measurement of
    test implications for, 25–27
    test nature for, 24–25
Maternal Rh alloimmunization, screening for, 476
Maternal syndrome of preeclampsia. *See* Preeclampsia
Maternal thrombocytopenia
  abnormal test for, 470–71
  normal test result for, 471
  peripartum coagulopathy and, 467
Maternal thromboprophylaxis, APS and, 295
Maternal thyroid antibody screen, costs of, 282
Maternal thyroid autoantibody screen, 282
Maternal thyroid function tests
  costs of, 285–86
  implications of, 285
  nature of, 285
  purpose of, 285
Maternal thyroid peroxidase autoantibodies, neonatal thyroid function and, 284
Maternal transfusion, incidence/prevalence of, 15, 19
Maternal vessels, test characteristics of, IUGR and, 364, *364*
Maternal viral load, HIV and, 114
Maternal weight
  AFP values and, 235
  gain, normal test result with, 401–2
  low birthweight infants with, 321
    screening for, *323*
MCAD. *See* Medium-chain acyl-coa dehydrogenase deficiency
MCAPI. *See* Middle cerebral artery PI
MCH. *See* Mean corpuscular hemoglobin
Mean corpuscle volume (MCV) levels, testing for, 35
Mean corpuscular hemoglobin (MCH), thalassemia, 141
Meat, Toxoplasma infection and, 63
Meconium aspiration syndrome, post term pregnancy and, 192
Meconium ileus, CF and, 514
Medical prevention, breast cancer and, 583
Medical Research Council on Congenital Dislocation of Hip, 517–18

Medications
  hearing impairment and, 520
  maternal, hyperthyroidism and, 281
Mediterranean community, disorders in,
  high-prevalence of, 147–48, *148*
Medium-chain acyl-CoA dehydrogenase
  deficiency (MCAD)
  conclusions for, 513
  incidence/prevalence of, 511
  PKU screening and, 506
  screening for, 511–13
  sequelae of, 511
  tests for, 512
Menstrual period
  gestational age dating and, 194, 327
  serum CA-125 screening and, 631
Mental health outcomes, GDM and, 305
Mental retardation
  CH and, 507
  fragile X syndrome and, 163
  PKU and, 504
Mental status, ABE and, 492
Metabolic disorders
  OCs and, 560
  TMS and, 506
Metabolic syndrome, 422
Metastases, breast cancer and, 592–93
Methylation mosaics, 165
Methylation status, fragile X syndrome and,
  168
MFMU. *See* Maternal Fetal Medicine Unit
MG. *See* Myasthenia gravis
Middle cerebral artery Doppler index, 455
Middle cerebral artery PI (MCAPI), 442
Midtrimester uterine artery Doppler, APS
  and, 294
Mineralocorticoid therapy, CAH and, 509
Miscarriage
  APS and, 293
  Huntington disease and, 179
Molar pregnancy, 326
  gestational trophoblastic neoplasia and,
  327
Molecular tests
  chromosome abnormalities with, detection of, *259*
  colon and, 652
  comparing laboratory throughput
  for, *260*
  conclusions and recommendations for,
  265–66
  fetal aneuploidy and, 253–66
  fetal cells and, 254–55
  FH and, 544
  with karyotyping, high-risk cases and,
  263
  karyotyping v., *256*
  LDL receptor genes and, 539
MoM value (multiple of median AFP value),
  234
Monoclonal antibody FDC-6, fFN and, 380

Monoclonal anti-FMRP antibodies, fragile
  X syndrome and, 166
Morphology scoring systems, 624, *625*
Mortality, colorectal cancer and, colonoscopy
  and, 652
MRI. *See* Magnetic resonance imaging
*MUC*16, ovarian cancer and, 630
Mucopurulent cervicitis, IUDs and, 568
Multiorgan dysfunction, preeclampsia
  and, 421
Multiple fetal pregnancy
  AFP values and, 235–36
  IUGR and, 327
Multiple gestations
  amniotic fluid embolism and, 470
  gestational age dating and, 193
Multiple of median AFP value. *See* MoM
  value
Multiplex ligation-dependent probe
  amplification (MLPA), fetal cells and, 255
Multiplex ligation-dependent probe
  hybridization, (MAPH), fetal cells and,
  255
Multisystem failure, CFand, 513
Mutation analysis of beta-globin gene,
  β thalassemia and, 156–57
Myasthenia gravis (MG), 298
Myelomeningocele, *in utero* repair of, 234
Myocardial infarctions, 658, *659*
  OCs and, 559
  statins and, 545
Myriad Genetics Laboratories, genetic testing
  and, 575

N
National Diabetes Data Group (NDDG),
  GDM prevalence and, 303, *304*
National Institute of Child Health and
  Human Development (NICHD), PTD
  and, 379
National Polyp study, 652
NDDG. *See* National Diabetes Data Group
Necrotizing enterocolitis, PTD and, 379
Negative predictive values (NPVs), 7, *7*
  preeclampsia and, 398
  uterine Doppler waveforms and, 414
Neonatal complications, prediction of, 445
Neonatal death, 344
Neonatal ferritin levels, 24
Neonatal genetic disorders
  screening for, 503–23
  summary for, 522–23
Neonatal goiter, 281
Neonatal group B streptococcal disease
  (GBS), 48–53
  incidence/prevalence of, 48
  public health and, *49*
  sequelae of, 48–49
  testing implications for, 50–51
    costs of, 51
  tests for, 49–51

Neonatal HBV infection, 82
Neonatal hearing screening, 522
Neonatal hemolytic anemia. *See* Hemolytic
    disease of newborn
Neonatal hyperbilirubinemia, 491–501
    normal test result and, 497
    post-discharge, 498
    risk factors, *495*
    sequelae of, 491–92
    systems strategies for, *497*
    tests for, 493–500
        costs, *497*, 500
Neonatal hypoglycemia
    abnormal test result for, 486–87
    clinical signs of, 485, *486*
    etiology of, *486*
    GDM and, 305
    incidence/prevalence of, 483–84
    initial management of, *487*
    normal test result and, 487
    recommendations for, 488
    screening for, 483–89
    sequelae of, 484
    summary of, 488–89
    tests for, 485–88
        costs, 488
Neonatal intensive care unit (NICU), hour
    specific bilirubin nomogram and, 497
Neonatal jaundice, kernicterus and, 491
Neonatal lupus syndrome, features of, 290
Neonatal morbidity
    Ponderal Index and, 361
    PTD and, 379
Neonatal mortality
    placental dysfunction and, 442
    prediction of, 445
    PTD and, 379
Neonatal screening
    benefits of, 510
        CAH and, 510
    CF and, 124
    tandem mass spectrometry and, 503
Neonatal thyroid function, maternal thyroid
    peroxidase antibodies and, 284
Neonates
    GBS and, 48
    Graves disease and, 280
    umbilical cord blood samples and, 479
Neural tube defects
    fetal sonographic biometry and, 193
    incidence/prevalence of, 232–33
    recommendations for, 239
    summary for, 240–41
    test costs and, 238–39
Neurodegenerative syndrome, fragile
    X syndrome and, 165
Neurodevelopment
    compromise
        CH and, 507
        chronic hypoxemia and, 429
    fetal behavioral responses and, 445–46

hypoglycemia and, 484
Neuromotor anomalies, CBE and, 493
Neuronal injury, kernicterus and, 491, 492
Newborn. *See also* Infants
    hypoglycemia in, screening of, 483
    infectious syphilis and, 94
    screening, fragile X syndrome and, 168
    syphilis and
Newborn Rh status, screening for, 480–81
NICHD. *See* National Institute of Child
    Health and Human Development
Niemann-Pick disease, 150
    test for, 155
Nitrite testing, 41
    costs for, 44
NNS. *See* Number of women needed to
    screen
Nonaneuploid syndromes, IUGR and, 433,
    433
Non-lactating women, iron postpartum
    in, 38
Nonsteroidal anti-inflammatory drugs
    (NSAIDs), gastroschisis and, 233
Nonstress test (NST), fetal distress
    and, 368
Nonsyndromic hearing loss, 152
    test for, 156
Nonvenereal diseases, pregnancy and, 61–67
Normal test results, 27
    amniotic fluid embolism and, 470
    APS and, 295
    asymptomatic bacteriuria in pregnancy
        and, 43
    BPS and, 452
    breast cancer and, 596
    CA-125 and, 639
    CF and, 129, 515
    Chlamydia infection, 106
    chromosomal screening, 208
    chromosome abnormalities with, 259
    CIN and, 606
    CMV and, 70
    CO and, 400
    for congenital rubella infection and, 57
    congenital toxoplasmosis and, 66
    CRS and, 59
    diabetic patients and, 552, *553*
    Doppler imaging and, fetal hypoxia and,
        439
    early-onset genetic diseases and, 158
    fetal arterial system, Doppler studies of, 443
    fetal hypoxia and, 450
    fetal movement and, 450
    fetal structural anomalies and, 248
    FHM and, *351*, 355
    FHM v. dating and, 337
    FHR and, 449
    fragile X syndrome and, 169
    GDM and, 307, 310
    gestational age dating and, 195–96
    gestational hypertension and, 398

gonorrhea and, 99
gynecologic cancers and, 583
hemoglobinopathies and, 143
hepatitis A virus infection and, 76
hepatitis B during pregnancy and,
    80–81
hepatitis C virus infection and, 85
HIV and, 116
Huntington disease and, 183
infectious syphilis and, 95
iron deficiency and, 30
IUFD and, 470
low birth weight infants and, maternal
    height screening, 322
maternal hyperthyroidism in pregnancy
    and, 282
maternal thrombocytopenia and, 471
maternal thyroid function tests and, 285
maternal weight, low birthweight infants
    with, *323*
maternal weight gain and, 401
MCAD and, 512
meaning of, 18, 20
    uterine Doppler waveforms and, 414
neonate GBS and, 51, 53
neural tube defects and, 238
ovarian size and, 624
peripheral edema, 402
peripheral vascular resistance and,
    preeclampsia and, 400
placental abruption and, 470
placental dysfunction and, 443, 445
preeclampsia and, 469
preterm birth and, 384–85
PTD and, 382, 384–85
serum uric acid concentration and,
    preeclampsia and, 424
sexually transmitted disease and, IUDs
    and, 568
SLE in pregnancy and, 291
thrombosis and, 273–74
thyroid disease in pregnancy and, 282
Toxoplasma infection and, 64
trisomy 18 and, 225
trisomy 21 fetus, 225
umbilical artery Doppler and, 369
NPV. *See* Negative predictive values
NSAIDs. *See* Nonsteroidal anti-inflammatory
    drugs
NT. *See* Nuchal translucency
Nuchal fold, second trimester, aneuploidy
    and, 220, 223
Nuchal translucency (NT), 208, 246
    trisomy 21 and, 204, *205*, 206
Nucleic acid amplification tests (GEN-PROBE)
    Chlamydia infection, 104, 105
    gonorrhea and, 98, 99
Nucleic acid hybridization. *See* Nucleic acid
    amplification tests
Number of women needed to screen (NNS),
    GDM and, 311, 312

O
OAEs. *See* Atoacoustic emissions
Obesity, serum uric acid and, 422
Obstetric care
    Doppler technology in, 362
    Toxoplasma infection and, 64
Obstetric hemorrhage, causes of, 467
Obstetric hypertension, 408
OC-associated venous thromboembolism, 562
OCs. *See* Oral contraceptives
Offspring health outcomes, GDM and, 304–5
Omphalocele, 232
    prevalence rate, 233
One-stop clinic for assessment of risk
    (OSCAR)
    chromosomal abnormalities and, 204
    chromosomal screening, 208
Open neural tube defect, 232
Open spina bifida, second trimester and,
    233–34
Oral contraceptives (OCs)
    estrogen-progestin, ovarian cancer and, 583
    medical complications with, 558–61, 561
    recommendations for, 563–64
Oral contraceptives (OCs) users
    screening tests for, 558–71
    summary on, 564–66
Oral glucose tolerance test (GTT)
    diabetes mellitus and, 554–56
    GDM and, 306
    OCs and, 560
Organ differentiation, third trimester and, 437
Organ-speicfic autoimmune disorders, 279
Ortolani and Barlow maneuvers, DDH and,
    517
OSCAR. *See* One-stop clinic for assessment of
    risk
Osteopenia, 673
Osteoporosis, 673–80. *See also* Post-
    menopausal osteoporosis
    conclusions and recommendations for,
        677–78
    incidence/prevalence of, 673
    screening summary for, 678–80
    sequelae of, 673–74
    tests for, 674–77
Outwards-in model, CF and, 124
Ovarian cancer. *See also* Familial ovarian
    cancer
    asymptomatic women and, 634
    *BRCA*1 mutations and, 576
    *BRCA*2 mutations and, 575
    cluster region, 581
    conclusions on, 625–26, 640–42
    incidence/prevalence of, 622, 629
    IUGR and, 361
    morphology index for, *625*
    sequelae of, 529–30, 622–23, 629–30
    Stage 1 disease and, 630–31
    summary of, 626–27, 642–44
    tests for, 530–33, 576–84, 623–25, 630–42

Ovarian cancer screening studies, CA125 and, ultrasound and, *632, 633*
Ovarian carcinomas. *See* Ovarian cancer
Ovarian cysts, pyelogram and, 668
Ovary, pre v. postmenopausal women and, 530–31
Oxidase (XO), 421
Oxidative stress, 421
Oxytocin, neonatal hyperbilirubinemia and, 494

P
Pacemaker, 662
PAH gene, mutations in, 505
Palpable pelvic mass, serum CA-125 and, 636, *636*
Pancreas, CF and, 122, 513
Panel sensitivity, molecular tests and, 255, 257
    karyotyping v., *257*
Panel specificity, molecular tests and, 255, 257
    karyotyping v., 257, *257*
Panhypopituitarism, neonates and, 484
Pap smear
    cervical cancer and, 603–9
    HIV and, 116
    negative, risk reduction for, *607*
Papillomavirus-induced condylomata acuminata, 612
PAPP-A levels, 208
Pariputum bleeding abnormalities, 466
Paroxysmal tachycardias, 658
Partial evaluation, 13
PCR assays. *See* Polymerase chain reaction assays
PD. *See* Pulsed Doppler
Pelvic brim, pyelogram and, 668
Pelvic examination, ovarian cancer syndrome and, 635
Pelvic inflammatory disease (PID)
    Chlamydia infection and, 104
    HIV and, 113
    incidence/prevalence of, 566–67
    IUD user, tests for, 567–69
    recommendations for, 569–70
    sequelae of, 567
    serum CA-125 screening and, 631
Penicillin
    infectious syphilis and, 92, 95
    neonatal GBS and, 51
Perforation, flexible sigmoidoscopy and, 651
Perinatal death
    Doppler velocimetry v., 442
    uterine artery Doppler indices and, 411–12, *412, 413*
Perinatal infection, positive fFN and, 380
Perinatal morbidity, 367
    post term pregnancy and, 193
    ultrasonography and, 248

Perinatal mortality (PNM)
    GDM and, 309
    gestational age dating and, 195
    incidence of, 244
    IUGR and, 327
    low birth weight infants and, 321
    post term pregnancy and, 192
    preeclampsia and, 409
    ultrasonography and, 248
Perinatal outcomes, Doppler and, 443
Perinatal transmission risk
    hepatitis C virus infection and, 85, 86–87
    HIV and, 115
Peripartum coagulopathy, 466–73
    incidence of, 466
    summary of, 472–73
Peripheral edema, preeclampsia and, 402
Peripheral vascular resistance
    tests for, preeclampsia, 400–401
Peritoneal cancers, 635
Permanent hypoglycemia, neonates and, 484
PET. *See* Positron emission topography
Peutz-Jeghers syndrome, STK11 and, 578
PGD. *See* Preimplantation genetic diagnosis
Phenylalanine hydroxylase, PKU and, 504
Phenylketonuria (PKU)
    incidence/prevalence of, 504
    recommendations for, 506
    screening for, 503, 504–6
    sequelae of, 504
    tests for, 504–6
Phototherapy, neonatal hyperbilirubinemia and, 491
PI. *See* Pulsatility index
PID. *See* Pelvic inflammatory disease
PKU. *See* Phenylketonuria
Placebo, uterine Doppler waveforms and, 414
Placental abruption
    abnormal test for, 470
    APS and, 294
    coagulation cascade and, 467
    coagulopathy and, 470
    peripartum coagulopathy and, 466
Placental dysfunction
    fetal arterial system and, Doppler studies of, 442–43
    fetal growth restriction, 345, *345*
    fetal hypoxemia and, 455
    IUGR and, 429, 453
    maternal circulation and, 438–39
    mechanisms of, 437–38
    pathophysiology of, 437
Placental nutrition, 430
Placental perfusion, 409
Placental position, uterine artery Doppler indices and, 410–11

Plasma glucose, fetal, neonatal hypoglycemia and, 483
Plasma glucose concentrations
    diabetes mellitus and, 550–51
    neonatal hypoglycemia, 485
    neonates and, 484
Platelet count, 471
    maternal thrombocytopenia, 471
    preeclampsia and, 469
PLCO trial. *See* Prostate, Lung, Colon, Ovary trial
PNM. *See* Perinatal mortality
Point-of-care glucose meters, neonatal hypoglycemia and, 485
Polycythemia, GDM and, 305
Polymerase chain reaction (PCR) assays
    CF and, 123
    Chlamydia infection, 104, 105
    congenital rubella infection and, 57
    fragile X syndrome and, 165
    Huntington disease and, 178
    maternal GBS and, 49
    OC users and, screening tests and, 562
    Toxoplasma infection and, 63
Ponderal Index, 361
    birth weight v., 364
Population screening programs, 1, 2
Positive fetal fibronectin (fFN), PTD and, 379
Positive predictive values (PPV), 7, 7
    PTD and, 379
    uterine artery waveforms and, 412
Positron emission topography (PET), Huntington disease and, 176
Postmenopausal osteoporosis, 673
    BMD t-score and, 676–77
Postmenopausal women
    CA125 and, 640, 641
    serum CA-125 screening and, 631
    TVS and, 623
Postpartum anemia
    abnormal test result and, 35–36
    tests for, 35–36
Postpartum hemorrhage, 34–35, 36
    LGA and, 328
Postpartum thyroiditis
    incidence/prevalence of, 287
    sequelae of, 287
    summary of, 288–89
    testing for, 288
Postpartum umbilical cord, blood testing for, 476–89
Post-term fetuses, erroneous dating of pregnancy and, 328
Post-term pregnancy
    dating of pregnancy and, 337
    incidence/prevalence of, 191–92
    sequelae of, 192–93
    summary of, 197–99
    ultrasound during, 191, 196
PPV. *See* Positive predictive values

Preconception counseling, Huntington disease and, 180, *180*
Preconceptual carrier screening, CF and, 125
Predicted birth weight, actual v., 360
Predictive test, Huntington disease and, 177–78, 179
Predictive values, 7
Preeclampsia, 394–404, 448, 467. *See also* Severe preeclampsia
    CO, 400
    established, maternal uric acid and, 422–23
    fetal growth restriction, 345
    FH and, 543
    GDM and, 308
    incidence/prevalence of, 408, 420
    maternal mortality and, 467
    pathogenesis of, 394–96, *395*
    peripartum coagulopathy and, 466
    peripheral vascular resistance and, 400
    polycythemia and, 24
    predicting, maternal uric acid and, 423
    recommendations and conclusions, 402–3
    sequelae of, 270–71, 394–96, 408–9
    serum uric acid measurement and
        conclusions and recommendations for, 424
        summary of, 425–26
    summary of, 403–4
    testing implications for, 469
    tests for, 396–402, 409–15, 420–24
        nature of, 396–97
    uric acid and, 420–26
    uterine artery Doppler and, 408–17, *412*, *413*
    weight gain and, 400–401
Preeclampsia-eclampsia syndrome, 420
    incidence/prevalence of, 394
Pregestational diabetes, maternal glucose levels and, 303
Pregnancy. *See also* Post-term pregnancy
    asymptomatic bacteriuria screening in, 44
    autoimmune diseases in, 279–98
    BP and, 397
    Chlamydia infection and, 104
    congenital Toxoplasma infection and, 61
    FH and, 453
    fibrinogen levels in, 469
    GBS and, 48
    gonorrhea and
    HBsAg and, 83
    hemoglobin values in, 22–23, *23*
    hepatitis A virus infection and, 77
    hepatitis B infection, 79
    hepatitis C virus infection and, 84, 85
    HIV and, 115
    hypercoagulability and, 467
    hyperthyroidism and, 280–84
    hypertriglyceridemia and, 542–43

Pregnancy *(Continued)*
    hypothyroidism in, 284–89
    iron supplementation in, 28, 31
    neonatal GBS and, 49
    nonvenereal diseases during, 61–67
    OCs and, 558
    preeclampsia and, 270, 394
    serum CA-125 screening and, 631
    thrombophilia and, 268–77
    ultrasound during, 191–99
    uric acid, 421–22
    venous thrombosis during, 270
    weight gain during, 400
Pregnancy outcomes
    GDM and, 303
    thrombosis and, 269
Pregnancy termination
    anencephaly and, 233
    fetal anomaly and, 246
    fetal structural anomalies and, 246
    fragile X syndrome and, 166, 168, 169
    hemoglobinopathies and, 143
    neural tube defects and, 237
    trisomy 13 fetuses and, 220
    ultrasonography and, 248
Pregnancy-related hypertension, 270
    excessive weight gain and, 401
    hyperuricemia and, 421
Preimplantation genetic diagnosis
    (PGD)
    fragile X syndrome and, 168
    Huntington disease and, 182
Premalignant adenomas, 650
Premature atrial beats, 659
Premature delivery. *See* Preterm delivery
Premature ventricular beats, 659
Premenopausal women
    CA-125 and, 631, 640, 641
        normal test result and, 639
        ultrasound and, 633
    TVS and, 623
Preterm birth. *See* Preterm delivery
Preterm delivery (PTD), 45. *See also* Preterm
    fetuses; Preterm infants
    APS and, 294
    asymptomatic bacteriuria in pregnancy
        and, 40
    conclusions and recommendations for,
        388–89
    fetal hypoxia and, 431
    GDM and, 305
    implications of testing for, 384
    incidence/prevalence of, 378–79
    normal test results for, 384–85
    perinatal mortality and, 244
    positive fFN and, 380
    screening for, 26–27, 378–90
    sequelae of, 379
    summary of, 389–90
    test costs for, 385
    testing for, 379–88

week of gestation when, 381, *382*
Preterm fetuses
    amniotic fluid embolism and, 470
    erroneous dating of pregnancy
        and, 328
Preterm infants, GBS and, 49
Preterm labor (PTL), 378
    fetal growth restriction and, 345
Pretest odds, prevalence v., 8
Prevalence, characteristics of, 3–4, *4*
Primary dyslipidemia
    conclusions on, 545
    gynecology and, 544
Progesterone supplementation
    PTD and, 380
    short cervix and, 386
Prolonged hypoglycemia, neonates
    and, 484
Prophylactic bilateral mastectomy, 584
    gene mutation and, 582, 583
Proportionality growth curve, 349
Propylthiouracil
    fetal hyperthyroidism and, 280
    maternal hyperthyroidism in pregnancy
        and, 282
Prostate, Lung, Colon, Ovary (PLCO) trial,
    ovarian cancer and, 641
Protein C deficiency, 270
    intrauterine fetal death and, 271
    tests for, 272
Protein S deficiency
    intrauterine fetal death and, 271
    tests for, 272
Proteinuria
    preeclampsia and, 270, 394, 408
    third trimester and, 398
Prothrombin, 270
    mutations, 272
Prothrombin time (PT)
    clotting pathways and, 468
    DIC and, 471
Psychological costs, screening and, 10, 11
PTD. *See* Preterm delivery
PTEN, Cowden syndrome and, 578
PTL. *See* Preterm labor
Public health
    hepatitis B during pregnancy and, *62*
    maternal GBS and, *49*
    maternal rubella infection and,
        55–56, *56*
Puerperium, Graves disease and, 280–81
Pulmonary emboli, atrial fibrillation and,
    658–59
Pulmonary hypertension, CF and, 513
Pulmonary infection, CF and, 514
Pulsatility index (PI)
    Doppler and, 409
    early diastolic notch and, 439
Pulsed Doppler (PD), 362, 410
    fetal arterial system, 442
    fetal hypoxia and, 432

Purine metabolism, 422
Pyelectasis, second trimester, aneuploidy and, 221
Pyelonephritis, 40
Pyridostigmine, MG and, 298
Pyrimethamine with sulfadiazine and folic acid, Toxoplasma infection and, 63–64

Q
Q waves, MI and, 660–61
Q-PCR. *See* Quantitative polymerase chain reaction
Quad test, 238
Quantitative McCaman-Robins Fluorometric test, PKU and, 504
Quantitative polymerase chain reaction (Q-PCR), 264
    antenatal diagnosis and, 255
    karyotyping fetal tissue, 206
    molecular methods v., *256*
    tests costs and, 260–61
Quiet sleep, fetal movement and, 450

R
RA. *See* Rheumatoid arthritis
RAD51 genes, 577
Radioimmune assay (RIA)
    21-hydroxylase deficiency test and, 510
    hepatitis A virus infection and, 76
Radioimmunoassay for T4, normal test result for, 508
Radioimmunoprecipitation assay (RIPA), HIV and, 113
Radioiodine, maternal hyperthyroidism in pregnancy and, 282
Radiologic testing. *See also* Abdominal radiographs
    colorectal cancer and, 650
Random plasma glucose, diabetes mellitus and, 551
Randomized controlled trials (RCTs), 10
    GDM and, 308, 309
    placental dysfunction and, 433
    twenty-four hour BP monitoring device and, 397
    umbilical artery Doppler and, 365
        IUGR and, *366*
Rapid antigen detection tests
    maternal GBS and, 49
    neonate GBS and, 52
Rapid eye-movement (REM) sleep, fetal acidemia and, 451
Rapid fetal karyotype, fetal aneuploidy and, 253
Rapid plasma reagent (RPR) tests, infectious syphilis and, 91
RBC antibody screening tests
    costs, 18–19
    normal test results for, 18
    purpose of, 17
    testing implications for, 17–18

RBCs. *See* Red blood cells
RCTs. *See* Randomized controlled trials
Receiver operating characteristic curve (ROC), 6
    predischarge total serum bilirubin level and, *496*
ReCoDe (Relevant Condition at Death), fetal growth restriction and, stillbirths and, 345, *346*
Recombinant immunoblot assay (RIBA), hepatitis C virus infection and, 84, 85, 86
Rectal swabs, maternal GBS and, 49, 50
Recurrent positive immune serology, APS and, 295
Red blood cells (RBCs)
    alloimmunization, 15, 476
    antibody screen, 477
        testing for, 15
    antigens, screening for, 15–20
    masses, postpartum women and, 36
    SCD and, 518
    transfusion, incidence/prevalence of, 15
Red cell mass testing, 35
    cost of, 27–28
Reference test, diabetes mellitus and, 551
Relevant Condition at Death. *See* ReCoDe
Reliability, test performance and, 9
Reliability/reproducibility of test, FHM and, 336
REM. *See* Rapid eye-movement sleep
Reminder system, screening program and, 10
Renal function testing, SLE in pregnancy and, 290
Renal tubular pathophysiology, preeclampsia and, 421
Reproduction choices, Huntington disease and, *180*
Resistance index (RI)
    Doppler and, 409
    early diastolic notch and, 439
Respiratory depression, colonoscopy and, 652
Respiratory failure, ABE and, 492
Retinopathy of prematurity, PTD and, 379
Reverse transcriptase-polymerase chain reaction (RT-PCR), hepatitis C virus infection and, 84, 85, 86
Reye-like features, MCAD and, 511
Rh (D)-negative typing, Rh positive child and, 478
Rh (D)-positive typing, tests for, 19
Rh (D) typing, 17
    costs of, 18–19
    testing implications for, 17–18
Rh(D) antigen, testing for, 17
Rheumatoid arthritis (RA), 297–98
Rh-negative women, umbilical cord blood samples and, 479
RI. *See* Resistance index
RIA. *See* Radioimmune assay
RIBA. *See* Recombinant immunoblot assay

Riley-Day disease, 150–51
RIPA. *See* Radioimmunoprecipitation assay
Risk index by Newman score, neonatal
  hyperbilirubinemia and, 494
Risk of malignancy index (RMI), 641
  ovarian cancer and, 637
  performance of, *638*
ROC. *See* Receiver operating characteristic
Routine dating of pregnancy with ultrasound
  advantages of, 196–97
  early pregnancy, 197
Routine testing
  APS and, 295
  iron supplementation and, 28
Routine ultrasonography, fetal structural
  anomalies and, 244–50
RPR tests. *See* Rapid plasma reagent tests
RT-PCR. *See* Reverse transcriptase-poly-
  merase chain reaction
Rubella during pregnancy, 55–60
Rubella infection, 57
Rubella-specific IgM antibodies, 57

S
Salt losing, CAH and, 509
Sarcoma, TP53 and, 578
SCD. *See* Sickle cell disease
Schistocytes, DIC and, 471
Screening procedures, demanding aspects
  of, 9–10
Screening program
  characteristics for, *3*
  community choice and, 4
Screening service, 211
Screening summary
  anemia secondary to delivery and, 34
  anemia secondary to pregnancy and, 34
  antiphospholipid syndrome and, 296–97
  asymptomatic bacteriuria in pregnancy
    and, 45–46
  BIND and, 500–501
  breast cancer, 598–600
  cardiac pathology and, 663–65
  cervical cancer, 608–9, 618–19
  Chlamydia infection and
  chromosomal abnormalities and, 212–13
  CMV infection and, 71–72
  colorectal cancer and, 654–56
  congenital Toxoplasma infection and,
    61–64
  congenital toxoplasmosis and, 65–66
  CRS and, 59–60
  CVD and, 545–47
  diabetes mellitus and, 554–56
  dyslipidemia, 545–47
  epidemiologic considerations in, 1–13
  fetal aneuploidy and, 265–66
  fetal growth restriction, 355–57
  fetal hypoxemia and, 455–57
  fetal structural anomalies and, 249–50
  fragile X syndrome and, 170

GDM and, 313–14
gynecologic malignancy and, 533–34
hepatitis A virus infection and, 77
inherited thrombophilias and, 275–77
IUGR, 373–75
IVP and, 670–71
maternal hyperthyroidism and, 283–84
maternal hypothyroidism and, 286–87
neonatal genetic disorders and, 522–23
neonatal hypoglycemia and, 488
neonate GBS and, 52–53
newborn Rh status and, 480–81
objective of, 13
OCs users and, 564–66
osteoporosis and, 678–80
ovarian cancer, 626–27, 642–44
perinatal outcome, 197–99
perinatal transmission of hepatitis B
  and, 81–83
peripartum coagulopathy and, 472–73
PID and, 570–71
postpartum thyroiditis, 288–89
preeclampsia, 420–26, 425–26
PTD, 389–90
SLE and, 292–93
summary of, 29–31
Screening tests
  GDM and, 307
  nature of result in, 2
  validity and, 5
S/D. *See* Systolic to diastolic ratio
Second trimester
  biochemical screening, 208
  BP measurement and, 397, 402
  MAP, 398
  placental dysfunction and, 437
  sonographic markers, aneuploidy and,
    220
  ultrasound, clinical management
    of, 222
Secondary osteoporosis, 673
Seizures, ABE and, 492
Sensitivity
  molecular tests and, 255, 257
  screening test and, 5, *6*
Serial human chorionic gonadotropin
  (hCG) measurements, trophoblastic
  disease and, 337
Serologic testing, hepatitis A virus infection
  and, 78
Serum AFP, trisomy 21 and, 219
Serum CA-125. *See* Cancer antigen-125
Serum ferritin
  levels, 35
  postpartum assessment of, 34–38
Serum grouping tests, accuracy of, 16–17
Serum lipid levels, OCs and, 560–61
Serum screening, gestation period
  and, 220
Serum uric acid
  cardiovascular risk factors and, 422

preeclampsia and, 420–26
Serum uric acid measurement
    preeclampsia and
        conclusions and recommendations
            for, 424
        test costs for, 424
17-hydroxy-progesterone (17-OHP), 510
Severe hyperbilirubinemia, 491, 536
Severe preeclampsia, 398
Sex chromosomal aneuploidy
    molecular tests for, 258
    sequelae of, 203
Sexual intercourse, high risk HPV and, 613
Sexually transmitted diseases (STDs).
        See also Chlamydia infection; Gonorrhea;
        Nonvenereal diseases
    gonorrhea and, 97
    syndromes
        infectious syphilis and, 91
        IUDs and, 568
SGA. *See* Small-for-gestational age
Short synacthen test, Addison disease and, 298
Sickle cell anemia, 518
Sickle cell detection test, costs of, 519–20
Sickle cell disease (SCD), 139, 153
    incidence of, 518
    sequelae of, 140
    testing for, 157
Sickle hemoglobinopathies, 518
Sickle screening test, hemoglobinopathies
        and, 140
Silent myocardial infarction, 660, 661, *661,*
    662
Size for dates discrepancy
    FHM and, 337
    size of uterine fundus and, summary
        of, 339–40
Skeletal dysplasia, IUGR and, 433, *433*
SLE. *See* Systemic lupus erythematosus
SMA. *See* Spinal muscular atrophy
Small-for-gestational age (SGA)
    abnormal fetal heart rate pattern, 365
    adverse perinatal outcome v., *349*
    BP and, 397
    Doppler velocimetry, 371
    IUGR v., 360
    preeclampsia and, 409
    third trimester and, 398
Sonographic ear length, second trimester,
        aneuploidy and, 221
Sonographic tests, chromosomal abnormali-
        ties and, 204–6
Southern blot, fragile X syndrome and, 165,
    166
Specificity
    molecular tests and, 255, 257
    screening test and, 5, *6*
Spina bifida, 232, 239
    amnionic fluid AFP and, 236
    high resolution ultrasound and, 237
    sequelae of, 233

test costs for, 248
Spinal muscular atrophy (SMA), screening
    for, 148
Spiral arteries, 409, 410, 437
Spiral CT scanning, colon and, 652
Spontaneous abortion, congenital
    toxoplasmosis and, 65
Spontaneous preterm delivery (PTD),
    378, 386
SRY PCR, fragile X syndrome and,
    167
SSA. *See* Anti-Ro
SSB. *See* Anti-La antibodies
Stage 1 ovarian cancer, 630–31
    CA-125 measurement and, 640
Stage 2 ovarian cancer, 635
Standard reference tests, GDM
    and, 306
Statin therapy
    homozygosity and, 538
    pregnancy and, 544
Station, 383
STDs. *See* Sexually transmitted diseases
Steroid biosynthesis, Addison disease,
    298
Steroids, APS and, 294
Stillbirth, 344
    BPS and, 452
    chronic hypoxemia and, 429
    fetal acidemia and, 453, *454*
    fetal growth restriction, 345
    GDM and, 310
    IUGR and, 361
    prediction of, 443–44
STK11 gene, Peutz-Jeghers syndrome
    and, 578
Stool DNA test, commercial, 652–53
Stool samples, FOBT and, 651
Stroke, BMD and, 674
Stroke volume (SV), CO and, 399
Subcutaneous mastectomy, gene mutation
    and, 582
Surgery
    benign gynecologic, ureteral injury
        and, 666
    breast cancer and, 593
    cardiac pathology screening and,
        663
    DIC and, 471
    prophylactic, ovarian carcinomas
        and, 640
    pyelogram and, 668
Surveillance, gene mutation and, *581*
Survival rates
    CA-125 measurement and, 641
    cancer stage and, colorectal cancer,
        649–50
    ovarian cancer and, 629
SV. *See* Stroke volume
fFN swab, cervical canal, 380
Sweat test, CF and, 122

Syndrome X, 422
Syphilis, 90–95. *See also* Congenital syphilis;
    Latent syphilis
    incidence/prevalence of, 90, 93, 100
    sequelae of, 90–91, 94, 100
    summary, 92–95
    tests for, 91, 94–95, 100–101
        implications of, 91–92
        nature of, 91
Systemic lupus erythematosus (SLE),
    289–93
    coexistent APS and, 290
    incidence/prevalence of, 289
    in pregnancy
        conclusions and recommendations
            for, 291
        tests for, 290–92
    sequelae of, 289–90
    summary of, 292–93
Systolic to diastolic ratio (S/D ratio)
    Doppler and, 409
    early diastolic notch and, 439

T
T. pallidum immobilization (TPI) test,
    infectious syphilis and, 91
Tachycardias, 658, 659
TAFI. *See* Thrombin activatable fibrinolysis
    inhibitor
TAG 72.3 assay, 634
Tamoxifen, breast cancer and, 583
Tandem mass spectrometry
    MCAD and, 512
    neonatal screening with, 503
Target condition, 4, 29
    anemia secondary to delivery, 34
    anemia secondary to pregnancy
        and, 34
    asymptomatic bacteriuria in pregnancy
        as, 40
    early treatment of, 10
Targeted screening programs, 2
    fetal structural anomalies and, 24 weeks
        gestation and, 245
    GDM and, 307
Tay-Sachs disease (TSD), 149, *149*
    test for, 154–55
TBS. *See* Total serum bilirubin
TcB. *See* Transcutaneous bilirubin
Term fetuses, erroneous dating of pregnancy
    and, 328
Term optimal weight, 349
Tertiary syphilis, 94
Test accuracy, serum grouping tests and,
    16–17
Test panels, CF and, 123
Test reliability, technology assessment and,
    IUGR and, 362
Test screening, low birthweight infants and,
    321
Testes, CF and, 122

Testing centers, CF and, 123
Testing costs, 30
    anemia during pregnancy and, 38
    anemia secondary to delivery and, 38
    aneuploidy and, 225
    antenatal FHR monitor, 449
    antepartum screening and, 36
    APS and, 296
    asymptomatic bacteriuria in pregnancy
        and, 43
    bimanual examination and, 532–33
    BPS and, 452
    breast cancer and, 596–97
    CAH and, 510
    cardiac pathology screening and, 662
    cervical cancer, 607
    CF and, 129–32, 515
    Chlamydia infection and, 106, 107
    chromosomal screening, 209
    chromosome abnormalities and, 260
    CMV and, 70–71
    colorectal cancer screening and, 653, *654*
    for congenital rubella infection and, 57–58
    congenital toxoplasmosis and, 66
    CRS and, 60
    DDH and, 517
    DEXA reading and, 677
    diabetes mellitus type 2 and, 553
    Doppler imaging and, fetal hypoxia and,
        439
    early-onset genetic diseases and, 158
    enzyme immunoassays for Immunoglob-
        ulin G antibodies and, 57–58
    fetal structural anomalies and, 248
    fFN and, 382–83
    FH and, 544–45
    FHM and, 337
    fragile X syndrome and, 169
    GDM and, 310–11
    gonorrhea and, 99
    gynecologic cancers and, 583
    hearing impairment, 521–22
    hepatitis A virus infection and, 76
    hepatitis B and, 80
    hepatitis B during pregnancy, 82
    hepatitis C virus infection and, 85, 87
    high-risk HPV screening
    HIV and, 116
    Huntington disease and, 183
    infectious syphilis and, 92–93, 95
    iron supplementation and, 30
    IUGR and, 369, 436–37
    IVP and, 669
    low birthweight infants and, maternal
        height and weight v., 323
    maternal thyroid function tests and, 285
    MCAD and, 512
    neonatal GBS and, 51
    neonatal hyperbilirubinemia and, 497, 500
    neural tube defects and, 238
    ovarian carcinomas and, 640

PKU and, 505–6
preterm birth and, 384–85
radioimmunoassay for T4 and, 508
serum uric acid measurement and, 424
sexually transmitted disease and, IUDs
    and, 569
sickle cell detection test and, 519–20
SLE in pregnancy and, 291
syphilis and, 92, 95
Toxoplasma infection and, 64
trisomy 21, 225
TSH test, 508
TVS and, 624
uterine Doppler waveforms and, 414
Testing implications, asymptomatic bacteri-
    uria in pregnancy and, 41, 43–44
Tests. *See also* Screening summary
    aberrant placental implantation and, 272
    anemia during pregnancy and,
        37–38
    anemia secondary to delivery and,
        37–38
    antepartum abnormalities of RBC mass
        and
        implications of, 30
        nature of, 29
        purpose of, 29
    asymptomatic bacteriuria in pregnancy
        and, 45–46
    Chlamydia infection, 108–9
    chromosomal abnormalities, 204–6
    CMV and, 69–70, 72
    for congenital rubella infection, 56–58
    congenital toxoplasmosis and, 65–66
    CRS and, 59–60
    fetal aneuploidy and, 253–54, 257–61,
        263–64
    fetal structural anomalies and, 245–48
    glucose intolerance, 306
    gonorrhea and, 98–99
    hemoglobinopathies and, 140
    hepatitis A virus infection and, 77–78
    hepatitis C virus infection and, 84–85,
        86–87
    HIV and, 117–18
    Huntington disease and, 176
    hyperthyroidism and, 281–82
    implications of, 17–18
    infectious syphilis and, 91, 94–95
    IUGR and, 361
    neonatal GBS and, 49–53
    open neural tube defect and, 234–39
    for postpartum anemia, 35–36
    postterm pregnancy, 198
    results
        abnormal, 13
        urine samples, *42*
    SLE in pregnancy and, 290
    syphilis and
    trisomy 18 and, 220
    trisomy 21 and, 220

Tetracycline
    Chlamydia infection and
        infectious syphilis and, 92
Tetrahydrobiopterin (BH4),
    hyperphenylalaninemia and, 505
Thalassemia
    diagnosis of, 141–42
    gene arrangements for, 141, *142*
Thalassemia major. *See* Cooley anemia
Thalassemia trait, 152
α-Thalassemia, 153
    carrier, 140
    SCD and, 518, 519
    testing for, 157
β-Thalassemia, 152
    hemoglobinopathies and, 141
    screening tests for, 156–57
    universal screening savings and, *144*
Thayer-Martin media, gonorrhea and,
    98, 99
Third trimester
    BP, 398
    placental dysfunction, 437
    scans, FHM and, 350
Thrombi-generation potential, preeclampsia
    and, 387
Thrombin, thrombophilia and, 268
Thrombin activatable fibrinolysis inhibitor
    (TAFI), 270
Thrombocytopenia, 467
    DIC and, 471
    testing and, 468
Thromboembolism, heritable thrombophilias
    and, *269*
Thrombophilia
    markers of, 270
    OC users and, screening tests and, 562
    OCs and, 563
    pregnancy complications and, 268–78
    prevalence of, 268, *269*
Thrombophylaxis, pregnancy and, 273
Thrombosis
    APS and, 296
    conclusions and recommendations
        for, 274
    sequelae of, 271–72
Thyroid antibody testing, costs of, 285–86
Thyroid disease, associated problems with,
    screening, 280–89
Thyroid disease in pregnancy, normal test
    result and, 282
Thyroid function tests
    abnormal test result with, 281
    costs of, 282, 285–86
    hyperthyroidism and, 281
Thyroid hormone, CH and, 507
Thyroid stimulating hormone (TSH)
    hyperthyroidism and, 281
    test, 508
        CH and, 507
Thyroid storm, pregnancy and, 280

Time-velocity curve, CO and, 399
Tissue culture isolation, Chlamydia infection and, 104
Tissue ischemia, sickle cell disease and, 153
Tissue sampling, flexible sigmoidoscopy and, 651
TMS. *See* Mass spectrometry screening
Total peripheral resistance (TPR), preeclampsia and, 400
Total serum bilirubin (TSB), 496
    kernicterus and, 491, *492*
    neonatal hyperbilirubinemia and, 493
    ROC and, *496*
Total to transcutaneous bilirubin (TSB/TcB), neonatal hyperbilirubinemia and, 494, *495*
TP53, breast cancer and, 578
TPI test. *See T. pallidum* immobilization test
TPR. *See* Total peripheral resistance
TRAM flap, breast reconstruction and, 582
Transcription-mediated amplification of RNA, Chlamydia infection, 104
Transcutaneous bilirubin (TcB)
    neonatal hyperbilirubinemia and, 493
    testing, 496
Transfusion support, β-thalassemia and, 144
Transient fetal/neonatal hyperthyroidism, 280
Transient hypoglycemia, neonates and, 483–84
Translabial imaging, 385
Transport mechanisms, fetal hypoxia, 430
Transvaginal cervical length measurements, PTD and, 387
Transvaginal sonography (TVS), ovarian cancer and, 623
Transvaginal ultrasound, 385, *385, 386, 387*
    cysts and, 532
    measurement of cervical length, nature of test for, 385–86
    ovarian cancer and, 584, 622–27
Treponema pallidum, 90
    sequelae of
Trial of umbilical and fetal flow in Europe (TRUFFLE), 455
Trichomonas vaginalis, PTD and, 380
Trichomoniasis, IUDs and, 568
Triglycerides
    ATP III classification of, *540*
    measurement of, 538–39
Triple marker program, neural tube defects and, 239
Triple screen risk, trisomy 21 and, 219, 220
Triple test, neural tube defects and, 238
Triploidy, sequelae of, 206
Trisomy 13
    fetuses, 220
    molecular tests for, 258
    sequelae of, 203

Trisomy 18
    antenatal sonography and, 223
    conclusions on, 226–27
    CPCs and, 224
    molecular tests for, 258
    prevalence/incidence of, 217–18
    second-trimester screening, 217–29
    sequelae of, 203
    summary of, 228–29
Trisomy 18 fetuses
    antenatal sonography and, 223
    sequelae of, 220
Trisomy 21, 201, 220, 264
    conclusions on, 226–27
    configurations for, 261
    detection rate for, *207,* 208
    early screening for, 211
    false positive rate for, *207*
    fetal sonographic biometry and, 193
    incidence/prevalence of, 217–18
    molecular tests for, 258
    second-trimester screening, 217–29, 219
    sequelae of, 202–3, 220
    summary of, 228–29
    test costs for, 248
Trisomy 21 fetus, ultrasound and, 222–23
Trophoblast, 409, 410
Trophoblastic disease, hCG measurements and, 337
Trophoblastic invasion, Doppler waveform and, 439
Trophoblastic migration, 410
TRUFFLE. *See* Trial of umbilical and fetal flow in Europe
TSB/TcB. *See* Total to transcutaneous bilirubin
TSD. *See* Tay-Sachs disease
TSH. *See* Thyroid stimulating hormone
Tumor marker(s), 636
    measurement, cysts and, 532
    ovarian cancer and, 641
        CA-125 and, 634
Tumor-specific gene therapy
Turner syndrome, 203
TVS. *See* Transvaginal sonography
Twenty-four hour BP monitoring device, pregnancy and, 397
21-hydroxylase deficiency, CAH and, 509, 511
Two-step screening
    CF and, 125, 132, 134
    CF carrier status and, 125, *127*

U

Ubiquitin, Huntington disease and, 176
U/C ratio. *See* Umbilical artery/cerebral artery Doppler ratio
U.K. Collaborative Trial for Ovarian Cancer Screening (UKCTOCS), 641
UKCTOCS. *See* U.K. Collaborative Trial for Ovarian Cancer Screening

Ultrasonography (US). *See also* High
 resolution ultrasound
  AFP MoM values and, 236
  amniocentesis v., 237
  anencephaly and, 233
  breast and, 594
  CA-125 measurement and, 640
  chromosomal abnormalities and, 205
  cost-effectiveness of, prenatal genetic
   screening and, 226, *227*
  costs of, 282
  DDH and, 517
  fetal growth, from 26-28 weeks, 350, *351*
  FHM and, costs of, 337
  FHM v. dating and, 336
  FHR and, 446
  GDM and, 310
  gestational age dating and, 193
  ovarian cancer screening studies and,
   ultrasound and, *632, 633*
  perinatal morbidity and, 248
  pregnancy and, 191–99
  routine, normal test result, 195–96
  sensitivity of, fetal structural anomalies
   and, 244–45
  trisomy 21 fetus and, 222
Ultrasound markers
  cost-effectiveness of, prenatal genetic
   screening and, 226, *227*
  second trimester, practice guidelines for,
   227
Ultrasound scoring systems, ovarian cancers
  and, 641–42
Umbilical and uterine artery resistance
  indices, 362
Umbilical artery
  delivery and, 454
  flow velocity profile, Doppler and, 441
  placental dysfunction and, 429
  pulsatility index, 365
  test costs for, 369, *370*
Umbilical artery Doppler, 365
  normal test result for, 369
  waveform, placental dysfunction and, 443
Umbilical artery/cerebral artery (U/C)
  Doppler ratio, 362
  fetal growth restriction and, 363, *363*
  IUGR and, 436
Umbilical cord. *See also* Postpartum umbilical
  cord
  compression, 369
  phenylalanine levels and, 505
Umbilical cord blood, testing of, 477, 478, 479
Umbilical vein, 437
Universal screening
  fetal structural anomalies and, 24 weeks
   gestation and, 245
  GDM and, 307
Urate, 422
Ureter, preoperative intravenous pyelogram
  and, 666–69

Ureteral deviation, pyelogram and, 668
Ureteral injury, benign gynecologic surgery
  and, 666
Uric acid, testing for, 421–22
Urinalysis, costs for, 43
Urinary tract
  abnormality, pyelogram and, 668
  anatomic distortion, normal test result
   and, 669
  infection, 43
   asymptomatic bacteriuria in preg-
    nancy and, 40
Urine. *See also* Dipstick testing
  culture, 45
   asymptomatic bacteriuria in preg-
    nancy and, 41
   costs for, 43
  samples
   nucleic acid amplification tests
    test results for, *42*
Urogenital tract Chlamydia infection. *See*
  Chlamydia infection
US. *See* Ultrasonography
Uterine arteries, Doppler and, 362
Uterine artery blood flow velocity waveforms
  first trimester and, 410
  indices measuring, 410, 411–12, *412, 413*
Uterine artery Doppler. *See* Uterine Doppler
  ultrasound
Uterine contraction monitoring, PTD and,
  380
Uterine Doppler ultrasound
  conclusions and recommendations for,
   415
  indices
   placental position and, 410–11
   testing implications using, 411–12, *412,
    413*
  preeclampsia and, 408–17
  waveforms, test costs for, 414–15
Uterine fundus
  measurement
   estimated gestational age and, 328
   height, 326–40
   issues in, 328–29
  size-for-date discrepancy in,
   incidence/prevalence of, 326–27
Uterine leiomyomas, 530
Uterine prolapse, pyelogram and, 668
Uteroplacental artery Doppler, IUGR and,
  364
Uteroplacental circulation, 410
Uteroplacental dysfunction, 362
  Doppler ultrasound and, 369

V

V Leiden mutation, OC users and, 562, 563
Vaccination
  CRS and, 58, 60
  HPV and, 604

Vaginal bleeding, fFN and, 380
Vaginal fluid, fFN and, 380
Vaginal swabs
    maternal GBS and, 49, 50
    neonate GBS and, 52
Validity of test
    FHM and, 336
    screening test and, 5
Vancomycin, gonorrhea and, 98, 99
Vascular disease, IUGR and, 361
Vascular occlusion, sickle cell disease and, 153
VDRL. *See* Venereal Disease Research Laboratory
Venereal Disease Research Laboratory (VDRL) test, infectious syphilis and, 91
Venous Doppler indices
    blood volume and, 441
    fetal heart failure and, 364
Venous flow velocity waveform, 441
Venous thromboembolism
    OCs and, 559–60
    pregnancy and, 271
Venous thrombosis
    APS and, 293
    inherited thrombophilias and, 269–70
    OC users and, screening tests and, 562
    tests for, 272–74
Ventilation, hearing impairment and, 520
Ventricular tachycardia, 659
Vertebral body fractures, back pain and, 674
Very low birth weight (VLBW) infants, 378
Viral infection, IUGR and, 433, *433*
Virilization, CAH and, 509
Virtual colonoscopy with CT, 652
    colorectal cancer and, 650
Vital signs, neonatal hyperbilirubinemia and, 493
Vitiligo, pregnancy and, 298

VLBW. *See* Very low birth weight infants
Vomiting, Addison disease and, 298
von Willebrand disease, 469

W
Warfarin, APS and, 294
a-wave, 444
WB. *See* Western blot
Weight gain, 402
    preeclampsia and, 400–401
    pregnancy and, 400
Weight loss
    Addison disease and, 298
    diabetic patients and, 552
Western blot (WB), HIV and, 113, 114
White-coat hypertension, BP and, 397
WHO. *See* World Health Organization
Whole-blood glucose concentrations, plasma glucose v., 485
World Health Organization (WHO)
    anemia during pregnancy criteria for, 22
    GDM prevalence and, 303, *304*
    GTT and, *304*, 306
    hepatitis B during pregnancy and, 79
    osteoporosis and, 673
    peripheral edema in pregnancy and, 402

X
Xanthine dehydrogenase/oxidase (XDH/XO), 421
Xanthine oxidoreductase (XOR) activity, uric acid and, 421, 422
XO. *See* Oxidase
XOR. *See* Xanthine oxidoreductase activity
X-ray mammography, digital mammography v., 593–94

Z
Zidovudine, HIV and, 115, 118

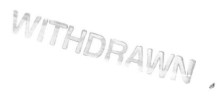